Manual of
Medical
Therapeutics

Manual of Medical Therapeutics

28th Edition

Department of Medicine
Washington University
School of Medicine
St. Louis, Missouri

Gregory A. Ewald, M.D.
Clark R. McKenzie, M.D.
Editors

Little, Brown and Company
Boston/New York/Toronto/London

Editorial: Nancy Chorpenning
Production Editor: Elizabeth Willingham
Copyeditors: Sharon Cloud Hogan, Elizabeth Willingham
Indexer: Elizabeth Willingham
Cover: Louis C. Bruno, Jr.

To Michael Karl, M.D., and Joseph Levitt, M.D., two master clinicians, who have devoted many years to teaching the principles of internal medicine to the medical students and house officers at Washington University

Contents

Preface

This is the 28th edition of the *Washington University Manual of Medical Therapeutics,* which, since its inception in 1943–44, has served as an up-to-date authoritative reference on medical therapy. This publication was originally devised by the Department of Internal Medicine at Washington University to facilitate a rational, conservative approach to a broad array of clinical problems in medicine for medical students and house officers. It has grown to become the leading reference manual on medical therapeutics. Advances in both diagnosis and treatment are reported at an ever-increasing rate in internal medicine, and it is increasingly difficult to incorporate these changes into medical practice. This manual presents a logical approach to diagnostic evaluation and therapeutics, but it is not designed to be an exhaustive reference in internal medicine. Discussions of pathophysiology and differential diagnosis are necessarily limited. Many disease processes in medicine may have multiple effective therapies, but an attempt has been made to present a concise approach to the clinical problem often reflecting opinions of the physicians at Washington University.

This edition has been updated to reflect ongoing changes in standards of clinical practice. It includes a new chapter on the immunocompromised host with an emphasis on the patient with HIV-related illness. A new chapter on critical care and medical emergencies consolidates concepts previously covered in various chapters in previous editions. An appendix of common formulas and reference values used by the internist has been included. The remaining chapters have been updated and extensively revised. Publication of the 28th edition has been accomplished by the combined efforts of many people. As in past editions, most chapters have been written by senior subspecialty fellows and assistant professors at Washington University with significant input from senior faculty members. Final content of all chapters has received extensive internal review, including important input from the medicine house staff at Barnes Hospital.

We are grateful for the invaluable assistance of the clinical pharmacy staff, particularly Robyn A. Schaiff, Pharm.D. We also thank Alison J. Whelan, M.D., an editor of the 27th edition of the manual, for her help and encouragement, and the house staff at Barnes Hospital for their continued interest and energy in making this book a success. We also appreciate the editorial assistance of Laura Berendson and Elizabeth Willingham, and our continued publishing relationship with Little, Brown and Company.

We have had the privilege of serving as chief residents in the Department of Medicine at Washington University under the guidance of John Atkinson, M.D., whose continued enthusiasm for both the art and science of internal medicine serves as an inspiration.

G. A. E.
C. R. M.

Manual of
Medical
Therapeutics

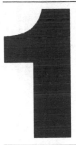

Patient Care in Internal Medicine

Alison J. Whelan

General Care of the Patient

This chapter reviews principles of general patient care, particularly those not covered in subsequent chapters. Although a general approach to common problems is outlined, **therapy must be individualized**. All diagnostic and therapeutic procedures should be carefully explained to the patient, including the potential risks, benefits, and alternatives. This explanation will minimize anxiety and give both the patient and physician the appropriate expectations.

I. **Preventive care.** The integration of preventive care into clinical practice should be done carefully. The benefit of preventing a target disease in asymptomatic patients, the accuracy and acceptability of available screening tests, and the cost of the screening tool must all be considered.

A. **Practice guidelines** reflect different targets, different objectives, and different rationales for decision making. Figure 1-1 is a compilation of preventive care guidelines from various North American health agencies. The guidelines are for persons who do not have a family history, signs, symptoms, or other diseases that place them at increased risk for the preventable target disease. Strategies for a wider range of preventive services and for patients at increased risk for certain target diseases are beyond the scope of this manual but are available from the major health agencies (*Ann Intern Med* 114:758, 1991; *Guide to Clinical Preventive Services, US Preventive Services Task Force Manual.* Baltimore: Williams & Wilkins, 1989).

B. **Individualized implementation** is based on an assessment of the risk profile, which is developed from the patient's personal and family history. A record-keeping method to track screening test results and interventions over several years is useful.

II. **Hospital orders**

A. **Admission orders** should be written promptly after evaluation of the patient. Each set of orders should bear the **date and time** written and the legible signature of the physician. All orders should be clear, concise, organized, and legible.

B. **The content and organization of admission orders** should follow a routine (e.g., the mnemonic ADC VAAN DISML) to ensure that no important therapeutic measures are overlooked.

1. Admitting diagnosis, location, and physician responsible for the patient.
2. Diagnosis pertinent to nursing care.
3. Condition of the patient.
4. Vital signs: type (T, HR, RR, BP), frequency, and parameters for notification of the physician (e.g., systolic BP < 90) should be specified.
5. Activity limitations.
6. Allergies, sensitivities, and previous drug reactions.
7. Nursing instructions (e.g., Foley catheter to gravity drainage, wound care, daily weights).
8. Diet.
9. Intravenous fluids including composition and rate.
10. Sedatives, analgesics, and other per request medications.
11. Medications, including dose, frequency, and route of administration.
12. Laboratory tests and radiographic studies.

A blackened square indicates that the service is recommended. An empty square indicates that either a recommendation has been made to not provide the service or that no recommendation has been made for or against the service by the particular authority. The placement and spacing of squares indicate a suggested age range and frequency for testing rather than actual ages at which services should be provided.

ACP	USPSTF
CTF	OTHER

ACP	American College of Physicians
USPSTF	US Preventive Services Task Force
CTF	Canadian Task Force on the Periodic Health Examination
Other	Immunization Recommendations – CDC Immunization Practices Advisory Committee.
	Cholesterol Recommendations – National Cholesterol Education Program Panel on Detection, Evaluation, and Treatment of High Blood Cholesterol in Adults.
	Hypertension Recommendations – Joint National Committee on Detection, Evaluation, and Treatment of High Blood Pressure.
	Cancer Screening Recommendations – American Cancer Society.

Hayward, Steinberg, Ford, Roizen, Roach.
© 1991 American College of Physicians

1. This list shows selected, age-specific preventive care services recommended by at least one of the ACP, CTF, or USPSTF, which should be offered to persons who do not have a family history, symptoms, signs, or other diseases that place them at increased risk for preventable target conditions. All authorities stress the importance of determining each person's unique risks for preventable disease in order to individualize preventive care. Strategies for the selective provision of a wider range of services to persons at low and increased risk for particular target conditions are found in Tables 2 through 5.

2. The CTF recommends screening at least every 5 years and at every clinical encounter. Others agree or suggest screening every 2 years.

3. The CTF recommends periodic serum cholesterol testing in men between the ages of 30 and 59 years. The USPSTF recommends determinations in middle-aged men and suggests that testing of young women, men, and the elderly may be clinically prudent.

4. ACP and USPSTF recommend a Papanicolaou smear for women over 65 years of age who have had consistently normal smears in the previous decade. CTF suggests Papanicolaou smears every 3 years before 35 years of age and every 5 years for 74 years of age, after two normal annual smears following the onset of sexual activity.

5. CTF and USPSTF concluded that there is insufficient evidence to recommend for or against fecal occult blood testing.

6. ACP recommends sigmoidoscopy every 3 to 5 years or air contrast barium enema every 5 years. Neither the CTF nor the USPSTF recommends for or against screening sigmoidoscopy.

7. American Cancer Society recommends annual or biennial mammography for women from 40 to 49 years of age.

8. ACP, USPSTF, and CTF emphasize that all adults should be routinely counseled about tobacco use, nutrition, exercise, sexual behavior, substance abuse, injury prevention, and dental care.

Fig. 1-1. Preventive care guidelines for asymptomatic, low-risk adults: Recommendations from various North American health organizations. (From RSA Hayward et al. Preventive care guidelines: 1991. *Ann Intern Med* 114:758, 1991.)

C. **Orders should be reevaluated frequently** and altered as the patient status dictates. **When changing an order,** the old order must be specifically canceled before a new one is written.

D. **Orders for medications to be taken as needed (prn)** require careful consideration to avoid adverse drug interactions. The minimum dosing interval should be specified (e.g., q4h). Drug orders should be reviewed frequently.

III. **Drug therapy**

A. **Prescriptions** should include the name of the patient, date, name of the drug, dosage, route of administration, amount dispensed, dosage schedule instructions, and signature of the physician. The number of refills should be limited, especially in patients who appear to be self-injurious. **For narcotics,** write out all numbers in parentheses [e.g., disp. #30 (thirty), refills 2 (two)].

B. **Adverse drug reactions** occur frequently, and the rate increases in proportion to the number of drugs taken. Adverse reactions may be allergic, idiosyncratic, or dose-related magnification of known effects. Following these principles may decrease the incidence of adverse drug reactions:

1. **Take a careful history** of previous drug reactions and record the drug and adverse reaction clearly on the chart.
2. **Use as few drugs as possible.**
3. **Drug interactions.** A new medication should be added only after careful consideration of the patient's current medical regimen. See Appendix B for a list of commonly used medications and their interactions.
4. **Consider the metabolism,** route of excretion, and major adverse effects associated with each drug used. Individualize dosages according to the patient's age, weight, and kidney and liver function.
5. **Report unusual drug reactions** to the U.S. Food and Drug Administration.

IV. **Fever** accompanies many illnesses and is a valuable marker of disease activity. The cause should be ascertained as quickly as possible. Infection is of primary concern; a drug reaction and fever secondary to malignancy or infarction are other possibilities but are diagnoses of exclusion.

A. **Fever may cause** increased tissue catabolism, dehydration, exacerbation of heart failure, delirium, and convulsions. Treatment of fever is indicated to prevent these harmful effects and for patient discomfort. Heat stroke and malignant hyperthermia are medical emergencies requiring prompt recognition and treatment (see Chap. 9).

B. **Treatment**

1. **Antipyretic drugs** may be given regularly until the underlying disease process has been controlled. Aspirin and acetaminophen are the drugs of choice (325–650 mg q4h). Aspirin should be avoided in adolescents with possible viral infections because this combination has been associated with Reye's syndrome.
2. **Hypothermic (cooling) blankets** may be effective but require careful monitoring of rectal temperatures and may produce excessive shivering and patient discomfort. The blanket should be discontinued when the patient's temperature falls below 39°C.
3. **Ice baths** are reserved for extreme cases of hyperthermia, such as heat stroke (see Chap. 9).

V. **Relief of pain**

A. **General**

1. **Pain** is always subjective, and therapy should be individualized. **Objective measurements** such as tachycardia are not reliable. A placebo response does not distinguish organic from psychogenic pain.
2. **Acute pain** usually requires only temporary therapy.
3. **Chronic pain** may occur in many situations. Nonnarcotic preparations should be used to treat it when possible. Occasionally, pain is refractory to conventional therapy, and nonpharmacologic modalities such as nerve blocks, sympathectomy, and relaxation therapy may be appropriate.

B. **Acetaminophen** has antipyretic and analgesic actions but does not have antiinflammatory or antiplatelet properties.

1. **Preparations and dosage.** Acetaminophen, 325–1,000 mg q4–6h (maximum dose 4 g/24h), is available in tablet, caplet, elixir, and rectal suppository form.
2. **Adverse effects.** The principal advantage of acetaminophen is its lack of gastric toxicity. Hepatic toxicity may be serious, however, and acute overdosage with 10–15 g can cause fatal hepatic necrosis (see Chap. 9).

C. **Aspirin** has analgesic, antipyretic, and antiinflammatory effects.
1. **Preparations and dosages.** Aspirin is given in a dose of 325–1,000 mg PO q4h for relief of pain. Rectal suppositories (300–600 mg q3–4h) may be irritating to the mucosa and have variable absorption. Enteric-coated tablets and nonacetylated salicylates (see Table 24-2) may cause less injury to the gastric mucosa than buffered or plain aspirin. The nonacetylated salicylates also lack antiplatelet effects.
2. **Adverse effects**
   a. **Dose-related side effects** include tinnitus, dizziness, and hearing loss.
   b. **Dyspepsia and GI bleeding** are often encountered and may be severe.
   c. **Hypersensitivity reactions,** including bronchospasm, laryngeal edema, and urticaria, are uncommon, but patients with asthma and nasal polyps are susceptible. Patients with allergic or bronchospastic reactions to aspirin should not be given nonsteroidal antiinflammatory drugs.
   d. **Antiplatelet effects** may last for up to 1 week after a single dose. **Aspirin should be avoided** in patients with known bleeding disorders, in those receiving anticoagulant therapy, and during pregnancy.
   e. **Chronic excessive use** may result in interstitial nephritis and papillary necrosis. Aspirin should be used with caution in patients with hepatic or renal disease.

D. **Nonsteroidal antiinflammatory drugs (NSAIDs)** are commonly prescribed for nonrheumatologic pain such as dental pain, menstrual cramping, headache, postoperative pain, and musculoskeletal pain. **NSAIDs should be used with caution in patients with impaired renal or hepatic function.**
1. **Preparations.** Ibuprofen (200–400 mg PO q4–6h) is an appropriate drug for most mild to moderate pain. Occasionally 600–800 mg PO q6–8h may be more effective (maximum dose 2,400 mg/24h). Many other **oral preparations are** available (see Table 24-2). They vary in lipid solubility, delivery to synovial tissue, half-lives, dosing schedules, and cost. **Ketorolac tromethamine may be administered IM or PO;** 30–60 mg IM is administered as a loading dose, followed by 15–30 mg IM q6h for short-term use. Analgesia peaks at 30–45 minutes.
2. **Adverse effects.** The most common adverse effects are GI and renal. All of these agents can cause dyspepsia. **Gastric** erosion, peptic ulceration, and major GI bleeding may occur (see Chap. 15). NSAIDs alter the autoregulation of renal blood flow and may cause reversible impairment of glomerular filtration, acute renal failure, interstitial nephritis, and papillary necrosis. **Renal function** should be monitored in patients who are receiving chronic NSAID therapy.

E. **Opioid analgesics**
1. **Opioid** describes drugs that are pharmacologically similar to opium or morphine. They are the drugs of choice when analgesia without antipyretic action is desired but should be used with caution in patients with impaired hepatic function.
2. **Dosing and administration** (Table 1-1)
   a. **Constant pain** requires continuous analgesia (around-the-clock) with supplementary (prn) doses for breakthrough pain. Each patient should be maintained at the lowest dosage that provides adequate analgesia. The amount of analgesia needed is frequently underestimated and the duration of action overestimated. If frequent prn doses are required, the regular dose should be increased or the dosing interval decreased.
   b. **If adequate analgesia** cannot be achieved at the maximum recommended dose of one narcotic, or if the side effects are intolerable, the patient should

Table 1-1. Analgesic potency of selected opioid drugs

Drug	Oral-parenteral potency ratio	Potency relative to equivalent parenteral dose of morphine	Usual analgesic dose range and dosing interval (hr)
Morphine	1:6	1.0	5–15 mg IM/SC (q4–5)
Hydromorphone	1:5	6.0	2–4 mg PO (q4–6) 1–2 mg IM/IV/SC (q4–6)
Meperidine	1:3	0.15	50–150 mg PO/SC/IM (q2–3)
Methadone	1:2	1.0	5–15 mg PO (q4–6)
Oxycodone	1:2	1.0	5 mg PO (q6)
With acet			5 mg/325 mg acet (q6)
With asa			4.5 mg/325 mg asa (q6)
Codeine	1:1.5	0.1	30–60 mg PO/IM/SC (q4–6)
Propoxyphene	*	<0.1	50 mg/325 mg acet (q4)
With acet			100 mg/650 mg acet (q4)

acet = acetaminophen; asa = aspirin.
* Not available in parenteral form.

be changed to another preparation beginning at one-half the equianalgesic dose (see Table 1-1).

   c. Oral medications should be used when possible. Parenteral administration is useful in the setting of dysphagia, emesis, and decreased GI absorption. The lowest initial dose should be given, with a gradual increase in the amount of drug given until adequate analgesia is obtained.

   d. Continuous IV administration provides steady blood levels and allows rapid dose adjustment. Agents with short half-lives, such as morphine, should be used. **Patient-controlled analgesia (PCA)** is often used to control pain in the postoperative or terminally ill patient. PCA often improves pain relief, decreases anxiety, and allows less total drug to be given.

3. Selected drugs

   a. Immediate (MSIR) and sustained-release (MS Contin) morphine preparations (MSIR, 5–30 mg PO q2–8h; MS Contin, 15–120 mg PO q12h or a rectal suppository) may be used. **MS elixir** may be useful in patients with dysphagia. Larger doses of morphine may be necessary to control pain as tolerance develops.

   b. Hydromorphone is a potent morphine derivative. It can be given IV with caution. It is also available as a 3-mg rectal suppository.

   c. Meperidine causes less biliary spasm and constipation than morphine. **It is contraindicated in patients taking monoamine oxidase inhibitors (MAOIs) and in patients with renal failure** (accumulation of active metabolites causes CNS excitement and seizures). Repetitive dosing is more likely to cause seizures; therefore, chronic administration is not recommended. **Coadministration of hydroxyzine** (25–100 mg IM q4–6h) may decrease nausea and potentiate the analgesic effect of meperidine.

   d. Methadone is very effective when administered orally and suppresses the symptoms of withdrawal from other opioids (due to its extended half-life). Despite its long elimination half-life, its analgesic duration of action is much shorter.

   e. Oxycodone and propoxyphene are usually prescribed orally in combination with aspirin and acetaminophen.

    f. Codeine can also be given in combination with aspirin or acetaminophen. It is an effective **cough suppressant** at a dosage of 10–15 mg PO q4–6h.

    g. Mixed agonist-antagonist agents (butorphanol, nalbuphine, oxymorphone, pentazocine) offer few advantages and more adverse effects than the other agents.

4. Precautions

    a. Opioids are contraindicated in acute disease states in which the pattern and degree of pain are important diagnostic signs (e.g., head injuries, abdominal pain). They may also increase intracranial pressure.

    b. Opioids should be used with caution in patients with hypothyroidism, Addison's disease, hypopituitarism, anemia, respiratory disease (e.g., chronic obstructive pulmonary disease, asthma, kyphoscoliosis, severe obesity), severe malnutrition, debilitation, or chronic cor pulmonale.

    c. The dosage should be adjusted for patients with impaired **hepatic function.**

    d. Drugs that potentiate the **adverse effects** of opioids include phenothiazines, antidepressants, benzodiazepines, and alcohol.

    e. Tolerance develops with chronic use and coincides with the development of physical dependence.

    f. Physical dependence is characterized by a withdrawal syndrome (anxiety, irritability, diaphoresis, tachycardia, GI distress, and temperature instability) when the drug is abruptly stopped. It may occur after only two weeks of therapy. Administration of an opioid antagonist (e.g., naloxone) may precipitate withdrawal after only 3 days of therapy. Withdrawal can be minimized by slowly tapering the medication over several days.

5. Adverse and toxic effects. While individuals may tolerate some preparations better than others, at equianalgesic doses there are few differences.

    a. CNS effects include sedation, euphoria, and pupillary constriction.

    b. Respiratory depression is dose-related and is especially pronounced after IV administration. Opioids should be used cautiously and at decreased doses in patients with respiratory impairment.

    c. Cardiovascular effects include peripheral vasodilatation and hypotension, especially after IV administration.

    d. The most common GI effect is constipation. Patients receiving opioid medications should be provided with stool softeners and laxatives. Opioids may precipitate toxic megacolon in patients with inflammatory bowel disease. **Nausea and vomiting** may be limited by keeping the patient in a recumbent position.

    e. Opioids increase bladder, ureter, and urethral sphincter tone, which may cause **urinary retention.**

    f. Allergic reactions (urticaria, rash, and anaphylaxis) are uncommon.

Sedative and Psychoactive Drug Therapy

I. Sedative-hypnotic and anxiolytic drugs are among the most widely prescribed medications in the United States, primarily due to the popularity of benzodiazepines in the treatment of insomnia and anxiety.

A. Principles of management

    1. Insomnia may be attributed to a variety of underlying medical or psychiatric disorders (e.g., depression). Behavioral and relaxation techniques should be attempted before drug therapy is initiated.

    2. Anxiety may be part of the symptom complex seen in major depression, panic disorder, drug toxicity or withdrawal, and metabolic disturbances. These underlying causes require specific therapy. The use of antianxiety medications for transient anxiety-provoking situations should be short-term.

    3. Physical dependence develops with regular use of barbiturates and benzo-

Table 1-2. Selected benzodiazepines

Drug	Route	Dosage	Half-life (hr)
Alprazolam	PO	0.75–4.00 mg/24 hr (in 3 doses)	11–15
Chlordiazepoxide	PO	15–100 mg/24 hr (in divided doses)	6–30
Clorazepate	PO	7.5–60.0 mg/24 hr (in 1–4 doses)	30–100
Diazepam	PO	6–40 mg/24 hr (in 1–4 doses)	20–50
	IV	2.5–20.0 mg (slowly)	
Flurazepam	PO	15–30 mg qhs	50–100
Lorazepam*	PO	1–10 mg/24 hr (in 2–3 doses)	10–20
	IV/IM	0.05 mg/kg (4 mg max)	
Midazolam	IV	0.035–0.100 mg/kg	1–12
	IM	0.08 mg/kg	
Prazepam	PO	20–60 mg/24 hr (in divided doses or qhs)	36–70
Oxazepam*	PO	30–120 mg/24 hr (in 3–4 doses)	5–10
Temazepam*	PO	15–30 mg qhs	9–12
Triazolam*	PO	0.125–0.250 mg qhs	2–3

* Metabolites are inactive.

diazepines. Abrupt termination of prolonged treatment at usual therapeutic doses can result in a withdrawal syndrome consisting of agitation, irritability, insomnia, tremor, headache, GI distress, and perceptual disturbance. Seizures and delirium may occur with sudden discontinuation of barbiturates or benzodiazepines.

4. **Sedative-hypnotic** medications potentiate the effects of other CNS depressants such as alcohol.

B. **Benzodiazepines** are effective as anxiolytics, hypnotics, anticonvulsants, and muscle relaxants. They are relatively safe in combination with most other medications and in patients with many medical illnesses. They are generally not lethal when taken alone in overdoses. Use should be short-term since they produce tolerance and dependence. The potential for abuse is considerable. Certain primary anxiety disorders may warrant longer-term use. Table 1-2 provides a list of selected benzodiazepines and their dosages.

1. **Pharmacology.** Most benzodiazepines undergo oxidation to active metabolites in the liver. However, the metabolites of lorazepam, oxazepam, triazolam, and temazepam are inactive and are therefore useful in patients with liver disease. **Benzodiazepine toxicity** is increased by advanced age of the patient, hepatic disease, and concomitant use of alcohol and other CNS depressants, disulfiram, and cimetidine. **Benzodiazepines with long half-lives** accumulate during repeated dosage intervals and may accumulate substantially even with single-daily dosing. This effect is of particular concern in the elderly, in whom the half-life may be increased two- to fourfold.

2. **Indications and dosage**
   a. **Relief of anxiety and insomnia** is achieved at the doses outlined in Table 1-2.
   b. **The acute treatment of status epilepticus** includes diazepam (see Chap. 25). It is used to abort prolonged seizure episodes while other longer-

acting anticonvulsants are administered. Diazepam, 1–2 mg/minute IV, is given to a total dose of 5–10 mg. **Extreme caution** should be used to avoid cardiac or respiratory compromise.

  c. **Skeletal muscle spasm** is relieved by benzodiazepines. Diazepam, 2–10 mg PO tid–qid, may be used for brief periods in the treatment of sciatica, temporomandibular joint pain, and other disorders with associated muscle spasm.

  d. **Before procedures** such as cardioversion, diazepam, 2–5 mg IV, or midazolam, 1–3 mg IV, over 2–5 minutes will relieve anxiety and reduce the patient's memory of the procedure.

  e. **Delirium tremens** and early signs of alcohol withdrawal may require large doses of chlordiazepoxide (see Chap. 25).

  3. Toxicity

    a. **Side effects** include drowsiness, dizziness, fatigue, and incoordination. Clinicians must warn patients about psychomotor impairment and the hazard of driving after even a single dose of these agents. Patients should also be warned about the possibility of the development of anterograde amnesia.

    b. **The elderly** are more sensitive to these agents and may also experience paradoxic agitation and delirium.

    c. **Respiratory depression** can occur with oral doses in patients with respiratory compromise. **Intravenous administration of diazepam and midazolam** can be associated with hypotension and respiratory or cardiac arrest in individuals without underlying disease.

    d. **Tolerance** develops to the benzodiazepines. **Benzodiazepine dependence** may develop after only four weeks of therapy. The **withdrawal syndrome** begins one to 10 days after abrupt cessation of therapy and may last for several weeks. Short-acting and intermediate-acting drugs should be decreased by 5–10% every 5 days. Dosages for patients who have been taking long-acting preparations can be tapered more quickly.

C. **Buspirone** is an anxiolytic agent with few side effects. It is associated with limited psychomotor impairment and interaction with ethanol. No tolerance or withdrawal occurs. The usual starting dosage is 5 mg PO tid, titrating to 10 mg tid as needed. It requires chronic administration to exert its anxiolytic effect. Buspirone has no sedative or hypnotic effect.

D. **Barbiturates** have a narrow therapeutic index and have generally been supplanted by the safer benzodiazepines for the treatment of anxiety and insomnia. Barbiturates are used more often in the treatment of seizures. **Acute barbiturate overdose** or poisoning is a medical emergency (see Chap. 9).

E. **Chloral hydrate** is a rapidly effective hypnotic that seldom produces excitement or hangover. It should be avoided in patients with hepatic or renal disease. **Common side effects** include gastric irritation and skin reactions. Toxic doses cause both CNS and respiratory depression. Tolerance, addiction, and withdrawal syndromes can be seen with chronic ingestion. A fatal interaction with ethanol and a short-term increase in the anticoagulant effect of warfarin have been reported. The usual hypnotic dose is 500–1,000 mg PO qhs.

F. **Some antihistamines** have sedative effects.

II. **Antipsychotic drugs** (Table 1-3) are used in the treatment of psychotic symptoms and to control nausea, vomiting, and intractable hiccups. These agents vary widely in their potency and side effects. Addiction does not occur, and overdosage rarely results in death.

A. **Pharmacologic properties.** These drugs have anticholinergic and anti–alpha-adrenergic effects. The plasma half-life is 10–20 hours for most drugs in this class. These agents should be used cautiously in patients with impaired hepatic function.

B. **Clinical use, preparations, and dosage** (see Table 1-3)

  1. **Acute psychotic symptoms.** The usual drug of choice is haloperidol, 1–5 mg PO or IM. This dose can be repeated hourly until the desired effect is achieved.

Table 1-3. Selected antipsychotic medications

Drug	Daily oral dose range (mg)
Chlorpromazine	300–800
Clozapine	250–450
Thioridazine	200–600
Thiothixene	6–30
Molindone	50–150
Perphenazine	8–32
Haloperidol	6–40
Fluphenazine	1–20
Trifluoperazine	6–20
Risperidone	2–10

2. **Chronic antipsychotic therapy.** These medications are used in the treatment of schizophrenia, schizoaffective disorder, psychotic depression, mania, and dementias with psychotic manifestations. These drugs may also be used in depression and anxiety disorders. Dosages and length of treatment vary tremendously depending on the clinical setting, response, and side effects. Furthermore, individuals differ widely in their metabolism of these drugs.
3. **Nausea and vomiting.** Prochlorperazine is usually given in a dosage of 5–10 mg PO, IM, or IV qid, or as a rectal suppository, 25 mg bid. Dystonic reactions may occur.
4. **Intractable hiccups** may be controlled with **chlorpromazine** in the lowest effective dosage (i.e., 10–25 mg PO q4–6h, 25–50 mg IM q3–4h, 25–100 mg rectal suppository q6–8h).
5. **Delirium and dementia**
   a. **In the management of agitation and psychosis** in patients with delirium or dementia, high-potency antipsychotic agents are useful in conjunction with behavioral interventions. Benzodiazepines and barbiturates produce CNS depression, contributing to behavioral problems and clouding etiologic assessment. **Haloperidol** is the drug of choice. Begin using 0.25 mg PO or IM and titrate up as needed to the lowest effective dose. Haloperidol rarely causes hypotension, cardiovascular compromise, or excessive sedation in low dosages, and it may be given to elderly patients. Gradual withdrawal of the medication should be attempted once the target symptoms respond and the patient's condition is stable.
   b. **Sundown syndrome** refers to the appearance of worsening confusion in the evening and is associated with dementia, delirium, and unfamiliar environments. If behavioral intervention such as increased lighting and attention and maintenance of a familiar environment are ineffective, short-term antipsychotic therapy may be beneficial.
C. **Adverse reactions.** In general, lower-potency drugs, such as chlorpromazine and thioridazine, are more sedating and produce more anticholinergic side effects; high-potency agents, such as haloperidol, produce less sedation and fewer anticholinergic effects but cause more extrapyramidal reactions.
   1. **Postural hypotension** may occasionally be acute and severe after IM administration. If significant hypotension occurs, administering IV fluids and placing the patient in the Trendelenburg position is usually sufficient. If **vasopressors** are required, norepinephrine or phenylephrine should be used. Dopamine may exacerbate the psychotic state.
   2. **Anticholinergic effects** include dry mouth, blurred vision, urinary retention, constipation, and tachycardia.
   3. **Extrapyramidal reactions**
      a. **Acute dystonic reactions**, characterized by torticollis, opisthotonos, tics,

grimacing, dysarthria, or oculogyric crisis may occur soon after therapy is initiated. **Diphenhydramine,** 25–50 mg PO, IM, or IV, is effective treatment. Repeat doses may be required.

  b. Parkinsonian reactions occur early in therapy and may require treatment with antiparkinsonian drugs such as benztropine (1–2 mg PO or IM).

  c. Akathisia is a sense of motor restlessness in which the patient feels a constant need to move about. It occurs early in therapy and may be managed with dose reduction or substitution of a less potent agent. Beta-adrenergic antagonists, benzodiazepines, and anticholinergics have also been used in combination with the antipsychotic agent.

  d. Tardive dyskinesia is a late adverse effect characterized by involuntary movement of the lips, tongue, jaw, and extremities. The condition may reverse over time if the antipsychotic can be stopped.

4. Neuroleptic malignant syndrome is an infrequent, potentially lethal complication of antipsychotic drug therapy. Clinical manifestations include rigidity, akinesia, altered sensorium, fever, tachycardia, and alteration in blood pressure. Severe muscle rigidity can cause rhabdomyolysis and acute renal failure. Laboratory abnormalities include elevations in creatine kinase, liver function tests, and white blood cell count.

5. Photosensitivity, urticaria, and maculopapular rashes may occur. These usually resolve after the offending agent is discontinued.

6. Cholestatic jaundice occurs rarely, most often during the first month of therapy. It generally subsides after withdrawal of the drug.

7. Transient leukopenia may develop; however, agranulocytosis is rare during the first 3 months of therapy. Leukocyte counts should be obtained when infections develop in patients who are taking these medications.

8. Galactorrhea, pigmentary retinopathy, keratopathy, and lowering of the seizure threshold have also been reported.

D. Clozapine is an antipsychotic drug that binds to dopamine receptors and may be effective in schizophrenics who fail to respond to conventional treatment. Initial dosage is 25 mg PO bid titrated to a maximum dose of 300 mg qd. Toxicity includes tachycardia, hypotension, seizures, and agranulocytosis. Patients taking clozapine must be enrolled in the Clozaril program, which includes weekly monitoring of the white blood cell count.

III. Antidepressants (Table 1-4)

A. Tricyclic antidepressants

  1. Pharmacologic properties. These drugs block the uptake of norepinephrine and serotonin. They are potent antihistamines and anticholinergics and should be used with caution in patients with glaucoma or prostatic hypertrophy. These compounds are metabolized by the liver, and individuals may differ greatly in their metabolism of these agents.

  2. Indications and dosage. Choice of drug should be individualized based on the side effect profile and the degree of sedation associated with the drug.

    a. Amitriptyline is useful for depressed patients who may benefit from sedation. However, this agent should not be used to treat insomnia unless the symptom is a manifestation of depression. The usual starting dosage of amitriptyline is 50 mg PO, given as a single bedtime dose. This dosage can be increased by 25–50 mg every 2–3 days to a daily dose in the therapeutic range. Patients usually require 2–4 weeks to achieve a significant clinical response. The drug can be increased as tolerated to the maximum therapeutic dose (200–300 mg/day).

    b. Desipramine or nortriptyline may be the preferred agent when it is important to minimize sedation and anticholinergic side effects. Plasma levels of specific tricyclic agents may aid in patient management, particularly in the elderly. A reasonable approach is to begin nortriptyline at 10 mg PO qhs, increasing by 10 mg every 3 days to a total of 30–40 mg PO qhs.

    c. Maprotiline has been associated with a higher incidence of seizures than the other tricyclic antidepressants.

Table 1-4. Selected antidepressant medications

Drug	Usual first-day dose (mg)	Daily dose range (mg)
Tricyclics		
Amitriptyline	50	100–300
Desipramine	50	100–300
Imipramine	50	100–300
Nortriptyline	25	75–150
Protriptyline	15	15–60
Dibenzoxapine tricyclics		
Amoxapine	150	200–400
Doxepin	50	100–300
Tetracyclic		
Maprotiline	75	150–225
Serotonin reuptake inhibitor		
Fluoxetine	20	20–80
Paroxetine	20	50
Sertraline	50	200
Others		
Trazodone	150	150–400
Bupropion	100	450
Venlafaxine	75	75–375

   d. Clomipramine can be effective in treating obsessive-compulsive disorder. It also has antidepressant properties, can be highly sedating, and is strongly anticholinergic.
   3. **Tricyclic antidepressants are now the leading cause of drug overdose death** in the United States. Because they are given to patients at high risk of suicide, prescriptions should be limited to a total of 1 g, without refills, in the early stages of therapy and when the patient appears to be suicidal.
   4. **Side effects and toxicities** (see Chap. 9 for management of overdosage).
      a. Anticholinergic effects include blurred vision, constipation, dry mouth, tachycardia, and urinary retention. These effects are increased by drugs that impair hepatic metabolism and other anticholinergic drugs such as antihistamines (e.g., diphenhydramine).
      b. Cardiovascular effects include postural hypotension and myocardial depression. Arrhythmias, tachycardia, and electrocardiographic changes such as prolongation of the QRS or QT intervals and ST-T wave changes may occur. **These drugs should be used with caution in patients with cardiovascular disease.**
      c. Tricyclic antidepressants have potential interactions with many drugs (see Appendix B).
      d. Hypersensitivity reactions include rashes, leukopenia, and cholestatic jaundice.
      e. Sedation occurs in varying degrees depending on the specific preparation. Other CNS effects include anxiety, confusion, tremor, and lowering of the seizure threshold.
   B. **Serotonin uptake inhibitors** (see Table 1-4) are chemically unrelated to the tri- and tetracyclic antidepressants. Serotonin uptake inhibitors **should not be used in combination with monoamine oxidase inhibitors (MAOIs) or within 14 days of MAOI use** as fatal reactions may occur. Morning dosing is generally recommended. Common side effects include anxiety, headache, insomnia, nausea, and weight loss. **Fluoxetine** may be used in the treatment of depression and may also be useful in the treatment of obsessive-compulsive disorder. The onset of action occurs 2–4 weeks after initiation of therapy. Because of its long

half-life, fluoxetine should be **discontinued 5 weeks prior to the initiation of MAOIs.** Urticaria and rashes require discontinuation of the drug. **Manifestations of toxicity** include agitation, seizures, and vomiting. Death has not been associated with fluoxetine alone. **Sertraline and Paroxetine** are newer serotonin uptake inhibitors useful in the treatment of depression.

C. Trazodone may be useful for the treatment of severe anxiety or insomnia. It is generally not used for depression. It is highly sedating, causes postural hypotension, and is associated with ventricular ectopic activity. No deaths or cardiovascular complications have been reported in patients taking trazodone alone. There are a number of potential drug interactions with trazodone (see Appendix B).

D. Bupropron is a phenylethylamine compound. The initial dosage is 100 mg PO bid, which may be increased to a maximum dose of 450 mg qd. Side effects include agitation, restlessness, and insomnia. It has fewer anticholinergic effects than tricyclic antidepressants. It may cause increased seizure activity.

E. Psychostimulants (methylphenidate, dextroamphetamine) do not exert a primary effect on mood. They are reportedly useful for short-term management of social withdrawal or psychomotor retardation in the depressed elderly patient.

F. Other agents

1. Monoamine oxidase inhibitors (phenelzine, tranylcypromine, isocarboxazid) are used to treat depression and anxiety disorders. MAOIs may interact with tyramine-containing foods and other drugs to produce a **hypertensive crisis.** Drugs that precipitate this reaction include sympathomimetic amines (e.g., those in decongestants and anorectal preparations), meperidine, methyldopa, and levodopa. Foods include beer, broad beans, canned figs, certain cheeses, chicken livers, chocolate, herring, processed meats, red wines, and yeast. **Treatment** requires immediate administration of an alpha-adrenergic antagonist such as phentolamine, 5 mg IV given slowly q4–6h, until the blood pressure is stabilized. Norepinephrine should be available in case of an exaggerated hypotensive response. MAOIs should not be used in combination with CNS depressants. **Seizures,** hyperpyrexia, circulatory collapse, and death have been reported after a single dose of **meperidine** in patients receiving MAOIs.

2. Lithium is used to treat bipolar affective disorders. It has a narrow therapeutic index, mandating cautious monitoring of serum levels during therapy. Renal function must be monitored, and the dose must be reduced in patients with impaired renal function. The therapeutic range is 0.6–1.2 mEq/liter. **Common side effects** include tremor, polydipsia, polyuria, weight gain, GI discomfort, and benign reversible T-wave depression on ECG. **Adverse reactions** include goiter, nephrogenic diabetes insipidus, leukocytosis, hypercalcemia, and multiple drug interactions (see Appendix B). Serum levels above 1.5 mEq/liter are accompanied by ataxia, CNS depression, seizures, GI disturbance, arrhythmias, and hypotension. Treatment of toxicity is supportive. If renal function is adequate, excretion can be accelerated with osmotic diuresis and sodium bicarbonate infusion. Dialysis should be reserved for severe toxicity.

IV. Electroconvulsive therapy (ECT) is the most effective treatment of major depression, catatonia, and mania, although its use is generally reserved until pharmacologic therapy has failed. It can be safely administered to all age groups and in the presence of most medical illnesses. The only **absolute contraindication is increased intracranial pressure.** Recent myocardial infarction, severe pulmonary disease, severe congestive heart failure, severe hypertension, and venous thrombosis are considered to be relative contraindications, and the risks must be weighed against those of suicide, starvation, and immobility. ECT is performed under anesthesia. **Adverse effects** include headaches, confusion, memory loss, myalgias, and minor arrhythmias. Death occurs in approximately 1 in 10,000 patients and is generally associated with cardiac disease, advanced age, and hypertension (*Anesthesiology* 67:367, 1987).

Pregnancy and Medical Therapeutics

Table 1-5 is a partial list of drugs used during pregnancy at Barnes Hospital in St. Louis, Missouri. **All drugs should be avoided during the first trimester of pregnancy (and, if possible, during the last half of the menstrual cycle in any sexually active fertile female) unless absolutely necessary.** As few drugs as possible should be used throughout pregnancy (*Drugs in Pregnancy and Lactation.* Baltimore: Williams & Wilkins, 1986; *Mayo Clin Proc* 59:707, 755, 1984).

Dermatologic Therapy

I. **Principles of management**
Skin disorders are characterized by pruritus, inflammation, alterations in hydration, and susceptibility to irritation. Identification and treatment of specific underlying conditions should always be attempted.
  A. **Restoration of proper hydration**
    1. **Dry skin** is a common problem in older patients and in many patients with dermatoses.
      a. **Bathing** should be kept to a minimum, followed by application of a bath oil immediately after blotting dry with a towel. Extrafatted soaps such as Basis should be used. Soap should be used only on the face, axillae, crural areas, feet, and obviously dirty areas.
      b. **Lubricating emollients** should be applied frequently and should be thoroughly rubbed into the skin. Available products include Aquaphor, Eucerin, lanolin, Nivea, white petrolatum, and urea-containing products.
    2. **Excessive moisture** in intertriginous areas requires careful drying followed by application of a powder or dry dressing of absorptive material. In severe cases with maceration, exudation, and erosion, wet-to-dry dressings should be applied. The skin surfaces should be kept separated with absorptive materials (see sec. II.E).
  B. **Pruritus** and burning can lead to uncontrolled scratching and perpetuate an underlying condition.
    1. **Topical agents** can be used to control symptoms.
      a. **Camphor** 1–3% and **menthol** provide a cooling sensation and can be used up to four times/day.
      b. **Phenol** 0.25–2.00% causes local hypoesthesia. It should not be used on raw or ulcerated skin.
      c. **Calamine** lotion may be helpful.
    2. **Systemic antihistamines** (H_1-receptor antagonists) are most useful in the treatment of urticaria but are also useful adjuncts in other skin disorders characterized by pruritus. Commonly used drugs include diphenhydramine, 25–50 mg PO q6–8h, and hydroxyzine, 10–50 mg PO q6–8h. While these agents are effective and inexpensive, their major drawback is sedation. Terfenadine (60 mg PO bid), astemizole (10 mg PO qd), and loratadine (10 mg PO qd) are not sedating and can be used for daytime dosing, with one of the other agents used at night. Both terfenadine and astemizole may prolong the QT interval and have rarely been associated with serious cardiac arrhythmias. Maximum recommended doses should not be exceeded, and concomitant use of erythromycin, ketoconazole, or troleandomycin should be avoided.
  C. **Control of inflammation.** Table 1-6 categorizes commonly used topical steroid preparations by the type of base and strength of preparation.
    1. **Base.** Ointments and creams are more lubricating than gels, lotions, and solutions. Ointments are more occlusive and therefore more potent. A lubricating ointment is best for dry eczema, whereas a cream would be more

Table 1-5. Partial list of drugs used during pregnancy at Barnes Hospital

Type of medication	Safe to use in pregnancy[a]	Limited information, relatively safe[b]	Risks associated with use[c]	Avoid in pregnancy[d]
Analgesics	Acetaminophen	Hydromorphone[e] Codeine[e] Meperidine[e] Oxycodone with aspirin[e] Morphine[e]	Salicylates Ibuprofen Indomethacin	
Antibiotics	Ampicillin Erythromycin Penicillin Carbenicillin Amphotericin B Nitrofurantoin Ethambutol	Amikacin Ampicillin with sulbactam Chloroquine[f] Isoniazid Metronidazole[g] Miconazole Aztreonam Ticarcillin Oxacillin Cephalosporins Clindamycin Gentamicin	Streptomycin Sulfonamides[h] Rifampin Trimethoprim Kanamycin Amoxicillin with clavulanic acid Tobramycin Chloramphenicol	Ciprofloxacin Norfloxacin Tetracyclines
Anticoagulants		Dipyridamole Heparin		Warfarin
Antiemetics	Meclizine	Prochlorperazine Trimethobenzamide Metoclopromide Scopolamine	Triethylperazine	
Antiepileptics		Ethosuximide Clonazepam	Phenytoin Valproic acid Primidone Phenobarbital	Trimethadione

Antihistamines	Tripelenamine Chlorpheniramine	Brompheniramine	Terfenadine Astemizole Diphenhydramine Hydroxyzine	
Antihypertensives		Atenolol Hydralazine Methyldopa Labetalol Metoprolol Propranolol	Nitroprusside Diazoxide Timolol Nadolol Clonidine Prazosin Albuterol Isoproterenol Metaproterenol	Captopril Reserpine Enalapril Lisinopril
Asthma preparations		Beclomethasone Aminophylline Cromolyn sodium Terbutaline Ipratropium bromide		
Cardiac drugs	Digoxin	Procainamide Atropine Quinidine Lidocaine Verapamil Disopyramide	Diltiazem Nifedipine	
Cough preparations		Terpin hydrate Guaifenesin		
Diuretics[1]		Furosemide Mannitol	Bumetanide Ethacrynic acid Acetazolamide Hydrochlorothiazide Spironolactone	

Table 1-5. (continued)

Type of medication	Safe to use in pregnancy[a]	Limited information, relatively safe[b]	Risks associated with use[c]	Avoid in pregnancy[d]
Hypoglycemics[j]	Insulin			Chlorpropamide[g] Tolbutamide[g] Glyburide[g]
Laxatives	Milk of magnesia Psyllium	Docusate		
Sedatives				Barbiturates Benzodiazepines
Thyroid preparations	Thyroxine		Methimazole Propylthiouracil Iodide	
Other drugs	Ferrous sulfate Kaopectate Probenecid Antacids	Allopurinol Clofibrate H$_2$-antagonists Vaccines (influenza, polio, rabies, tetanus) Bromocriptine	Glucocorticoids Amphetamines EDTA General anesthetics Haloperidol Penicillamine Phenothiazines Tricyclic antidepressants	Antineoplastic agents Lithium Disulfiram Estrogens, DES Isotretinoin Quinine Vaccines (rubella, mumps, measles, smallpox) Misoprostol

[a] Although no drug can be used with certainty that there will be no adverse effects, drugs listed in this column are used at Barnes Hospital.

[b] Many drugs in this column are new and data are limited, but no consistent adverse effect has been attributed to their use.

[c] These drugs have some associated risk when used in pregnancy. The potential benefit must be weighed against possible adverse effects.

[d] These drugs have been well documented to produce adverse fetal effects and this risk outweighs any possible benefit.

[e] Possible neonatal addiction and withdrawal may occur after long-term use. Neonatal depression may occur with intrapartum use.

[f] Drug of choice for malaria treatment and prophylaxis in pregnancy.

[g] Avoid in first trimester.

[h] Avoid near term.

[i] Diuretics can deplete maternal intravascular volume and, in rare instances, can be associated with neonatal thrombocytopenia. Diuretics are not indicated in pregnancy-induced hypertension as first-line agents.

[j] There is no place for oral hypoglycemic agents in the treatment of diabetes in pregnancy. Oral hypoglycemic agents have been associated with prolonged hypoglycemia in newborn infants. Insulin and dietary control are indicated to bring blood sugar under rigid control.

Table 1-6. Commonly used topical glucocorticoids

Ointments and creams	Lotions and solutions
Low strength	
Hydrocortisone 1%	Hydrocortisone lotion 1%
Desonide 0.05%	
Medium strength	
Triamcinolone acetonide 0.1%	Triamcinolone acetonide lotion 0.1%
Flurandrenolide 0.05%	Fluocinolone acetonide solution 0.01%
Fluocinolone acetonide 0.025%	Betamethasone valerate lotion 0.1%
Betamethasone valerate 0.1%	
Betamethasone dipropionate 0.05%	
High strength	
Halcinonide 0.1%	
Fluocinonide solution 0.05%	
Fluocinonide 0.01% and 0.025%	
Desoximetasone 0.25%	
Highest strength*	
Clobetasol propionate 0.05%	
Betamethasone dipropionate 0.05% in optimized vehicle (e.g., Diprolene)	

* May produce adrenal suppression.

appropriate for a weeping, eczematous dermatitis. Lotions, gels, and solutions are easy to use in hairy areas, including the scalp.

2. **Strength.** Lower-strength preparations are indicated for facial use. Higher-strength preparations are used for palmar or plantar involvement, or for severe and resistant lesions not responsive to lower-strength products. **Fluorinated steroids** are significantly more potent than hydrocortisone or nonfluorinated preparations and **should never be used on the face.** The most potent topical steroids can cause suppression of the pituitary-adrenal axis.

3. **Dosage** of topical steroids depends on the clinical situation. Application should be performed bid–qid. When cream or ointment is used, roughly 25–40 g is needed to cover the entire body of an adult.

4. **Occlusion** with plastic wrap increases the potency of the products but should be reserved for severe, resistant lesions. Occlusion can cause sweat retention, atrophy, maceration, folliculitis, and suppression of the pituitary-adrenal axis if extensive areas of skin are involved.

D. **Protection**

1. **Cotton and rubber gloves** can be used to avoid excessive contact with water or chemical irritants. Cotton absorbs palmar sweat and should be cleaned or changed frequently.

2. **Barrier creams and ointments** containing silicone may prevent contact of irritating chemicals with sensitive skin but are not substitutes for mechanical barriers.

3. **Sunscreens** are useful adjuncts to long sleeves and wide-brimmed hats for fair-skinned people or patients with dermatoses activated by exposure to ultraviolet light. UVB (280–320 nm) is the principal ultraviolet wavelength responsible for sunburn. Sunscreens for UVB are sufficient for routine use. Certain light-sensitive disorders (e.g., systemic lupus erythematosus) and photosensitizing drugs (e.g., tetracycline, sulfonamides, thiazides, norfloxacin) cause a response to UVA (320–400 nm), and combination sunscreens (UVA and UVB) are necessary. All sunscreens are most effective if applied 30–60 minutes before exposure and should be reapplied after bathing or excessive sweating.

a. **Para-aminobenzoic acid (PABA)** and its esters absorb UVB and are ideal for preventing sunburn. Allergic and photosensitivity reactions occur, however, especially in patients sensitive to benzocaine, procaine, thiazides, and sulfonamides.

   b. Benzophenone derivatives (oxybenzone, dioxybenzone) absorb UVB and some UVA.

   c. Titanium dioxide and zinc oxide are opaque sunscreens that shield against both UVA and UVB. They are particularly useful on the nose and lips.

II. Specific therapy of selected disorders

   A. Acne vulgaris. Routine treatment includes topical medications, possibly with oral antibiotics. Refractory cases should be referred to a dermatologist for isotretinoin and acne surgery. Routine dietary restrictions are not helpful.

   1. Benzoyl peroxide, 5–10% qhs or bid, has antibacterial and drying effects. Therapy should begin with a 5% aqueous base to minimize irritation. More potent alcohol-based gels can be used.

   2. Retinoic acid, 0.05–0.10% cream or 0.010–0.025% gel, inhibits comedone formation. Mild facial erythema should be expected. It is applied once daily (e.g., one-half hour after cleansing) and can be alternated cautiously with benzoyl peroxide in patients who do not respond sufficiently to either medication alone.

   3. Topical antibiotic preparations include clindamycin, erythromycin, and tetracycline. They can be used alone (e.g., in patients who experience excessive irritation with benzoyl peroxide) or in combination with other topical agents.

   4. Systemic antibiotics are used for moderate or severe inflammatory acne, usually in combination with topical therapy. Tetracycline or erythromycin, 500 mg PO bid, should be given until improvement occurs, then gradually reduced as tolerated. **Tetracycline should not be given to children or pregnant women.**

   5. Isotretinoin is a vitamin A derivative effective for refractory nodulocystic acne. It should be prescribed only by a physician experienced in its use.

   a. The usual dosage is 1 mg/kg/day in two divided doses with meals. Therapy is continued for 15–20 weeks. Improvement occurs within 1 month, and long remissions may occur.

   b. Cheilitis, dry skin, dry nose and mouth, and pruritus are commonly observed with its use.

   c. Serious complications include arthralgias, diffuse idiopathic skeletal hyperostosis, pseudotumor cerebri, hyperkalemia, and corneal opacification. **Major fetal abnormalities have been reported. A pregnancy test should be performed before therapy is initiated, and contraception should be used during therapy and for one month after discontinuation.** Liver function tests and serum lipoprotein levels should be monitored monthly.

   6. Other therapies include regular drainage of cysts, nodules, and pustules and removal of closed comedones. Intralesional steroids are used for severe cases.

   B. Eczematous dermatitis. Contact dermatitis, atopic dermatitis, and dyshidrotic eczema are common disorders.

   1. Acute dermatitis (e.g., poison ivy dermatitis) is characterized by erythematous, edematous papules and plaques. Vesicle and bulla formation is common. The rash from poison ivy will begin 24–48 hours following exposure. However, new areas may erupt for up to 4 days. Washing with soap and water will remove unbound antigen and prevent further spread. While mild dermatitis will respond to high-potency topical glucocorticoids, more extensive cases and those involving the face should be treated with prednisone, 40–80 mg/day for the first 3 days and tapered over 10 days. Pruritus may be severe (see sec. **I.B** for treatment of pruritus).

   2. Chronic dermatitis (e.g., atopic or stasis dermatitis, dyshidrotic eczema) is characterized by lichenification, scaling, intense pruritus, and hyperpigmentation. It is often worsened by scratching. Effective therapy includes hydration, reduction of pruritus, and control of inflammation. The frequent use of

emollients, systemic antihistamines, and topical steroid ointments is beneficial. Successful treatment of stasis dermatitis requires reduction of lower-
extremity edema. Stasis ulcers form as a result of trauma in the area of the
dermatitis. The utility of topical and systemic antibiotics is controversial.

3. **Seborrheic dermatitis** is an erythematous, scaly, frequently oily and yellow
   eruption that most often involves the scalp, face, and intertriginous areas. It
   is less pruritic than contact or atopic dermatitis. The scalp is most effectively
   treated by vigorous washing with 2.5% selenium sulfide shampoo 3
   times/week. A keratolytic gel can be used for thick scales. Hydrocortisone 1%
   cream applied qd or bid is effective for lesions of the face, intertriginous areas,
   and more inflamed scalp lesions.

C. **Psoriasis** is a common disorder. Treatment is guided by the extent of skin
   involvement and location of the lesions.
   1. **Mild to moderate psoriasis**
      a. **Topical glucocorticoid creams or ointments** (of medium to high strength)
         should be applied to affected areas tid–qid (see Table 1-6). Overnight
         occlusion of the steroid-treated areas with plastic wrap will hasten
         resolution of the lesions.
      b. **Ultraviolet light (UVL)**, including sunlight, is very effective therapy.
      c. **Tar compounds** may be beneficial when alternated with glucocorticoids.
      d. **Keratolytic agents** can initially be alternated with topical steroids when
         marked hyperkeratosis is present. Salicylic acid, 5% gel or cream, com-
         bined with overnight occlusion is effective.
      e. **Glucocorticoid solutions and tar shampoos** can be used for scalp lesions.
         If scaling is prominent, treatment can be continued overnight with a
         keratolytic preparation or anthralin 0.1–1.0% ointment. In the morning,
         these are washed out with a tar shampoo.
   2. **Severe psoriasis.** Chemotherapeutic agents and long-wave UVL should be
      administered only by a dermatologist. These treatments should be reserved
      for patients who are incapacitated by their disease and who are resistant to
      less toxic forms of treatment.

D. **Urticaria** is characterized by raised erythematous, pruritic plaques that are
   transient in nature. Individual lesions may appear, change shape, and disappear
   within hours. Urticaria accompanied by **anaphylaxis** (wheezing, stridor, hypotension, abdominal or uterine cramping) is a medical emergency.
   1. **Recognition of the precipitating factor** is an important step toward elimi-
      nating the rash. Urticaria may represent a reaction to a medication, food,
      cosmetic, insect sting, or physical factor (pressure or cold). Urticaria may
      accompany a connective tissue disease, malignancy, or infection. Suspected
      etiologies should be eliminated. All unnecessary medications (including
      over-the-counter) should be stopped. Frequently implicated medications
      (beta-lactam antibiotics, sulfonamides, NSAIDs) should be stopped if possi-
      ble; frequently an alternate drug that is less commonly associated with
      urticaria may be substituted.
   2. **Antihistamines** are the mainstay of therapy in the absence of systemic
      symptoms. Hydroxyzine, 10–25 mg PO q6–8h, should be increased to the
      maximum tolerated dose. If the lesions persist, an H_2-antagonist should be
      added. Glucocorticoids should be used for facial involvement and for lesions
      refractory to H_1- and H_2-antagonists. Medications should be used around-the-
      clock for the first 48 hours.
   3. **Chronic urticaria and angioedema** persisting for longer than three weeks
      warrant a thorough evaluation to identify and eliminate the causative agent.
      Tricyclic antidepressants are potent antihistamines and in low doses tend to
      cause less sedation than traditional antihistamines. Doxepin (Sinequan),
      10–25 mg tid, is well tolerated. The evening dose can be increased to 30–50
      mg, as tolerated. A combination of traditional and nonsedating antihista-
      mines (terfenadine, astemizole, and loratadine) can be used to maximize
      control of hives and minimize daytime sedation.

E. **Intertrigo** is an eruption in the body folds resulting from skin rubbing on skin and may be colonized by yeast or bacteria. The skin surfaces must be kept clean, separated, cool, and dry. Topical steroids and powders are helpful. The lesions should be cultured.

F. Fungal skin infections. Clinical diagnosis should be confirmed by culture or by microscopic visualization of fungal forms with 10% potassium hydroxide (KOH).

1. **Candidiasis**
   a. **Intertriginous.** Nystatin cream, 100,000 units/g; miconazole 2% cream or lotion; or clotrimazole 1% cream or solution should be applied bid. Ketoconazole cream can be used once a day for two weeks or until the rash is completely resolved.
   b. **Periungual.** Thymol 2–4% in absolute alcohol applied bid–tid is useful.

2. **Dermatophyte infections** of small areas of glabrous skin and feet (tinea corpora, tinea cruris, tinea pedis) respond to miconazole, clotrimazole, haloprogin, and tolnaftate cream or ointment applied bid. Ketoconazole cream can be used once a day. Nystatin is not effective.

3. **Tinea capitis,** onychomycosis, and widespread dermatophyte infections respond to micronized griseofulvin, 500–1,000 mg PO daily in divided doses. Therapy is continued until the infection is culture-negative and clinically resolved (4–6 weeks for tinea capitis, 6–8 months for fingernail infections). Toenail infections are often resistant to all therapy and may best be treated with removal of the nail and destruction of the nail bed. If cosmesis is of major importance, a trial of griseofulvin and topical medication (1–2 years) may be effective. Headache, nausea, and vomiting are the most common side effects of griseofulvin. The complete blood count and liver function tests should be monitored during therapy. Nail changes may recur after griseofulvin is discontinued. Oral ketoconazole, 200–400 mg/day, is a broad-spectrum antifungal agent that may be effective in resistant cases or in patients not tolerating griseofulvin.

4. **Tinea versicolor.** Regardless of the mode of therapy, this condition recurs.
   a. **Selenium sulfide** 2.5% suspension may be applied as a lotion for 20 minutes, then washed off and reapplied daily for 7 days, then once weekly for 6–8 weeks. Pigmentary changes are slow to resolve. Further applications (several times monthly) may prevent relapse.
   b. **Clotrimazole,** econazole, haloprogin, ketoconazole, miconazole, and tolnaftate are effective but more expensive.

G. Scabies

1. **Permethrin 5% cream** should be applied to the entire body, except the eye area, with attention to the intertriginous areas, skin folds, and finger webs. It is allowed to remain 8–14 hours, after which the patient should shower and dress in clothes that are known to be uncontaminated. One application is curative. Pruritus may persist for 3–4 days and is not a sign of treatment failure.

2. **Lindane** can be used in patients with hypersensitivity to permethrin. **Lindane is contraindicated in young children and pregnant women.** Crotamiton 10% cream can be substituted.

3. **To avoid reinfestation,** all household contacts should be inspected and treated if indicated. All clothes and bed linens should be washed in very hot water or dry-cleaned.

H. Warts

1. **Common warts** are most reliably treated with liquid nitrogen cryotherapy. It can be repeated in several weeks if necessary. Daily treatment with a preparation containing 17% salicylic acid and 17% lactic acid in a flexible collodion is often effective and painless but produces a slower response.

2. **Plantar warts** can be treated with salicylic acid 40% plaster, cut to fit the lesion. It should be applied daily under adhesive tape occlusion followed by debridement of the macerated skin. Daily application of 17% salicylic acid and 17% lactic acid in a flexible collodion is also effective.

3. **Condylomata acuminata** require application by the physician of podophyllin 20–25% in tincture of benzoin, avoiding normal skin. It should be washed off

after 4 hours. Repeat applications on a weekly basis may be necessary. Liquid nitrogen cryotherapy is also effective.

Therapy of Surgical Patients

Medical care of the surgical patient includes appropriate management of underlying illnesses and assistance in avoiding perioperative medical complications. Elective surgery has less risk of postoperative complications than emergency surgery, since the patient's general medical condition can be improved by treating malnutrition, metabolic and electrolyte abnormalities, hypoxemia, and anemia. However, in emergency situations, the disadvantages of delaying surgery may offset the benefit of stabilizing the patient.

I. **Cardiovascular considerations**
  A. **Preoperative assessment of risk** for perioperative cardiac complications in patients undergoing noncardiac surgery is frequently performed. An appropriate assessment of cardiac risk allows a rational assessment of risks and benefits in elective surgery.
  1. **Clinical risk assessment.** The risk of **perioperative myocardial infarction or cardiac death** is greatly increased in patients with the following characteristics, often referred to as the "**Goldman criteria**": (1) decompensated heart failure, (2) myocardial infarction within the last 6 months, (3) more than five ventricular premature contractions (VPCs)/minute, (4) frequent atrial premature contractions (APCs) or more complex atrial arrhythmias, (5) age greater than 70 years, (6) illness requiring emergency procedures, (7) evidence of hemodynamically significant aortic stenosis, and (8) poor general medical condition (*Med Clin North Am* 71:413, 1987). Table 1-7 may be used to calculate a cardiac risk index (CRI). The CRI is a useful predictor of the relative risk of cardiac death or nonfatal cardiac complications associated with surgery (Table 1-8). Additional factors that may be **independent risk factors** for significant perioperative cardiac morbidity include angina and a history of heart failure (*J Gen Intern Med* 1:211, 1986). Preoperative evaluation and intraoperative management should be aimed at eliminating these factors and reducing the risk of a cardiac event.
  2. **Noninvasive tests of cardiac function in the preoperative evaluation** are most useful when the presence, type, or severity of coronary artery disease (CAD) is unknown (*The Medical Consultant*. Baltimore: Williams & Wilkins, 1989). Exercise stress testing may be helpful in sedentary patients with multiple CAD risk factors who are to undergo major surgery. Dipyridamole thallium or dobutamine echocardiographic testing can be used to further stratify patients with an intermediate CRI. It can also be useful in patients with a low CRI but who have multiple CAD risk factors and who are to undergo major vascular surgery (*Ann Intern Med* 110:859, 1989). Preoperative cardiac catheterization should be performed in patients with markedly positive stress tests and in patients with a high CRI.
  B. **Hemodynamic monitoring** with pulmonary artery or intraarterial catheters aids in the management of high-risk patients with a history or presence of congestive heart failure (including S3 gallop or jugular venous distention), aortic stenosis, recent angina, or myocardial infarction. It is prudent to invasively monitor elderly patients and those at risk to develop intraoperative hypotension (i.e., those having vascular procedures). Monitoring should be continued for 48 hours postoperatively until fluids have been mobilized into the vascular space.
  C. **Medical therapies**
  1. **Angiotensin-converting enzyme inhibitors** should be considered in patients with signs and symptoms of heart failure.
  2. **Digoxin** may also be initiated preoperatively to treat patients with signs and symptoms of heart failure.

Table 1-7. Cardiac risk assessment in the preoperative evaluation of noncardiac surgery candidates*

Item	Points
History	
Age >70 years	5
Myocardial infarction within 6 months	10
Physical	
S3 gallop or JVD	11
Important aortic valvular stenosis	3
Electrocardiogram	
Rhythm other than sinus or APCs on preoperative ECG	7
>5 VPCs per minute at any time before surgery	7
Poor general medical status	3
PO_2 <60 or PCO_2 >50 mm Hg	
K^+ <3.0 or HCO_3 <20 mEq/liter	
BUN >50 or creatinine >3 mg/dl	
Abnormal SGOT	
Chronic liver disease	
Bedridden due to noncardiac cause	
Operation	
Intraperitoneal, intrathoracic, aortic surgery	3
Emergency surgery	4
Total points	53

JVD = jugular venous distention; APC = atrial premature contraction; VPC = ventricular premature contraction.
* Once point total of risk is assessed, see Table 1-8 to characterize the percentage risks of different possible complications (e.g., from minor to life-threatening complication).
Source: Modified from HH Weitz, L Goldman. Noncardiac surgery in the patient with heart disease. *Med Clin North Am* 71:416, 1987.

Table 1-8. Risks of cardiac complications in unselected patients older than 40 years who underwent major noncardiac surgery

Class by cardiac risk index	Point total	No or only minor complication (n = 2048) (%)	Life-threatening complication* (n = 60) (%)	Cardiac deaths (n = 33) (%)
I (n = 1127)	0–5	1118 (99)	7 (0.6)	2 (0.2)
II (n = 769)	6–12	735 (96)	25 (3)	9 (1)
III (n = 204)	13–25	175 (86)	23 (11)	6 (3)
IV (n = 41)	≥26	20 (49)	5 (12)	16 (39)

* Life-threatening complications were perioperative myocardial infarction, pulmonary edema, or ventricular tachycardia without progression to cardiac death.
Source: Compiled from numerous sources and modified from HH Weitz, L Goldman. Noncardiac surgery in the patient with heart disease. *Med Clin North Am* 71:416, 1987.

    3. Antiarrhythmic drugs. Patients with a history of arrhythmias should receive their usual dose of antiarrhythmic medication on the morning of surgery. Prophylactic lidocaine should be reserved for patients with a history of sudden death or symptomatic ventricular arrhythmias. The half-life of lidocaine is prolonged by most general anesthetics, and toxicity may occur. Serum levels of lidocaine should be monitored in most cases.

4. **Antianginal drugs** should be continued in the perioperative period. If oral medications cannot be taken, alternative routes of administration should be used (e.g., topical nitrates or IV administration of nitrates or beta-adrenergic antagonists).

D. **Specific conditions**
   1. **Aortic stenosis.** Patients with suspected aortic stenosis should have preoperative echocardiographic evaluation. In cases of symptomatic stenosis, aortic valve replacement should precede elective surgery.
   2. **Permanent transvenous pacemakers** should be placed when indicated, before elective surgery (see Chap. 7). **Temporary transvenous pacemakers** should be used preoperatively in patients at risk for transient bradyarrhythmias or in those who will require a permanent pacemaker but in whom intraoperative bacteremia is likely to develop.
   3. **Stable hypertension** with diastolic blood pressures less than 110 mm Hg does not increase the risk of cardiovascular complications (*Anesthesiology* 50:285, 1979). Antihypertensive medication, especially beta-adrenergic antagonists, should be continued through the morning of surgery. If oral medications cannot be taken for a prolonged period, IV alternatives can be substituted (see Chap. 4).
   4. **Patients with prosthetic valves** are at risk for complications of chronic anticoagulation (see Chap. 17) and bacterial endocarditis (see Chap. 13).

E. **Common postoperative complications**
   1. **Hypertension. Sedation, analgesia, and oxygen** are most effective for the treatment of hypertension in the immediate postoperative period. Marked hypertension should be controlled with IV nitroprusside or nitroglycerin (see Chap. 4). Enalaprilat, 0.625–1.250 mg IV; labetalol, 20–40 mg IV; nicardipine, 5 mg IV; or hydralazine, 5–10 mg IV or IM, may also be effective. Diuretics may be used 24–48 hours postoperatively after mobilization of fluid into the vascular space has occurred.
   2. **Ventricular premature contractions** are best treated by correcting fluid and electrolyte abnormalities. Specific antiarrhythmic therapy is reserved for patients with hemodynamic compromise or life-threatening arrhythmias. Lidocaine or procainamide is the drug of choice (see Chap. 7).
   3. **Supraventricular tachycardias** are best treated by correcting the precipitating causes, such as medications, fever, hypoxemia, and electrolyte abnormalities. Acute management may require the use of adenosine or DC cardioversion (see Chap. 8). Digoxin or verapamil, used perioperatively in patients without underlying heart disease, can usually be discontinued before hospital discharge.
   4. **Heart failure** is usually caused by exogenous fluid administration. Diuretics are the treatment of choice. The possibility of postoperative myocardial ischemia or infarction should be considered.
   5. **Myocardial infarction** tends to occur within 6 days of the procedure. Painless infarction is common. ECGs should be monitored on postoperative days 1, 3, and 6, particularly in patients at high risk for infarction.

II. **Pulmonary complications**
   A. **The risk of pulmonary complications** is greatest in the setting of acute or chronic lung disease, cigarette smoking, obesity, abdominal or thoracic surgery, and anesthesia time longer than 3 hours. Patients should be advised to quit smoking 3–4 weeks before an elective procedure.
   B. **Preoperative evaluation** of patients with pulmonary disease or symptoms should include spirometry, arterial blood gas analysis, and occasionally radioisotope determination of regional lung function. General anesthesia can induce bronchospasm; therefore, patients with reactive airway disease should be treated preoperatively with aggressive bronchodilator therapy to maximize lung function.
   C. **Postoperative management** should include frequent monitoring of oxygen saturation, arterial blood gases, incentive spirometry in patients with asthma and chronic obstructive pulmonary disease. **Sedative and narcotic medications should be used cautiously** to minimize respiratory depression. Chest physical

therapy, postural drainage, deep breathing exercises, and encouragement of coughing are useful in the management of atelectasis. Antibiotics and bronchodilators may be required to treat infection and bronchospasm.

III. **Anticoagulation** (see Chap. 17). The incidence of deep venous thrombosis (DVT) is greatest in patients undergoing major orthopedic procedures and is also increased in patients who are older than 40 years, who have a history of previous pulmonary embolus or DVT, who have secondary risk factors (i.e., obesity, immobilization, varicose veins, estrogen use, paralysis, coagulopathy), or who are undergoing pelvic or abdominal cancer surgery. Perioperative anticoagulation is effective in decreasing the incidence of DVT. The risk of clinically important bleeding with moderate-intensity regimens is relatively low, and recent reports indicate that low molecular weight heparin may minimize this complication (*Ann Intern Med* 114:545, 1991).
   A. **High-risk patients** may be treated with warfarin to a target international normalized ratio (INR) of 2.0–3.0, adjusted low-dose heparin to a target activated partial thromboplastin time (APTT) at the upper limits of normal ± 4 seconds, or external pneumatic compression sleeves (*Med Clin North Am* 77:397, 1993; *Chest* 102: 3125, 1992). Low molecular weight heparin may also be used (see Chap. 17).
   B. **Early postoperative ambulation** reduces the risk of thromboembolic complications but is not a substitute for anticoagulation in high-risk patients.
   C. **In patients requiring prolonged bed rest** but who are not in the high-risk groups, pressure gradient stockings, pneumatic compression, and heparin SC are effective alternatives.
   D. **Patients receiving long-term anticoagulation.** Oral agents can generally be discontinued 48 hours before surgery. Alternatively, oral anticoagulants can be discontinued 3–5 days before surgery, with initiation of full-dose heparin until 4–6 hours before surgery. Heparin is resumed 12–24 hours postoperatively, and oral anticoagulation is restarted when oral intake resumes.

IV. **Patients receiving chronic glucocorticoid therapy** require stress doses of hydrocortisone perioperatively (see Chap. 21).

General Eye Care

I. **Ophthalmologic assessment**
   A. **A complete physical examination** should include assessment of the external eye and eyelid; pupillary size, shape, and reactivity; extraocular muscle function; and visual fields and acuity. A direct fundoscopic examination should also be performed.
   B. **Disturbances of vision** should be evaluated by an ophthalmologist. **Sudden, severe, painless loss of vision requires evaluation by an ophthalmologist in the first few hours.**
   C. **Burning and itching** are usually caused by relatively minor eye disorders. A foreign body sensation should first be evaluated by eversion of the upper lid and examination of the lids, sclera, and conjunctiva for a foreign body, which can be carefully removed with a cotton swab dipped in saline. If no foreign body is seen, the eye should be irrigated with normal saline and patched for 24 hours. If the sensation persists, the patient should be referred to an ophthalmologist.
   D. **Ocular trauma** requires urgent ophthalmologic evaluation (see sec. **IV**).

II. **The red eye** is a common problem. The differential diagnosis includes conjunctivitis, corneal injury or ulceration, foreign body, acute glaucoma, endophthalmitis (intraocular infections), iritis, scleritis, and episcleritis. If alterations in visual acuity are present, the patient should be referred to an ophthalmologist. Patients with corneal injury or ulceration, acute glaucoma, endophthalmitis, iritis, or scleritis also require referral.
   A. **Conjunctivitis** refers to inflammation with or without infection of the ocular mucosa manifested by itching, burning, and discharge without decreased vision. Prolonged or severe cases should be referred to an ophthalmologist.

  1. **Viral conjunctivitis** is characterized by watery discharge and preauricular adenopathy with an associated upper respiratory infection and is often bilateral. Symptoms usually resolve in 7–10 days but may last up to three weeks. Individuals should be cautioned to avoid contact with other people (e.g., avoid shaking hands, sharing towels or pillows).
     a. **Warm compresses** provide symptomatic relief.
     b. **Ocular decongestants** such as naphazoline or tetrahydrazoline are not generally recommended due to the side effects of rebound hyperemia and hypersensitivity.
     c. **Eye makeup** is frequently contaminated and should be discarded.
     d. **Contact lenses** should be washed thoroughly and sterilized.
  2. **Bacterial conjunctivitis** presents with purulent discharge and is usually unilateral.
     a. **Broad-spectrum antibiotic preparations** (e.g., Polytrim drops qid or Polysporin ophthalmic ointment qid) are usually effective. **Sulfacetamide,** 10% ophthalmic drops (e.g., sodium sulamyd) q3h, can also be used but is associated with a much higher incidence of allergic reaction. Tobramycin or gentamicin eye drops should be reserved for more serious infections.
     b. **Gonococcal** conjunctivitis requires parenteral antibiotics (see Chap. 13). Appropriate cultures should be obtained if gonococcal infection is suspected.
  3. **Allergic conjunctivitis** presents with itching, whitish mucus discharge, and boggy conjunctival edema. Allergic upper-respiratory symptoms may also be present.
     a. **Cold compresses** provide symptomatic relief.
     b. **Naphazoline combined with an antihistamine** (e.g., pheniramine) may relieve the itching.
     c. **Intraocular glucocorticoid drops or systemic glucocorticoids should not be used.**
     d. **Systemic antihistamines** may decrease pruritus.
  4. **Toxic or hypersensitive conjunctivitis** mimics viral and allergic inflammations. Antibiotics, ocular decongestants, contact lens solutions, and eye makeup are common causes. Treatment involves discontinuation of the offending agent.
B. **Corneal injury** may be caused by trauma or infection.
  1. **Corneal and conjunctival abrasions** should be assessed with fluorescein staining.
     a. **A sterile fluorescein strip** is placed under the lower lid. The fluorescein will spread across the eye in the tears. After a minute, the strip is removed and the eye rinsed with sterile saline or eyewash. Defects in the conjunctiva or corneal layer will stain bright green when examined with a Wood's lamp.
     b. **Minor defects** should be irrigated, treated with ophthalmic ointment, and covered with an eye patch. **Referral to an ophthalmologist should take place within 24 hours.** Analgesics may be required.
     c. **Extensive abrasions require urgent evaluation.**
     d. **Abrasions from vegetable matter or contaminated material** must be evaluated daily by an ophthalmologist for signs of infection until healing occurs.
     e. **Any abrasion in contact lens wearers should be evaluated by an ophthalmologist.**
     f. **Topical glucocorticoids or anesthetic drops should never be used for treatment of abrasions.**
  2. **Corneal ulcerations** are of two types.
     a. **Bacterial ulceration** is actually a corneal abscess characterized by a ground glass haziness or whitish opacification of the cornea. **Vision is decreased,** but pain can be variable. A predisposing cause, such as an untreated abrasion, inappropriate use of steroid-containing medication, contact lens wear, poor eyelid function, or diabetes mellitus, is almost always present. **The patient should be referred to an ophthalmologist immediately.** Antibiotics should be withheld until the ophthalmologic evaluation occurs. **Under no circumstances should steroid drops be prescribed.**

      b. Herpes simplex keratitis presents with a red eye, blurred vision, and a dendritic ulcer on the cornea. Any patient with suspected herpetic keratitis should be referred to an ophthalmologist.

III. External eye and eyelid problems

    A. Blepharitis refers to inflammation, and occasionally infection, of the eyelid margin. The patient has normal vision but complains of itching, burning, scratchiness, and mattering of the eyelids. Scales, crusting, and sticking together of the lashes are noted clinically. **Treatment** relies on warm compresses qid, lid hygiene with dilute baby shampoo scrubs of the lid margin, and application of ophthalmic antibiotic ointment qhs. Referral to an ophthalmologist is indicated only if the patient's condition fails to improve.

    B. Styes (hordeolum) are acute purulent infections of the marginal eye glands. **Chalazion** is a chronic granulomatous inflammation of the eyelid glands. Treatment for both is the same as for blepharitis. Failure to improve requires referral to an ophthalmologist.

    C. Exposure keratopathy is due to corneal drying and results from failure of eyelid closure in several disease states. The eyelid can be patched or taped closed, and artificial tears (e.g., Refresh, Hypotears) or ophthalmic antibiotic ointments can be prescribed as frequently as q2h. If this treatment proves inadequate, ophthalmologic evaluation should be obtained for the use of a moisture chamber or tarsorrhaphy.

    D. Dry eye states are exacerbated by wind, cold air, and smoke in patients with keratoconjunctivitis sicca (e.g., Sjögren's syndrome, atrophy of the accessory tear glands in the elderly). **Artificial tear replacements** (i.e., Hypotears, Refresh) given qid or more often provide symptomatic relief. Referral to an ophthalmologist is necessary only in refractory cases.

    E. Contact lens care

        1. Soft lenses can be temporarily stored in normal saline. The patient must not replace the soft lenses until they have been properly sterilized.

        2. Hard lenses can be stored dry or in saline and can be replaced after careful rinsing.

    F. Prosthetic eye care includes removal (once weekly to once monthly), cleansing with a mild soap (e.g., Enuclene, baby shampoo), and rinsing before replacement. Prolonged removal of the prosthesis (i.e., for weeks) can lead to contracture of the socket and failure to properly fit.

IV. Ocular trauma

    A. Major injury. Chemical injury, ruptured globe, corneal laceration, and hyphema (blood in the anterior chamber) threaten vision and require immediate recognition and urgent ophthalmologic evaluation (*N Engl J Med* 325:408, 1991).

        1. Chemical injuries (especially after alkali exposure) require immediate profuse irrigation with saline or water until the pH is approximately 7.0, followed by ophthalmologic evaluation.

        2. A ruptured globe may not be readily apparent on physical examination, and vision may remain intact. Patients who were hammering or using power tools at the time of the injury should be carefully evaluated. Intraocular foreign body should be ruled out with CT scan or plain orbital radiograph. Broadspectrum parenteral antibiotic coverage should be administered. The eye should be protected with a metal shield until ophthalmologic evaluation is performed. No drops or ointments should be placed in the eye. Tetanus toxoid administration should be considered (see Appendix E).

        3. Blunt trauma to the globe may result in hyphema, iritis, retinal detachment, disruption of intraocular tissues, or glaucoma. **Hyphema or visual loss necessitates immediate ophthalmologic evaluation**.

    B. Minor trauma

        1. Superficial foreign bodies can be safely removed with a soft cotton swab. Topical anesthesia may be required.

        2. Corneal abrasions (see sec. II.B).

V. Glaucoma can be generally subdivided into two categories.

    A. Open-angle glaucoma is usually treated with drops, but occasionally laser therapy or surgery is required.

    B. Closed- (or narrow) angle glaucoma can be cured by laser iridectomy, but patients often require medications.

    C. Acute angle-closure attacks can rarely be induced by pupillary dilation and usually occur several hours after instillation of the mydriatic drops.

      1. This problem can be avoided by using weak agents such as one drop of Neo-Synephrine 2.5% or tropicamide 0.5%.

      2. An acute angle-closure attack should be treated promptly with acetazolamide, 250 mg PO, and miotic drops such as pilocarpine 2% ophthalmic solution (2 gtts every 15 minutes).

      3. Ophthalmologic referral is necessary within 12 hours.

    D. Many glaucoma medications can have systemic side effects (see sec. **XI**). Since alternatives are often available, an ophthalmologist should be consulted before any medication is discontinued.

VI. Diabetic eye care. See Chap. 20.

VII. The immunocompromised host frequently has eye problems (see Chap. 14).

VIII. Varicella zoster ophthalmitis includes keratitis, uveitis, retinitis, optic neuropathy, or orbital inflammation.

    A. Acyclovir, 200 mg PO 5 times/day for 10 days, reduces the ocular complications in nonimmunocompromised patients when it is administered within 7 days of eruption of the skin lesions.

    B. Ophthalmic antibiotic ointment applied to eyelid vesicles can prevent bacterial superinfection.

    C. Topical and systemic steroids are occasionally required to control inflammatory complications and should be administered only in consultation with an ophthalmologist.

IX. Optic nerve swelling is caused by a variety of entities that are differentiated by vision, visual field, and afferent pupillary defects.

    A. Papilledema is a bilateral phenomenon, with normal vision and pupils.

    B. Optic neuropathy is usually unilateral, with decreased vision and an afferent pupillary defect.

      1. Ischemic optic neuropathy, which occurs after ischemic infarction of the optic nerve, has two forms.

        a. Arteritic optic neuropathy (e.g., giant cell arteritis) is associated with catastrophic visual loss and is suggested by an elevated erythrocyte sedimentation rate (ESR). It is confirmed by a positive temporal artery biopsy. **Polymyalgia rheumatica** is related to this disorder, and any patient with visual disturbances, jaw claudication, or scalp or jaw tenderness should be urgently referred to an ophthalmologist. **Prednisone,** 100 mg PO qd, should be initiated immediately on suspicion of the diagnosis (i.e., after the ESR is obtained and before the biopsy) to protect the contralateral eye and to perhaps preserve residual function in the affected eye. Treatment can be stopped 7–10 days later if the temporal artery biopsy is normal. High-dose steroids (e.g., methylprednisolone, 1–2 g/day) can rarely restore vision in the involved eye.

        b. Nonarteritic optic neuropathy is associated with hypertension. It is analogous to cerebral lacunar infarction and does not require treatment. Associated hypertension should be treated.

      2. Optic neuritis is usually idiopathic and strongly associated with multiple sclerosis. There is no effective treatment.

      3. Other causes include malignant hypertension, compressive orbital lesions, intraocular diseases, toxic neuropathies, and infiltrative lesions; all require ophthalmologic evaluation.

X. Prescribing ophthalmic medications

    A. Ophthalmic antibiotics are available as drops or ointments. Topical ophthalmic Polytrim (trimethoprim, sulfate, and polymyxin) or sodium sulfacetamide 10% drops (e.g., sodium sulamyd), 1 drop qid, or ointment qid, is usually sufficient. Polysporin ointment (polymyxin and bacitracin) is a good alternative. Tobramycin and gentamicin drops should be reserved for specific indications. Neosporin ointment causes ocular hypersensitivity and should be avoided.

B. **Ophthalmic steroids should only be prescribed by an ophthalmologist.** They can cause cataracts, glaucoma, ocular perforation, and exacerbation of infections.

C. **Dilating drops** include a single drop of tropicamide 0.5%, which is usually adequate for direct bedside ophthalmoscopy. Ophthalmologists generally use three drops of tropicamide 1% and phenylephrine 2.5%.

D. **Artificial tear substitutes** provide symptomatic relief and are nonirritating. They are available in a variety of over-the-counter preparations.

E. **Ocular decongestants.** Tetrahydrazoline and naphazoline are mild adrenergic agents and are available in combination with an ocular antihistamine (pheniramine) or with phenylephrine. They relieve minor irritation and vasoconstrict surface blood vessels. Overuse may result in hypersensitivity reactions or rebound hyperemia. Pupillary dilation may precipitate an acute angle-closure glaucoma attack.

XI. **Systemic side effects from ocular medication.** Ophthalmic medications are often an unsuspected cause of patient complaints.

A. **Cholinergic agonists for glaucoma** (pilocarpine, carbachol) usually cause a dull aching in the brow. Rarely, cholinergic toxicity can cause rhinorrhea, salivation, diaphoresis, cramping and other GI complaints, and, rarely, CNS effects.

B. **Anticholinesterases** for glaucoma and strabismus (echothiophate, isoflurophate) can cause side effects similar to those of the cholinergics. Many patients experience mild side effects, especially paresthesias. **Echothiophate inhibits serum pseudocholinesterase; therefore, it must be discontinued several weeks before surgery** to avoid possible succinylcholine toxicity. RBC pseudocholinesterase levels can be measured if necessary.

C. **Adrenergic agonists** for glaucoma (epinephrine, dipivefrin) can cause adrenergic activation with cardiovascular side effects, especially arrhythmias. Dipivefrin is a prodrug that is activated mostly in the eye and therefore produces fewer of these complications.

D. **Beta-adrenergic antagonists** for glaucoma (timolol, levobunolol, betaxolol) are absorbed through the mucosa, and many patients achieve significant plasma levels after a topical dose. Typical **side effects** include bronchospasm, bradycardia, congestive heart failure, mood alterations, and neurologic findings. Betaxolol is cardioselective and has fewer systemic side effects.

E. **Carbonic anhydrase inhibitors** for glaucoma (acetazolamide, methazolamide) almost always cause a metabolic acidosis and paresthesias. Mood disturbances, fatigue, anorexia, GI upset, and diarrhea are common. Occasionally, renal calculi can occur, and these agents should not be used in patients with a history of nephrolithiasis. Hypokalemia may occur, particularly if used concomitantly with thiazide diuretics. Rarely, idiosyncratic aplastic anemia has been reported. Methazolamide causes less of a metabolic acidosis than acetazolamide.

F. **Cycloplegics** for uveitis (atropine, scopolamine, cyclopentolate) are parasympathetic antagonists that can produce systemic toxicity. Facial flushing, disorientation, GI upset, and tachycardia are rarely encountered. Small children are more likely to absorb a toxic dose of atropine when it is used for cycloplegia of the lens and ciliary body before refraction.

G. **Adrenergics** used for dilating the pupil (phenylephrine) can have a high level of systemic absorption. Hypertension following dilation of the pupil occurs in a small percentage of patients receiving the 10% solution. Rarely, hemorrhagic complications secondary to a hypertensive crisis have been associated with phenylephrine.

XII. **Presurgical evaluation of eye patients.** Most eye surgery is done using local retrobulbar anesthesia. Since retinal procedures and orbital surgery can require 2–6 hours and are often done under general anesthesia, cardiac risk assessment is important (see Tables 1-7 and 1-8). **Complications of the local anesthetic agent** include seizures, hypotension, bradycardia, cardiovascular collapse, and respiratory depression or arrest. Coagulopathies can result in retrobulbar hemorrhage, a potentially disastrous complication.

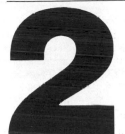

Nutritional Therapy

Stephen J. Bickston

Basic Concepts

I. **Introduction.** As multidisciplinary nutrition teams take a growing role in medical centers, the role of the physician in nutrition management is changing. This chapter is intended to acquaint the reader with the fundamentals of nutritional therapy with an emphasis on disease states requiring specialized therapy.

II. **Patient selection** begins by identifying individuals with significant deficiencies of macronutrients (carbohydrate, protein, and fat) or micronutrients (vitamins, minerals, trace elements).

    A. **Identifying macronutrient deficiency.** Technical means of assessing the nutritional state of patients have not been superior to bedside examination. Commonly used assessments include measuring body weight and immune competence and biochemical testing, though each has limitations. Ideal body weight (IBW) is an estimate derived from actuarial tables providing values associated with longevity. Usual body weight (UBW) relies on patient or family recall and may be a more reliable estimate. Useful biochemical measurements include transferrin, albumin, and pre-albumin. Immune competence, as estimated by lymphocyte count and cutaneous cell-mediated immunity, is not often used. Of all the parameters mentioned, **weight loss over time is probably the most helpful in identifying significantly malnourished patients** (Table 2-1).

    B. **Micronutrient evaluation.** When nutrient consumption exceeds supply, deficiency states occur. Micronutrient deficiencies are generally multiple, but individual deficiencies may be seen as a manifestation of a specific disease or drug effect. Laboratory evaluation has limited utility, as circulating levels of many vitamins and minerals often do not reflect body stores. Discussions of iron, calcium, and vitamin B_{12} deficiency are found in other chapters.

III. **Requirements.** The body's needs for continued existence must be met by exogenous foodstuffs or by tissue catabolism. Adequate nutrient supply is necessary to avoid catabolism, but nutrient excess can be expensive and toxic, causing hypermetabolism, fatty liver, uremia, and encephalopathy. Metabolizing nutrients consumes approximately 10% of the energy they supply. Recommended daily allowances (RDAs) are calculated for healthy individuals taking all nourishment by mouth and have limited application to hospitalized patients.

    A. **Energy needs** are estimated from **basal energy expenditure (BEE)** adjusted for the stress of various conditions and level of activity. This gives an estimate of caloric needs, which can then be met with enteral or parenteral therapy. The Harris-Benedict equations estimate BEE:

Male: BEE (kcal) = $66 + (13.7 \times \text{wt in kg}) + (5 \times \text{ht in cm}) - 6.8 \times \text{age}$ (1)
Female: BEE (kcal) = $655 + (9.6 \times \text{wt in kg}) + (1.85 \times \text{ht in cm}) - 4.7 \times \text{age}$ (2)

A steady state dry weight should be used for volume overloaded patients. As excess fat is metabolically inactive, an adjusted value for patients weighing more than 125% of IBW should be used:

Adjusted weight = $\text{IBW} + [(\text{ABW} - \text{IBW}) \times 0.025]$ (3)

(ABW is actual body weight in kg.) This estimate is then modified by applying

Table 2-1. Estimation of protein-calorie deficiency

	Mild	Moderate	Severe
Percent IBW*	80–90%	70–79%	<70%
Percent UBW	90–95%	80–89%	<80%
Albumin (g/dl)	2.8–3.4	2.1–2.7	<2.1
Transferrin (mg/dl)	150–200	100–149	<100
Weight loss			>5% over 1 mo >7.5% over 3 mos >10% over 6 mos
Total lymphocyte count (mm³)	1,200–2,000	800–1,199	<800
Cell-mediated immunity	Reactive	Reactive	Anergic

UBW = usual body weight.
* Ideal body weight (IBW) can be estimated using the Hamwi method:
  Males: 106 lb for first 5 ft plus 6 lb for each additional inch.
  Females: 100 lb for first 5 ft plus 5 lb for each additional inch.
Note that for patients whose actual body weight (ABW) is more than 125% of IBW, an adjusted IBW should be calculated as follows: IBW + [(ABW − IBW) × 0.25].
Source: Adapted from JP Grant. *Handbook of Total Parenteral Nutrition* (2nd ed). Philadelphia: Saunders, 1992. P. 20.

Table 2-2. Disease stress factors used in calculation of total energy expenditure

Clinical condition	Stress factor
Starvation	0.8–1.0
Elective operation	1.0–1.1
Peritonitis or other infections	1.05–1.25
ARDS or sepsis	1.3–1.35
Bone marrow transplant	1.2–1.3
Cardiopulmonary disease without sepsis, dialysis, or surgery	0.8–1.0
Cardiopulmonary disease with dialysis or sepsis	1.2–1.3
Cardiopulmonary disease with major surgery	1.3–1.55
Acute renal failure	1.3
Liver failure	1.3–1.55
Liver transplant	1.2–1.5
Pancreatitis	1.3–1.8

ARDS = adult respiratory distress syndrome.
Source: Adapted from *Barnes Hospital Nutrition Support Handbook*. St. Louis, 1992. P. 16.

an activity factor (AF) and stress factor (SF) (Table 2-2), yielding **total energy expenditure (TEE).**

$$\text{TEE (kcal)} = \text{BEE} \times \text{AF} \times \text{SF} \qquad (4)$$

For hospitalized patients an AF of 1.2 is generally appropriate, though a factor of 1.0 may be appropriate for paralyzed intubated patients. Simplified estimates of TEE for general disease states are provided in Table 2-3.
  B. **Protein requirements** in various disease states are estimated based on IBW in Table 2-4. A simplified estimate of daily protein requirement for general degrees of metabolic stress is also provided.
IV. **Continuous monitoring** of the patient is required to ensure that the prescribed regimen adequately meets the patient's needs and avoids toxicity.

Table 2-3. Simplified estimates to calculate daily energy expenditure

Simplified estimates	Energy requirement (kcal/kg/day)	Disease examples
Mild stress	25	Elective surgery, mild infection
Moderate stress	35	Fracture, severe infection
Severe stress	45	Severe burn, hepatic failure

Source. Adapted from *Barnes Hospital Nutrition Support Handbook*. St. Louis, 1992. P. 16.

A. **General parameters** include daily weight, vital signs, and physical findings. Increased body water can cause a deceptive weight gain.
B. **Standard laboratory testing** focuses on circulating proteins— namely albumin, pre-albumin, and transferrin. Like weight, all of these protein levels can fluctuate with changes in body water. Albumin has a half-life of approximately 20 days, limiting its use in short-term monitoring. Transferrin has an intermediate half-life of approximately 8 days. Pre-albumin has a shorter half-life of 2–3 days and may be preferable in determining a patient's response to nutritional therapy. Dramatic changes in the concentrations of these proteins may also be seen as part of the acute phase response to illness.
C. **Special studies** may be required in patients whose response cannot be determined by the above measures. The nitrogen balance offers a day-to-day indirect measure of protein catabolism, with the goal being a positive balance. A 24-hour urine sample is collected for urinary urea nitrogen (UUN), and **nitrogen balance** is calculated using equation 5.

$$N_2 \text{ balance} = (\text{protein intake} / 6.25) - ([\text{UUN} / 0.8] + 2 \text{ g}) \tag{5}$$

Negative values indicate net catabolism. Indirect calorimetry using respiratory gas exchange to estimate energy utilization is another method available in some centers, but maintenance of the required metabolic cart is expensive.

Table 2-4. Estimated protein requirements in various disease states

Clinical condition	Protein requirements (g/kg IBW/day)
Healthy, nonstressed	0.8
Bone marrow transplant	1.4–1.5
Liver disease without encephalopathy	1.0–1.5
Liver disease with encephalopathy	0.5–0.75 (advance as tolerated)
Renal failure without dialysis	0.6–1.0
Renal failure with dialysis	1.0–1.3
Pregnancy	1.3–1.5
Simplified estimates:	
Mild metabolic stress (elective hospitalization)	1.0–1.1
Moderate metabolic stress (complicated postoperative care, infection)	1.2–1.4
Severe metabolic stress (major trauma, pancreatitis, sepsis)	1.5–2.5

Source: Adapted from *Barnes Hospital Nutrition Support Handbook*. St. Louis, 1992. P. 19.

Specialized Nutrient Delivery

I. **Nutrition delivery systems**
   A. **Oral feeding is the preferred route.** Restrictive diets and other conditions may preclude adequate caloric intake of exogenous foodstuffs. A variety of palatable flavored commercial formulas (e.g., Ensure) can be added, at one to three cans a day, to meet a patient's requirements of nutrients and calories.
      1. **Protein supplements** are available with modified amino acid profiles intended to benefit particular conditions. Renal formulas, such as Travasorb Renal, are rich in essential amino acids and have restricted electrolyte contents. Travasorb Hepatic is rich in branched-chain amino acids to minimize encephalopathy in patients with liver disease. The usual prescribed amount of such supplements is 2–4 prepared packets/day.
      2. **Medium-chain triglyceride** (MCT) oil is derived from coconut oil and is absorbed without requiring significant amounts of pancreatic enzymes or bile salts. Daily doses of 3–4 tablespoons (45–60 ml) supply approximately 400 kcal and can be administered to patients with fat malabsorption from a variety of causes. MCT oil lacks essential linoleic acid, so another lipid source must also be supplied.
   B. **Enteral feedings** can be delivered through a flexible nasoduodenal tube placed at the bedside or with fluoroscopic guidance. Metoclopramide, 10 mg PO, IM, or IV, or cisapride, 20 mg PO or per tube, can assist proper positioning. The tube should have adequate slack and the patient should rest in the right lateral decubitus position to facilitate advancement of the tip. Proper placement should be confirmed with fluoroscopy or abdominal radiography before use of the tube, particularly in obtunded patients. Nasogastric or nasoenteric tubes are suitable when 4–6 weeks of enteral feeding is anticipated. Longer periods require percutaneous feeding routes. Percutaneous gastrostomy tubes may be placed endoscopically, surgically, or radiographically. Surgical placement is attended by a slightly higher rate of complications. Surgically placed jejunostomy tubes are less prone to mechanical difficulties than those placed endoscopically as gastrojejunostomy (GJ) tubes. Such endoscopically placed tubes have a reported dysfunction rate of 36% (*GI Endoscopy* 36:261, 1990).
      1. **Commercial products** for oral or tube feeding are available with varied characteristics (Table 2-5). Standard solutions supply 1 kcal/ml and are suitable as complete diets. **With such products, the goal intake in milliliters/day equals the TEE as calculated above.** Volume-restricted products generally supply more calories as fat and have higher osmolality.
      2. **Enteral feeding** in healthy patients can often begin with a full-strength product, because the osmolality is no higher than that of foodstuffs included in a clear liquid diet (*J Parenter Enteral Nutr* 10:588, 1986). Hypertonic (>300 mosm) solutions may need to be given at half-strength initially, or full strength but at a lower rate.
         a. **Intermittent feeding** is generally reserved for tubes with their tips in the stomach, as the small intestine lacks a reservoir function. Feeding generally begins with 50–100 ml of full-strength product given q3h, increasing the amount by 50-ml increments with each feeding until the desired intake (240–480 ml) is reached. The patient's head should be elevated during and for several hours after feeding, and residual gastric volume should be checked before each feeding. Enteral feeding should be withheld for at least 1 hour if a residual volume of more than 100 ml is present.
         b. **Continuous feeding** is delivered at a set rate over some cyclic period (8, 12, 16, 24 hours), generally using a feeding pump. The feeding begins with a rate of 25–50 ml/hour, advancing by 25 ml/hour with each cycle. Elevation of the head is advised.
         c. **Flushes.** Tubes should be flushed with 30 ml of warm water after each

Table 2-5. Barnes Hospital enteral nutrition product formulary

Product	Description	Kcal/ml	mosm	Per 1,000 ml									
				Protein (g/%)	Carbohydrates (g/%)	Fat (g/%)	H₂O	Na (mEq)	K (mEq)	Ca (mg)	PO₄ (mg)	Vitamin K (μg)	U.S. RDAs (ml)
STANDARD													
Ensure	Lactose free, low residue, flavored	1.06	470	37.2/14	145/54.5	37.2/31.5	845	36.8	40	530	530	43	1887
Osmolite	Isotonic, lactose free, low residue	1.06	300	37.2/14	145/54.6	38.5/31.4	841	27.6	25.9	533	530	43	1887
Jevity	Isotonic, lactose free, high dietary fiber (14.4 g/liter), higher nitrogen content	1.06	310	44.4/16.7	151.7/53.3	36.8/30	833	40.4	40	909	756	61	1321
Gluerna	Lactose free, low carbohydrates, high fiber (14.4 g/liter), vanilla flavor	1	375	41.8/16.7	93.7/33.3	55.7/50	873	40.3	40	703	703	57	1422
VOLUME RESTRICTED													
Ensure Plus	Lactose free, low residue, flavored	1.5	690	54.9/14.7	200/53.3	53.3/32	769	45.9	49.7	734	704	57	1420
Magnacal	Lactose free, low residue, vanilla flavor	2.0	590	70/14	250/50	80/34	690	43.5	32	1000	1000	300	1000
VOLUME RESTRICTED–HIGH NITROGEN													
Ensure Plus HN	Lactose free, low residue, flavored	1.5	650	62.6/16.7	199.9/53.3	50/30	769	51.5	46.5	1056	1056	85	947
Perative*	Lactose free, low residue, unflavored	1.3	425	66.6/20.5	177/54.5	37.3/25	789	45.2	44.3	867	867	70	1155
VERY HIGH NITROGEN													
Replete with Fiber	Lactose free, high fiber (14 g/liter), unflavored	1.0	300	62.5/25	113/45	34/30	840	21.7	40	1000	1000	80	1000
Sustacal	Lactose free, low residue, flavored	1.01	650	61/24	140/55	23/21	840	40	54	1010	930	240	1060
ELEMENTAL													
Vivonex TEN	Elemental, low fat, low residue	1	630	38.2/15.3	205.6/82.2	2.77/2.5	845	20	20	500	500	22.3	2000
PUDDING (per 5-oz serving)													
Ensure Pudding	Contains lactose	250		6.8	34	9.7		10.4	8.5	200	200	12	
MODULARS (analysis per tablespoon)													
Polycose Liquid	Glucose polymer	30			7.5								
ProMod	Protein supplement	17		3	0.4	0.4		0	1	15.6	15.6		
Microlipid	Fat supplement	67.5				7.5							
MCT Oil	MCT supplement	115.5				14							

* May be contraindicated in transplant patients.
RDA = recommended daily allowance; MCT = medium-chain triglyceride.

feeding or after each 4 hours of continuous feeding. This volume can be increased if additional free water is needed.

3. **Metabolic complications** are rare, but several **nonmetabolic complications** warrant discussion.

a. **Diarrhea** is frequently caused by factors other than tube feeding, but it may be secondary to product characteristics (high osmolarity, high fat, lactose) or to rate of delivery. Diarrhea may also be related to drugs or supplements (e.g., antibiotics, magnesium) or sorbitol and other additives in elixir formulations (*Am J Med* 88:91, 1990). If removing offending medications and reducing formula strength and/or rate does not cause improvement, another formula should be tried. Some authors advocate fiber-containing formulas such as Jevity. If antibiotics have been used, stool samples should be sent for *Clostridium difficile* toxin assay. Further stool microbiologic studies are costly and unlikely to reveal the cause of the diarrhea in hospitalized patients unless mitigating conditions such as malignancy or AIDS are present (*JAMA* 263:979, 1990). Antidiarrheals such as loperamide or deodorized tincture of opium, 6–10 drops q6–12h, can be used once major diagnostic possibilities are excluded.

b. **The risk of aspiration is equal in patients with nasogastric or nasoduodenal tubes** (*J Parenter Enteral Nutr* 16:59, 1992). The addition of several drops of methylene blue to the feeding solution and checking respiratory secretions for color can assist in diagnosis. Respiratory secretions can also be tested for the presence of feeding solution with glucose strips; a positive test for glucose in secretions indicates aspiration of feeding solution. Elevation of the head of the bed remains the mainstay of treatment. Surgical jejunostomy may be required in some aspiration-prone patients (*Ann Surg* 215:140, 1991), as no clear benefit is evident from the conversion of percutaneous gastrostomy tubes to GJ tubes. **No form of tube feeding eliminates the risk of aspiration of the patient's own pharyngeal secretions.**

c. **Obstruction** of the feeding tube can result from improper flushing, thick solutions, or inappropriate medication use. Remedies include infusion of 30–60 ml of diet carbonated soda, cranberry juice, or a solution of 1 teaspoon of papain (meat tenderizer) in 30 ml of warm water. Vigorous stylet use may perforate the tube and should not be attempted.

d. **High gastric residual** volumes may result from mechanical problems such as gastric outlet obstruction, partial small bowel obstruction, disordered motility, or ileus. Fats can also slow gastric emptying. If delayed or reduced feeding does not result in residual volumes less than 100 ml, an obstructive series should be performed. Medications that slow GI motility (e.g., narcotics, anticholinergic drugs) should be discontinued if possible.

e. **Esophagitis** secondary to pressure and reflux may persist despite precautions and should be treated with appropriate doses of H_2-antagonists (ranitidine, 300 mg PO qhs; famotidine, 40 mg PO qhs) or omeprazole, 20 mg PO qd. Omeprazole is delivered in coated granules that should be gently stirred into juice rather than crushed. This procedure may preclude its use in fine-bore tubes.

4. **Transition to oral feeding** is performed by offering increasing amounts of oral foods. Tapering the tube feeding or administering feeding in a nocturnal cycle may increase the patient's appetite. Discontinuation of tube feeding should proceed only after calorie count documentation that the patient is meeting at least 75% of his or her energy requirements with oral intake.

5. **Administration** of oral medications is often performed via feeding tubes. When solid forms of medications are given through tubes placed distal to the stomach (e.g., nasoduodenal, nasojejunostomy tubes), normal drug dissolution may not occur. Liquid drug preparations should be used when possible. Some medications may be incompatible with enteral feeding products and should not be used.

C. **Parenteral nutrition** is indicated for patients in whom more than 5–7 days of

Table 2-6. Sample formulation for peripheral parenteral nutrition

Nutrient	Volume concentration
Dextrose 70%	135 ml
Amino acid 10%	400 ml
Lipid emulsion 20%	260 ml
Sterile water	625 ml
Sodium	40 mEq
Potassium	30 mEq
Chloride	35 mEq
Phosphate	6 mmol
Magnesium (as sulfate)	4 mEq
Calcium (as acetate)	4.6 mEq
Acetate	124 mEq
Multivitamin	10 ml
Trace element solution	1 ml
Total volume	1,450 ml/1,000 kcal
Calculated osmolarity	760 osm

bowel rest are anticipated, in those with intestinal dysfunction precluding enteral feeding, and in those whose nutritional requirements cannot be met enterally. **It is invasive care and should be consistent with an overall treatment plan for the patient.**

1. **Peripheral parenteral nutrition (PPN)** can be delivered through ordinary peripheral catheters that are moved to a different site every 72 hours. Partial calorie and protein supplementation through this route may provide limited support for patients who will be able to resume enteral intake after temporary abstinence, or who require a supplement to enteral feeding. Solutions with osmolarity less than 900–1000 mosm are recommended to avoid phlebitis. A sample formula delivering 1,000 kcal is provided in Table 2-6.

2. **Total parenteral nutrition (TPN)** is usually administered through a central venous catheter although peripherally inserted central catheters (PICC) have been used successfully. Single-lumen catheters should be used when possible. If multilumen catheters are used, a dedicated TPN port should be clearly labeled. This port should not be used to draw blood, and its use for the administration of medications or blood products should be avoided.

   a. **Solutions** deliver macronutrients in three major categories: protein, as amino acids; carbohydrate, as dextrose; and fat, as lipid emulsions. Micronutrients and electrolytes are added and adjusted according to particular disease states. Table 2-7 lists the caloric value of dextrose and lipid solutions. Standard solutions use D_{70}, which yields 3.4 kcal/g; this is generally used to supply 40–65% of total calories, though special formulas may vary. Standard 20% lipid emulsions yield 2 kcal/ml and can supply up to 65% of total calories. The standard concentration of amino acids in nutritional solutions is 10%. **Three-in-one** admixtures combine all three solutions in a single daily bag, facilitating administration, particularly for patients requiring long-term, cyclic, or home therapy. Sample formulation of standardized TPN solutions is provided in Table 2-8.

   b. **Additives** include nutrients and medications. Typical nutrient additives and medications that may be added to TPN are also shown in Table 2-9. Some additives—namely iron and albumin—are not approved for 3-in-1 solutions. Insulin, when used as a TPN additive, may bind to the plastic bag and tubing and higher doses may be required.

   c. **The initial infusion** of a 3-in-1 solution should be with one-third to one-half

Table 2-7. Caloric value and osmolarity of parenteral solutions

Solution	Caloric value (kcal/dl)	Osmolarity (mosm/liter)
Dextrose (%)		
5	17	250
10	34	500
20	68	1,000
50	170	2,500
70	237	3,500
Lipid emulsions (%)		
10	110	280
20	200	330–340

of the total daily caloric requirement administered over 24 hours. For TPN using individual solutions, no more than one liter of the amino acid–dextrose solution should be administered over the first 24 hours, and lipids should not be given on the first day of therapy. With both formulations, the amount of TPN given may be increased by up to one liter per day until total daily caloric requirements are met.

d. **Regular monitoring** is required because patients' metabolic responses vary as nutrition is supplied. The blood glucose level should be measured on blood samples obtained by finger stick four times daily. Baseline serum chemistries, blood counts, and lipid profiles should be performed prior to initiating therapy. These studies should be repeated following the first day of therapy and at least weekly thereafter. If triglycerides remain normal with continued therapy, their levels do not need to be followed closely. A prothrombin time should be performed periodically in patients on long-term therapy to exclude vitamin K deficiency. Nitrogen balance (see equation 5) should be followed weekly.

e. **Cyclic TPN** may be preferred in patients on home therapy, in those with fatty liver, or to allow increased activity in patients requiring long-term therapy. A sample schedule for converting from continuous to cyclic TPN is given in Table 2-10. Finger stick glucose levels should be monitored every 30 minutes for several hours following infusion of the TPN solution during the first few days of cyclic TPN to monitor patients for the development of hypoglycemia. Hyperglycemia may be present during the maintenance period of rapid infusion.

3. **Complications of parenteral nutrition** can be minimized by providing a dedicated parenteral nutrition service responsible for catheter placement and solution management. If such a team is not available, it may be preferable to have a single surgical service insert all TPN catheters.

a. **Mechanical complications** of catheter insertion occur in 5–7% of patients and include pneumothorax, hydrothorax, great vessel injury, and brachial plexus injury (*Am J Surg* 152:93, 1986). **A chest x-ray is recommended before using any new subclavian or internal jugular catheter for TPN.**

b. **Thrombosis** of central veins occurs in approximately one in 20 patients but is often clinically silent. Some authors advocate addition of 1,000–3,000 units of heparin/liter of TPN to prevent venous thrombosis, but this practice is not universally endorsed.

c. **Catheter-related sepsis** may be more common with multilumen catheters than with single-lumen catheters but can be minimized with meticulous catheter insertion and maintenance (*Arch Surg* 125:990, 1990). Staphylococcal infections are the most common, followed by infection with fungal (*Candida*) and gram-negative organisms. Judgment is required in balancing the risk of obtaining new access against the risk of attempting to sterilize an indwelling catheter with six weeks of antibiotic therapy.

Table 2-8. Sample formulation of central vein total parenteral nutrition solutions

Central formulas	Percentage of total calories provided as			Grams/1,000 kcal			Approximate volume per 1,000 kcal (ml)
	Dextrose	Amino acids	Fat	Dextrose	Amino acids	Fat	
Intermediate nitrogen							
Standard carbohydrates	60	16	24	176	40	24	771
Intermediate carbohydrates	49	16	35	144	40	35	780
Low carbohydrates, high fat	42	16	42	123	40	42.5	787
Standard, no fat	84	16	—	247	40	—	752
High nitrogen							
Standard carbohydrates, high nitrogen	60	20	20	176	50	20	850
Intermediate carbohydrates	50	20	30	147	50	30	860
High nitrogen, no fat	80	20	—	235	50	—	836
Very high nitrogen	56	24	20	165	60	20	935
Low nitrogen							
Standard carbohydrates, low nitrogen	65	12	23	191	30	23	688
Intermediate carbohydrates	55	12	33	162	30	33	696
Low nitrogen, high fat	50	10	40	147	25	40	660

Source: Adapted from Barnes Hospital formulary, St. Louis, MO.

Table 2-9. Total parenteral nutrition (TPN) additives and sample daily amounts

Additive	Daily amount[a]	Comments
Electrolytes		
Sodium	20–80 mEq	As acetate or chloride salt
Potassium	30–60 mEq	As acetate or chloride salt
Chloride	80–100 mEq	Balanced with acetate
Magnesium	8.1–20 mEq	
Calcium	4.6–9.2 mEq	Sum of calcium mEq and phosphorus mmol should be <30
Phosphorus	12–24 mmol	
Vitamins	10-ml multivitamin	Meets 1979 AMA recommendations
A	3,300 IU	As retinol
D	5 µg	As ergocalciferol
E	10 mg	
C	100 mg	Single dose of 500 mg/ml available[b]
B_1 (thiamine)	3 mg	Single dose of 100 mg/ml available[b]
B_2 (riboflavin)	3.6 mg	
B_6 (pyridoxine)	4 mg	Single dose of 100 mg/ml available[b]
B_{12} (cobalamin)	5 µg	Single dose of 1 mg IM or SQ for deficiency[b]
Pantothenic acid	15 mg	
Niacin	40 mg	
Biotin	60 µg	
Folate	0.4 mg	Single dose of 5 mg/ml available
Vitamin K	10 mg weekly	In patients who are not anticoagulated
Trace elements		
Zinc	2–8 mg	
Copper	0.3–1.5 mg	
Chromium	10–15 µg	
Manganese	0.15–0.8 mg	
Iron	1–3 mg	50 mg/month as 1 ml iron dextran
Iodine	50–75 µg	
Selenium	40–120 µg	
Molybdenum	20 µg	
Medications		
Ranitidine	150 mg	
Famotidine	20–40 mg	
Cimetidine	300 mg	Not approved for 3-in-1 use
Heparin	3,000–5,000 units	Not recommended for short-term TPN
Insulin (regular humulin)	5–10 units/liter D_{25}	

[a] Dosages described are for patients who are not pregnant and who do not have renal or hepatic failure.
[b] Larger doses may be necessary to correct individual deficiency states.

Table 2-10. Cyclic total parenteral nutrition schedule providing 2 liters over 12 hours

Time	Rate
0600–0700	120 ml/hr
0700–0800	80 ml/hr
0800–2000	Off
2000–2100	80 ml/hr
2100–2200	120 ml/hr
2200–0600	200 ml/hr

Source: Adapted from *Barnes Hospital Nutrition Support Handbook*. St. Louis, 1992. P. 61.

d. **Metabolic complications** are particularly common when initiating TPN therapy. The laboratory studies described above should allow the clinician to detect and correct complications promptly. **Hyperglycemia** may lead to hyperosmolarity with subsequent coma or death. Finger stick blood samples for glucose level should be performed four times daily to guide an adjusted-dose insulin regimen until a stable insulin requirement is established. The addition of regular insulin to the TPN solution is recommended at 5–10 units/liter of D_{25} (see sec. **I.C.2.b**). Hyperglycemia in a previously normoglycemic patient should raise one's suspicion of infection. **Hypoglycemia** may occur following abrupt discontinuation of TPN. Hypoglycemia can be treated by infusion of $D_{10}W$ solution or tapered discontinuation of the TPN solution. **Electrolyte abnormalities** can be corrected by adjusting the electrolyte content of daily solutions or by infusion of supplemental IV solutions. Specific electrolyte disturbances and their treatment are discussed in Chap. 3.
e. **The refeeding syndrome** is characterized by hypophosphatemia and fluxes in electrolytes, glucose, and water in severely malnourished patients who are fed enterally or with TPN. Carbohydrate refeeding stimulates insulin secretion, which in turn increases cellular uptake of phosphorus and glucose. This can cause severe hypophosphatemia, associated with possible cardiac dysfunction and death. Like other metabolic derangements, this syndrome is best avoided by carefully monitoring the patient's volume status, electrolytes, and serum phosphorus and magnesium concentrations. An initial regimen matching baseline caloric intake and replenishing protein at 1.2–1.5 g/kg (IBW) is suggested (*J Parenter Enteral Nutr* 14:90, 1990). This can then be advanced slowly.
f. **Hepatic dysfunction** is common in patients receiving TPN. Laboratory abnormalities may be seen in up to 61% of these patients (*J Parenter Enteral Nutr* 14:618, 1990). Steatosis (hepatic fat accumulation without inflammation) is the most frequently documented pathologic liver abnormality in patients receiving TPN. It is characterized by the early appearance of modest increases in transaminases, sometimes with mild increases of alkaline phosphatase and bilirubin, and generally relates to excessive caloric intake, particularly of carbohydrates. Steatosis is considered a benign condition that can be remedied by **reducing daily calories** and supplying them in a balanced solution of protein, dextrose, and fat.
g. **Biliary disease** is also common in parenterally fed patients. The incidence of cholelithiasis and biliary sludge increases with duration of parenteral feeding and may rarely require cholecystectomy. Stimulation of gallbladder contraction with small enteral meals or administration of Sincalide (c-terminal octapeptide of cholecystokinin), 0.02 µg/kg daily given IV over 30–60 seconds, may help avoid bile stasis.

h. **Individual micronutrient deficiencies** occur frequently in patients receiving TPN for long periods. Zinc, iron, and vitamin B_{12} deficiencies are common. Many deficiencies will require larger initial dosages for repletion followed by usual maintenance dosing (see Table 2-9).

i. **Elevation of BUN** may reflect intravascular volume depletion, tissue catabolism, or excessive feeding. If parameters such as orthostatic blood pressure changes or increasing hematocrit or creatinine suggest volume depletion, additional crystalloid should be administered. If caloric requirements are being met and volume depletion is not present, then the infusion rate of the base solution should be decreased.

4. **Home TPN** (HPN) may be indicated in patients with radiation enteritis, short-bowel syndrome, motility disorders (e.g., scleroderma), inflammatory bowel disease, or cancer. Patients should be selected with care, because HPN patients with malignancy or AIDS have substantially higher mortality rates than patients with other illnesses (*J Parenter Enteral Nutr* 15:384, 1991).

a. **Administration** is usually by a 3-in-1 solution providing approximately 1.2 × BEE (20–30% of calories as fat and approximately 1 g/kg/day of protein), generally given as a nocturnal cycle. Multivitamin, mineral, and trace element supplements are added to each daily bag. Vitamin K (10 mg) is added to one bag each week in patients who are not receiving systemic anticoagulation. Patients must be educated in the use of a volumetric pump, catheter care, and the daily injection of a low-concentration (100 U/ml) heparin solution.

b. **Complications of HPN** include those discussed for TPN patients but also include an increased risk of metabolic bone disease, venous thrombosis, and micronutrient deficiencies. Because of the 10–20% incidence of venous thrombosis, warfarin, 2.5 mg/day, has been advocated. Patients may also suffer severe **muscle cramping** during the first few hours of infusion secondary to compartmental fluxes of magnesium and calcium. Empiric trials of increased magnesium, calcium, saline, phosphorus, or quinine sulfate (200–300 mg PO one hour prior to infusion) may decrease the incidence of cramping. Depression is also common in HPN patients and may warrant psychiatric consultation.

II. Specialized therapy

A. **Pancreatic disease.** Acute pancreatitis frequently requires administration of TPN, which can decrease pancreatic secretion and provide nutritional support. Standard mixtures are generally well tolerated, but restriction of lipids may be necessary if pancreatitis is secondary to hyperlipidemia (*World J Surg* 14:572, 1990). Triglyceride levels should be determined prior to starting TPN and monitored to maintain levels less than 1.5 times the upper limit of normal. Serum glucose and calcium levels also require close monitoring. Patients with alcoholic pancreatitis are frequently malnourished and have additional micronutrient requirements. **Folic acid (1 mg/day) and a water-soluble vitamin preparation including thiamine (50–100 mg/day)** should be added. Patients with severe pancreatitis requiring surgical exploration should be considered for feeding jejunostomy placement. Low-fat enteral feeding (e.g., Vital HN, Vivonex High Nitrogen) can then begin when bowel function allows (*Surg Gynecol Obstet* 175:275, 1992).

B. **Inflammatory bowel disease (IBD).** Decreased oral intake, a restricted diet, malabsorption, bacterial overgrowth, and diarrhea can cause protein, calorie, and micronutrient deficiencies in IBD patients (*Nutr Clin Pract* 7:51, 1992). Ileal involvement or resection can result in malabsorption of fats and fat-soluble vitamins; ileal disease also impairs vitamin B_{12} absorption. Dosages for these and other supplements are given in Table 2-9.

1. **Drug intervention** in IBD patients can also cause nutrient deficiencies. Cholestyramine administration to alleviate bile salt–induced diarrhea may exacerbate fat-soluble vitamin deficiencies. Sulfasalazine can cause folate deficiency. Calcium supplementation may be necessary for patients with prolonged glucocorticoid use (see Chap. 23).

2. **Crohn's disease** may improve with trial of a lactose-free diet or with low-residue enteral feeding. TPN as primary therapy can induce remission, but relapse is common. Short-term (5–10 days) preoperative use of TPN can decrease surgical complications in patients requiring bowel resection (*Am J Surg* 143:139, 1982). Data are lacking about longer use of preoperative TPN in these patients.

3. **Patients with ulcerative colitis** may require TPN for nutritional support, though this is not presently considered primary therapy.

C. **Short bowel syndrome** generally results from massive resection of the small bowel and/or colon leaving 150 cm or less of functional small bowel. A detailed review of the variety of resulting disorders is beyond the scope of this chapter, but several universal principles apply. Enteral feeding should be initiated as early as possible to facilitate intestinal adaptation and should be accompanied by antacids or H_2-antagonists to combat the effect of postsurgical hypergastrinemia. Long-term antacid therapy may not be necessary. Early parenteral nutrition is often necessary and can decrease mortality (*Dig Dis Sci* 31:718, 1986). Lifelong TPN is required in some patients, but TPN may be discontinued after prolonged treatment in others as adaptation appears to occur for years following bowel resection. Deficiencies of iron, B_{12}, and fat-soluble vitamins are common, as are other micronutrient deficiencies. A daily trace element supplement should also be provided. Exogenous foodstuffs should be given as frequent small meals.

D. **Renal failure.** Acute renal failure (ARF) is associated with increased tissue catabolism, which can cause increases in BUN of 30–50 mg/dl/day. This catabolism may be increased in patients requiring dialysis. A positive cumulative calorie balance is associated with decreased mortality in ARF. Parenteral nutrition is frequently required. Balanced solutions supplying essential and nonessential amino acids should be used to supply approximately **1 g protein/ kg/day**. Hypertonic dextrose and a lipid solution can supply the remaining calories while minimizing volume expansion. Daily water-soluble vitamin supplements and trace metals should be given, but fat-soluble vitamin preparations containing vitamin A should be avoided because of the possibility of achieving toxic vitamin A levels.

E. **AIDS** patients are candidates for nutritional intervention before clinical deficiency states occur. Protein-calorie deficiency, as well as trace element and other micronutrient deficiencies, are common in these patients. These deficiencies may be caused by poor oral intake, associated disease, or metabolic derangement. Anorexia may improve with administration of megestrol acetate, 240 mg PO qd, up to 800 mg/day in divided doses, or dronabinol, 2.5–5.0 mg bid (*Ann Pharmacother* 27:827, 1993). Enteral feeding may help patients with inadequate oral intake secondary to oral or pharyngeal lesions. Patients with inadequate intake may also benefit from standard formula supplements (e.g., Ensure) between meals. Specific oral supplements recommended are a daily multivitamin and zinc sulfate, 200 mg PO bid. Patients intolerant of enteral feeding (e.g., because of severe diarrhea) may require TPN. Multivitamins and a trace element supplement should be added daily (*Gastrointest Clin North Am* 17:545, 1988). Phosphorus and magnesium supplementation may also be necessary. Benefit from TPN without marked risk of sepsis has been described (*J Parenter Enteral Nutr* 16:165, 1992). **The administration of TPN must be consistent with the overall level of medical care.**

F. **Malignancy.** A large number of studies have failed to demonstrate any clear benefit from the routine use of parenteral nutrition in cancer patients. Although enteral or parenteral support may be required in patients who meet the indications for therapy, there does not appear to be a role for the routine use of specialized nutritional treatment. **Narcotics** such as morphine, meperidine, hydromorphone, and levorphanol are compatible with standard lipid-free TPN solutions and may be coadministered in patients with limited IV access. Maximum compatible doses reported are given in Table 2-11.

G. **Respiratory illnesses.** Patients with chronic obstructive pulmonary disease

Table 2-11. Narcotic compatibility with total parenteral nutrition

Agent	Maximum compatible dose described
Morphine	2 mg/ml
Meperidine	100 mg/liter
Hydromorphone	80 mg/liter

Source: Adapted from JP Grant. *Handbook of Total Parenteral Nutrition* (2nd ed). Philadelphia: Saunders, 1992. P. 212.

have increased energy requirements but may lack adequate ventilatory reserve to compensate for increased CO_2 production from increased intake. Data suggest that **avoiding excess calories** is far more important than specialized manipulations of lipids, protein, and carbohydrates (*Chest* 102:551, 1992). In the patient with a particularly tenuous respiratory status, specialized regimens favoring fat over carbohydrates may be helpful. Regimens supplying 1.2 × BEE are recommended.

H. Perioperative nutrition. Prompt nutritional support is necessary for the malnourished patient who requires surgery. Early pre- and postoperative TPN can reduce complications in patients with significant malnutrition (*N Engl J Med* 325:525, 1991). Early enteral feeding should be considered to reduce the rate of septic complications (*Ann Surg* 216:172, 1992).

Fluid and Electrolyte Management

Bruce J. Lippmann

General Management of Fluids

I. **Maintenance therapy**
   A. **Minimum water requirements** for daily fluid balance can be estimated from the sum of the urine output necessary to excrete the daily solute load (500 ml/day if the urine concentrating ability is normal) plus the insensible water losses from the skin and respiratory tract (500–1,000 ml/day), minus the amount of water produced from endogenous metabolism (300 ml/day). It is customary to administer 2,000–3,000 ml of water daily to produce a urine volume of 1,000–1,500 ml/day since there is no advantage to minimizing urine output. **Weighing the patient daily** is the best means of assessing net gain or loss of fluid, since the GI, renal, and insensible fluid losses of the hospitalized patient are unpredictable. Table 3-1 lists commonly used IV fluid preparations.
   B. **The electrolytes** that are usually administered during maintenance fluid therapy are the cations **sodium** and **potassium**, accompanied by **chloride** as the anion. The kidneys are normally capable of compensating for wide variations in sodium intake; urinary sodium excretion can be reduced to less than 5 mEq/day in the absence of sodium intake. It is customary to supply 50–150 mEq of sodium daily. Some potassium supplementation should be given, due to continued obligatory potassium excretion. Usually, 20–60 mEq/day is given if renal function is adequate. **Carbohydrate** in the form of dextrose (100–150 g/day) is necessary to minimize protein catabolism and prevent ketosis. **Dextrose does not contribute effectively to the osmolality of the administered fluid** since it is quickly metabolized to CO_2 and H_2O. Solutions such as lactated Ringer's are designed to more closely duplicate the composition of the extracellular fluid. However, there is no evidence of any clinical benefit of lactated Ringer's solution over standard isotonic solutions. Lactate-containing solutions should not be used in patients with lactic acidosis.
   C. **A maintenance IV fluid regimen** can be provided by the administration of 2,000–3,000 ml (90–125 ml/hour) of 0.45% NaCl with 5% dextrose and 20 mEq KCl/liter. Calcium, magnesium, phosphorus, vitamins, and protein replacement may be necessary after 1 week of parenteral therapy (see Chap. 2).
II. **Replacement of abnormal water and electrolyte losses**
   A. **Insensible water losses** from the skin and respiratory tract average 500–1,000 ml/day and depend on respiratory rate, ambient temperature, humidity, and body temperature. Water losses increase by 100–150 ml/day for each degree of body temperature over 37°C. Fluid losses from sweating can vary enormously (0–2,000 ml/hour) and depend on physical activity and body and ambient temperature. Mechanical ventilation with humidified gases eliminates losses from the respiratory tract. Replacement of insensible water losses should be with 5% D/W or hypotonic saline.
   B. **GI losses** vary in composition and volume depending on the source. Laboratory measurement of fluid composition can be performed to increase the accuracy of electrolyte replacement.
   C. **Urinary losses of sodium** may be significant, particularly in the setting of diuretic use, the recovery phase of acute tubular necrosis, postobstructive

Table 3-1. Commonly used parenteral solutions

IV solutions	Osmolality (mosm/kg)	Glucose (g/liter)	Na (mEq/liter)	Cl (mEq/liter)
5% D/W	252	50	—	—
10% D/W	505	100	—	—
50% D/W	2520	500	—	—
0.45% NaCl	154	a	77	77
0.9% NaCl	308	a	154	154
3% NaCl	1026		513	513
Ringer's lactate[b]	272	a	130	109

[a] Also available with 5% dextrose.
[b] Also contains K^+ (4 mEq/liter), Ca (3 mEq/liter), and lactate (28 mEq/liter).
One ampule (50 ml) of 7.5% $NaHCO_3$ contains 44.6 mEq each of Na and HCO_3^-.

diuresis, moderately severe renal failure (glomerular filtration rate of 10–25 ml/minute), renal tubulointerstitial diseases, or aldosterone deficiency. Urinary loss of **potassium** may occur with the recovery phase of acute tubular necrosis, renal tubular acidosis, diuretic use, and various states of mineralocorticoid excess. If prolonged losses occur, measurement of the urine sodium and potassium may help guide replacement (see also Salt and Water, sec. **V.C.2**, and Potassium, sec. **I.B.4**, respectively).

   D. **Rapid internal fluid shifts** may occur with peritonitis, pancreatitis, portal vein thrombosis, extensive burns, fulminant nephrotic syndrome, ileus or intestinal obstruction, bacterial enteritis, crush injuries, and internal bleeding (ruptured abdominal aortic aneurysm, retroperitoneal bleeding, femoral or pelvic fractures), as well as during the postoperative period. Replacement of sequestered fluid with isotonic saline is necessary in these situations.

Salt and Water

   I. **Total body water (TBW)** constitutes about 60% of the body weight in males and 50% in females. Approximately two-thirds of TBW is intracellular fluid (ICF) and one-third is extracellular fluid (ECF). Of the ECF, three-fourths is interstitial fluid and one-fourth is in plasma. The most important determinant of ECF volume is its sodium content. Changes in ECF volume are dictated by net gain or loss of sodium with an accompanying gain or loss of water.
   II. **ECF volume depletion** occurs with losses of both sodium and water. The character of the fluid lost will dictate the clinical picture. If the loss is isotonic (e.g., blood loss), the osmolality of the ECF is unaffected and intracellular volume will change minimally. However, loss of hypotonic fluid (e.g., nasogastric suction, sweating) will lead to an increase in plasma osmolality. As plasma osmolality rises, intracellular water moves to the ECF as a result of osmotic equilibration across cell membranes. Thus, larger volumes of hypotonic fluid loss may occur before clinical manifestations of ECF volume depletion present themselves. The plasma sodium concentration will depend on the volume of fluid lost, its electrolyte composition, and the kidneys' ability to maintain homeostasis. (Disorders of plasma sodium are discussed in secs. **V** and **VI**.)
      A. **Manifestations of ECF volume depletion** depend on its magnitude and on the plasma osmolality. Symptoms include anorexia, nausea, vomiting, apathy, weakness, orthostatic lightheadedness, and syncope. **Weight loss** is not only an important sign of volume contraction but also provides an estimate of the

magnitude of the volume deficit. Other physical findings include orthostatic hypotension, poor skin turgor, sunken eyes, absence of axillary sweat, oliguria, and tachycardia. With severe volume depletion, shock and coma may occur. If hyponatremia or hypernatremia is present, symptoms referable to the change in plasma osmolality may also be present (see secs. **V** and **VI**). There are no laboratory tests that will accurately determine the degree of volume depletion; measurement of the urine sodium, fractional excretion of sodium, and serum BUN-creatinine ratio may, however, provide additional diagnostic information (see Chap. 11). A rise in hematocrit, uric acid, and serum protein concentration may also be seen.

B. **Causes of ECF volume depletion** include GI losses (vomiting, diarrhea, fistula drainage, nasogastric suction), diuretics, renal or adrenal disease (renal sodium wasting), blood loss, and sequestration of fluid (ileus, burns, peritonitis, pancreatitis).

C. **Treatment** should be directed at restoration of the ECF volume with solutions containing the lost water and electrolytes. During replacement, daily assessment of weight, ongoing fluid losses, and serum electrolyte concentrations are necessary to evaluate the progress of therapy. Mild degrees of volume depletion can be corrected orally (4–8 g Na diet and 2–4 liters of water/day). If more severe deficits accompanied by circulatory compromise are present, the **initial treatment** should be IV isotonic fluid replacement (0.9% saline) until hemodynamic stability has been restored. One to two liters of fluid should be given over the first hour. Further therapy should be guided by the symptoms and signs as outlined in sec. **II.A.** Central venous or pulmonary capillary wedge pressure monitoring should be considered. Colloid solutions have no clear advantage over electrolyte solutions except in the setting of hypoalbuminemia. Sodium can also be given as sodium bicarbonate if acidosis is present. Three ampules of $NaHCO_3$ (44.6 mEq each of Na and HCO_3/ampule) mixed in one liter of 5% D/W produces a solution with a sodium concentration of 134 mEq/liter.

III. **ECF volume excess**

A. **Manifestations.** Weight gain is the most sensitive and consistent sign of ECF volume excess. Edema, another important manifestation, is usually not apparent until 2–4 kg of fluid have been retained. Other clinical findings include dyspnea, tachycardia, jugular venous distention, hepatojugular reflux, the presence of rales on pulmonary examination, and auscultation of an S3.

B. **Causes** of ECF volume excess such as in heart, liver, or renal failure and the nephrotic syndrome, have in common excessive renal sodium and water retention. The problem can be further aggravated by unnecessary salt administration (e.g., IV line flushes, parenteral drug solutions, dietary excess).

C. **Treatment** must address not only the ECF volume excess but also the underlying pathologic process. Treatment of the nephrotic syndrome and the cardiovascular volume overload associated with renal failure are discussed in Chap. 11. Treatment of heart failure and cirrhosis is discussed in Chaps. 6 and 16, respectively.

IV. **Plasma osmolality and the osmolal gap.** The normal range of plasma osmolality is 280–295 mosm/kg. The calculated plasma osmolality accounts for the most prevalent solutes contributing to the osmolality:

$$Osmolality \ (mosm/kg) = 2[Na^+ \ (mEq/liter)]$$
$$+ \ [glucose \ (mg/dl)/18] + [BUN \ (mg/dl)/2.8]$$

Urea, unlike Na^+ and K^+, freely crosses cell membranes and reaches osmotic equilibrium quickly. Fluid shifts from the ICF to the ECF do not occur and elevation of BUN does not affect the plasma Na^+ concentration; urea is an ineffective osmole. Plasma osmolality can also be directly measured by the laboratory and can be compared with the calculated osmolality. If the measured plasma osmolality exceeds the calculated plasma osmolality by more than 10 mosm/kg, significant quantities of unmeasured solutes are present (**the osmolal gap**). The conditions that may cause an osmolal gap include those discussed in secs. **V.A** and **V.B** below (mannitol, glycine, lipids, proteins) as well as the toxic alcohols (ethanol, isopropyl alcohol, methanol, and ethylene glycol) (see Acid-Base Disturbances, secs. **III.D.1.d** and **e**). The former are effective osmoles and can affect the plasma sodium, while the alcohols are ineffective osmoles and do not affect the plasma sodium concentration.

V. **Hyponatremia.** As sodium and its attendant anions are the primary determinants of ECF osmolality, hyponatremia is usually accompanied by hypo-osmolality. However, hyponatremia may be associated with a normal or elevated plasma osmolality. Therefore, initial evaluation should include a clinical estimate of the ECF volume status and both a measured and a calculated plasma osmolality. Measurement of the urine sodium and urine osmolality is often helpful both in determining etiology and in guiding therapy.

A. **Hyponatremia with an increase in plasma osmolality** occurs when there is an accumulation of large amounts of solutes restricted primarily to the ECF space. The increase in ECF osmolality results in a shift of water from the ICF to the ECF, thereby diluting the ECF sodium. **Hyperglycemia** is the most common cause, resulting in a 1.6 mEq/liter decrement in plasma sodium for each 100 mg/dl increment in glucose concentration. The osmotic diuresis that ensues may further raise the plasma osmolality. **Manifestations** of hyperosmolality are similar to those of hypernatremia (see sec. **VI.A**). **Treatment** is directed at correction of the hyperglycemia. The use of hypertonic **mannitol** as a diuretic in patients with renal insufficiency can produce similar findings. Rarely, hyponatremia may result from the use of isotonic or hypotonic **genitourinary irrigants** (e.g., mannitol, sorbitol, or glycine) (*Br J Urol* 66:71, 1990; *Am J Kidney Dis* 4:80, 1984).

B. **Hyponatremia with a normal plasma osmolality (pseudohyponatremia)** is usually caused by severe **hyperlipidemia** (as in uncontrolled diabetes mellitus) and **hyperproteinemia** (>10 g/dl) (as in multiple myeloma). The serum may be reported as lactescent in hyperlipidemia. These two disorders increase the nonaqueous, non–sodium-containing fraction of plasma (normally, 5–7% of plasma volume). The sodium concentration and osmolality of plasma water are normal despite a reduced whole plasma sodium concentration. **Treatment** of the hyponatremia is not required.

C. **Hyponatremia associated with decreased plasma osmolality (hypotonic hyponatremia). Manifestations** of hyponatremia usually do not occur until the plasma sodium falls below 120 mEq/liter but may occur at higher concentrations if the rate of fall is rapid. Those with acute hyponatremia are much more likely to develop symptoms than those in whom the hyponatremia develops more slowly. Premenopausal women, who are prone to develop the syndrome of inappropriate antidiuretic hormone secretion (SIADH) during the postoperative period, appear to be at greatest risk (*N Engl J Med* 314:1529, 1986; *Ann Intern Med* 117:891, 1992). Initial findings include headache, nausea, malaise, lethargy, and cramps, which can progress to delirium, psychosis, seizures, and coma. Permanent neurologic damage may occur. **Urgent treatment** is required if symptoms are present or the plasma sodium is less than 110 mEq/liter. However, **caution should be exercised when treating hyponatremia** because too rapid a rate of correction may also cause acute and permanent neurologic damage characterized by paraparesis, dysphagia, dysarthria, and coma. **The rate of correction depends on the severity of symptoms and the acuity of the process.** In general, the rate of increase in the plasma sodium should not exceed 0.5 mEq/liter/hour and 12 mEq/liter/day in asymptomatic patients. In patients who are exhibiting severe symptoms, particularly if the process is acute, a more rapid rate of increase of 1.0–1.5 mEq/liter/hour for the first 3–4 hours should be undertaken. The total daily increment in the plasma sodium should still not exceed approximately 12 mEq/liter (*Am J Med* 88:161, 1990; *Crit Care Clin* 7:127, 1991). Frequent monitoring of the plasma sodium as often as hourly is required.

1. **Hypotonic hyponatremia with ECF volume excess** and a **urine sodium greater than 20 mEq/liter** can occur with advanced renal failure, whereas a **urine sodium less than 20 mEq/liter** is characteristic of heart failure, hepatic cirrhosis, and the nephrotic syndrome. However, diuretics used in these disorders may elevate urinary Na^+. In these conditions, renal excretion of both sodium and water is impaired but the rise in total body water exceeds that of the rise in sodium. Symptomatic hyponatremia is unusual, and

therefore urgent treatment is rarely necessary. **Treatment** consists of judicious sodium (1–3 g/day) and water (1.0–1.5 liters/day) restriction in conjunction with nonthiazide diuretics. Water intake must be less than the urine output to raise the plasma sodium. However, water restriction may be difficult in these patients because of increased thirst. In heart failure, the use of an angiotensin-converting enzyme inhibitor along with a loop diuretic is often effective in raising the plasma sodium.

2. **Hypotonic hyponatremia with decreased ECF volume** occurs when total body sodium is depleted disproportionately to water losses or when a sodium deficit is replaced with hypotonic fluids. Hyponatremia in this setting may be due to **renal losses** that can result from an osmotic diuresis, salt-losing nephropathies (usually tubulointerstitial diseases such as pyelonephritis, urinary tract obstruction, medullary cystic kidney disease, polycystic kidney disease), diuretic therapy (see sec. **V.C.3.c**), proximal renal tubular acidosis, or adrenal insufficiency. A **urine sodium greater than 20 mEq/liter** is typical. This condition can also arise from **extrarenal loss** of sodium and water (e.g., by vomiting, diarrhea, skin losses, and third-space sequestration). The **urine sodium is usually less than 20 mEq/liter** in this case. However, when vomiting results in a metabolic alkalosis, bicarbonaturia may cause an obligate urinary sodium loss and an elevated urine sodium despite the presence of volume depletion. In this case, the urine chloride will still be low. The clinical **manifestations** are usually due to the volume depletion rather than to the hyponatremia. The **treatment** is re-expansion of the ECF volume with isotonic (rarely hypertonic) saline and correction of the underlying disorder. Care must be exercised as the patient's volume status nears repletion since antidiuretic hormone (ADH) levels will become suppressed and a rapid rise in the plasma sodium may result. Any potassium deficit must also be corrected since it contributes to the hyponatremia (see sec. **V.C.3.c**).

3. **Hypotonic hyponatremia with clinically normal ECF volume** can be seen in primary polydipsia in which the **urine osmolality and the urine sodium are low** (<100 mosm/kg and <20 mEq/liter, respectively) and those states (sec. **V.C.3.b–e**) in which the **urine osmolality and the urine sodium are inappropriately high** (usually >200 mosm/kg and >20 mEq/liter, respectively).

   a. **Primary polydipsia** is most often seen in patients with psychiatric illness, particularly in those taking phenothiazines that may cause a dry mouth. Psychosis itself may increase ADH production and potentiate its effect. Diseases that cause hypothalamic disorders (e.g., sarcoidosis) may also cause polydipsia and subsequently hyponatremia by affecting the regulation of thirst. If daily solute intake is normal and the diluting ability of the kidneys is intact, water intake must be greater than the maximum urine volume of 10–15 liters/day to produce significant hyponatremia. In clinical situations where dietary solute intake is poor (e.g., heavy beer drinkers), hyponatremia may develop with less water intake because maximal urine volume is proportionally decreased. **Treatment** is water restriction with close monitoring of the plasma sodium level. If the hyponatremia begins to correct more rapidly than is desired, the water restriction should be liberalized somewhat. More aggressive efforts to raise serum Na$^+$ should be used if severe symptoms are present (see sec. **V.C.3.b.(2)**).

   b. **SIADH** is characterized by (1) hypotonic hyponatremia, (2) less than maximally dilute urine (urine osmolality usually >100 mosm/kg), (3) elevated urine sodium (typically >20 mEq/liter), (4) clinical euvolemia, and (5) normal renal, adrenal, and thyroid function. A low serum uric acid and BUN are commonly associated findings. Although these patients are clinically euvolemic, this condition actually represents a state of free water excess. Therapy is directed at decreasing total body water.

      (1) **Causes** of SIADH are many and include neuropsychiatric disorders (meningitis, subarachnoid hemorrhage, neoplasm, psychosis), nausea, drugs (IV cyclophosphamide, chlorpropamide, oxytocin, vasopressin), pulmonary disease (pneumonia, acute asthma, tuberculosis), carci-

noma causing ectopic production of ADH (oat cell of lung), and the postoperative state (especially in premenopausal women).

(2) Acute treatment of SIADH should be reserved for those patients who are symptomatic or in whom the hyponatremia is severe. Chronic SIADH may be well tolerated, and rapid normalization of serum Na^+ may result in neurologic dysfunction. Correction of hyponatremia may be accomplished by initiating and maintaining a rapid diuresis with IV furosemide to decrease urine osmolality, followed by IV replacement of urinary sodium and potassium losses. Isotonic saline is usually sufficient as replacement fluid, and 3% saline is rarely required. The urine osmolality must be lower than the osmolality of the replacement fluid for the plasma sodium to rise. Acute therapy is directed at decreasing TBW and consists of the following steps:

(a) Calculate the free water excess using the following formula:

Current total body water (TBW) (liters) = 0.6 × current body weight (kg) (use 0.5 in female, elderly, or cachectic)

Free H_2O excess (liters) = TBW × $\{1 - [Na^+/140]\}$

(b) Choose the rate of correction based on clinical circumstances; usually 0.5 mEq/hour rise in plasma $[Na^+]$ is the target (see sec. **V.C**).

(c) The total change in plasma Na^+ (140 minus measured Na^+) divided by 0.5 mEq/liter/hour will yield the period of time over which correction should occur (in hours).

(d) The free water excess divided by the period of time calculated in step (c) yields the target rate of free water removal in liters/hour.

(e) Establish urine output with IV furosemide, 40 mg, and titrate dose to achieve a urine output (ml/hour) equal to the rate of free water removal in (d).

(f) Replace urine output with isotonic saline.

These rates must be adjusted based on close monitoring of the plasma Na^+, and treatment should be tapered when the plasma $[Na^+]$ reaches 120 or symptoms resolve (see sec. **V.C.3.b.(3)**).

(3) Chronic treatment of SIADH may not be necessary after recovery from an acute precipitating illness (e.g., meningitis or pneumonia) or discontinuation of an offending drug. **Water restriction** to 500–1,000 ml daily is the mainstay of chronic management. Increased salt and protein intake may be effective when water restriction alone is unsuccessful. A loop diuretic can be used to lower urine osmolality. Demeclocycline (300–600 mg/day) antagonizes the effect of ADH and may be used in chronic treatment. Demeclocycline may be nephrotoxic in patients with liver disease (*JAMA* 243:2513, 1980).

c. Thiazide diuretics commonly cause hyponatremia, particularly in older women. These patients are usually euvolemic but may be volume depleted. Hypokalemia often coexists and contributes to the hyponatremia by causing Na^+ to shift intracellularly to compensate for decreased K^+. A metabolic alkalosis also may be present. **Treatment** consists of discontinuing the diuretic and replacing a potassium deficit if present. The hyponatremia usually resolves quickly, but occasionally it may take 1–2 weeks. Volume deficits should be replaced if present. Urgent therapy should be considered if hyponatremia is severe and symptoms are present.

d. Hypothyroidism may produce hyponatremia. The impaired free water excretion may be due to increased ADH levels or to a reduction in GFR and effective renal plasma flow. The **treatment** is thyroxine replacement and water restriction.

e. Adrenal insufficiency causes hyponatremia. This is probably largely secondary to glucocorticoid deficiency, which causes an effective volume depletion and thereby an increase in ADH release. True volume depletion due to mineralocorticoid deficiency may also contribute. **Treatment** consists of adrenal replacement therapy and correction of volume deficits if present.

VI. Hypernatremia. All hypernatremic states are hyperosmolar. As plasma osmolality exceeds 280-285 mosm/kg H_2O, there is a linear increase in ADH release by the posterior pituitary. ECF volume depletion potentiates ADH release, whereas ECF volume expansion may blunt it. The renal response to ADH is conservation of free water, characterized by low urine volumes (<500 ml/day) and a high urine osmolality (>1,000 mosm/kg H_2O). In addition, an increase in plasma osmolality above a threshold probably 5–10 mosm/kg higher than that for ADH release should stimulate thirst and thereby an increase in free water intake.

A. Manifestations. The most common symptoms in hypernatremia can often be attributed to the underlying cause. Signs of volume overload or volume depletion may be prominent and provide a clue to diagnosis. Clinical manifestations attributable to the hypernatremia include tremulousness, irritability, ataxia, spasticity, confusion, seizures, and coma. Symptoms are more likely to occur with acute rises in plasma sodium concentration. Chronic hypernatremia is characterized by increased CNS intracellular osmolality due to uptake and generation of solutes (idiogenic osmoles) beginning about 4 hours after the onset of hypernatremia and stabilizing in 4–7 days. This increase in CNS osmolality prevents cellular dehydration and mitigates the effects of the hypernatremia. However, it must also be accounted for when considering the therapy of hypernatremia, since **rapid correction may cause cerebral edema**.

B. Causes and treatment. Hypernatremic states arise from net sodium gain, net water loss, or failure to replace obligate water losses, as in the case of patients unable to obtain water due to an altered mental status or severe debilitating disease. The diagnostic approach is based on an assessment of the ECF volume, urine volume, urine osmolality (U_{osm}) and urine sodium.

1. **Hypernatremia with ECF volume expansion** signifies net sodium gain. It is usually seen in patients receiving hypertonic saline or $NaHCO_3$. The urine volume, urine osmolality, and urine sodium will be elevated. Mild hypernatremia can be seen with primary hyperaldosteronism and Cushing's syndrome. **Therapy** is directed at allowing a spontaneous diuresis or removal of the excess sodium with diuretics or dialysis (if renal failure is present). The latter maneuvers are followed by replacement of fluid losses with 5% D/W.

2. **Hypernatremia with ECF volume depletion** occurs with hypotonic fluid loss, typically in patients who are unable to obtain water in the face of ongoing losses.

   a. **Extrarenal losses** include GI (diarrhea) and insensible losses (sweating, burns, respiratory). Urine volume is decreased, U_{osm} is high (>800 mosm/kg H_2O), and urine sodium is low.

   b. **Renal losses** due to the presence of a diuretic, an osmotic diuresis (glucose, high-protein tube feedings, prolonged mannitol infusion), or partial diabetes insipidus should be suspected if both urine volume and osmolality are high. If urine volume is high but U_{osm} is low (<250), diabetes insipidus, either central (CDI) or nephrogenic (NDI), is the most likely diagnosis (see sec. **VII.B**).

   c. **Redistribution** into cells causing hypernatremia can occur with strenuous exercise, seizures, and rhabdomyolysis.

   d. **A disorder of the thirst mechanism** should be suspected in an alert patient with hypernatremia who has access to free water. Granulomatous, vascular, and neoplastic hypothalamic diseases all may produce this.

3. The **acute treatment** of hypovolemic hypernatremia depends on the degree of volume depletion. If there is evidence of hemodynamic compromise (e.g., orthostatic hypotension, marked oliguria), treatment should initially be with isotonic saline. Once hemodynamic stability is achieved, the remaining free water deficit can be estimated as follows:

   Current TBW (liters) = $0.5 \times$ current body weight (kg)

   (use 0.4 for females, the elderly, and cachectic patients)

   Body water deficit (liters) = TBW $\times \{$(plasma $[Na^+]/140) - 1\}$

The approximate rate of free H_2O replacement initially required = $\{TBW/(\text{plasma } [Na^+])\} \times$ desired rate of decrease in plasma $[Na^+] \times$

$$1,000 \text{ (mEq/liter/hour)}$$

The rate of free water replacement will change with changes in the TBW and the plasma Na^+. The free water deficit should be corrected either orally or with 5% D/W; one-fourth or one-half normal saline should be used if sodium depletion is present or if there are ongoing GI or renal solute losses. However, one-fourth and one-half normal saline contain only 750 ml and 500 ml of free water per liter, respectively, while 5% D/W is equivalent to free water. Any potassium that is added also contributes to the osmolality of the replacement solution. Ongoing insensible losses of free water (25–50 ml/hour) must also be replaced. If the hypernatremia is due to renal losses (see sec. **VI.B.2.b**) and these losses are continuing, additional free water to replace that lost in the urine must be given. **Excessively rapid correction is dangerous,** particularly in patients with hypernatremia for more than 24 hours, as it may lead to lethargy and seizures secondary to cerebral edema. The plasma sodium should be corrected at a rate not greater than 0.5 mEq/liter/hour in asymptomatic patients or 1 mEq/liter/hour in symptomatic patients. The plasma sodium concentration and ECF volume status should be monitored closely.

VII. Polyuria is generally defined as a urine output greater than 3–4 liters/day. It is useful to classify polyuric states into those that involve a water diuresis (U_{osm} <250 mosm/kg) and those that involve a solute diuresis (U_{osm} >300 mosm/kg). Note that polyuric states may be associated with either hyponatremia or hypernatremia, depending on the cause.

  A. A solute (osmotic) diuresis is most often caused by uncontrolled diabetes mellitus. Iatrogenic causes include excessive saline infusion, prolonged hypertonic mannitol infusion, and high-protein tube feedings. A postobstructive diuresis is a solute diuresis that is appropriate, as the kidneys eliminate accumulated solute and fluid. Only rarely will a postobstructive diuresis lead to volume depletion.

  B. A water diuresis may be due to infusion of large amounts of dilute solutions, primary polydipsia (see sec. **V.C.3.a**), loop diuretics, or diabetes insipidus. Patients with polyuria secondary to iatrogenic infusion or primary polydipsia tend to have plasma sodium in the low normal range (135–140 mEq/liter), though frank hyponatremia may occur if water intake is very high. Patients with diabetes insipidus (DI) tend to have a plasma sodium in the high normal range (140–145 mEq/liter). However, true hypernatremia may occur if there is inadequate access to free water or coexisting impairment of the thirst mechanism.

  1. Central DI (CDI) is due to a complete or partial deficiency of ADH secretion. The causes include hypoxic or ischemic encephalopathy, head trauma, posthypophysectomy, tumor, anorexia nervosa, granulomatous disease (sarcoidosis, histiocytosis X), infection, and idiopathic causes.

  2. Nephrogenic DI (NDI) is due to complete or partial renal resistance to ADH and/or impairment of the countercurrent mechanism in the loop of Henle. The causes include congenital defects, hypercalcemia, severe hypokalemia, drugs (e.g., lithium, demeclocycline, amphotericin, propoxyphene, methoxyflurane), sickle cell disease, Sjögren's syndrome, and amyloidosis. Rarely, the third trimester of pregnancy is associated with NDI due to increased breakdown of ADH.

  3. Evaluation is usually performed to distinguish among primary polydipsia and central and nephrogenic DI. It should be noted that partial forms of CDI and NDI do not usually result in polyuria. This is because the maximum U_{osm} is high enough so that the daily solute load can be excreted in a urine volume less than 3 liters. These patients will mainly complain of nocturia. Initial testing involves water deprivation under direct physician supervision. Close monitoring is required because of the risk of severe volume depletion in patients with complete DI. Failure to appropriately concentrate the urine suggests the diagnosis. A subsequent rise in urinary concentrating ability after SC or IV injection of aqueous arginine vasopressin (5 units) (AVP) confirms the diagnosis of CDI. Lack of a response to AVP indicates NDI. However, patients with primary polydipsia may behave in an identical manner to those with a partial NDI due to washout of the medullary concentration gradient.

4. **Treatment of DI.** If hypernatremia or volume depletion is severe, acute treatment is indicated as outlined in sec. **VI.B.3.** Chronic treatment of DI depends on the cause. CDI is most often physiologically treated with vasopressin administration. The preparation of choice is desamino-D-arginine vasopressin (dDAVP), a long-acting vasopressin analog given intranasally at a dose of 5–10 µg once or twice a day (*Ann Intern Med* 103:228, 1985; *Hosp Prac* 24:114, 1989). It should be given cautiously in patients with coronary artery disease. The smallest dose needed to decrease the urine output to an acceptable volume must be used to avoid the development of water retention and hyponatremia. Unfortunately, dDAVP is very expensive, and other measures may be useful. Moderate protein restriction will decrease the daily solute intake and therefore decrease the minimum daily urine volume. Thiazide diuretics and a low sodium diet produce mild volume depletion, thereby reducing delivery of filtrate to diluting segments of the nephron and decreasing urine output. Chlorpropamide potentiates the action of ADH and may be used in conjunction with dDAVP but may produce hypoglycemia. NDI is unresponsive to vasopressin, but most cases have a treatable cause. Hypercalcemia and hypokalemia should be corrected, and offending drugs should be discontinued if possible. The effect of lithium is usually reversible if discontinued. If lithium must be continued, the K^+-sparing diuretic amiloride may be used. It blocks uptake of lithium in the collecting tubule cells, preventing interference with ADH effect. However, caution must be used in treating patients with diuretics who are also taking lithium. Volume depletion will increase both proximal Na^+ and Li^+ absorption and may result in increased Li^+ levels. For other causes of NDI, nonspecific measures such as protein and sodium restriction and thiazide diuretics are used.

Potassium

The total body potassium of a normal adult is approximately 40–50 mEq/kg body weight. Only about 1.5% is present in the ECF. A typical daily potassium intake is 1.0–1.5 mEq/kg body weight; about 10% of this is excreted in the stool and sweat and the remainder by the kidneys. The normal kidney can excrete up to 6 mEq/kg/day of potassium. The serum potassium concentration is a general indicator of total body potassium, but various factors can affect its transcellular distribution (acid-base abnormalities, increased extracellular osmolality, insulin deficiency). For example, one may expect an inverse change of variable magnitude (0.1–0.7 mEq/liter) in serum potassium concentration for each 0.1 unit change in serum pH.

I. **Hypokalemia.** Assuming a normal pH, a normal serum potassium concentration may actually belie a total body deficit of up to 200 mEq. In general, however, each 1 mEq/dl decrease in serum potassium concentration reflects a deficit of approximately 200–400 mEq. Serum potassium concentrations less than 2 mEq/dl may reflect total body potassium deficits of greater than 1,000 mEq.

A. **Manifestations of hypokalemia** usually occur at potassium concentrations below 2.5 mEq/liter, but there is much individual variability. A rapid decrease in the serum concentration may induce symptoms at a higher potassium level. Signs and symptoms include malaise, fatigue, neuromuscular disturbances (e.g., weakness, hyporeflexia, paresthesias, cramps, restless legs syndrome, paralysis, respiratory failure), GI disorders (e.g., constipation, ileus, vomiting), rhabdomyolysis, and worsening of hepatic encephalopathy. Cardiovascular abnormalities, such as orthostatic hypotension, arrhythmias (particularly with digitalis therapy), and ECG changes (T wave flattening, prominent U waves, decreased QRS voltage, and ST segment depression), may occur. Renal and electrolyte abnormalities include metabolic alkalosis, urinary concentrating defects with polyuria, decreased GFR, and glucose intolerance.

B. Causes. A 24-hour urine measurement for K^+ may be helpful in determining the etiology of hypokalemia. A concurrent measurement of total urine sodium should be performed. Na^+ excretion less than 100 mEq/day suggests inadequate intake of potassium as well as sodium. Na^+ excretion greater than 100 mEq/day and K^+ excretion less than 25 mEq/day suggests extrarenal loss. A K^+ excretion greater than this suggests renal wasting. However, if the cause for the urinary K^+ loss has been removed (e.g., discontinuation of diuretic), then K^+ excretion will be low.

1. **Transcellular shifts** can occur due to increased beta-adrenergic activity (beta-agonist medications, physiologic stress, delirium tremens), alkalemia, insulin excess, acute glucose loads, hypokalemic periodic paralysis, hypothermia, ingestion of barium salts, and anabolic states. Pseudohypokalemia may be seen in leukemia with a very high white blood cell count due to uptake of K^+ intracellularly after the blood has been drawn.

2. **Inadequate intake** of potassium (<10–20 mEq/day) over a prolonged period may produce a significant deficit.

3. **Extrarenal losses** of potassium may be of GI origin (vomiting, nasogastric drainage, fistulas, diarrhea, laxative abuse) or in sweat. Hypokalemia in the setting of gastric losses is mostly due to GI losses as well as enhanced urinary excretion.

4. **Renal losses** of potassium may be due to use of loop or thiazide diuretics, mineralocorticoid excess, penicillin derivatives (especially carbenicillin), amphotericin B, metabolic acidosis, polyuria, and salt-wasting nephropathies (see Salt and Water, sec. **V.C.2**). Diabetic ketoacidosis may cause K^+ wasting because of the osmotic diuresis of hyperglycemia and the filtering of nonreabsorbable ketone anions. Other forms of metabolic acidosis (primarily mineral acids) may cause renal K^+ loss without causing hypokalemia because of the transcellular shifts of K^+ out of cells. Proximal and distal renal tubular acidoses may present with hypokalemia. States of mineralocorticoid excess that cause renal K^+ loss include primary hyperaldosteronism, exogenous mineralocorticoid (fludrocortisone, black licorice), congenital adrenal hyperplasia, renal artery stenosis, and Bartter's syndrome. States of glucocorticoid excess may cause hypokalemia because of the mineralocorticoid effect of cortisol.

C. Treatment

1. **Oral therapy.** Potassium supplements are usually given as potassium chloride. Other forms are available but are generally not as effective in increasing the plasma K^+. **Chloride is required** in cases in which the hypokalemia is associated with metabolic alkalosis and ECF volume contraction. Slow-release KCl tablets or capsules are useful in patients who are unable to tolerate liquid forms of potassium supplementation. The rare occurrence of GI tract ulcers has been reported with these preparations, particularly in the setting of intestinal dysmotility. Salt substitutes provide an economical alternative to prescription potassium supplements; they contain 7–14 mEq potassium/g (5 g equals approximately 1 teaspoon). If a patient consumes a diet that is deficient in potassium-rich foods (e.g., fruits, vegetables), dietary alterations may be attempted but are unlikely to be sufficient. Severe hyperkalemia can occur during oral potassium supplementation; hence, serum potassium levels should always be monitored during therapy. The plasma K^+ may transiently rise by up to 1.0–1.5 mEq/liter after a dose of 40–60 mEq PO. The potassium-sparing diuretics (spironolactone, triamterene, or amiloride) may be an alternative for patients in whom hypokalemia develops secondary to renal losses. These drugs should not be used in patients with renal insufficiency, in conjunction with potassium supplements, or with other agents that impair potassium secretion (e.g., angiotensin-

converting enzyme inhibitors); they should also be used with caution in diabetics.

2. **IV therapy.** The IV administration of potassium is appropriate in patients with severe hypokalemia and in those with hypokalemia who are unable to take oral supplements. However, large doses are difficult to administer because the limits on K^+ concentration in IV replacement solutions make large volumes necessary. An approximation of the potassium deficit can be obtained as discussed above, but frequent serum potassium determinations are necessary to guide therapy. If the serum potassium is greater than 2.5 mEq/liter and ECG changes are not present, potassium can be given at a rate of up to 10 mEq/hour and in concentrations up to 30 mEq/liter. A nondextrose solution is preferred because dextrose may actually decrease the plasma K^+ transiently by stimulating insulin secretion. If the serum potassium is less than 2.5 mEq/liter and accompanied by ECG abnormalities or severe neuromuscular complications, emergency treatment is required. In this setting, potassium can be given through a peripheral IV line at rates up to 40 mEq/hour and in concentrations up to 60 mEq/liter. Higher concentrations are very irritating to the peripheral vein and may cause sclerosis. However, in situations which are life threatening and where the potassium deficit is very large, concentrations as high as 200 mEq/liter at rates up to 100 mEq/hour have been used if administered through a large vein such as the femoral vein (*Arch Intern Med* 150:613, 1990). These high concentrations should be prepared in small volumes (e.g., 20 mEq in 100 ml isotonic saline) to avoid accidental infusion of large amounts of K^+. Administration through a central venous line in other than a femoral vein should be avoided because of the risk of locally high K^+ concentrations near the heart. Continuous ECG monitoring and measurement of the serum potassium concentration every four hours should be performed. Rapid replacement of K^+ can be dangerous even in severe hypokalemia. Once the indications for emergency treatment have resolved, less aggressive replacement should be undertaken as already described.

II. **Hyperkalemia**

A. **Manifestations of hyperkalemia** usually occur when the serum potassium concentration is greater than 6.5 mEq/liter. Neuromuscular manifestations include weakness, paresthesias, areflexia, and ascending paralysis. **Cardiac arrhythmias** include bradycardia that can progress to asystole, prolongation of atrioventricular (AV) conduction leading to complete heart block, and ventricular fibrillation. As the serum K^+ increases, the ECG manifests progressive changes. At a level of 5.5–6.0, the electrocardiogram shows **peaked T waves** and a shortened QT interval. At a level of 6.0–7.0, **lengthening of the PR interval** and **QRS widening occur.** When the serum K^+ reaches 7.0–7.5, the ECG shows flattening of the P waves and further widening of the QRS. When the K^+ level exceeds 8.0, a biphasic sine wave appears, representing fusion of the widened QRS and T wave. This signals imminent ventricular standstill. **The rate of progression is not predictable, and patients may progress from initial ECG changes to dangerous conduction disturbances or arrhythmias within minutes.** Also, the serum K^+ level at which these ECG changes occur shows wide individual variability. If the increase in K^+ level has been slow (e.g., chronic renal failure), these changes are less likely to develop at any given level. However, the ECG changes are exacerbated by coexisting hyponatremia, hypocalcemia, and acidosis (all of which may occur in renal failure).

B. **Causes**

1. **Redistribution of potassium from ICF to ECF** can result from acidosis. Because cell membranes are more permeable to organic acids (e.g., ketoacids, lactic acid), organic acids are much less likely to cause hyperkalemia than are mineral acids (NH_4Cl, HCl). Acutely, acidosis also inhibits distal potassium excretion. Other causes of potassium redistribution include hyperkalemic periodic paralysis, digitalis intoxication, succinylcholine administration, insulin deficiency, increased ECF osmolality (hyperglycemia), and heavy

exercise. Beta-adrenergic antagonists, which can block cellular potassium uptake mediated by beta$_2$-receptors, may cause hyperkalemia in patients with diabetes mellitus, those on dialysis, and those undergoing cardiopulmonary bypass. This effect should be less pronounced with beta$_1$-selective antagonists.

2. **A potassium load** can result from **exogenous** sources such as IV potassium administration, blood transfusions, high-dose potassium-salt penicillin therapy (1.7 mEq potassium/1 million units), and oral potassium supplements or salt substitutes. **Endogenous** potassium loads arise from tissue destruction as seen with rhabdomyolysis, hemolysis, tumor lysis, burns, major surgery, or GI bleeding.

3. **Pseudohyperkalemia** occurs when potassium is released from cells either during blood sample clotting in the presence of leukocytosis ($>$100,000/μl) or thrombocytosis ($>$1 million/μl), or with red blood cell hemolysis due to drawing through a small needle, delay in analysis, or a prolonged, excessively tight tourniquet with repeated fist clenching. A normal plasma (unclotted sample) potassium level will eliminate leukocytosis and thrombocytosis as causes.

4. **Decreased renal excretion** can result from the following:
   a. **Acute or chronic oliguric renal failure.** Acute renal failure, acute tubular necrosis, and acute interstitial nephritis are most likely to cause hyperkalemia. Patients with nonoliguric renal failure will usually not be hyperkalemic unless there is another exacerbating factor.
   b. **Decreased distal nephron sodium delivery** as is seen in volume depletion, heart failure, and hepatic cirrhosis.
   c. **Impairment of the renin-angiotensin system** including hyporeninemic hypoaldosteronism associated with mild to moderate renal insufficiency (GFR 25–75 ml/minute). The renal disease is usually secondary to diabetes or various forms of interstitial disease. AIDS also has been reported as a cause. Various drugs including nonsteroidal antiinflammatory agents, angiotensin-converting enzyme inhibitors, cyclosporine (see sec. **II.B.4.d** below), and pentamidine are also etiologies.
   d. **Decreased aldosterone production** secondary to primary adrenal insufficiency, congenital adrenal hyperplasia, or isolated hypoaldosteronism. Heparin decreases aldosterone production but only causes hyperkalemia in the setting of some other predisposing factor such as renal insufficiency. **Impaired response to aldosterone** is seen with the use of the potassium-sparing diuretic spironolactone and in pseudohypoaldosteronism. The latter has a congenital form and an acquired form associated with various tubulointerstitial renal diseases. Cyclosporine also diminishes the response to aldosterone administration (see sec. **II.B.4.c**).
   e. **Inhibition of tubular secretion of potassium** independent of aldosterone effect is seen with the potassium-sparing diuretics amiloride and triamterene. This also occurs in the hyperkalemic form of distal renal tubular acidosis that is most often seen in obstructive uropathy or sickle cell disease (though they more often cause hyporeninemic hypoaldosteronism). The use of trimethoprim in the treatment of *Pneumocystis carinii* infections in AIDS patients has also been reported to cause hyperkalemia by this mechanism (*N Engl J Med* 328:703, 1993).

C. **Acute treatment.** The goals in the treatment of hyperkalemia are (1) to protect the heart from the effects of potassium by antagonizing the effect on cardiac conduction (calcium administration), (2) to shift potassium from the ECF to the ICF (sodium bicarbonate, beta-adrenergic agonists, insulin, and glucose), and (3) to reduce total body potassium (cation exchange resins, diuretics, dialysis). The need for treatment is urgent if the serum potassium is greater than 7 mEq/liter or if the ECG shows changes of hyperkalemia. Life-threatening arrhythmias may occur at any time during therapy; hence, continuous ECG monitoring is required. The serum potassium should be followed closely during therapy. In patients with hyperkalemia due to tissue destruction or increased total body potassium, therapy directed at net removal of potassium from the body should be initiated simultaneously with acute measures.

1. **Calcium administration** will temporarily antagonize the cardiac and neuromuscular effects of hyperkalemia. Calcium gluconate (10 ml of a 10% solution or 1 g) should be given intravenously slowly over two to five minutes. A second dose can be given after five minutes if no response occurs. Slower infusion rates should be considered in patients receiving digitalis because of the danger of hypercalcemia-induced digitalis toxicity. Unless hypocalcemia is present, further calcium therapy is unlikely to be of benefit. The effect of calcium occurs within minutes and lasts for approximately 1 hour; hence, other modalities should be initiated as soon as possible. Calcium should not be given before or after bicarbonate in the same IV to avoid precipitation.

2. **Sodium bicarbonate administration** causes a shift of potassium from the ECF to the ICF. Treatment with bicarbonate is particularly important in patients with acidosis, since further therapy for hyperkalemia may not be required after correction of the acidosis. One ampule of 7.5% $NaHCO_3$ (44.6 mEq HCO_3) can be given slowly IV over 5 minutes and repeated at 10- to 15-minute intervals if ECG changes persist. The onset of action occurs within 30 minutes and the effect lasts for 1–2 hours. Circulatory overload and hypernatremia can occur when large volumes of hypertonic $NaHCO_3$ are given. If hypocalcemia is present, seizures and tetany may occur as blood pH rises and the ionized free Ca^+ decreases; hence, calcium should be given first. Hyponatremia will magnify the cardiac effects of hyperkalemia, and $NaHCO_3$ can be used to treat this as well. Bicarbonate is less effective in patients with renal failure.

3. **Glucose and insulin infusions** act to shift potassium from the ECF into cells. Ten units of regular insulin can be added to 500 ml of a 10% glucose solution and administered intravenously over 60 minutes. A response should be seen within 30–60 minutes, and the effect typically lasts for several hours. Spot blood glucoses should be followed over this time. The therapy may be repeated as needed. Alternatively, the insulin can be given at the same time as 1 ampule of 50% glucose (25 g) over 5 minutes. However, this may produce hyperglycemia and hyperosmolality, which will exacerbate the hyperkalemia. For the same reason, glucose should be omitted in patients who are already hyperglycemic. The $beta_2$-adrenergic agonist **albuterol** in nebulized form at a dose of 10–20 mg has been shown to be effective in treating hyperkalemia in hemodialysis patients by causing a shift of K^+ intracellularly (*Ann Intern Med* 110:426, 1989). In addition, the coadministration of albuterol may attenuate the hypoglycemic effect of insulin (*Kidney Int* 38:869, 1990).

4. **Cation exchange resins** bind potassium in exchange for another cation (usually sodium) in the intestinal tract, thereby removing potassium from the body. This method of therapy should be given as soon as possible if hyperkalemia results from decreased potassium excretion or an increased potassium load. Onset of action is 1–2 hours and duration is 4–6 hours. Fifty grams will decrease the serum K^+ level by approximately 0.5–1.0 mEq/liter. Each gram of **sodium polystyrene sulfonate** (Kayexalate) binds approximately 1 mEq K^+. Significant amounts of Ca^+ and Mg^{++} may be removed as well. This drug also exchanges about 1–2 mEq Na^+ for each 1 mEq K^+ removed and should therefore be used with caution in patients who are unable to tolerate sodium loads (e.g., because of heart failure, oliguric renal failure, or severe hypertension). Hypernatremia may also occur.

   a. **Oral administration** is the preferred route. Since this drug is constipating, it should be given with a poorly absorbed carrier (osmotic agent) such as sorbitol (commercially available as 15 g/60 ml with 23.5% sorbitol). The initial dose is 15–30 g of sodium polystyrene sulfonate. This dose can be repeated q3–4h up to 4–5 doses/day until the hyperkalemia has resolved. The side effects of nausea and vomiting may be seen. Intestinal necrosis has been reported in surgical patients during the first postoperative week (*Am J Kidney Dis* 20:159, 1992).

b. Rectal administration can be used if the oral route is not tolerated or if an ileus is present. A retention enema can be given as 50 g sodium polystyrene sulfonate powder, mixed in 200 ml of 20% D/W. Retention of the enema for at least 30–60 minutes may be facilitated by using an inflated rectal catheter. Enemas can be repeated q4–6h up to four doses/day. Sorbitol-containing preparations are not recommended for rectal administration. Colonic necrosis and perforation have been reported with the use of cation exchange resin enemas, especially in renal transplant patients (*Dis Colon Rectum* 36:607, 1993), and animal studies suggest sorbitol may be the offending agent. Non–sodium-containing cleansing enemas should be given after each dose to remove the resin.

5. Hemodialysis can remove potassium from the body very effectively but should be reserved for those clinical situations in which more conservative methods have failed or are inappropriate. Peritoneal dialysis is much less effective. Of importance, significant hyperkalemic rebound can occur after dialysis as potassium is mobilized from intracellular stores.

D. Chronic treatment. Treatment of the underlying disorder may obviate the need for specific therapy for hyperkalemia. Patients with renal failure (GFR <10 ml/minute) require restriction of dietary potassium to 40–60 mEq/day. Loop diuretics are efficacious in treating the hyperkalemia as well as the volume overload in renal failure. Sodium polystyrene sulfonate can also be given orally in lower doses (5–10 g two or three times/day) as chronic therapy. If metabolic acidosis is present, treatment with oral sodium bicarbonate may help to control serum K^+. In patients with aldosterone deficiency, treatment with fludrocortisone (Florinef, 0.2 mg/day) is appropriate. However, sodium retention, with its attendant side effects, may occur.

Acid-Base Disturbances

The regulation of pH in a narrow range is the function of the lungs, kidneys, and various buffers. Carbon dioxide, the final product of carbonic acid hydrolysis ($H^+ + HCO_3^- \rightleftarrows H_2CO_3 \rightleftarrows CO_2 + H_2O$), is removed by the lungs. Other acids are excreted by the kidneys, which have the ultimate role in correction of acid-base disorders. Approximately 1 mEq/kg body weight of fixed (nonvolatile) acid is produced daily from the metabolism of sulfur-containing amino acids and of carbohydrates and fats not completely oxidized to CO_2 and H_2O. This acid is excreted by the kidneys. Buffers defend against rapid changes in pH and include bicarbonate, phosphate, proteins, hemoglobin, and bone carbonate. The most important buffer is bicarbonate. The kidneys function to reclaim bicarbonate in the glomerular filtrate by reabsorption and to regenerate bicarbonate consumed in the buffering process by net excretion of acid. The kidneys excrete acid primarily as ammonium (H^+ buffered by NH_3) and titratable acid (H^+ buffered by HPO_4^{2-}). The kidneys are able to increase net acid excretion in certain pathophysiologic states mainly by enhanced ammonia production and excretion (urine pH to a low of approximately 4.5).

I. The arterial blood gases (ABGs). Normal ABG values are pH 7.36–7.44; PCO_2 35–45 mm Hg; and total CO_2 24–32 mEq/liter. Normal venous BG values are pH 7.32–7.38; PCO_2 42–50 mm Hg; and total CO_2 25–33 mEq/liter. When obtaining an ABG, the syringe should be coated with 1 ml heparin (1,000 units/ml) for anticoagulation. The excess heparin should be expelled to prevent factitious lowering of the pH. If drawn from a heparinized arterial line, the first 8–10 ml of blood must be discarded. The sample should be measured immediately to avoid the effects of cell metabolism. If the sample is cooled with ice, the results will remain accurate up to 2 hours after the blood was obtained.

II. The primary acid-base disturbances result from conditions that initially affect either the [HCO_3^-] (metabolic acidosis and alkalosis) or the PCO_2 (respiratory acidosis and alkalosis). Each of these primary disturbances causes the blood pH to shift away from normal and evokes compensatory responses that return pH toward,

Table 3-2. Summary of expected compensation for simple acid-base disorders

Disorder	Initial change	Compensatory response
Metabolic acidosis	Decrease in HCO_3	1.1–1.3 mm Hg decrease in PCO_2 for every 1 mEq/liter decrease in HCO_3^-
Metabolic alkalosis	Increase in HCO_3^-	0.6–0.7 mm Hg increase in PCO_2 for every 1 mEq/liter increase in HCO_3^-
Respiratory acidosis Acute	Increase in PCO_2	1 mEq/liter increase in HCO_3^- for every 10 mm Hg increase in PCO_2
Chronic		3.0–3.5 mEq/liter increase in HCO_3^- for every 10 mm Hg increase in PCO_2
Respiratory alkalosis Acute	Decrease in PCO_2	2.0–2.5 mEq/liter decrease in HCO_3^- for every 10 mm Hg decrease in PCO_2
Chronic		4.0–5.0 mEq/liter decrease in HCO_3^- for every 10 mm Hg decrease in PCO_2

but not completely to, normal. Table 3-2 shows the expected compensatory responses. The acid-base template in Fig. 3-1 illustrates these relationships in graphic form. Caution should be exercised in interpreting these values since what may appear to be a simple disorder may in fact represent a mixed acid-base disturbance (see sec. **VII**). It is sometimes useful to verify that the values for pH, PCO_2, and HCO_3^- are consistent with one another by using the Henderson-Hasselbalch equation, which defines the relationship between pH, PCO_2, and HCO_3^- in blood:

$$pH = 6.1 + \{[HCO_3^-]/(0.031 \times PCO_2)\}$$

An alternative way to express the same relationship is:

$$[H^+] = 24 \times (PCO_2/[HCO_3^-])$$

where the H^+ concentration in nEq/liter can easily be obtained:

pH	6.90	7.00	7.10	7.20	7.30	7.40	7.50	7.60	7.70
$[H^+]$	125	100	80	64	51	40	32	25	20

Note that the H^+ falls by 20% for each 0.1 pH unit increment over the entire range. Intermediate values can be interpolated with accuracy.

A. **Metabolic acidosis** is defined by a reduction in HCO_3^- that reflects either the accumulation of fixed acids or the loss of alkali. The compensatory response is increased ventilation, leading to a fall in PCO_2. The compensatory response begins in 1–2 hours and reaches maximum within 12–24 hours.

B. **Metabolic alkalosis** is defined by a primary increase in HCO_3^- arising either from a loss of acid or, less commonly, from a gain of bicarbonate. The compensatory response is hypoventilation, leading to a rise in PCO_2. The degree of hypoventilation may be reduced if hypoxia is present.

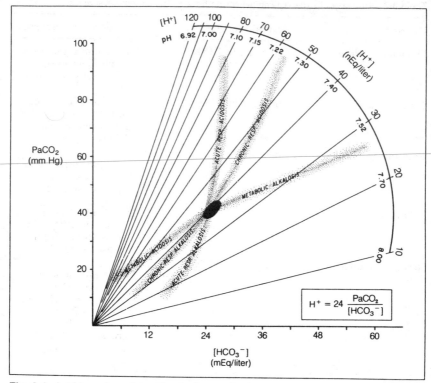

Fig. 3-1. Acid-base template. The dark area in the center represents the normal range. The shaded areas are consistent with, but not necessarily diagnostic of, simple acid-base disorders. The values outside the shaded areas represent mixed acid-base disorders. (From JT Harrington, JJ Cohen, JP Kassirer. Mixed Acid-Base Disturbances. In JJ Cohen, JP Kassirer [eds], *Acid-Base*. Boston: 1982. P. 379. Published by Little, Brown and Company.)

    C. Respiratory acidosis is characterized by a primary increase in PCO_2 due to processes that interfere with the pulmonary excretion of CO_2. The compensatory response that occurs over several days is an increase in renal reabsorption and generation of bicarbonate, leading to a rise in serum HCO_3^-.

    D. Respiratory alkalosis is characterized by a decreased PCO_2 due to primary hyperventilation. The compensatory response that occurs over several days is increased renal bicarbonate excretion leading to a fall in serum HCO_3^-.

III. Metabolic acidosis

    A. Manifestations of acute metabolic acidosis are often hard to separate from the primary disease process but may involve the respiratory, cardiovascular, neurologic, and skeletal systems. The respiratory compensation causes deep (Kussmaul) respirations. There may be an increase in the respiratory rate, which can result in fatigue and ultimately respiratory failure. An increased respiratory rate without obvious pulmonary pathology can often be an important clinical clue to metabolic acidosis. There is also an increased susceptibility to cardiac arrhythmias, a decrease in myocardial contractility, and a decreased response to inotropic agents. A secondary decrease in intracerebral pH may cause a decrease in the level of consciousness, though this often is hard to separate from the effects of cerebral hypoperfusion in shock, hyperosmolality in diabetic ketoacidosis, or the toxic effects of ingested alcohols. Chronic metabolic acidosis causes loss of calcium from bone, as well as skeletal muscle breakdown.

B. **The anion gap (AG)** (*Kidney Int* 27:472, 1985) can aid in the differential diagnosis of metabolic acidosis. The AG is an indirect measurement of those plasma anions not measured by routine laboratory screening. It is defined as the difference between the plasma sodium concentration and the sum of the plasma chloride and bicarbonate concentrations:

$$AG = [NA^+] - ([Cl^-] + [HCO_3^-])$$

Normal AG = 12 ± 4 mEq/liter

Negatively charged plasma proteins account for most of the normal AG. Nonhyperchloremic acidoses produce unmeasured anions that increase the AG. When the increase in the AG is small, assays for unmeasured anions may be negative. Other conditions without acidosis may elevate the AG, such as hyperalbuminemia or a decrease in nonsodium cations. Conversely, hypoalbuminemia or an increase in nonsodium cations may decrease the AG and may mask a nonhyperchloremic metabolic acidosis.

C. **Treatment of acute metabolic acidosis** with parenteral bicarbonate therapy may be considered in patients with a pH below 7.2. **Bicarbonate must be administered cautiously,** however, because overalkalinization can induce tetany, seizures, cardiac arrhythmias, and increased lactate production. Since the distribution of bicarbonate is about 50% of lean body weight, an approximation of the amount of bicarbonate necessary to return the serum concentration to normal can be estimated as follows:

$$HCO_3^- \text{ deficit (mEq)} = 0.5 \times \text{lean body wt (kg)}$$
$$\times (\text{desired } [HCO_3^-] - \text{measured } [HCO_3^-])$$

Since the degree of respiratory compensation, ECF volume status, and progression of the underlying disease may vary from patient to patient, alkali therapy must be guided by frequent assessment of acid-base status and electrolyte levels. Usually, 2–3 ampules of 7.5% $NaHCO_3$ (44.6 mEq/ampule) are added to 1,000 ml of 5% D/W to provide a solution with a Na^+ concentration of 89–134 mEq/liter. One-half the calculated deficit may be replaced in three to four hours if severe heart failure is not present. **No further bicarbonate therapy should be given once the pH reaches 7.2.** Because correction of acidosis without correction of a potassium deficit may lead to profound hypokalemia (due to intracellular shift of potassium), potassium supplementation should be undertaken if the serum potassium concentration begins to fall during correction of the acidosis. Serum calcium should also be monitored and hypocalcemia treated because a relative alkalosis may decrease the ionized calcium concentration. In lactic acidosis, correction of serum pH to greater than 7.2 can result in "overshoot alkalosis" since oxidation of lactate and endogenous regeneration of bicarbonate occurs once the cause of the lactic acidosis has been corrected.

D. **Causes and chronic treatment**
   1. **Increased AG metabolic acidosis.** Serum ketones, lactate, and plasma osmolality should be measured and an **osmolal gap should be calculated.** If an osmolal gap is present (see Salt and Water, sec. **IV**), blood tests for toxic alcohols (ethanol, methanol, ethylene glycol) should be performed.
      a. **Diabetic ketoacidosis (DKA)** (see Chap. 20). **Lactic acidosis** can also be seen in acutely ill diabetic patients, especially those with DKA. When lactic acidosis occurs in DKA, ketoacid formation is shifted from acetoacetate to beta-hydroxybutyrate, which is not measured by the nitroprusside reaction.
      b. **Lactic acidosis** may be seen in any condition that results in **tissue hypoperfusion or impaired oxygenation.** Examples include cardiopulmonary arrest, shock of any type, pulmonary edema, severe hypoxemia, carbon monoxide poisoning, or vascular insufficiency (mesenteric or limb ischemia). Hyperphosphatemia, hyperuricemia, and moderate hyperkalemia can accompany the acidosis. Conditions that cause a marked **increase in the metabolic rate** may also cause a lactic acidosis. These include

generalized seizures, strenuous exercise, severe asthma, and hypothermic shivering. **Other conditions** associated with lactic acidosis include malignancy, diabetes mellitus (usually with DKA; see sec. **III.D.1.a**), hypoglycemia, D-lactate–producing bacteria in the short bowel syndrome, and various intoxications. Among the latter are cyanide (including from metabolism of the drug nitroprusside), alcohol, methanol, and salicylate. Patients with renal and, particularly, liver failure are predisposed to lactic acidosis since these are the organs responsible for lactate metabolism.

   c. **Renal failure** results in an AG acidosis when the GFR falls below 20–30 ml/minute. The AG is due to retained sulfate, phosphate, and organic anions. The AG will not account for the entire decrease in the serum HCO_3^- because the acidosis is in part secondary to decreased ammoniagenesis and impaired bicarbonate regeneration. The serum HCO_3^- usually will not be less than 12 mEq/liter because of bone buffering, unless another etiology for metabolic acidosis is superimposed, including a hypoaldosterone state (see sec. **III.D.2.d** and Potassium, secs. **II.B.4.c** and **d**). When the bicarbonate concentration is less than 17–18 mEq/liter, bicarbonate replacement is necessary to prevent osteopenia and skeletal muscle breakdown. **Treatment** should be in the form of **sodium bicarbonate.** Tablets are available in 325- and 650-mg sizes containing approximately 12 mEq of alkali/g. These may be given in divided doses for a total of 2–4 g/day. Caution must be used in those patients who are unable to tolerate a volume load. **Shohl's solution should not be used** in renal failure because the citrate contained in it can increase aluminum absorption and lead to aluminum intoxication.

   d. **Alcoholic ketoacidosis** occurs after the abrupt discontinuation of ethanol consumption and is usually due to vomiting, malnutrition, and volume depletion. If enough ethanol remains in the blood, an **osmolal gap**, along with the increase in the AG, will be present (see Salt and Water, sec. **IV**). The osmolal gap should be equal to ethanol (in mg/dl)/4.6 unless there is an associated ingestion of another toxic alcohol. Beta-hydroxybutyrate initially predominates in the serum; hence, the nitroprusside ketone reaction (Acetest), which detects acetoacetic acid, can underestimate severity. As beta-hydroxybutyrate is metabolized to acetoacetate, the Acetest becomes increasingly positive, giving the false impression of worsening ketosis. **Lactic acidosis** may coexist, but lactate levels usually do not exceed 3 mEq/liter. Serum glucose is typically normal or low. **Treatment** is directed at replacement of volume and glucose with 0.45% saline with 5% dextrose. The acidosis, unless severe, usually corrects with these measures. Hypokalemia, hypophosphatemia, and hypomagnesemia may occur, especially after 12–24 hours of therapy.

   e. **Toxic ingestion** of other alcohols such as **methanol** and **ethylene glycol** causes an increased AG metabolic acidosis along with an osmolal gap. **Toluene** and **paraldehyde** may cause an increased AG acidosis, but without an osmolal gap (see Chap. 9).

   f. **Salicylate intoxication** can result in respiratory alkalosis and metabolic acidosis. The metabolic acidosis may be due to increased lactate and ketoacid levels, as well as, to a minor degree, salicylic acid and its acid intermediates themselves. A significant osmolal gap will usually not be present. Diagnosis and treatment are described in Chap. 9.

   g. **Starvation,** if prolonged, may produce a mild ketoacidosis ($[HCO_3^-] \geq 18$ mEq/liter).

2. **Normal AG (hyperchloremic) acidosis** may be of GI origin (loss of bicarbonate), of renal origin (loss of bicarbonate or retention of acid), or due to the administration of acidic or acid-producing substances. The measurement of urine electrolytes and calculation of the **urine anion gap** ($[Na^+] + [K^+] - [Cl^-]$) can be helpful in determining if the acidosis is of renal origin (*Am J Nephrol* 10:89, 1990). A negative gap signifies normal renal NH_4^+ excretion and therefore a nonrenal cause for the acidosis. A positive gap indicates

impaired renal NH_4^+ excretion and an acidosis of renal origin. However, if there is concurrent volume depletion due to GI losses, distal acidification may be impaired due to a decrease in distal Na^+ delivery and therefore the urine anion gap may be positive. The urine anion gap should not be used when an elevated serum anion gap acidosis is present because the unmeasured anions may also be present in the urine, causing a positive urine anion gap despite a nonrenal origin for the acidosis

a. **GI loss of bicarbonate** may be due to diarrhea, ureteral diversions (ureterosigmoidostomy, long or obstructed ileal conduit), cholestyramine (especially in the presence of renal failure), or ingestion of calcium or magnesium chloride. GI losses may also be due to small bowel, biliary, or pancreatic drainage or fistulas.

b. **Proximal (type II) renal tubular acidosis** (RTA) is due to a reduction in the capacity of the proximal tubule to reclaim filtered bicarbonate. Initially, the urine pH is greater than 5.5, but as the serum bicarbonate concentration falls, proximal tubular bicarbonate reabsorption increases and the **urine pH becomes less than 5.5.** The plasma HCO_3^- is usually between 14 and 20 mEq/liter. The plasma K^+ may be normal or decreased. Causes include certain inherited disorders, multiple myeloma, autoimmune disorders (Sjögren's syndrome, systemic lupus erythematosus, chronic active hepatitis), interstitial nephritis, carbonic anhydrase inhibitors (acetazolamide), heavy metals, ifosfamide, and outdated tetracycline. Osteopenia is a common complication. The bicarbonate wasting may occur as part of a generalized defect in proximal tubular transport (Fanconi's syndrome) with associated glucosuria, aminoaciduria, hypophosphatemia, and hypouricemia. **Treatment** should include attempts to correct the underlying cause. Large amounts of **alkali** (5–15 mEq/kg/day) are required. Citrate may cause fewer GI side effects than bicarbonate. Alkali therapy can produce **severe hypokalemia,** and a portion of the alkali should be given as the potassium salt. **Thiazide** diuretics can be used to increase proximal tubule bicarbonate reabsorption by inducing a mild ECF volume depletion.

c. **Distal (type I) RTA** is due to a defect in distal nephron acidification and results in hypokalemia and a **urine pH greater than 5.5.** The plasma $[HCO_3^-]$ is variable but may be less than 10 mEq/liter. It is also manifested by hypokalemia, hypercalciuria, hyperphosphaturia, osteomalacia, nephrolithiasis (calcium phosphate or struvite stones), and nephrocalcinosis. In some cases, hypercalciuria (either idiopathic or familial) is thought to be the etiology of the RTA. Other causes include autoimmune disorders (Sjögren's syndrome, rheumatoid arthritis), multiple myeloma, primary hyperparathyroidism, marked volume depletion, and drugs (amphotericin B, lithium, toluene, ifosfamide). There is also a **hyperkalemic form** of distal RTA usually seen with obstructive uropathy, sickle cell nephropathy, and SLE. **Treatment** consists of **bicarbonate** replacement (usually 1–2 mEq/kg/day is required), which can also correct calcium wasting and osteomalacia. Any potassium deficit should be corrected acutely. As with a proximal RTA, chronic potassium replacement may be necessary, but losses are decreased with treatment of the acidosis. Potassium citrate may be necessary for stone disease or nephrocalcinosis.

d. **Type IV RTA** is usually caused by insufficient urinary buffers—usually NH_3. It is commonly seen with the syndrome of hyporeninemic hypoaldosteronism associated with mild to moderate renal insufficiency. However, it may be seen with any cause of hypoaldosteronism or resistance to its effects (see Potassium, secs. **II.B.4.c** and **d**). The plasma $[HCO_3^-]$ is usually greater than 15 mEq/liter. Hyperkalemia is often present, but the plasma K^+ concentration may be normal. Urine pH is usually less than 5.5. **Treatment** consists of dietary **potassium restriction** to 40–60 mEq/day and usually a loop diuretic. Control of the serum K^+ alone may result in a sufficient improvement in the acidosis, but **bicarbonate supplementation,** 1.5–2.0 mEq/kg/day, may be required. Chronic Kayexalate therapy may also be necessary. **Fludrocortisone** (Florinef), 0.1–0.2 mg PO qd, should be considered in patients with primary adrenal insufficiency and those with hyperkalemia, normal BP, and no edema.

   e. **Administration of non–bicarbonate-containing IV fluids** in large amounts may cause a dilutional acidosis. If normal kidney function is present, it will be quickly corrected. **Hyperalimentation** fluids may cause a hyperchloremic acidosis, which can be treated by balancing the cations with acetate rather than bicarbonate.

IV. **Metabolic alkalosis** may occur secondary to ingestion of exogenous alkali, HCl losses (renal, GI), or ECF volume contraction around a fixed blood content of bicarbonate. The kidneys are normally capable of excreting excess bicarbonate, but this ability may be impaired as a result of ECF volume contraction, hypokalemia, chloride depletion, or excess mineralocorticoid or glucocorticoid states. Measurement of the urine chloride concentration can help differentiate the causes of the metabolic alkalosis. This, in turn, has therapeutic implications since it indicates whether or not the alkalosis can be corrected by the administration of chloride (chloride-responsive vs. chloride-resistant alkalosis).

A. **Manifestations of metabolic alkalosis** are often due more to the coexisting volume depletion and hypokalemia, but the alkalemia may produce impaired mentation, hypotension, cardiac arrhythmias, hypoventilation, and decreased ionized calcium.

B. **Causes and treatment**

   1. **Chloride-responsive alkalosis** with a **urine chloride less than 10 mEq/liter** is the more common form of metabolic alkalosis. It is usually, but not necessarily, accompanied by ECF volume depletion ("contraction alkalosis"). It most commonly occurs with GI HCl losses (vomiting, nasogastric suction, villous adenoma) or with diuretic use. Acutely, diuretic therapy may raise the urine chloride. Measurement after the duration of the diuretic effect (12–24 hours) will then reveal a low urine chloride. Hypokalemia often accompanies these disorders and helps perpetuate the alkalosis. Other causes include the post-hypercapnic state and cystic fibrosis. **Treatment** should be directed at correction of the underlying disorder. Correction of the chloride depletion can be achieved by administration of NaCl tablets or, if significant volume contraction is present, IV saline. Hypokalemia should be treated with potassium chloride. In edematous states where there is effective circulatory volume depletion (left-sided heart failure, cor pulmonale, liver cirrhosis), NaCl administration will worsen the volume overload. Therefore, if adequate renal function is present, a carbonic anhydrase inhibitor (acetazolamide) is often useful. This is also effective in the post-hypercapnic state. The usual dosage of acetazolamide is 250–500 mg PO or IV q8h. Gastric HCl losses may be attenuated with the use of either IV or PO H_2-receptor antagonists or omeprazole.

   2. **Chloride-resistant alkalosis** with a **urine chloride greater than 20 mEq/liter** is much less common. Causes include those associated with hypertension, such as primary hyperaldosteronism, Cushing's syndrome, renal artery stenosis, licorice, and Liddle's syndrome; and those without hypertension, such as Bartter's syndrome, severe hypokalemia (K^+ <2 mEq/liter), and perhaps hypomagnesemia. Hypokalemia of a less severe degree often accompanies many of the other disorders and helps perpetuate the alkalosis. **Treatment** is directed at the underlying disorder. Potassium deficits should be corrected. In states of mineralocorticoid excess, spironolactone or amiloride may be helpful.

   3. **Exogenous administration of alkali** including massive blood transfusions containing citrate, bicarbonate administration, milk-alkali syndrome, and ingestion of antacids along with cation exchange resins in renal failure all may cause metabolic alkalosis.

   4. **Miscellaneous causes** include hypercalcemia of nonparathyroid origin (malignancy, sarcoidosis, hypervitaminosis D), refeeding alkalosis (prolonged fasts broken with high-carbohydrate meals), and high-dose carbenicillin or penicillin.

C. Treatment of severe metabolic alkalosis (pH >7.55) with clinically evident systemic effects should employ acid therapy, particularly if a contraindication to NaCl administration exists (e.g., heart failure, renal failure). **This therapy should be done with extreme caution.** The amount of acid that would theoretically correct the alkalosis is given by the following formula:

$$H^+ \text{ deficit (mEq)} - 0.5 \times \text{lean body wt (kg)}$$
$$\times \text{ (measured } [HCO_3^-] - \text{ desired } [HCO_3^-])$$

One-half of the deficit can be replaced over the first 12 hours and the remainder over the next 24 hours, as the clinical situation dictates. A HCl solution consisting of 150 ml of 1.0 N HCl in 1 liter of sterile water (H^+ = 130 mEq/liter) can be administered via a central line at a rate no greater than 0.2 mEq/kg/hour (*Surgery* 75:194, 1974). Acid should not be infused directly into the right atrium. The infusion should be accompanied by frequent measurements of ABGs and serum electrolytes (at least q4h). In patients with renal failure, alkalosis can be corrected with hemodialysis.

V. Respiratory acidosis is caused by inadequate pulmonary excretion of CO_2. **Causes** include CNS depression (drugs, infection, brain injury, obesity), neuromuscular disorders (myopathy, Guillain-Barré syndrome, myasthenic crisis, hypokalemia), and pulmonary diseases (chronic obstructive pulmonary disease, sleep apnea, asthma, kyphoscoliosis, pneumothorax). **Manifestations** include agitation, asterixis, papilledema, headache, somnolence, hypertension, tachycardia, heart failure, and cardiac arrhythmias.

A. The diagnosis should be made when the ABGs reveal a decreased pH and an elevated PCO_2. It is important to determine whether the change in pH is appropriate for the change in PCO_2 in order to differentiate acute from chronic respiratory disturbances and to detect the presence of a mixed disorder (see Table 3-2). Renal compensation occurs over several days. In general, the compensated serum bicarbonate does not exceed 35 mEq/liter; if it does, a concomitant metabolic alkalosis may be present.

B. Treatment of respiratory acidosis is directed at improving ventilation (see Chap. 9). Administration of bicarbonate to correct the acidosis may be harmful since the low pH is an important stimulus for ventilation. However, in patients on mechanical ventilation because of severe status asthmaticus and in whom the respiratory acidosis cannot be corrected quickly, small doses of bicarbonate may be beneficial for (1) improvement in the response to adrenergic bronchodilators and (2) avoiding barotrauma by allowing less vigorous ventilation without exacerbating the acidemia (*Am J Med* 74:898, 1983).

VI. Respiratory alkalosis is due to excessive pulmonary CO_2 excretion (hyperventilation). **Causes** include CNS disorders (anxiety, brainstem tumors, infection), drugs (salicylates, theophylline, catecholamines, progesterone), hypoxemia, pulmonary disease (pneumonia, pulmonary emboli, pulmonary edema, interstitial lung disease), gram-negative sepsis, liver disease, pregnancy, and excessive ventilation from mechanical ventilators. Rapid correction of chronic metabolic acidosis can also produce a respiratory alkalosis because of the persistent and more slowly corrected CNS acidosis causing persistent hyperventilation. **Manifestations** include lightheadedness, paresthesias, cramps, tetany, syncope, seizures, and cardiac arrhythmias.

A. The diagnosis should be made when the ABGs reveal an increased pH and a decreased PCO_2. One should determine whether there has been appropriate renal compensation; if not, a mixed disorder is present (see Table 3-2). The serum bicarbonate usually does not fall below 15 mEq/liter unless a concomitant metabolic acidosis is present.

B. Treatment should be directed at the underlying disorder. Acute therapy is usually not necessary, unless the pH is greater than 7.5. If hypoxemia is not present, symptoms of acute hyperventilation may be relieved by reassurance and rebreathing into a paper bag. If PCO_2 is rapidly corrected in chronic respiratory alkalosis (as in readjustment of mechanical ventilator settings or rebreathing), metabolic acidosis will ensue because of the previous compensatory decrease in the serum bicarbonate concentration. If persistent hyperventilation occurs (such as in CNS disease or paradoxical CNS acidosis), use of a CO_2 rebreathing apparatus may be warranted.

VII. **Mixed acid-base disturbances** (*Medicine* 59:161, 1980; *Clin Endocrinol Metab* 13:333, 1984) are common in the acutely ill patient and can often be predicted based on the clinical scenario. Comparison of the actual with the expected compensatory changes of the pH, PCO_2, and HCO_3^- is necessary (see Table 3-2 and Fig. 3-1). However, values within the expected range for a simple disorder may still represent a mixed disorder, and therefore careful attention must be paid to the possible underlying clinical disorders. Measurement of serum electrolytes and calculation of the anion gap must also be performed. Probably the most common example of a mixed acid-base disorder is respiratory acidosis and metabolic acidosis. This may be seen in cardiorespiratory arrest, lung disease with severe hypoxemia, and shock with respiratory failure. Other examples are salicylate intoxication, gram-negative sepsis, liver failure (respiratory alkalosis and metabolic acidosis); treatment of cor pulmonale with diuretics (respiratory acidosis and metabolic alkalosis); treatment of liver cirrhosis with diuretics (respiratory alkalosis and metabolic alkalosis); and vomiting with severe volume depletion causing lactic acidosis (metabolic alkalosis and metabolic acidosis).

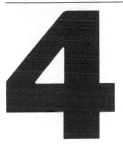

Hypertension

Clark R. McKenzie and
Linda K. Peterson

Definitions and Diagnostic Evaluation

Hypertension is the presence of an elevated blood pressure that places patients at increased risk for target organ damage (TOD) (Table 4-1) in several vascular beds including the retina, brain, heart, and kidneys. Hypertension is the most common condition for which patients receive prescription medication in the United States, and it is estimated that approximately 50 million Americans are hypertensive as defined by a BP greater than 140/90 mm Hg, but only 35% are aware of their condition (*Arch Intern Med* 153:154, 1993). Hypertension affects nearly 20% of the white and 30% of the black U.S. population older than 18 years of age; essential hypertension accounts for approximately 90% of these cases. The remainder are afflicted with secondary hypertension caused by renal parenchymal disease, renovascular disease, pheochromocytoma, Cushing's syndrome, primary hyperaldosteronism, and coarctation of the aorta. The prevalence of disease-associated morbidity and mortality, including atherosclerotic cardiovascular disease, stroke, heart failure (HF), and renal insufficiency, increases with higher levels of both systolic and diastolic BP (*Ann Intern Med* 119:329, 1993; *Arch Intern Med* 153:156, 1993). It is important to recognize that both systolic and diastolic BP elevations are important in diagnosis and therapy and that isolated systolic hypertension of the elderly is associated with increased cardiovascular and cerebrovascular complications.

Patients with a recent substantial increase in BP above their baseline value sufficient to cause acute damage to retinal vessels (hemorrhage, exudates, papilledema) are considered to have accelerated malignant hypertension, regardless of the absolute level of BP (*Br Med J* 292:235, 1986).

I. **Detection and classification.** It is important to perform BP measurements on multiple occasions under nonstressful circumstances (i.e., rest, empty bladder, comfortable temperature, sitting) to obtain an accurate assessment of BP in a given patient. Hypertension should not be diagnosed on the basis of one measurement alone, unless it is greater than 210/120 mm Hg or accompanied by TOD. Three or more abnormal readings should be obtained, preferably over a period of several weeks, before consideration of therapy. Care should also be used to exclude pseudohypertension, which usually occurs in elderly individuals with stiff, noncompressible vessels. A palpable artery that persists after cuff inflation (Osler's sign) should alert the physician to this possibility. Home and ambulatory BP monitoring can be used to assess a patient's true average BP, and there is evidence that the risk for TOD correlates better with these measurements (*Am Heart J* 114:925, 1987; *Arch Intern Med* 153:158, 1993). Circumstances in which ambulatory BP monitoring might be of value include (1) suspected "white coat hypertension" (increases in BP associated with the stress of physician office visits), (2) high normal BP (130–139 mm Hg systolic; 85–89 mm Hg diastolic) with TOD, (3) evaluation of possible drug resistance, (4) episodic hypertension, and (5) hypotension symptoms associated with medication or autonomic dysfunction (*Arch Intern Med* 150:2276, 1990). It is important to note the presence or absence of other cardiovascular risk factors (e.g., diabetes mellitus, hyperlipidemia, cigarette smoking, obesity) and TOD when considering therapy for hypertensive patients. Hypertension is present if a patient's

Table 4-1. Manifestations of target organ disease

Organ system	Manifestations
Cardiac	
Acute	Pulmonary edema
Chronic	Clinical or electrocardiographic evidence of CAD; LVH by ECG or echocardiogram
Cerebrovascular	
Acute	Intracerebral bleeding, coma, seizures, mental status changes, TIA, stroke
Chronic	TIA, stroke
Renal	
Acute	Hematuria, azotemia
Chronic	Serum creatinine >1.5 mg/dl, proteinuria >1 + on dip-stick
Retinopathy	
Acute	Papilledema, hemorrhages
Chronic	Hemorrhages, exudates, arterial nicking

CAD = coronary artery disease; LVH = left ventricular hypertrophy; TIA = transient ischemic attack.

average BP is greater than 140 mm Hg systolic and greater than 90 mm Hg diastolic (Table 4-2) (*Arch Intern Med* 153:154, 1993).

II. **Initial clinical evaluation.** Elevated BP is usually discovered in asymptomatic individuals during screening. Optimal detection and evaluation of hypertension requires accurate noninvasive **BP measurement,** and this should be obtained in a seated patient with his or her arm level with the heart. A calibrated, appropriately fitting BP cuff should be used because falsely high readings can be obtained if the cuff is too small. Two readings should be taken, separated by two minutes. Systolic BP should be noted with the appearance of Korotkoff sounds (phase I) and diastolic BP with the disappearance of sounds (phase V). In certain patients, the Korotkoff sounds do not disappear but will be present to 0 mm Hg. In this case, phase IV (the initial muffling of Korotkoff sounds) should be taken as the diastolic BP (*Hypertension* 11:211A, 1988). One should be careful to avoid spuriously low BP readings due to an auscultatory gap, which is caused by the disappearance and reappearance of Korotkoff sounds in hypertensive patients, and may account for up to a 25-mm Hg gap between true and measured BP. Hypertension should be confirmed in both arms and the higher reading used. The **history** should seek to discover secondary causes of hypertension and note the presence of medications that may affect BP (e.g., decongestants, oral contraceptives, appetite suppressants, nonsteroidal antiinflammatory agents [NSAIDs], exogenous thyroid hormone, and recent alcohol consumption). The **physical examination** should include investigation for TOD or a secondary cause of hypertension by noting the presence of carotid bruit, an S3, an S4, cardiac murmurs, neurologic deficits, elevated jugular venous pressure, rales, retinopathy, unequal pulses, enlarged kidneys, cushingoid features, and abdominal bruits. A diagnosis of secondary hypertension should be considered in the following situations: (1) age of onset less than 30 or greater than 60, (2) hypertension that is difficult to control after therapy has been initiated, (3) stable hypertension that becomes difficult to control, (4) accelerated or malignant hypertension, and (5) the presence of signs or symptoms of a secondary cause.

III. **Laboratory evaluation of the patient with newly diagnosed hypertension.** All newly diagnosed hypertensive patients should have a laboratory assessment, including a urinalysis, hematocrit, plasma glucose, serum potassium, creatinine, calcium, uric acid, chest x-ray, and electrocardiogram. Fasting serum cholesterol and triglycerides should be obtained to screen for hyperlipidemia (see Chap. 22). This battery of tests helps identify patients with possible TOD and provides a

Table 4-2. Classification of blood pressure for adults aged 18 years and older[a]

Category	Systolic (mm Hg)	Diastolic (mm Hg)
Normal[b]	<130	<85
High normal	130–139	85–89
Hypertension[c]		
Stage 1 (mild)	140–159	90–99
Stage 2 (moderate)	160–179	100–109
Stage 3 (severe)	180–209	110–119
Stage 4 (very severe)	≥210	≥120

[a] Not taking antihypertensive drugs and not acutely ill. When systolic and diastolic pressures fall into different categories, the higher category should be selected to classify the individual's BP status. Isolated systolic hypertension is defined as a systolic BP of 140 mm Hg or more and a diastolic BP of less than 90 mm Hg and staged appropriately (e.g., 170/85 mm Hg is defined as stage 2 isolated systolic hypertension).

In addition to classifying stages of hypertension on the basis of average BP levels, the clinician should specify presence or absence of target organ disease and additional risk factors. This specificity is important for risk classification and management.

[b] Optimal blood pressure with respect to cardiovascular risk is less than 120 mm Hg systolic and less than 80 mm Hg diastolic. However, unusually low readings should be evaluated for clinical significance.

[c] Based on the average of two or more readings taken at each of two or more visits after an initial screening.

Source: The Fifth Report of the Joint National Committee on Detection, Evaluation, and Treatment of High Blood Pressure. *Arch Intern Med* 153:161, 1993.

baseline for assessing adverse effects of therapy. Assessment of cardiac function or left ventricular hypertrophy by echocardiogram may be of value for certain patients (*N Engl J Med* 322:1561, 1990; *Br Med J* 303:81, 1991).

Therapeutic Considerations

I. General considerations and goals. The goal of treatment for hypertension is to prevent the long-term sequelae of this disease (i.e., TOD). Unless there is an overt need for immediate pharmacologic therapy, most patients should be given the opportunity to achieve a reduction in BP over an interval of 4–6 months by applying nonpharmacologic modifications. The primary goal is to reduce BP to less than 140/90 mm Hg while concurrently controlling other modifiable cardiovascular risk factors. Treatment should be more aggressive for those patients in whom TOD or other cardiovascular risk factors are present (*Ann Intern Med* 119:329, 1993). Protection from stroke, myocardial infarction (MI), IIF, progression to severe hypertension, and all-cause mortality has been demonstrated with antihypertensive therapy. As much as a 42% reduction in stroke has been achieved with a decrease in diastolic BP of only a few points (*Lancet* 335:827, 1990). Discretion is warranted when prescribing medication to lower BP that may adversely affect cardiovascular risk in other ways (e.g., glucose control, lipid metabolism, uric acid levels). Since isolated systolic hypertension is also associated with increased cerebrovascular and cardiac events, the therapeutic goal in this subset of patients should be to lower BP to less than 160 mm Hg systolic. In the absence of hypertensive crisis, BP should be reduced gradually to avoid cerebral ischemia. Patient education is an essential component of the treatment plan and promotes patient compliance. Physicians should emphasize that (1) lifelong treatment is usually required, (2) symptoms are an unreliable gauge of severity of hypertension, and (3) prognosis improves with proper management. Cultural and other individual differences among patients must be considered when planning a therapeutic regimen. Table 4-2 includes a recent classification for hypertension.

A. Stages 1 and 2 hypertension. After establishing a mean BP of greater than 140/90 mm Hg, a trial of nonpharmacologic therapy should be initiated with close follow-up for 3–6 months. If this is not effective, antihypertensive medication should be initiated. In patients without other cardiovascular risk factors or evidence of TOD, mild elevations in BP (diastolic BP 90–94 mm Hg) can be followed closely without therapy. If the BP continues to increase, antihypertensive therapy should then be initiated.

B. Stages 3 and 4 hypertension. Treatment for these grades of hypertension should be similar to that in stages 1 and 2 with shorter intervals of follow-up. Patients with BPs of greater than 180/110 mm Hg should be treated with medication and will often require more than one drug before adequate control is achieved. Those with diastolic BPs greater than 120 mm Hg require immediate drug therapy.

C. Isolated systolic hypertension. Isolated systolic hypertension, defined as a systolic BP greater than 160 mm Hg, occurs frequently in the elderly (beginning after the fifth decade and increasing with age). Nonpharmacologic therapy should be attempted initially. If it fails, medication should be used to lower systolic BP to less than 160 mm Hg if it is initially greater than 180 mm Hg, and to lower the systolic BP by 20 mm Hg in those with a systolic BP of 160–180 mm Hg. Patient tolerance of antihypertensive therapy should be frequently assessed.

II. Individual patient considerations. A vast array of effective antihypertensive agents is available. A patient's pathogenic derangement of renin secretion, sympathetic tone, and renal sodium excretion should be considered, as well as the attendant changes in cardiac output, peripheral vascular resistance, and volume status to make logical therapeutic choices.

A. The young hypertensive patient (≤35 years) is generally characterized as an active individual with increased sympathetic tone and elevated plasma renin activity. Diuretics, angiotensin-converting enzyme (ACE) inhibitors, calcium channel antagonists, combined alpha- and beta-adrenergic antagonists, and alpha-adrenergic antagonists are effective in this population. Beta-adrenergic antagonists alone are also effective but may adversely affect high-density lipoprotein (HDL) cholesterol, cause sexual dysfunction, or impede physical and athletic performance by decreasing cardiac output.

B. The elderly hypertensive patient (≥60 years) is generally characterized by increased vascular resistance, decreased plasma renin activity, and greater left ventricular hypertrophy (LVH) than younger patients. They often have coexisting medical problems that must be considered when initiating antihypertensive therapy. When making adjustments in a therapeutic regimen, drug doses should be increased slowly to avoid adverse effects and hypotension. Diuretics are often chosen as initial therapy and have been shown to decrease the incidence of stroke, fatal MI, and overall mortality in this age group (*JAMA* 265:3255, 1991; *Lancet* 1:1349, 1985). Calcium channel antagonists decrease vascular resistance, have no adverse effects on lipid levels, and are also good choices for elderly patients. Even though elderly patients tend to have low plasma renin activity, ACE inhibitors may be effective agents in this population (*N Engl J Med* 328:914, 1993). Long-term studies have documented the safety and efficacy of beta-adrenergic antagonists, especially after acute MI; however, they should be used with caution as they may increase peripheral resistance, decrease cardiac output, and decrease HDL cholesterol (*Ann Intern Med* 110:901, 1989). Agents that produce postural hypotension (i.e., prazosin, guanethidine, guanadrel) should be avoided. Central alpha-adrenergic agents are generally effective in elderly patients but commonly cause sedation. In elderly patients with isolated systolic hypertension, the same approach to initiating therapy should be used, but smaller doses should be given, and adjustments should be made less frequently.

C. Black hypertensive patients generally have a lower plasma renin level, higher plasma volume, and higher vascular resistance than white patients. Thus, black patients respond well to diuretics, alone or in combination with calcium channel antagonists. ACE inhibitors and labetalol (an alpha- and beta-adrenergic antagonist) have also been shown to be effective agents in this population.

D. **The obese hypertensive patient** is characterized by more modest elevations in vascular resistance, higher cardiac output, expanded intravascular volume, and lower plasma renin activity at any given level of arterial pressure. Even though these patients respond to diuretics, weight reduction is the primary goal of therapy and has been shown to bo effective in reducing BP and causing regression of LVH.

E. **The diabetic patient with nephropathy** may have significant proteinuria and renal insufficiency, which can complicate their management (see Chap. 20). Control of BP is the most important intervention shown to slow loss of renal function (*Arch Intern Med* 151:1280, 1991). ACE inhibitors should be used as first-line therapy as they have been shown to decrease proteinuria and slow progressive loss of renal function independent of their antihypertensive effects (*N Engl J Med* 329:1456, 1993). Hyperkalemia is a common side effect in diabetic patients treated with ACE inhibitors, especially in those with moderate to severe impairment of their glomerular filtration rate (GFR). Calcium channel antagonists are also effective in diabetic patients.

F. **The hypertensive patient with LVH** is at increased risk for sudden death, MI, and all-cause mortality (*N Engl J Med* 322:1561, 1990). Although there is no direct evidence, regression of LVH could be expected to reduce the risk for subsequent complications. Sodium restriction, weight loss, and all drugs except direct-acting vasodilators have been shown to decrease left ventricular mass and wall thickness (*N Engl J Med* 14:998, 1992). ACE inhibitors in one study showed the greatest effect on regression (*Am J Hypertension* 4:95, 1992).

G. **The hypertensive patient with coronary artery disease** is at increased risk for unstable angina and MI. Beta-adrenergic antagonists may be used as first-line agents in these patients, as they have been shown to decrease cardiac mortality and subseqent reinfarction in the setting of acute MI, and to decrease progression to MI in those presenting with unstable angina. Beta-adrenergic antagonists also have a role in secondary prevention of cardiac events and increasing long-term survival after MI (*JAMA* 260:2088, 1988). Care should be exercised in those with cardiac conduction system disease. Calcium channel antagonists should be used with caution in the setting of acute MI as studies have shown conflicting results from their use (*Arch Intern Med* 153:345, 1993; *N Engl J Med* 319:385, 1988). Nitrates and ACE inhibitors also may be useful in patients with coronary artery disease (see Chap. 5).

H. **The hypertensive patient with chronic renal insufficiency** has hypertension that is usually in part volume-dependent. Retention of sodium and water exacerbate the existing hypertensive state, and diuretics are important in the management of this problem. With a serum creatinine greater than 2.5 mg/dl, loop diuretics are the most effective class. BP control in this patient group has been shown to decrease progression to end-stage renal disease (*Arch Intern Med* 151:1280, 1991).

I. **The hypertensive patient with congestive heart failure** is at risk for progressive left ventricular dilatation and sudden death. In this population, ACE inhibitors decrease mortality (*N Engl J Med* 327:685, 1992), and in the setting of acute MI, they may decrease the risk of recurrent MI, hospitalization for HF, and mortality in patients with ejection fractions of less than 40% (*N Engl J Med* 327:669, 1992). Nitrates and hydralazine have also been shown to decrease mortality in those with HF irrespective of hypertension, but hydralazine may cause reflex tachycardia and worsening ischemia in patients with unstable coronary syndromes and should be used with caution. Calcium channel antagonists should be used with caution in patients in whom negative inotropic effects will adversely affect their status (see Chap. 6).

III. **Nonpharmacologic therapy.** Life-style modifications should be encouraged in all hypertensive patients whether or not they require medication (*Arch Intern Med* 153:163, 1993). These changes may have beneficial effects on other cardiovascular risk factors. Although smoking has not been shown to cause hypertension, physicians should advise their patients who smoke that cessation is an effective measure in reducing cardiovascular risk and TOD. At minimal cost, nonpharmacologic therapy is effective in lowering BP and may be of benefit in primary prevention of the development of subsequent hypertension.

A. **Weight reduction** should be strongly encouraged in patients who weigh more than 10% over their ideal body weight. Reduction in body weight, especially male pattern obesity involving the trunk and upper body, may obviate the need for drug therapy or decrease the amount of medication required to control hypertension. In addition, improvements in cholesterol profile and regression of LVH have been documented in hypertensive patients managed with weight reduction (*N Engl J Med* 314:334, 1986). Truncal and abdominal obesity have also been associated with increased coronary mortality (*Arteriosclerosis* 10:497, 1990). Weight loss is not recommended for pregnant patients with hypertension (see Special Considerations, sec. **V**).

B. **Alcohol consumption** should be decreased to 1 oz or less/day. In large amounts, ethanol clearly has a direct vasopressor effect. Moderation in drinking should be encouraged in all hypertensive patients.

C. **Regular dynamic exercise** should be advised if the clinical status permits. Repeated periods of exercise, such as walking, running, or swimming, result in a significant reduction in BP independent of weight loss or altered sodium excretion (*Lancet* 2:473, 1986), decreasing all-cause risk and cardiovascular morbidity and mortality (*JAMA* 262:2395, 1989). Systolic BP reduction of up to 10 mm Hg has been documented in patients who exercise regularly. Exercise should be performed at least three times/week for at least 30 minutes, achieving 65–70% of a patient's predicted maximum heart rate. Patients with known or suspected coronary artery disease and those over 40 years of age with multiple coronary risk factors should undergo exercise stress testing before beginning an exercise program.

D. **Dietary modifications.** Sodium restriction is an effective and safe means of modestly lowering BP in hypertensive patients. Sodium restriction may also decrease drug resistance and enhance efficacy. Total sodium chloride intake should be limited to less than 6 g/day. The use of potassium as a therapeutic agent is controversial. Normal serum potassium levels should be maintained in patients with spontaneous or drug-induced hypokalemia. Dietary intake of cholesterol and saturated fat should be reduced to lessen hyperlipidemia and facilitate weight loss.

E. **Primary prevention.** Application of certain life-style modifications to a population as a whole might be expected to decrease the incidence of subsequent development of hypertension. Individuals with high normal BP, a family history of hypertension, high-sodium diet, obesity, and excessive alcohol intake (*Arch Intern Med* 153:160, 1993) are candidates for primary preventive measures.

IV. **Pharmacologic therapy**

A. **Adrenergic antagonists**

1. Beta-adrenergic antagonists (Table 4-3) are effective antihypertensive agents and are part of medical regimens proven to decrease the incidence of stroke, MI, and HF. These agents may offer advantages in selected populations, including patients with increased adrenergic drive (i.e., those with a wide pulse pressure and tachycardia), LVH, and a previous MI (*Am J Cardiol* 66:251, 1990). There are also data to suggest that low doses of beta-adrenergic antagonists can be used in patients with stable HF; however, because of the potential for clinical deterioration, use should be limited to physicians experienced in cardiac care in a closely supervised setting (see Chap. 6).

a. **The mechanism of action** of beta-adrenergic antagonists is competitive inhibition of the effects of catecholamines at beta-adrenergic receptors, which decreases heart rate and cardiac output. These agents also decrease plasma renin and cause a resetting of baroreceptors to accept a lower level of BP. Beta-adrenergic antagonists cause release of vasodilating prostaglandins, decrease plasma volume, and may also have a CNS-mediated antihypertensive effect.

b. Classes of beta-adrenergic antagonists can be subdivided into those that are **cardioselective**, with primarily $beta_1$-blocking effects, and those that are **nonselective**, with $beta_1$- and $beta_2$-blocking effects. At low doses, the cardioselective agents can be given with caution to patients with mild bronchospastic disease, diabetes mellitus, and peripheral vascular disease. At higher doses, these agents lose their $beta_1$ selectivity and may cause unwanted effects in these patients. Beta-adrenergic antagonists can also be categorized according to the presence or absence of **intrinsic sympathomimetic activity (ISA)**. Beta-adrenergic antagonists with ISA cause less bradycardia than those without it.

c. Side effects include high-degree atrioventricular block, HF, Raynaud's phenomenon, and impotence. Lipophilic beta-adrenergic antagonists such as propranolol have a higher incidence of CNS side effects, such as insomnia and depression, than the more hydrophilic agents. Propranolol can also cause nasal congestion. Beta-adrenergic antagonists can cause adverse effects on the lipid profile; increased triglyceride and decreased HDL levels occur mainly with nonselective beta-adrenergic antagonists but generally do not occur when beta-adrenergic antagonists with ISA are used (*J Hypertension* 3:297, 1985). Pindolol, a selective beta-adrenergic antagonist with ISA, may actually increase HDL and nominally increase triglycerides (*Am Heart J* 121:1029, 1991). Since beta-receptor density is increased with chronic antagonism, abrupt withdrawal of these agents can precipitate angina pectoris, increases in BP, and other effects attributable to an increase in adrenergic tone (*Br Heart J* 45:637, 1981).

2. Alpha-adrenergic antagonists. Selective $alpha_1$-adrenergic antagonists (e.g., prazosin, terazosin, doxazosin) have replaced nonselective alpha-adrenergic antagonists, such as phentolamine (see Table 4-3), in the treatment of essential hypertension. Nonselective alpha-adrenergic antagonists are no longer used routinely in the treatment of hypertension (except in special situations, such as the treatment of pheochromocytoma) because of their lack of long-term efficacy and frequent occurrence of side effects. Selective $alpha_1$-adrenergic antagonists may improve lipid profiles by decreasing total cholesterol and triglyceride levels and increasing HDL levels (*Am Heart J* 121:251, 1991). In addition, these agents can improve the negative effects on lipids induced by thiazide diuretics and beta-adrenergic antagonists (*Am Heart J* 121:1307, 1991).

a. The mechanism of action of selective $alpha_1$-adrenergic antagonists is to block postsynaptic alpha-receptors, producing arterial and venous vasodilation.

b. Side effects of these agents include a "first dose effect" resulting from a greater decrease in BP with the first dose than with subsequent doses. Selective $alpha_1$-adrenergic antagonists may cause syncope, orthostatic hypotension, dizziness, headache, and drowsiness. In most cases, side effects are self-limited and do not recur with continued therapy.

3. Labetalol is an agent with both alpha- and beta-adrenergic antagonist properties (see Table 4-3). It is effective in both white and black patients with hypertension. Reflex tachycardia may rarely occur because of its initial vasodilatory effect. Labetalol has negligible effects on lipids.

a. The mechanism of action of labetalol is to antagonize the effects of catecholamines at beta-receptors and peripheral $alpha_1$-receptors. The effects on alpha-receptors decrease with chronic administration and are essentially gone within a few months (*Drugs* 28 (Suppl 2):35, 1984).

b. Side effects of labetalol include hepatocellular damage, paresthesias, postural hypotension, a positive antinuclear antibody test (ANA), a lupus-like syndrome, tremors, and potential hypotension in the setting of halothane anesthesia.

4. Centrally acting adrenergic agents (see Table 4-3) are potent antihypertensive agents. In addition to its oral dosage forms, clonidine is available in a transdermal patch that is applied weekly.

Table 4-3. Commonly used antihypertensive agents by functional class

Drugs by class	Properties	Initial dose	Usual dosage range
Beta-adrenergic antagonists			
Atenolol[a, b]	Selective	50 mg PO qd	25–100 mg
Betaxolol	Selective	10 mg PO qd	5–40 mg
Bisoprolol[a]	Selective	5 mg PO qd	5–20 mg
Metoprolol	Selective	50 mg PO bid	50–200 mg
Metoprolol XL	Selective	50–100 mg PO qd	50–200 mg
Nadolol[a]	Nonselective	40 mg PO qd	20–240 mg
Propranolol[b]	Nonselective	40 mg PO bid	40–240 mg
Propranolol LA	Nonselective	80 mg PO qd	60–240 mg
Timolol[b]	Nonselective	10 mg PO bid	20–40 mg
Acebutolol[a]	ISA, selective	200 mg PO bid, 400 mg PO qd	200–1,200 mg
Carteolol[a]	ISA	2.5 mg PO qd	2.5–10.0 mg
Penbutolol	ISA	20 mg PO qd	20–80 mg
Pindolol[b]	ISA	5 mg PO bid	10–60 mg
Labetalol	Alpha- and beta-antagonist properties	100 mg PO bid	200–1,200 mg
Calcium channel antagonists			
Amlodipine	DHP	5 mg PO qd	2.5–10.0 mg
Diltiazem		30 mg PO qid	90–360 mg
Diltiazem CD		60–120 mg PO bid	120–360 mg
Diltiazem XR		180 mg PO qd	180–360 mg
Felodipine	DHP	5 mg PO qd	5–20 mg
Isradipine	DHP	2.5 mg PO bid	2.5–10.0 mg
Nicardipine[b]	DHP	20 mg PO tid	60–120 mg
Nicardipine SR	DHP	30 mg PO bid	60–120 mg
Nifedipine	DHP	10 mg PO tid	30–120 mg
Nifedipine XL	DHP	30 mg PO qd	30–90 mg
Verapamil[b]		80 mg PO tid	80–480 mg
Verapamil SR		120–240 mg PO qd	120–480 mg
Angiotensin-converting enzyme inhibitors			
Benazepril[a]		10 mg PO bid	10–40 mg
Captopril[a]		25 mg PO bid–tid	12.5–150.0 mg
Enalapril[a]		5 mg PO qd	2.5–40.0 mg
Fosinopril		10 mg PO qd	10–40 mg
Lisinopril[a]		10 mg PO qd	5–40 mg
Quinapril[a]		10 mg PO qd	5–80 mg
Ramipril[a]		2.5 mg PO qd	1.25–20.00 mg

Table 4-3. (continued)

Drugs by class	Properties	Initial dose	Usual dosage range
Diuretics			
Bendroflumethiazide	Thiazide diuretic	5 mg PO qd	2.5–5.0 mg
Benzthiazide	Thiazide diuretic	50 mg PO qd	12.5–50.0 mg
Chlorothiazide	Thiazide diuretic	500 mg PO qd (or IV)	125–500 mg
Chlorthalidone	Thiazide diuretic	25 mg PO qd	12.5–50.0 mg
Hydrochlorothiazide	Thiazide diuretic	25 mg PO qd	12.5–50.0 mg
Hydroflumethiazide	Thiazide diuretic	50 mg PO qd	12.5–50.0 mg
Indapamide	Thiazide diuretic	1.25 mg PO qd	2.5–5.0 mg
Methyclothiazide	Thiazide diuretic	2.5 mg PO qd	2.5–5.0 mg
Metolazone	Thiazide diuretic	2.5 mg PO qd	0.5–5.0 mg
Polythiazide	Thiazide diuretic	2.0 mg Po qd	1–4 mg
Quinethazone	Thiazide diuretic	50 mg PO qd	25–100 mg
Trichlormethiazide	Thiazide diuretic	2.0 mg PO qd	1–4 mg
Bumetanide	Loop diuretic	0.5 mg PO qd (or IV)	0.5–5.0 mg
Ethacrynic acid	Loop diuretic	50 mg PO qd (or IV)	25–100 mg
Furosemide	Loop diuretic	20 mg PO qd (or IV)	20–320 mg
Torsemide	Loop diuretic	5 mg PO qd (or IV)	5–10 mg
Amiloride	Potassium-sparing diuretic	5 mg PO qd	5–10 mg
Spironolactone	Potassium-sparing diuretic	50 mg PO qd	25–100 mg
Triamterene	Potassium-sparing diuretic	100 mg PO qd	50–150 mg
Alpha-adrenergic antagonists			
Doxazosin		1 mg PO qd	1–16 mg
Prazosin		1 mg PO bid–tid	1–20 mg
Terazosin		1 mg PO qd	1–20 mg
Centrally acting adrenergic agents			
Clonidine[b]		0.1 mg PO bid	0.1–1.2 mg
Clonidine patch		TTS 1/weekly (equivalent to 0.1 mg/day release)	0.1–0.3 mg
Guanfacine		1 mg PO qd	1–3 mg
Guanabenz		4 mg PO bid	4–64 mg
Methyldopa[b]		250 mg PO bid	250–2,000 mg
Direct-acting vasodilators			
Hydralazine		10 mg PO qid	50–300 mg
Minoxidil		5 mg PO qd	2.5–80.0 mg
Miscellaneous			
Reserpine[b]		0.1 mg PO qd	0.05–0.25 mg

ISA = intrinsic sympathomimetic activity; DHP = dihydropyridine.
[a] Adjusted in renal failure.
[b] Available in generic form.

    a. The mechanism of action of centrally acting adrenergic agents is to stimulate the presynaptic alpha$_2$-adrenergic receptors in the CNS. This stimulation leads to a decrease in peripheral sympathetic tone, which reduces systemic vascular resistance. It also causes a modest decrease in cardiac output and heart rate. Renal blood flow is not compromised by centrally acting adrenergic agents, but fluid retention may occur.

    b. Side effects may include bradycardia, drowsiness, dry mouth, orthostatic hypotension, galactorrhea, and sexual dysfunction. Transdermal clonidine causes a rash in up to 20% of patients. These agents may precipitate HF in patients with decreased LV function, and abrupt cessation may precipitate an **acute withdrawal syndrome** of elevated BP, tachycardia, and diaphoresis (see Special Considerations, sec. **II**). Methyldopa produces a positive direct Coombs' test in up to 25% of patients, but significant hemolytic anemia is much less common (*N Engl J Med* 313:596, 1985). If a patient develops a hemolytic anemia secondary to methyldopa, the drug should be withdrawn. Severe cases of hemolytic anemia may require treatment with glucocorticoids. Methyldopa causes positive ANA test results in approximately 10% of patients and may cause an inflammatory reaction in the liver that is indistinguishable from viral hepatitis; fatal hepatitis has been reported. Guanabenz and guanfacine both decrease total cholesterol levels, and guanfacine can also decrease serum triglyceride levels (*Clin Pharm Ther* 44:297, 1988; *Am J Cardiol* 57:27E, 1986).

  5. Other adrenergic antagonists. These agents (see Table 4-3) were among the first effective antihypertensive agents available. Currently, these drugs are not regarded as first- or second-line therapy because of their significant side effects.

    a. The mechanism of action is to inhibit the release of norepinephrine from peripheral neurons. **Reserpine,** which is more lipophilic than other drugs in this class, also affects the CNS. It has been postulated that reserpine inhibits norepinephrine release by preventing it from being packaged into storage vesicles within neurons, thereby allowing norepinephrine to be degraded by cytoplasmic monoamine oxidase. **Guanethidine and guanadrel** directly inhibit the release of norepinephrine from peripheral nerve terminals.

    b. Side effects of reserpine include severe depression in approximately 2% of patients. Sedation and nasal stuffiness are also potential side effects. **Guanethidine** can cause severe postural hypotension by effecting a decrease in cardiac output, a decrease in peripheral resistance, and venous pooling in the extremities. Patients on guanethidine with orthostatic hypotension should be cautioned to arise slowly and wear support hose. Guanethidine may also cause ejaculatory failure and diarrhea.

B. Diuretics (see Table 4-3) are effective agents in the therapy of hypertension, and data have accumulated to demonstrate their safety and benefit in reducing the incidence of stroke and HF. Therefore diuretics are considered first-line agents in the treatment of hypertension. However, diuretics have shown a less consistent decrease in the incidence of ischemic cardiac events, and at higher doses (e.g., >50 mg of hydrochlorothiazide may increase ventricular arrhythmias).

  1. The mechanism of action is to initiate a natriuresis and subsequently to decrease intravascular volume. Diuretics may cause an increase in peripheral resistance and a decrease in cardiac output, but with chronic administration, these parameters return to normal. Diuretics may also produce mild vasodilation by inhibiting sodium entry into vascular smooth muscle cells. Indapamide in particular has a pronounced vasodilating effect.

  2. Several **classes of diuretics** are available and are generally categorized by their site of action in the kidney. **Thiazide diuretics** (e.g., hydrochlorothiazide, chlorthalidone) block sodium reabsorption predominantly in the distal convoluted tubule. **Loop diuretics** (e.g., furosemide, bumetanide, ethacrynic acid, and torsemide) block sodium reabsorption in the thick ascending loop of Henle and are the most effective agents in patients with renal insufficiency (creatinine > 2.5 mg/dl). Spironolactone, a **potassium-sparing** agent, acts by competitively inhibiting the actions of aldosterone on the kidney. Triamterene and amiloride are potassium-sparing drugs that act on the distal convoluted tubule to inhibit secretion of potassium ions. Potassium-sparing diuretics are weak agents when used alone and are often combined with a thiazide for added potency.

3. **Side effects** of diuretics vary by class. Thiazide diuretics may produce weakness, muscle cramps, and impotence. Metabolic side effects include hypokalemia, hypomagnesemia, hypercholesterolemia (with an increase in LDL levels), hypercalcemia, hyperglycemia, hyperuremia, hyponatremia, and, rarely, azotemia. Thiazide-induced pancreatitis has also been reported. Metabolic side effects may be limited when thiazides are used in low doses (e.g., hydrochlorothiazide, 12.5–25.0 mg/day). Loop diuretics may cause electrolyte abnormalities such as hypomagnesemia, hypocalcemia, and hypokalemia and can also produce ototoxicity (usually with IV dosing). Spironolactone may produce hyperkalemia; gynecomastia may occur in men, and breast tenderness has been noted in women. Triamterene (usually in combination with hydrochlorothiazide) may cause renal tubular damage and renal calculi. Unlike thiazides, potassium-sparing diuretics do not cause adverse lipid effects. Ethacrynic acid may cause fewer allergic side effects than other loop diuretics or thiazides due to absence of a sulfhydryl moiety.

C. **Calcium channel antagonists** (see Table 4-3) may be used as first-line agents in the treatment of hypertension. They are generally effective in both black and white hypertensive patients, have no significant CNS side effects, and can be used to treat diseases such as angina pectoris that can coexist with hypertension. Calcium channel antagonists have no significant effects on glucose tolerance, electrolytes, or lipid profiles.

1. **The mechanism of action** is to cause arteriolar vasodilation by selectively blocking the slow inward calcium channels in vascular smooth muscle cells. These agents also cause an initial natriuresis, potentially obviating the need for concurrent diuretic therapy.

2. **Classes of calcium channel antagonists** include diphenylalkylamines (verapamil), benzothiazepines (diltiazem), and dihydropyridines (nifedipine). The dihydropyridines include many newer "second-generation" drugs (e.g., felodipine, nicardipine, isradipine, amlodipine), which are more vasoselective and have longer plasma half-lives than nifedipine. Verapamil and diltiazem have negative cardiac inotropic and chronotropic effects. Nifedipine also has a negative inotropic effect, but in clinical use, it is much less pronounced than that of verapamil or diltiazem because of the increase in peripheral vasodilatation and tachycardia the drug causes. Less negative inotropic effects have been observed with the second-generation dihydropyridines. All calcium channel antagonists are metabolized in the liver; thus, in patients with cirrhosis, the dosing interval should be adjusted accordingly. Some of these drugs also inhibit the metabolism of other hepatically cleared medications (e.g., cyclosporine). Verapamil and diltiazem should be used with caution in patients with cardiac conduction abnormalities and can cause HF in patients with decreased LV function.

3. **Side effects** of verapamil include constipation, nausea, headache, and orthostatic hypotension. Diltiazem can cause nausea, headache, and rash. Dihydropyridines may cause lower-extremity edema, flushing, headache, and rash. In general, calcium channel antagonists should not be given to patients following MI because of the increased mortality risk in all but the most stable patients who have no evidence of HF (see Chap. 5).

D. **Angiotensin-converting enzyme inhibitors** (see Table 4-3) can be used as first-line antihypertensive agents and may have beneficial effects in patients with concomitant HF or diabetic nephropathy. ACE inhibitors can reduce hypokalemia, hypercholesterolemia, hyperglycemia, and hyperuricemia caused by diuretic therapy and are particularly effective in states of hypertension associated with a high renin state (e.g., scleroderma renal crisis) (*Med Clin North Am* 71:979, 1987). Fosinopril is unique in that 50% of the drug is eliminated by the liver under normal conditions, but this percentage increases in the presence of renal insufficiency.

1. One **mechanism of action** of ACE inhibitors is to block the production of angiotensin II, a vasoconstrictor, by competitively inhibiting ACE and producing arterial and venous vasodilation and natriuresis. ACE inhibitors also increase levels of vasodilating bradykinins, and some agents (e.g., captopril) directly stimulate production of renal and endothelial vasodilatory prostaglandins. Despite these vasodilating effects, ACE inhibitors do not cause significant reflex tachycardia, perhaps due to a resetting of the baroreceptor reflex (*Br J Clin Pharmacol* 21:338, 1986).

2. **Few metabolic side effects** are associated with use of ACE inhibitors. They do not cause levels of lipids, glucose, or uric acid to increase. ACE inhibitors can cause a dry cough (perhaps because of elevated levels of bradykinins), angioneurotic edema, and hypotension. ACE inhibitors that contain a sulfhydryl group (such as captopril) may cause a glomerulopathy with proteinuria, taste disturbance, and leukopenia. Because ACE inhibitors cause preferential vasodilation of the efferent arteriole in the kidney, worsening of renal function may occur in patients who have decreased renal perfusion or who have preexisting severe renal insufficiency. These drugs are **contraindicated in patients with significant bilateral renal artery stenosis.** ACE inhibitors can cause hyperkalemia and should be used with caution in patients with a decreased GFR, taking potassium supplements, or on potassium-sparing diuretics. ACE inhibitors are contraindicated in pregnancy (see Special Considerations, sec. **V**).

E. **Direct-acting vasodilators.** These potent antihypertensive agents (see Table 4-3) are now reserved for refractory hypertension or specific circumstances, such as the use of hydralazine in pregnancy (see Special Considerations, sec. **V**). Hydralazine in combination with nitrates is useful in treating patients with hypertension and HF (see Chap. 6).

1. **The mechanism of action** of these agents (e.g., minoxidil, hydralazine) is to produce direct arterial vasodilation. Although these drugs lower BP when used alone, their sustained antihypertensive action is limited because of reflex sodium and fluid retention and sympathetic hyperactivity producing tachycardia. Concomitant diuretic or beta-adrenergic antagonist use is often required in addition to a direct-acting vasodilator to ameliorate these unwanted effects. These agents should be used with caution or avoided in patients with ischemic heart disease because of the reflex sympathetic hyperactivity they induce.

2. **Side effects** of hydralazine therapy may include headache, nausea, emesis, tachycardia, and postural hypotension. Asymptomatic patients may have a positive ANA test result, and a hydralazine-induced systemic lupus–like syndrome may develop in approximately 10% of patients. Patients who may be at increased risk for this latter complication include (1) those treated with excessive doses (e.g., >400 mg/day), (2) those with impaired renal or cardiac function, and (3) those with the slow acetylation phenotype. Hydralazine should be discontinued if clinical evidence of a lupus-like syndrome develops and a positive ANA result is present. The syndrome usually resolves with discontinuation of the drug, leaving no adverse long-term effects. Side effects of minoxidil include weight gain, hypertrichosis, ECG abnormalities, and pericardial effusions (*Arch Intern Med* 131:69, 1981).

F. **Parenteral antihypertensive agents.** The use of parenteral medications to immediately reduce BP is indicated in patients with (1) intracranial hemorrhage (but not uncomplicated stroke; see Chap. 25), (2) aortic dissection, (3) rapidly progressive renal failure, (4) eclampsia, or (5) accelerated malignant hypertension. Judicious administration of these agents (Table 4-4) to patients with hypertension complicated by HF or MI may also be appropriate. These drugs are also indicated for individuals with uncomplicated accelerated malignant hypertension who are perioperative or in need of emergency surgery. If possible, **an accurate baseline BP should be established before the initiation of therapy**. In the setting of hypertensive emergency, the patient should be admitted to an ICU for close monitoring, and an intraarterial monitor should be used when available (*Clinical Hypertension* [5th ed.]. Baltimore: Williams & Wilkins, 1990. P. 274). Although parenteral agents may be used in patients with uncomplicated accelerated malignant hypertension who are not perioperative or undergoing emergency surgery, oral agents may also be effective in this group (see sec. **IV.G**); the choice of drug and route of administration must be individualized (*Am Heart J* 111:211, 1986). If parenteral agents are used initially, oral medications should be administered shortly thereafter to facilitate rapid weaning from parenteral therapy.

1. **Sodium nitroprusside,** a direct-acting arterial and venous vasodilator, is the drug of choice for most hypertensive crises (see Table 4-4). It reduces BP rapidly and is easily titratable, and its action is short-lived when discontinued. Patients should be monitored very closely to avoid an exaggerated hypotensive response. Therapy for more than 48–72 hours with a high cumulative dose or renal insufficiency may cause accumulation of thiocyanate, a toxic metabolite. **Thiocyanate toxicity** may cause paresthesias, tinnitus, blurred vision, or delirium. Patients on high doses (>2–3 µg/kg/minute) or patients with renal dysfunction should have serum levels of thiocyanate drawn after 48–72 hours of therapy. In patients with normal renal function or on lower doses, levels may be drawn after 5–7 days. Hepatic dysfunction may result in accumulation of cyanide, which can cause metabolic acidosis, dyspnea, vomiting, dizziness, ataxia, and syncope. Hemodialysis should be considered for thiocyanate poisoning. Nitrites and thiosulfate can be administered intravenously for cyanide poisoning.

2. **Nitroglycerin,** given as a continuous IV infusion (see Table 4-4), may be appropriate in situations in which sodium nitroprusside is relatively contraindicated, such as in patients with severe coronary insufficiency or advanced renal or hepatic disease. It is the preferred agent for patients with moderate hypertension in the setting of acute coronary ischemia or after coronary artery bypass surgery because of its more favorable effects on pulmonary gas exchange and collateral coronary blood flow (*Circulation* 65:1072, 1982). In patients with severely elevated BP, sodium nitroprusside remains the agent of choice. Nitroglycerin reduces preload more than afterload and should be used with caution or avoided in patients with inferior MI with right ventricular infarction who are dependent on preload to maintain cardiac output.

3. **Labetalol** can be administered parenterally (see Table 4-4) in cases of severe hypertension or hypertensive crisis, even in patients in the early phase of an acute MI (*Int J Cardiol* 10:149, 1986). When given intravenously, the beta-adrenergic antagonist effect is greater than the alpha-adrenergic antagonist effect. Symptomatic postural hypotension may occur with IV use, suggesting that patients should be treated in a supine position. The use of labetalol may be of particular benefit in states of adrenergic excess (e.g., pheochromocytoma, monoamine oxidase inhibitor toxicity, clonidine withdrawal, cocaine intoxication, post–coronary bypass grafting). Since the half-life of labetalol is 5–8 hours, intermittent IV bolus dosing may be preferable to IV infusion. IV infusion may be discontinued 5–8 hours before one begins oral labetalol. When the supine diastolic BP begins to rise, oral dosing can be initiated at 200 mg PO, followed in 6–12 hours by 200–400 mg PO, depending on the BP response.

4. **Esmolol** is a parenteral, short-acting cardioselective beta-adrenergic antagonist (see Table 4-4) that can be used in the treatment of hypertensive

Table 4-4. Intravenous antihypertensive drug preparations

Drug	Administration	Onset	Duration of action	Dosage	Adverse effects and comments
Sodium nitro-prusside	IV infusion	Immediate	2–3 min	0.5–10.0 µg/kg/min (initial dose, 0.25 µg/kg/min for eclampsia and renal insufficiency)	Hypotension, nausea, vomiting, apprehension. Risk of thiocyanate and cyanide toxicity is increased in renal and hepatic insufficiency, respectively; levels should be monitored. Must shield from light.
Diazoxide	IV bolus	1–5 min	6–12 hr	50–100 mg q5–10min, up to 600 mg	Hypotension, tachycardia, nausea, vomiting, fluid retention, hyperglycemia. May exacerbate myocardial ischemia, heart failure, or aortic dissection. May require concomitant use of a beta-adrenergic antagonist.
	IV infusion			10–30 mg/min	
Labetalol	IV bolus	5–10 min	3–6 hr	20–80 mg q5–10min, up to 300 mg	Hypotension, heart block, heart failure, bronchospasm, nausea, vomiting, scalp tingling, paradoxic pressor response. May not be effective in patients receiving alpha- or beta-antagonists.
	IV infusion			0.5–2.0 mg/min	
	IV infusion	1–2 min	3–5 min	5–100 µg/min	Headache, nausea, vomiting. Tolerance may develop with prolonged use.

Drug	Route			Dose	Adverse effects
Esmolol	IV bolus IV infusion	1–5 min	10 min	500 µg/kg/min for first 1–4 min 50–300 µg/kg/min	Hypotension, heart block, heart failure, bronchospasm
Phentolamine	IV bolus	1–2 min	3–10 min	5–10 mg q5–15min	Hypotension, tachycardia, headache, angina, paradoxic pressor response
Trimethaphan	IV infusion	1–5 min	10 min	0.5–5.0 mg/min	Hypotension, urinary retention, ileus, respiratory arrest, mydriasis, cycloplegia, dry mouth. More effective if patient's head is elevated.
Hydralazine (for treatment of eclampsia)	IV bolus	10–20 min	3–6 hr	5–10 mg q20min (if no effect after 20 mg, try another agent)	Hypotension, fetal distress, tachycardia, headache, nausea, vomiting, local thrombophlebitis; infusion site should be changed after 12 hr.
Methyldopa (for treatment of eclampsia)	IV bolus	30–60 min	10–16 hr	250–500 mg	Hypotension
Nicardipine	IV infusion	1–5 min	3–6 hr	5 mg/hr, increased by 1.0–2.5 mg/hr q15min, up to 15 mg/hr	Hypotension, headache, tachycardia, nausea, vomiting.
Enalaprilat	IV bolus	5–15 min	1–6 hr	1.25–2.50 mg q6hr	Hypotension

Source: DA Calhoun, S. Oparil. Treatment of hypertensive crisis. *N Engl J Med* 323:1177, 1990.

emergencies. Esmolol is also useful for the treatment of aortic dissection. Beta-adrenergic antagonists may be ineffective when used as monotherapy in the treatment of accelerated malignant hypertension and are frequently combined with other agents (e.g., with sodium nitroprusside in the treatment of aortic dissection).

5. **Nicardipine** is an effective IV preparation (see Table 4-4) approved for use in postoperative hypertension. Side effects include headache, flushing, reflex tachycardia, and venous irritation. If administered peripherally, the IV site should be changed every 12 hours. Fifty percent of the peak effect is seen within the first 30 minutes, but the full peak effect is not achieved until 48 hours of administration.

6. **Enalaprilat** is the active deesterified form of enalapril (see Table 4-4) that results from hepatic conversion after an oral dose. Enalaprilat (as well as other ACE inhibitors) has been used effectively in cases of severe and malignant hypertension. However, variable and unpredictable results have also been reported. ACE inhibition can cause rapid BP reduction in hypertensive patients with high renin states such as with renovascular hypertension, concomitant use of vasodilators, and scleroderma renal crisis but should be used cautiously to avoid precipitating hypotension. Therapy can be changed to an oral preparation when IV therapy is no longer necessary.

7. **Diazoxide, hydralazine, and trimethaphan camsylate** are now rarely used in hypertensive crises and offer little or no advantage to the agents discussed above.

G. **Oral loading of antihypertensive agents.** Oral agents have been used successfully in patients with hypertensive crisis when urgent but not immediate reduction of BP is indicated.

1. **Sublingual nifedipine** has an onset of action within 30 minutes and has been used safely in patients with hypertensive urgencies. Reports of clinically significant myocardial ischemic events with the use of sublingual nifedipine suggest that it be used with caution in the setting of known coronary disease or ECG evidence of LVH (*Ann Intern Med* 107:185, 1987). A 10-mg capsule can be pierced or chewed and swallowed, which allows a similar onset of action as the sublingual route. The duration of action for the sublingually administered drug is 4–5 hours. During this time, therapy with oral agents can be administered. Side effects include facial flushing and postural hypotension.

2. **Oral clonidine** loading is achieved by using an initial dose of 0.2 mg PO followed by 0.1 mg PO q1h to a total dose of 0.7 mg or a reduction in diastolic pressure of 20 mm Hg or more. BP should be checked at 15-minute intervals over the first hour, 30-minute intervals over the second hour, and then hourly. After 6 hours, a diuretic may be added and an 8-hour clonidine dosing interval begun. Sedative side effects may be significant and should be anticipated.

V. **Initial drug therapy.** Currently, diuretics, beta-adrenergic antagonists, calcium channel antagonists, ACE inhibitors, and alpha-adrenergic antagonists are regarded as first-line agents. Data from long-term trials have shown decreased cardiovascular and cerebrovascular morbidity and mortality with the use of thiazide diuretics and beta-adrenergic antagonists; thus, these may be used as first-line agents unless a contraindication to their use exists (hyperlipidemia, glucose intolerance, or an elevated uric acid) or characteristics of a patient's profile (concomitant disease, age, race) mandate institution of a different agent. Calcium channel antagonists and ACE inhibitors have been shown to decrease BP to degrees similar to those observed with diuretics and beta-adrenergic antagonists (*N Engl J Med* 328:914, 1993) and are also good initial agents because of their low side effect profile. The majority of patients with stages 1 or 2 hypertension can attain adequate BP control with single-drug therapy. Initial drug choice may be affected by coexistent factors such as age, race, angina, congestive heart failure, renal insufficiency, LVH, obesity, hyperlipidemia, gout, and bronchospasm. Cost and drug interactions should also be considered. BP response is usually consistent within a given class of agents; therefore, if a drug fails to control BP, it is unlikely that another agent from the same class will be effective. At times, however, a change within drug class may be useful in reducing adverse effects. The lowest possible effective dosage should be used to control BP, adjusted every 1–3 months as needed.

VI. **Additional therapy.** More severe cases may require changing to a different class of drugs or the stepwise addition of drugs from different classes. When a second drug is needed, it can generally be chosen from among the other first-line agents. A diuretic should be added first, as this may enhance effectiveness of the first drug, yielding more than a simple additive effect.

VII. **Adjustments of a therapeutic regimen.** When considering a modification of therapy because of inadequate response to the current regimen, the physician should investigate other possible contributing factors. Poor patient compliance, use of antagonistic drugs (i.e., sympathomimetics, antidepressants, steroids, NSAIDs, cyclosporine, caffeine, thyroid hormones, cocaine, erythropoietin), or increased alcohol intake should be considered before antihypertensive drug therapy is modified. Unacceptable side effects from a particular agent may contribute to poor patient compliance. Excessive fluid retention should be evaluated and treated. Continued patient education is imperative. Secondary causes of hypertension need to be considered when a previously effective regimen becomes inadequate and other factors noted above are not present.

Special Considerations

I. **Hypertension associated with withdrawal syndromes.** Hypertension may be part of several important syndromes of withdrawal from drugs including alcohol, cocaine, and opioid analgesics. Hypertension and rebound increases in BP may also be seen in patients who abruptly discontinue antihypertensive therapy.

A. **Alcohol** withdrawal is associated with significant morbidity and mortality. For those patients who are not candidates for benzodiazepine therapy, clonidine (0.2 mg PO tid the first day, bid the second day, then tapered) or atenolol (100 mg PO qd for a heart rate >80; 50 mg PO qd for heart rate between 50–79; hold dose if heart rate <50) have been used effectively to treat the hypertension and sympathetic overactivity seen with alcohol withdrawal (*Arch Intern Med* 149:1089, 1989) (see Chap. 25).

B. **Cocaine** and other sympathomimetic drugs (e.g., amphetamines, phencyclidine hydrochloride) can produce hypertension in the setting of acute intoxication as well as when the agents are abruptly discontinued after chronic use. Hypertension is often complicated by other end-organ insults such as ischemic heart disease, cerebrovascular accident, and seizures. Labetalol and phentolamine are effective in acute management, and sodium nitroprusside can be used as an alternative (see Table 4-3).

C. **Narcotic analgesic** withdrawal may cause significant morbidity but rarely produces mortality. Symptoms of nausea, tremulousness, tachycardia, and hypertension can be effectively managed with clonidine beginning at a dose of 0.2 mg PO bid and increasing up to 17–25 µg/kg/day in two divided doses. Clonidine should be withheld if the diastolic BP is less than 60 mm Hg or if sedation occurs (*JAMA* 243:343, 1980).

D. **Monoamine oxidase (MAO) inhibitors** used in association with certain drug or food ingestion can produce a catecholamine excess state and accelerated hypertension. Interactions are common with tricyclic antidepressants, meperidine, methyldopa, levodopa, sympathomimetic agents, and antihistamines. Common tyramine-containing foods that have been causally associated with this syndrome include certain cheeses, red wine, beer, chocolate, chicken liver, processed meat, herring, broad beans, canned figs, and yeast. Nitroprusside, labetalol, and phentolamine have all been used effectively in the treatment of accelerated hypertension associated with MAO inhibitor use (see Table 4-4 and Chap. 1).

II. **Withdrawal syndrome associated with discontinuation of antihypertensive therapy.** Most patients experience a gradual return of hypertension following discontinuation of therapy. When substituting therapy in patients with moderate to severe hypertension, it is reasonable to increase doses of the new medication in small increments while tapering the previous medication to avoid excessive BP fluctuations. On occasion, an **acute withdrawal syndrome (AWS)** will develop, usually within the first 24–72 hours. In a few patients, BP may rise to levels much greater than baseline values. The most severe complications of AWS include encephalopathy, stroke, MI, and sudden death. The AWS is most commonly associated with centrally acting adrenergic agents (particularly clonidine) and beta-adrenergic antagonists but has been reported with other agents as well, including diuretics. Rarely should BP medications be withdrawn, but when discontinuing therapy, these drugs should be tapered over several days to weeks unless other medications are used to substitute in the interim. Discontinuation of antihypertensive medications should be done with caution in patients with preexisting cerebrovascular or cardiac disease. Management of AWS by reinstitution of the previously administered drug is generally effective. Sodium nitroprusside (see Table 4-3) is the treatment of choice when parenteral administration of an antihypertensive agent is required or when the identity of the previously administered agent is unknown (*Am Heart J* 102:415, 1981). **In the AWS caused by clonidine, beta-adrenergic antagonists should not be used** because unopposed alpha-adrenergic activity will be augmented and may exacerbate hypertension. Labetalol (see Table 4-3), however, may be useful in this situation.

III. **Hypertensive crisis** is defined as a substantial increase in BP, usually defined as a diastolic BP greater than 120–130 mm Hg (*N Engl J Med* 323:1177, 1990). This relatively rare event occurs in approximately 1% of hypertensive patients. Hypertensive crisis usually develops in patients with a previous history of elevated BP but may develop in patients previously normotensive. The severity of a hypertensive crisis correlates not only with the absolute level of BP elevation but also with the rapidity of development because autoregulatory mechanisms have not had sufficient time to adapt. Crises are further classified as either **urgencies** (i.e., elevated BP with associated symptoms but no acute or ongoing TOD) or **emergencies** (i.e., elevated BP with acute or ongoing TOD). Common manifestations of acute or ongoing TOD are classified as (1) retinal (hemorrhages, exudates, or papilledema), (2) cardiac (pulmonary edema, myocardial ischemia, or infarction), (3) CNS (mental status changes, seizures, coma), and (4) renal (hematuria, azotemia). When TOD is present, BP control with a parenteral agent with rapid onset should be accomplished as soon as possible (within 1 hour) to reduce permanent organ dysfunction and death. The presence of acute or ongoing TOD is more important than the absolute level of BP. **The goal of BP reduction needs to be individualized,** but it is reasonable to attempt a 25% reduction of mean arterial pressure or to reduce the diastolic pressure to 100–110 mm Hg over a period of minutes to hours. A precipitous fall in BP may occur in patients who are elderly, volume depleted, or receiving other antihypertensive agents, and caution should be used to avoid cerebral hypoperfusion. Hypertensive urgencies include those conditions with no ongoing TOD. In this situation, BP control can be accomplished more slowly. The initial goal of therapy should be to achieve a diastolic BP of 100–110 mm Hg; excessive or rapid decreases in BP should be avoided to minimize the risk of cerebral hypoperfusion or coronary insufficiency. Normal BP can be gradually attained over several days as tolerated by the individual patient (*N Engl J Med* 323:1177, 1990).

IV. **Aortic dissection.** Acute, proximal aortic dissection (type A) is a surgical emergency, whereas uncomplicated, distal dissection (type B) can be treated successfully with medical therapy alone. All patients, including those treated surgically, require both acute and chronic antihypertensive therapy to provide initial stabilization and prevent complications (e.g., aortic rupture, continued dissection).

A. **Sodium nitroprusside** is considered the initial drug of choice because of the predictability of response and absence of tachyphylaxis. The dose should be titrated to achieve a systolic blood pressure of 100–120 mm Hg or the lowest possible BP that permits adequate organ perfusion. Nitroprusside alone causes an increase in left ventricular dv/dt and subsequent arterial shearing forces, which contribute to ongoing intimal dissection. Thus, **when using sodium nitroprusside, adequate simultaneous beta-adrenergic antagonist therapy is essential, regardless of whether systolic hypertension is present.** Traditionally, propranolol has been recommended. Esmolol, a cardioselective IV beta-adrenergic antagonist with a very short duration of action, may be preferable to propranolol, especially in the presence of chronic obstructive pulmonary disease, asthma, or HF, by allowing closer titration of $beta_1$-adrenergic antagonist effect (i.e., target heart rate of 60–80 beats/minute) while minimizing unwanted concomitant $beta_2$-adrenergic antagonism.

B. **IV labetalol** has been used successfully as a single agent in the treatment of acute aortic dissection (*JAMA* 258:78, 1987). Labetalol produces a dose-related decrease in BP and lowers dv/dt. It has the advantage of allowing for oral administration after the acute stage of dissection has been successfully managed.

C. **Trimethaphan camsylate,** a ganglionic blocking agent, can be used as a single IV agent if sodium nitroprusside or beta-adrenergic antagonists cannot be tolerated. Unlike sodium nitroprusside, trimethaphan reduces left ventricular dv/dt. Because trimethaphan is associated with rapid tachyphylaxis and sympathoplegia (e.g., orthostatic hypotension, blurred vision, and urinary retention), other drugs are preferable.

D. **Hypotension** in the setting of aortic dissection may indicate that external rupture has occurred (rupture into the intraperitoneal or intrapleural spaces, or into the pericardium with tamponade). A proximal dissection may occlude the brachial arteries and prevent accurate determination of BP in one or both arms. Medical therapy of chronic stable aortic dissection should seek to maintain systolic BP at or below 130–140 mm Hg if tolerated. Antihypertensive agents with negative inotropic properties, including calcium channel antagonists, beta-adrenergic antagonists, methyldopa, clonidine, and reserpine, are preferred. Diuretics are an effective adjunctive therapy in the acute and chronic setting if fluid overload is present.

V. **Pregnancy and hypertension.** Hypertension in the setting of pregnancy is a special situation because of the potential for maternal and fetal morbidity and mortality associated with elevated blood pressure and the clinical syndromes of preeclampsia and eclampsia. The possibility of teratogenic or other adverse effects of antihypertensive medications on fetal development should also be considered. The American College of Obstetrics and Gynecology has proposed the following classification of hypertension during pregnancy: (1) preeclampsia-eclampsia, (2) chronic hypertension of any cause, (3) chronic hypertension with superimposed preeclampsia-eclampsia, and (4) transient or late hypertension (*Obstetric Gynecologic Terminology.* Philadelphia: Davis, 1972).

A. **Preeclampsia-eclampsia.** Preeclampsia is a condition defined by pregnancy, hypertension, proteinuria, generalized edema, and occasionally coagulation and liver function abnormalities. Eclampsia encompasses those physical signs, but in addition patients have generalized seizures.

B. **Chronic hypertension** is defined by a BP of >140/90 mm Hg before the twentieth week of pregnancy.

C. **Transient hypertension** is a condition in which increases in BP occur without associated proteinuria or CNS manifestations and in which BP returns to normal within ten days of delivery.

D. **Therapy.** Treatment for hypertension in pregnancy should begin if the diastolic BP is greater than 100 mm Hg (*Am J Obstet Gynecol* 163:1689, 1990). Nonpharmacologic therapy such as weight reduction and vigorous exercise is not recommended during pregnancy. Alcohol and tobacco use should be strongly discouraged. Pharmacologic intervention with methyldopa is recommended as first-line therapy because of its proven safety. Hydralazine is also safe and may be used as an alternative agent; it can also be used parenterally. Other antihypertensives have theoretical disadvantages, but none except the ACE inhibitors has been proven to increase perinatal morbidity or mortality (*Am J Med* 96:451, 1994). A theoretical disadvantage of using nonselective beta-adrenergic antagonists is that uterine contractility may occur with beta$_2$-receptor blockade; however, there are several studies showing the safety of using labetalol (*N Engl J Med* 323:1181, 1990). Rare side effects in the fetus and neonate from propranolol include hyperbilirubinemia, hypoglycemia, growth retardation, bradycardia, and delayed respiration (*Cardiol Clin* 5:651, 1987). Diuretics are generally not recommended during pregnancy because of the potential decrease in uterine blood flow, and there are reports of neonatal thrombocytopenia, jaundice, hyponatremia, and bradycardia with thiazides (*Principles of Medical Therapy in Pregnancy*. New York: Plenum, 1985. P. 646). Calcium channel antagonists can cause a decrease in uterine contractility, and nifedipine in particular is not recommended because, when combined with beta-adrenergic antagonists, there is a high rate of cesarean section, premature delivery, and small-for-date infants (*Br J Obstet Gynecol* 94:1136, 1987). Diazoxide may inhibit uterine contractions, and trimethaphan can cause meconium ileus. If a patient is suspected of having preeclampsia or ecclampsia, urgent referral to an obstetrician specializing in high-risk pregnancy is recommended.

Ischemic Heart Disease

Kenneth J. Winters and
Paul R. Eisenberg

General Considerations

Ischemic heart disease secondary to atherosclerosis of the coronary arteries remains the leading cause of morbidity and mortality in North America. **Risk factors** for the development of coronary artery atherosclerosis include a family history of premature coronary artery disease, cigarette smoking, hypercholesterolemia, hypertension, and diabetes mellitus. Obesity, physical inactivity, and stress may play a lesser role. Coronary artery disease (CAD) may be clinically silent but more frequently is associated with symptoms (e.g., myocardial infarction [MI], angina pectoris, sudden death) (*Am J Cardiol* 37:269, 1976).

Angina Pectoris

I. **Diagnosis.** Angina pectoris is the chest discomfort associated with myocardial ischemia that occurs when myocardial oxygen demand exceeds supply.
  A. **Clinical history.** Angina is typically described as a retrosternal pain, discomfort, heaviness, or pressure radiating to the neck, jaw, shoulders, or arms, and lasting two to five minutes. It is usually precipitated by exertion and relieved with rest. Associated symptoms include dyspnea, diaphoresis, nausea, vomiting, and occasionally palpitations or lightheadedness. Factors that increase myocardial oxygen demand or that decrease oxygen supply may precipitate or aggravate angina and should be excluded by history and appropriate laboratory evaluation. In men and older women, a history of typical angina, especially in the presence of other cardiac risk factors, is good evidence of ischemic heart disease (90% probability). In such patients, the role of invasive and noninvasive cardiac tests is to assess the severity of CAD, guide therapy, and estimate the risk of MI. In patients with chest pain not likely to be of cardiac origin and without significant cardiac risk factors, the prevalence of ischemic heart disease is low (25%), and further cardiac evaluation may be necessary to determine whether CAD is present. However, results of noninvasive tests in this group of patients are often falsely positive (*N Engl J Med* 300:1350, 1979). Noninvasive tests are particularly useful in patients with an intermediate probability of disease.
  B. **Noninvasive diagnosis of angina.** When the clinical history suggests the presence of angina, the diagnosis should be confirmed by invasive or noninvasive tests, and the need for further medical or invasive intervention should be assessed.
    1. **The resting ECG** may demonstrate the following: (1) significant Q waves (>40 msec) consistent with a prior MI, (2) resting ST segment depression or elevation, and/or (3) T-wave inversion suggestive of myocardial ischemia. Frequently, the resting ECG is normal, even in the presence of significant CAD. However, documentation of ST segment or T-wave abnormalities **during an episode of chest discomfort** can be invaluable for confirming the diagnosis of CAD and may limit the need for further noninvasive testing.
    2. **Exercise electrocardiography** (stress testing) is useful in establishing the diagnosis of CAD and allows risk stratification of patients with angina.

Exercise sufficient to increase the heart rate to 85% of the predicted maximum for age is necessary for optimal sensitivity. Patients who have a markedly positive test result should undergo cardiac catheterization to define the need for coronary revascularization. **A markedly positive test** indicative of severe CAD is defined as the presence of any of the following:

a. ST segment depression early after the start of exercise.

b. >2 mm of new ST segment depression in multiple leads.

c. New ST segment elevation.

d. Decreased systolic BP with exercise.

e. Inability to exercise for more than 2 minutes.

f. Development of heart failure with exercise.

g. Prolonged interval after exercise before ischemic ST segment changes return to baseline.

In contrast, in patients with known CAD, the ability to complete 7 minutes of a standard Bruce exercise protocol without development of significant ST segment depression is associated with an excellent 4-year survival rate (*J Am Coll Cardiol* 3:772, 1984).

3. **Exercise thallium imaging** and **radionuclide ventriculography** improve the sensitivity and specificity of exercise testing and are particularly useful in patients taking digoxin or those with preexisting ECG abnormalities, such as left ventricular hypertrophy, ST-T changes, left bundle branch block, or preexcitation (*Am J Cardiol* 45:674, 1980). Addition of an imaging modality to exercise stress testing has been reported to increase the sensitivity for detection of significant CAD from 70% to 80%, and the specificity from 80% to 90% (*Circulation* 83:363, 1991). The choice of the radionuclide procedure depends on the experience of individual centers.

4. **Exercise two-dimensional echocardiography** performed in experienced centers is useful in the diagnosis of CAD, with sensitivity and specificity similar to that of exercise radionuclide ventriculography (*J Am Coll Cardiol* 2:1085, 1983).

5. **Pharmacologic stress testing.** Dipyridamole thallium stress testing is useful in the evaluation of patients with suspected CAD who are unable to exercise (*N Engl J Med* 312:389, 1985). Two-dimensional echocardiography has also been used in conjunction with administration of IV dipyridamole, adenosine, or infusions of high doses of dobutamine to induce detectable cardiac ischemia in such patients.

6. **Resting two-dimensional echocardiography or radionuclide ventriculography** is warranted in patients with suspected CAD in whom the clinical assessment suggests left ventricular dysfunction. Patients with left ventricular ejection fractions of <50% and significant CAD have a better prognosis if treated with coronary artery bypass surgery compared with medical therapy (*N Engl J Med* 312:1665, 1985). Therefore, coronary angiography should be considered in patients with left ventricular dysfunction and suspected CAD to determine the extent of CAD and the patient's suitability for coronary artery bypass grafting (CABG).

C. **Coronary angiography** with left ventriculography is the definitive test for the diagnosis of CAD and can be performed with an incidence of serious morbidity and mortality of only 0.1–0.2%. Significant coronary obstruction is usually defined as greater than 70% narrowing of the luminal diameter. Coronary angiography can be combined with pharmacologic or exercise stress testing to assess the physiologic significance of observed coronary stenoses. Angiography can also exclude the presence of CAD in patients with equivocal symptoms and false-positive stress test results. Coronary angiography is generally indicated in high-risk patients, such as those with refractory unstable angina and those with spontaneous or exercise-induced ischemia after MI. In addition, this technique provides prognostic information about the number of significantly obstructed coronary arteries and the degree of left ventricular dysfunction.

II. **Therapy**

A. **General principles** in the management of angina pectoris include modification of

Table 5-1. Doses and action of commonly used nitrate preparations

Preparation	Dose	Onset	Duration
Sublingual nitroglycerin	0.3–0.6 mg	2–5 min	10–30 min
Aerosol nitroglycerin	0.4 mg	2–5 min	10–30 min
Sublingual/chewable isosorbide dinitrate	2.5–10.0 mg	10–30 min	1–2 hr
Oral isosorbide dinitrate	5–40 mg	30–60 min	4–6 hr
Oral isosorbide mononitrate	10–20 mg	30–60 min	6–8 hr
Oral sustained-release nitroglycerin	2.5–9.0 mg	30–60 min	2–8 hr
2% nitroglycerin ointment	0.5–2.0 in.	20–60 min	3–8 hr
Transdermal nitroglycerin patches	5–15 mg	>60 min	12–14 hr*

* Recommended maximum duration of application.

reversible cardiac risk factors. Cessation of cigarette smoking should be emphasized. Elevated serum cholesterol levels should be treated (see Chap. 22). Studies suggest that regression of atherosclerotic plaques is possible, but serum cholesterol must be decreased to 150–180 mg/dl (*JAMA* 257:3233, 1987). Specific treatment of angina is directed toward improving myocardial oxygen supply, reducing myocardial oxygen demand, and treating precipitating factors or concurrent disorders (e.g., anemia) that may exacerbate ischemia.

B. **Drug therapy.** The selection of an effective therapeutic regimen depends on the acuity and severity of symptoms, the presence of associated disease (e.g., pulmonary or renal disease), the patient's age and activity level, and the underlying pathophysiologic mechanism presumed to be responsible for the ischemia (e.g., arterial spasm, fixed stenosis). Because myocardial ischemia is often multifactorial, a combination of agents with different mechanisms of action is frequently more effective than monotherapy.

1. **Nitrates** are important first-line agents for the treatment of angina (*N Engl J Med* 316:1635, 1987). The primary antianginal effect is via an increase in venous capacitance, reducing ventricular volume and pressure, and improving subendocardial perfusion. Coronary vasodilation, improvement in collateral flow, and afterload reduction augment this primary effect.

   a. **Sublingual nitroglycerin** is available as 0.3-, 0.4-, and 0.6-mg tablets or as a metered-dose spray (0.4 mg). Usually, 0.4-mg tablets are prescribed, but occasionally lower doses are required. Peak pharmacologic action occurs within 2 minutes and continues for 15–30 minutes. Nitroglycerin can be repeated at 5-minute intervals if symptoms persist. Patients should be informed of possible side effects (e.g., headache, hypotension), the importance of taking the drug while seated, the need for airtight storage of the drug in the original amber bottle, and replacement of medication every 6 months. The patient should be advised to take nitroglycerin at the first indication of angina and prophylactically before situations that are known to precipitate angina. Medical attention should be sought promptly if angina occurs at rest or with increasing frequency, or if an anginal episode fails to respond by the third nitroglycerin tablet.

   b. **Long-acting nitrates** are indicated for long-term management of angina pectoris. High doses of oral nitrates must be used because extensive hepatic degradation occurs after intestinal absorption (first-pass effect). Several preparations of long-acting nitrates are available (Table 5-1). Although the optimal dosing interval for long-acting oral nitrates has not been established, administration of isosorbide dinitrate three times a day

Table 5-2. Doses and actions of selected beta-adrenergic antagonists

Agent	Oral dose	Half-life (hr)	Actions
Beta$_1$-selective			
Atenolol[a,b]	50–100 mg qd	6–9 h	Beta$_1$
Metoprolol[a,b]	50–100 mg bid	3–4 h	Beta$_1$
Acebutolol	200–600 mg bid	3–4 h	Beta$_1$, ISA
Nonselective			
Propranolol[a,b]	20–80 mg qid	4–6 h	Beta$_1$, beta$_2$
Propranolol-LA[a]	80–160 mg qd	10 h	Beta$_1$, beta$_2$
Nadolol[a]	40–160 mg qd	20–24 h	Beta$_1$, beta$_2$
Timolol[b]	10–20 mg bid	3–4 h	Beta$_1$, beta$_2$
Pindolol	5–20 mg tid	3–4 h	Beta$_1$, beta$_2$, ISA
Labetalol	100–600 mg bid	6–8 h	Alpha, beta$_1$, beta$_2$

ISA = intrinsic sympathomimetic activity; LA = long-acting.
[a] FDA-approved for treatment of angina.
[b] FDA-approved for treatment of MI.

with meals is convenient and allows for a 12-hour nitrate-free period to minimize development of tolerance.

c. **Topical 2% nitroglycerin ointment** is applied to the skin as a 1- to 2-inch measured dose by use of an occlusive dressing every 4–6 hours. The onset of action is approximately 30 minutes. Nitroglycerin ointment is an acceptable long-acting nitrate for patients who are unable to take oral medications. Because absorption of topical nitrates may be unpredictable, the IV route of administration should always be used when predictable nitrate levels and rapid control of dosage rate are required.

d. **Sustained-release transdermal nitroglycerin preparations** are limited by the failure of low-dose patches (2.5–5.0 mg/24 hours) to achieve therapeutic drug concentrations and by development of nitrate tolerance with the use of higher-dose patches. Patients should be instructed to remove the patch for 12 hours each day to minimize the development of nitrate tolerance.

e. **Nitrate tolerance,** resulting in reduced therapeutic response, may occur with all nitrate preparations including oral nitrates at fixed tid and qid intervals as well as transdermal preparations left in place for 24 hours. The use of a nitrate-free interval of at least 10–12 hours can enhance treatment efficacy (*N Engl J Med* 317:805, 1987; *J Am Coll Cardiol* 16:941, 1990). When nitrates cannot be discontinued, even for a short time, higher doses may be required to overcome tolerance.

2. **Beta-adrenergic antagonists** are also important in the management of stable angina. They reduce the frequency of episodes of angina and raise the exercise threshold for angina (*Am J Cardiol* 77:119, 1984).

a. **Selection.** Beta-adrenergic antagonists are generally classified with respect to their selectivity for cardiac beta$_1$-receptors compared with beta$_2$-receptors. There are no clear differences among the various beta-adrenergic antagonists in their antianginal efficacy (Table 5-2). However, beta$_1$-selective drugs (metoprolol and atenolol) at low doses are less likely to cause bronchospasm or to exacerbate peripheral vascular disease. At higher doses beta$_1$ selectivity is lost. Agents with intrinsic sympathomimetic activity (ISA), such as pindolol and acebutolol, may dilate peripheral vessels and have less effect on resting heart rate. Lipid-insoluble beta-adrenergic antagonists (atenolol and nadolol) have a longer duration of action and penetrate the CNS to a lesser extent, which may limit side effects. Labetalol has both beta- and alpha-adrenergic antagonist effects. Because of the additional vasodilation induced by alpha-adrenergic blockade, this agent is useful in hypertensive patients (see Chap. 4).

b. Dosage should be carefully titrated on an individual basis to achieve a resting heart rate of 50–60 beats/minute and an exercise heart rate that does not exceed 90–100 beats/minute. Asymptomatic resting bradycardia does not require a reduction in dosage. Resting heart rate cannot be used to evaluate therapy in patients taking agents with ISA. Increasing the dose of a beta-adrenergic antagonist may improve antianginal effects in some patients but may also increase the incidence of side effects. The patient should be observed for signs of bronchospasm or congestive heart failure (CHF) when beta-adrenergic antagonist therapy is initiated and when the dose is being adjusted.

c. Contraindications to the use of beta-adrenergic antagonists include clinical evidence of CHF, a history of bronchospasm, atrioventricular (AV) nodal block, severe peripheral vascular disease, and marked resting bradycardia. In patients with depressed left ventricular function, beta-adrenergic antagonist therapy can be attempted but should be initiated at a low dose, with gradual increases as tolerated. The use of beta-adrenergic antagonists in patients with depressed left ventricular ejection fractions can result in CHF; therefore, initiation of therapy should be supervised by clinicians experienced in using these agents.

d. Side effects of beta-adrenergic antagonists include bronchospasm, nausea, diarrhea, postural hypotension, claudication, impotence, fatigue, headache, nightmares, depression, hallucinations, deterioration in intellectual capacity, salt retention, and potential masking of hypoglycemia in insulin-dependent diabetics. Infrequently, abrupt withdrawal of these agents may precipitate unstable angina, arrhythmias, MI, and even sudden death; therefore, when beta-adrenergic antagonists must be stopped abruptly, patients at high risk for these events should be monitored for symptoms of sympathetic overactivity (see Chap. 4).

3. Calcium channel antagonists inhibit the uptake of calcium ions by myocytes, specialized cardiac conducting tissues, and vascular smooth muscle cells. The antianginal effect of these agents is due to direct coronary vasodilation and reduced peripheral vascular resistance. All calcium channel antagonists have potential negative inotropic effects, but in the absence of significant heart failure, cardiac performance is usually preserved by a reduction in afterload. Calcium channel antagonists are indicated in the management of both stable and unstable angina and are the agents of choice in patients unable to tolerate beta-adrenergic antagonists or nitrates (Table 5-3). Because these agents are potent coronary vasodilators, they are particularly effective in patients with coronary vasospasm (Prinzmetal's angina). Calcium channel antagonists can be used as initial single-agent therapy in many patients or in combination with nitrates or beta-adrenergic antagonists in those with angina refractory to single-drug therapy (*Mayo Clin Proc* 60:539, 1985; *J Am Coll Cardiol* 1:492, 1983).

a. Nifedipine (*Am J Cardiol* 71:645, 1981) is a dihydropyridine with more pronounced arteriolar vasodilating properties than verapamil or diltiazem. Although nifedipine has negative inotropic effects in vitro, the decrease in peripheral vascular resistance induced by pharmacologic doses usually results in a slight increase in cardiac output and heart rate. Bradycardia and AV block are not a common problem. Common side effects include dizziness, headache, hypotension, flushing, nausea, reflex tachycardia, and peripheral edema, all of which occur less frequently with the sustained-release preparation. Nifedipine is contraindicated in patients with hypotension and should not be used in those with unstable angina unless it is administered with a beta-adrenergic antagonist to minimize reflex increases in heart rate. In patients with decreased left ventricular ejection fraction, worsening heart failure may occur (*Circulation* 82:1954, 1990).

Table 5-3. Doses and actions of selected calcium channel antagonists

Agent	Oral dose	Half-life (hr)	Myocardial depression	Bradycardia, heart block
First generation				
Verapamil*	80–120 mg tid–qid	3–6	+ +	+/+ +
Verapamil-SR	120–240 mg bid	5–12	+ +	+/+ +
Diltiazem*	30–90 mg qid	3–4	+	+/+ +
Diltiazem-SR	60–180 mg bid	5–7	+	+/+ +
Diltiazem-CD	180–360 mg qd	5–8	+	+/+ +
Nifedipine*	10–30 mg tid–qid	2–3	0/+	0
Nifedipine-XL*	30–120 mg qd	—	0/+	0
Second generation				
Amlodipine*	2.5–10 mg qd	35	0/+	0
Felodipine	5–10 mg bid	10	0/+	0
Isradipine	2.5–10 mg bid	8	0/+	0
Nicardipine*	20–40 mg tid	2–4	0/+	0
Nicardipine-SR	30–60 mg bid	8	0/+	0

SR = sustained release; CD/XL = extended release; 0 = minimal effect; + = modest effect; + + = significant effect.
* FDA-approved for treatment of angina.

    b. Second-generation calcium channel antagonists, including amlodipine, felodipine, isradipine, and nicardipine, are members of the dihydropyridine class (see Table 5-3). Like nifedipine, these agents are potent coronary and peripheral vasodilators. Their side effects are similar to those of nifedipine. Bradycardia and AV block have not been reported. Uncontrolled studies have suggested that these newer agents have less negative inotropic effects in patients with mild-to-moderate depression of cardiac function. However, none of these agents is recommended as vasodilator therapy in the presence of CHF, and only amlodipine (*Am Heart J* 118:1137, 1989) and nicardipine (*Am Heart J* 116:254, 1988) have been approved by the U.S. Food and Drug Administration for use in patients with angina.

    c. Verapamil (*Circulation* 65:17, 1982), a papaverine derivative, has arteriolar vasodilating properties and slows AV nodal conduction. It has a greater negative inotropic effect than nifedipine or diltiazem, limiting its use in patients with significant left ventricular dysfunction. It is a valuable agent in the treatment of supraventricular tachyarrhythmias but may produce bradycardia and advanced AV block. Verapamil is contraindicated in patients with sick sinus syndrome, AV nodal disease, and CHF. Verapamil should be used cautiously with beta-adrenergic antagonists, which increases the potential for bradycardia or AV block. Verapamil increases serum digoxin levels and should be avoided in patients with digitalis toxicity. The most common side effect of verapamil is constipation (30%).

    d. Diltiazem (*Am J Cardiol* 54:738, 1984), a benzothiazine, is an arteriolar vasodilator that also prolongs AV nodal conduction and slows the sinus node rate. Concomitant use of beta-adrenergic antagonists may potentiate AV nodal conduction disturbances and sinoatrial nodal depression; therefore, combination therapy is rarely indicated. Despite data suggesting that the negative inotropic effects of diltiazem are modest, its use has been shown to increase mortality in patients with left ventricular dysfunction and recent MI (*N Engl J Med* 319:385, 1988).

  4. Aspirin prolongs survival in patients with unstable angina (*N Engl J Med*

309:396, 1983; *N Engl J Med* 313:1369, 1985) and is effective in the primary prevention of cardiovascular events (*N Engl J Med* 318:262, 1988). The beneficial effects of aspirin appear to be greater in men than in women in most studies. Inhibition of platelet function is presumed to be the mechanism of aspirin's effect. Most clinicians recommend daily use of aspirin in low doses (80–325 mg qd) for patients with known CAD or multiple risk factors.

C. **Invasive therapy.** Percutaneous transluminal coronary angioplasty (PTCA) and coronary artery bypass grafting (CABG) are invasive procedures designed to improve regional myocardial blood flow by dilating or bypassing stenotic coronary vessels.

1. **CABG** is beneficial in patients with angina refractory to medical management, even if only single-vessel disease is present. In addition, it appears to prolong life compared with medical therapy in patients with left main CAD and in those with triple-vessel disease, particularly in the presence of left ventricular dysfunction or easily inducible ischemia (*Circulation* 68:939, 1983).

   a. **Results.** Improvement of ischemic symptoms is achieved in 80–90% of patients, and 50–75% are asymptomatic for variable periods after bypass surgery (*Circulation* 65:225, 1982). Angina recurs at a rate of 10–20% each year in patients who initially benefit from CABG and correlates with graft occlusion or progression of native CAD. The use of internal mammary artery grafts is associated with 90% graft patency at 10 years, compared with 40% for saphenous vein grafts (*J Thorac Cardiovasc Surg* 89:248, 1985).

   b. **Medical versus surgical therapy.** The risks of CABG include a 1–3% operative mortality and a 5–10% incidence of perioperative MI. Approximately 15–20% of grafts close in the first year; over the next 5 years, 2% close per year, and subsequently 4% occlude each year. Previous data suggest that three-vessel disease can be successfully managed with medical therapy, with a 2–3% annual mortality. Because there are constant improvements in both the medical and surgical management of CAD, it is difficult to unequivocally recommend one therapy over the other except in patients with left main disease, in whom the mortality associated with medical treatment approaches 30% at 18 months (*Prog Cardiovasc Dis* 22:73, 1979). The best therapy for a given patient will depend on considerations of his or her life-style, severity of ischemia, evidence of silent ischemia, extent of the coronary artery lesions, and the amount of myocardium subtended by critical stenoses. After 10 years of follow-up in patients presenting with stable angina without left main CAD, survival was similar in patients randomly assigned to CABG and those assigned to medical therapy. However, a survival advantage was evident in surgically treated patients with three-vessel disease and left ventricular ejection fractions of 35–50% (*Circulation* 82:1629, 1990). In patients with more severe angina or easily induced ischemia, CABG may be indicated even in the absence of three-vessel disease (*J Am Coll Cardiol* 17:543, 1991).

2. **PTCA** is accomplished by positioning a balloon catheter across a stenotic coronary artery segment and inflating the balloon to increase the luminal diameter via atherosclerotic plaque rupture. Successful dilatation is initially achieved in more than 90% of patients. Approximately 30–50% of dilated vessels will develop restenosis within 3–6 months (*Am J Cardiol* 69:194, 1992), but repeat angioplasty of these lesions is highly successful (*N Engl J Med* 318:265, 1988). Patients undergoing PTCA should, in general, be candidates for CABG, since surgery may be necessary if PTCA fails or if complications arise. Patients undergoing PTCA should receive aspirin before the procedure, as well as heparin during and following the procedure, to minimize the risk of thrombosis. Calcium channel antagonists may decrease the risk of vasospasm. Potential complications of PTCA include coronary artery dissection and occlusion, as well as bleeding related to anticoagulation. In trials of elective PTCA, the risk of death was less than 1%, the

incidence of nonfatal MI was less than 5%, and emergency CABG was required in 3–5% of patients (*Circulation* 86:100, 1992).

3. **Newer nonsurgical techniques** for coronary revascularization include directional atherectomy, rotational atherectomy, excimer laser angioplasty, transluminal extraction catheters, and intracoronary stents. The role of these technologies in the treatment of CAD is being investigated. To date, none has eliminated the problem of restenosis, but they have expanded the range of coronary lesions that can be approached without surgery (*N Engl J Med* 329:221, 1993).

Unstable Angina

I. **Definition and diagnosis.** Unstable angina is a clinical syndrome characterized by angina of new onset, angina at rest or with minimal exertion, or a crescendo pattern of angina with episodes of increasing frequency, severity, or duration. Although the pathophysiology is heterogeneous, in most patients the transition from stable to unstable angina appears to be due to rupture or fissuring of atherosclerotic plaques, resulting in thrombus formation, increased platelet reactivity, and increased coronary vasomotor tone (*Circulation* 77:1213, 1988). In a small percentage of patients, unstable ischemic symptoms are precipitated by severe anemia, hypertension, or heart failure.

II. **Risk of MI.** The development of unstable symptoms carries a 10–20% risk of progression to acute MI. Patients who are thought to be at a higher risk for progression to acute infarction include those with new onset of pain at rest or a sudden change in anginal pattern, particularly when associated with labile ST-T changes on the ECG. Recurrent or persistent pain after initiation of treatment also increases the likelihood of subsequent infarction. Clinical evidence of left ventricular dysfunction, pulmonary edema, transient mitral regurgitation, or hypotension during episodes of ischemia identifies patients with extensive areas of myocardium at risk. The development of new ST segment depression or elevation or deep T-wave inversions in the anterior precordial leads in the absence of MI are findings that suggest severe underlying CAD (*Am Heart J* 103:730, 1982).

III. **Management** includes hospitalization, bed rest, sedation, and correction of precipitating conditions such as hypertension, anemia, and hypoxemia. The goals of treatment are to aggressively relieve ischemic symptoms with antianginal drugs, using IV preparations when necessary, and to inhibit thrombosis in high-risk patients.

A. **Treatment of ischemia.** In general, IV nitroglycerin is preferred to oral or cutaneous preparations because of the ability to rapidly achieve predictable blood levels of drug. Patients should receive a beta-adrenergic antagonist when not contraindicated or a calcium channel antagonist, preferably verapamil or diltiazem. Nifedipine generally should not be used without concomitant beta-adrenergic antagonist therapy in patients with unstable angina because of the potential for reflex tachycardia (*Circulation* 73:331, 1986; *J Am Coll Cardiol* 5:717, 1985). Due to similar pharmacologic effects, other dihydropyridines should also be avoided until evidence of their safety is available. The choice of a specific agent should be dictated by the underlying pathophysiology and associated hemodynamics.

B. **Narcotic analgesics** such as morphine sulfate are reserved for treatment of patients with pain that is refractory to aggressive medical therapy.

C. **Anticoagulants.** IV heparin decreases the incidence of MI in patients with unstable angina (*N Engl J Med* 319:1105, 1988; *Lancet* 1:1225, 1981).

D. **Aspirin** has been shown to reduce both mortality and the occurrence of nonfatal infarction in patients with unstable angina when administered either in low (325 mg qd) or high (325 mg q6h) dosages (*N Engl J Med* 309:396, 1983; *N Engl J Med* 313:1369, 1985). The combination of heparin and aspirin has not been shown to provide a greater reduction in the risk of MI but has been associated with increased bleeding complications (*N Engl J Med* 319:1105, 1988). To avoid reactivation of unstable angina, aspirin should be started before the discontinuation of heparin. Patients in whom PTCA is contemplated should be treated with aspirin, but this may be associated with more bleeding complications in patients referred for CABG.

   E. Intraaortic balloon counterpulsation is indicated in patients with ischemic symptoms that are refractory to medical therapy. Because this procedure is associated with a 10–15% risk of significant vascular complications, it should only be used to stabilize the patient's condition before CABG or PTCA.

IV. Prognosis. Most patients (75–85%) with unstable angina respond to aggressive medical management. After stabilization, these patients should undergo elective coronary angiography to evaluate the severity of CAD and their suitability for PTCA or CABG. Those who continue to experience angina at rest despite adequate medical therapy, including IV heparin and nitroglycerin, are candidates for emergency coronary angiography and subsequent PTCA or CABG. Although invasive evaluation is often indicated because of the risk of progression to MI, selected patients can be evaluated with noninvasive tests to assess their prognosis (see sec. I).

Coronary Vasospasm and Variant Angina

I. Definition. Prinzmetal's variant angina is characterized by episodes of chest pain occurring at rest associated with transient ST segment elevations on the ECG due to coronary artery vasospasm, without evolution to MI. Symptomatic coronary vasospasm typically occurs in association with a fixed atherosclerotic lesion but may occasionally be seen in normal arteries, in which case it is associated with a better prognosis (*Circulation* 65:825, 1982). Episodes of vasospasm may be accompanied by arrhythmia, such as ventricular tachyarrhythmia or heart block (*Am J Cardiol* 50:203, 1982) and may rarely progress to MI or sudden death. Sustained coronary vasospasm is also thought to play a role in MI associated with cocaine or amphetamine abuse.

II. Diagnosis. Transient ST segment elevation during chest pain is indicative of coronary vasospasm. Ambulatory ECG monitoring is often useful in detecting such episodes. Coronary angiography is indicated to evaluate the extent of underlying CAD, and the diagnosis can be confirmed by demonstrating coronary artery narrowing during a spontaneous or provoked episode of characteristic chest pain. IV ergonovine maleate (*Circulation* 69:690, 1984) or intracoronary acetylcholine (*J Am Coll Cardiol* 12:883, 1988) induces focal coronary vasospasm during coronary angiography in most patients with Prinzmetal's angina. Provocative testing carries a small risk of refractory spasm and MI.

III. Management. Acute episodes of coronary vasospasm generally respond to **sublingual nitroglycerin. Nifedipine** (10 mg), which is chewed and swallowed for more rapid onset of action, can be used for refractory spasm in the absence of hypotension. Long-acting nitrates or calcium channel antagonists have been shown to reduce the frequency of chest pain when used for long-term treatment of Prinzmetal's angina (*Am Heart J* 103:44, 1982; *J Am Coll Cardiol* 21:1365, 1993). Cigarette smoking should be discontinued because it appears to predispose the patient to coronary vasospasm. CABG or PTCA is of benefit only in the presence of significant fixed obstructions.

Silent Ischemia

I. Definition. Silent ischemia is defined as objective evidence of myocardial ischemia in the absence of angina or anginal equivalents. Silent ischemia may be documented by asymptomatic ST depression on ambulatory electrocardiography or during exercise stress testing. It occurs in 2.5% of middle-aged men without signs or symptoms of CAD and in approximately 40% of patients with angina (*Ann Intern Med* 109:312, 1988). The clinical significance and prognostic implications of silent ischemia are not well established, and there are no convincing data showing that reduction of silent ischemia is beneficial. However, in patients with unstable angina or those recovering from an MI, the presence of silent ischemia on ambulatory ECG monitoring identifies a population at high risk for subsequent cardiac events (*N Engl J Med* 314:1214, 1986; *JAMA* 259:1030, 1988). In these subgroups of patients, attempts to identify and treat silent ischemia may be warranted. Twenty-four-hour continuous ambulatory ECG monitoring and exercise stress testing, often combined with thallium perfusion imaging or echocardiography, may be used to diagnose silent ischemia.

II. **Therapy** for silent ischemia is similar to that for ischemia associated with symptoms. In a study of patients with stable angina and a high frequency of silent ischemia, propranolol was more effective than diltiazem or nifedipine (*Circulation* 82:1962, 1990). PTCA or CABG may also be effective. Therapeutic efficacy of various interventions can be assessed by ambulatory ECG monitoring.

Myocardial Infarction

I. **Definition.** MI constitutes a medical emergency requiring prompt hospitalization and careful medical management in an intensive care setting. Occlusive or near-occlusive thrombus overlying or adjacent to a ruptured atherosclerotic plaque is the cause of MI in the majority of patients. Rarely, infarction occurs with normal or minimally diseased coronary arteries as a result of coronary spasm or embolism. Mortality from MI is greatest within the first 2 hours after the onset of symptoms and can be significantly reduced by rapid transport to the hospital, institution of prompt pharmacologic or mechanical reperfusion, and treatment of ventricular arrhythmias.

II. **Diagnosis.** Definitive diagnosis of MI requires the presence of at least two of the following criteria: (1) a history of prolonged chest discomfort, (2) ECG changes consistent with ischemia or necrosis, or (3) elevated cardiac enzymes.

A. **History.** Chest pain associated with MI resembles that of angina pectoris but is typically more severe, longer in duration, and not relieved by rest or nitroglycerin. Accompanying symptoms include dyspnea, nausea, vomiting, fatigue, diaphoresis, and palpitations. MI may occur without chest pain, especially in postoperative patients, the elderly, and patients with diabetes mellitus or hypertension. In these patients, the symptoms may be isolated dyspnea, exacerbation of CHF, or acute confusion. Other causes of chest pain should also be considered (Table 5-4).

B. **Physical examination.** The initial examination should be directed at identifying hemodynamic instability and pulmonary congestion. Hypotension, cool extremities, diaphoresis, and confusion are often indicative of cardiogenic shock. Elevation in the jugular venous pulse indicates volume overload or right ventricular failure. Cardiac auscultation typically demonstrates an S4, reflecting decreased left ventricular compliance, and less commonly an S3, suggesting heart failure. Murmurs of various causes may be apparent, but new systolic murmurs are of particular importance, suggesting the presence of ischemic mitral regurgitation or a ventricular septal defect.

C. **Clinical stratification** of patients with acute MI into high- and low-risk subgroups is based on the initial physical examination. Those without evidence of pulmonary congestion or shock (Killip class I) have an excellent prognosis (mortality <5%) and generally require less aggressive management. The prognosis with only mild pulmonary congestion or an isolated S3 gallop (Killip class II) is also reasonably good. Patients with pulmonary edema (Killip class III) often have extensive left ventricular dysfunction or acute mitral regurgitation and require aggressive management. Patients with hypotension and evidence of shock

Table 5-4. Selected differential diagnosis of myocardial infarction (MI)

Diagnosis	ECG findings mimicking MI	Diagnostic evaluation
Pericarditis ·	ST elevation	Echocardiography
Myocarditis	ST elevation Q-waves	Echocardiography
Acute aortic dissection	ST elevation or depression or nonspecific	Chest CT or MRI, transesophageal echocardiography, aortography
Pneumothorax	New poor R-wave progression V1–V6 or acute QRS axis shift	Chest x-ray
Pulmonary embolism	Inferior ST elevation or ST shifts V1–V3	Ventilation-perfusion scan
Acute cholecystitis	Inferior ST elevation	Abdominal ultrasound

(Killip class IV) have a mortality approaching 80% unless the cause of shock is treatable. Cardiogenic shock due to right ventricular infarction occurs in patients with inferior wall infarction and is often clinically recognized by the presence of elevated jugular venous pressures without evidence of pulmonary congestion.

- D. **Electrocardiography.** Serial ECGs are essential; an ECG should be obtained on admission and daily during hospitalization in the cardiac care unit. ECGs should be repeated for evaluation of recurrent chest pain or arrhythmias. Although some patients initially have a normal ECG, the majority of patients with MI do not.
    1. **ST-T changes.** Convex ST segment elevation with either peaked upright or inverted T-waves is usually indicative of acute myocardial injury. ST segment depression, particularly when it persists, may also be indicative of a non–Q-wave MI.
    2. **Q-waves.** The development of new Q-waves (>40 msec) is generally considered diagnostic of MI but may occur in patients with prolonged ischemia and occasionally in patients with myocarditis.
    3. **MI may occur in the absence of Q-waves (non–Q-wave MI).** Although the extent of infarction in patients with non–Q-wave MI is often less than in patients with Q-wave infarction, they are at high risk of recurrent MI and have a similar long-term prognosis.
    4. **ECG changes that mimic MI.** ST segment elevation and evolution of Q-waves may on rare occasions result from preexcitation syndromes, pericarditis, cardiomyopathy, chronic obstructive pulmonary disease, and pulmonary embolism, among others (see Table 5-4).
- E. **Cardiac enzymes.** The plasma levels of aspartate aminotransferase (AST or SGOT), creatine kinase (CK), and lactate dehydrogenase (LDH) progressively increase as myocardial necrosis evolves. Although these enzymes are found in many organs, the MB isoenzyme of creatine kinase (MB-CK) and the LDH_1 isoenzyme are relatively specific for myocardial necrosis.
    1. **CK** (*N Engl J Med* 313:1050, 1985) exists in three plasma isoenzymes: MM, MB, and BB, found predominantly in muscle, heart, and brain, respectively.
        a. **Increased plasma MB-CK** activity has a greater than 95% sensitivity and specificity for myocardial injury when measured within 24–36 hours of the onset of chest pain. With MI, plasma MB-CK activity increases within 4–6 hours of chest pain, reaches a peak in 12–20 hours, and returns to baseline in 36–48 hours, depending on the extent of myocardial necrosis. Increased plasma concentrations of MB-CK are almost always indicative of myocardial cell death, although not always due to MI (Table 5-5).

Table 5-5. Selected causes of increased plasma MB-CK activity other than myocardial infarction (MI)

I. Myocardial injury other than MI
   a. Myocarditis
   b. Pericarditis (? due to associated myocarditis)
   c. Myocardial contusion/blunt chest trauma
   d. Defibrillation (>300 joules × 2)
   e. Cardiac surgery
II. Noncardiac muscle injury
   a. Low percentage MB-CK relative to total CK
      1. Extensive muscle trauma
      2. Rhabdomyolysis
   b. High percentage MB-CK to total CK
      1. Polymyositis
      2. Muscular dystrophy
      3. Myopathies
      4. Vigorous exercise in trained athletes (e.g., marathon runners)
      5. Patients with chronic renal insufficiency (? only with myopathy)
III. Nonmuscle sources of MB-CK or BB-CK
   a. Intracerebral hemorrhage (BB-CK)
   b. Extensive intracerebral infarction (BB-CK)
   c. Prostatic carcinoma (BB-CK)
   d. Bronchogenic carcinoma (BB-CK, MB-CK rare)
   e. Bowel infarction (BB-CK)
IV. Delayed clearance of CK
   a. Hypothyroidism (? only with myopathy)

   b. Increased MB-CK not due to MI. Infrequently, elevations in MB-CK occur as a result of release from noncardiac sources, delayed clearance of MB-CK, or cross-reactivity of some assays for MB-CK with BB-CK. A cause of increased MB-CK other than MI should be considered when elevations persist without change over serial samples, in contrast to the typical rise and fall that occur with MI.

2. **LDH,** which exists as five isoenzymes, is present in most body tissues. With acute MI, elevations in LDH levels become detectable by 12 hours after chest pain, reach a peak in 24–48 hours, and remain elevated for 10–14 days after infarction. An $LDH_1 : LDH_2$ ratio greater than 1.0 is consistent with MI. The diagnostic sensitivity and specificity of LDH isoenzymes are reduced in the presence of hemolysis, megaloblastic anemia, renal insufficiency, and various solid tumors that produce elevation of LDH_1. Measurement of plasma LDH isoenzymes is a valuable adjunct to CK determinations in patients presenting 24 hours or more after onset of symptoms.

3. **Use of cardiac enzymes.** In patients in whom MI is suspected, determinations of plasma CK and MB-CK should be performed on admission and two to three times thereafter (q12h). Plasma LDH should be measured in patients presenting 24 hours or more after the onset of symptoms, especially if the MB-CK isoenzyme levels are not diagnostic. If the LDH is elevated, LDH isoenzymes should be assayed. The assay should be repeated if the $LDH_1 : LDH_2$ ratio is only slightly less than 1.0 on admission (*Ann Intern Med* 102:221, 1986).

4. **Newer cardiac enzyme assays.** Despite the established utility of MB-CK in the diagnosis of MI, there are groups of patients in whom elevated MB-CK may be derived from skeletal muscle (see Table 5-5). Preliminary investigations of **cardiac troponin-I** demonstrate higher specificity and comparable sensitivity for cardiac injury compared with MB-CK (*Circulation* 88:101, 1993; *N Engl J Med* 330:707, 1994). Studies in which myoglobin or isoforms of MB-CK and MM-CK have been assayed suggest a potential for early detection of MI and coronary reperfusion (*Circulation* 82:759, 1990; *Circulation* 74:105, 1986).

F. Noninvasive cardiac imaging

1. **Technetium-99m-pyrophosphate scintigraphy** is generally used for the diagnosis of MI in patients hospitalized late after the onset of symptoms in whom cardiac enzymes are no longer elevated or are unreliable. Imaging is optimal 2–7 days after MI. Focal increases in technetium pyrophosphate uptake are generally diagnostic of infarction. This technique is highly sensitive (>90%) in detecting large transmural infarcts but is less reliable in the detection of small non–Q-wave MI (*Semin Nucl Med* 10:168, 1980).

2. **Radionuclide ventriculography (RVG)** allows for characterization of right and left ventricular ejection fraction and assessment of regional wall motion abnormalities. Because RVG provides less information regarding the cardiac structures, echocardiography is generally preferred in the initial evaluation of patients with MI. However, RVG is useful to assess regional wall motion or quantify ventricular function when echocardiographic studies are inadequate.

3. **Two-dimensional echocardiography** images the cardiac structures, pericardium, and ascending aorta, allowing identification of regional wall motion abnormalities, valvular abnormalities, and global left and right ventricular function. Doppler and color flow Doppler techniques characterize blood flow within the heart. In patients with MI, Doppler imaging is indicated in the evaluation of new or changed murmurs to define the presence or absence of valvular regurgitation or ventricular septal rupture (*Br Heart J* 47:461, 1982; *Mayo Clin Proc* 62:59, 1987). In patients in whom traditional echocardiographic and Doppler studies are inadequate, **transesophageal echocardiography** may be indicated.

III. Management. Mortality in patients with MI results from both cardiac arrhythmias and myocardial pump failure. Prompt detection and treatment of potentially lethal ventricular arrhythmias decreases in-hospital mortality. Most of the in-hospital mortality associated with MI is in patients with extensive left ventricular dysfunction and shock. Because myocardial necrosis evolves over several hours, early restoration of perfusion by thrombolysis or PTCA reduces infarct size and preserves left ventricular function. Large-scale clinical trials have shown that administration of fibrinolytic agents reduces mortality, particularly when therapy is started within 4 hours of the onset of symptoms (*Lancet* 1:398, 1986).

A. Goals of immediate management are to relieve ischemic pain, provide supplemental oxygen, and recognize and treat potentially life-threatening complications of infarction such as hypotension, pulmonary edema, and ventricular arrhythmias.

1. **Analgesia.** Adequate control of pain reduces oxygen consumption and decreases levels of circulating catecholamines.

a. **Sublingual nitroglycerin** (0.4 mg) should be administered to most patients with ischemic chest pain in the absence of hypotension and can be repeated every 5 minutes. If symptoms persist after three doses, morphine should be given. Hypotension may occur in patients with volume depletion or inferior MI complicated by right ventricular infarction and should be treated by elevation of the lower extremities and IV saline infusion. A vagotonic response occurs on rare occasions, particularly with IV nitroglycerin, and can be treated with atropine (see sec. **IV.A.3.a**).

b. **Morphine sulfate** is the analgesic of choice for the treatment of the pain of infarction. Morphine also induces modest venodilation, which decreases preload, has a modest arterial vasodilating effect, and has a vagotonic effect that can decrease heart rate. Morphine is given intravenously in doses of 2–4 mg and can be repeated every 5–10 minutes until pain is controlled or side effects develop. Nausea, vomiting, dizziness, hypotension, and respiratory depression are all potential adverse effects of morphine sulfate. Nausea and vomiting can be avoided by concomitant use of an antiemetic agent. Hypotension is prevented by adequate volume expansion, and the vagotonic effects of morphine can be treated with atropine sulfate in doses of 0.3–0.5 mg IV. **Naloxone hydrochloride,** administered in increments of 0.4 mg IV to a total dose of 1.2 mg, reverses the effects of morphine and can be used for treatment of respiratory depression. Due to the short half-life of naloxone (30–90 minutes), multiple doses may be required.

  c. **Meperidine hydrochloride**, given in doses of 10–20 mg IV, is an alternative to morphine.

  2. **Oxygen therapy**, 2–4 liters/minute via nasal cannula, is indicated in most patients with acute MI because mild hypoxemia is common. Patients in respiratory distress should be given oxygen by face mask, preferably at concentrations of 60–100%, until blood gas measurements are available. Arterial blood gas measurements should only be obtained on admission if the patient is in respiratory distress and is not a candidate for thrombolytic therapy. Subsequently, oxygen therapy should be adjusted to maintain a hemoglobin oxygen saturation greater than 90%. Increasing oxygen tension to supranormal levels is not indicated because it may produce an increase in blood pressure and systemic vascular resistance. **Intubation and mechanical ventilation** are indicated if persistent hypoxemia is documented (arterial O_2 saturation <90%) or there is ventilatory failure (PCO_2 >45–50 mm Hg) despite administration of 100% oxygen by mask. Prompt institution of mechanical ventilation when necessary decreases the work of breathing and reduces myocardial oxygen demand.

B. Reperfusion

  1. **Thrombolytic therapy.** Approximately 90% of patients with acute MI and ST segment elevation have complete thrombotic occlusion of the infarct-related coronary artery (*N Engl J Med* 303:897, 1980). Administration of fibrinolytic agents will induce clot lysis and restore blood flow in 60–90% of patients, depending on the agent used. In the absence of contraindications, thrombolytic therapy is the treatment of choice for restoring perfusion in patients with acute MI. Thrombolytic therapy offers the advantage of widespread availability and rapid administration.

    a. **Patient selection.** Thrombolytic therapy is indicated in patients with ischemic symptoms persisting more than 30 minutes that are associated with new ST segment elevation of at least 0.1 mV (>1 mm) in at least two leads in the inferior, anterior, or lateral location. Thrombolytic therapy is also indicated in patients with ST segment depression in the anterior leads due to posterior wall infarction or in those with prolonged chest pain and new left bundle branch block. Optimal myocardial salvage generally requires treatment to be initiated within 4–6 hours of the onset of chest pain (*Lancet* 1:398, 1986; *Circulation* 88:296, 1993). Thrombolytic therapy should also be considered in patients presenting up to 12 hours after MI if there is persistent chest pain and ST elevation. **Contraindications to thrombolysis** may be either **relative** or **absolute** (Table 5-6). The age of the patient should not be an absolute contraindication to thrombolysis because the prognosis after MI is worse in the elderly. Hypertension that responds rapidly to analgesia and nitrates should not preclude administration of thrombolytic therapy. In patients with relative contraindications, the decision to initiate thrombolytic therapy should be individualized based on an assessment of the risk of severe bleeding compared with the risk of complications of MI. Patients with contraindications for thrombolysis may be candidates for primary PTCA.

    b. **Specific agents.** Fibrinolytic agents can be classified based on the extent to which they have specificity for activating plasminogen bound to fibrin compared with circulating plasminogen. Agents such as streptokinase (SK) or anisoylated streptokinase (anistreplase, APSAC) induce a generalized fibrinolytic state characterized by extensive fibrinogen degradation (*N Engl J Med* 317:850, 1987). SK and APSAC both have the potential to cause allergic reactions. SK administration is associated with a higher incidence of hypotension that responds to volume expansion. SK and APSAC also induce the formation of neutralizing antibodies, which may

Table 5-6. Contraindications to thrombolytic therapy

Absolute contraindications	Relative contraindications
Active bleeding	Systolic BP ≥180 mm Hg
Defective hemostasis	Diastolic BP ≥110 mm Hg
Recent major trauma	Bacterial endocarditis
Surgical procedure ≤10 days	Hemorrhagic diabetic retinopathy
Invasive procedure ≤10 days	History of intraocular bleeding
Neurosurgical procedure ≤2 months	Stroke/TIA ≥12 months
GI/GU bleeding ≤10 days	Brief CPR ≤10 minutes
Prolonged CPR ≥10 minutes	Chronic warfarin therapy
Stroke/TIA <12 months	Severe renal or liver disease
History of cerebral tumor, aneurysm, or AVM	Menstrual bleeding
Acute pericarditis	
Suspected aortic dissection	
Active peptic ulcer disease	
Active inflammatory bowel disease	
Active cavitary lung disease	
Pregnancy	

TIA = transient ischemic attack; AVM = arteriovenous malformation.

limit the response to future administration of these agents. In comparison, recombinant tissue plasminogen activator (rt-PA) is more clot selective, does not cause allergic reactions or hypotension, and appears to result in a higher rate of early coronary reperfusion compared with SK (*Circulation* 76:142, 1987). It may also result in a modest mortality advantage over SK (*N Engl J Med* 329:673, 1993). IV doses of the currently available agents are listed in Table 5-7.

c. **Adjuvant therapy**

(1) **Adjunctive IV heparin** therapy has been shown to increase the rate of late coronary artery patency when administered in conjunction with rt-PA (*N Engl J Med* 323:1433, 1990). Heparin should be given as an IV bolus of 5,000 units, followed by a 1,200-unit/hour continuous infusion titrated to maintain the activated partial thromboplastin time (aPTT) at twice the control value (see Chap. 17). Heparin should be started with initiation of thrombolytic therapy, particularly with rt-PA, and should be continued for 3–5 days. Subcutaneous heparin, 12,500 units q12h, may also be effective in decreasing mortality in patients treated with SK or rt-PA. Newer anticoagulants such as hirudin are currently under investigation.

(2) **Aspirin** has been shown to decrease mortality in patients treated with SK (*Lancet* 2:349, 1988). Chewable aspirin, 160 mg, should be given when fibrinolytic therapy is initiated with any agent, and oral aspirin should be continued at a dose of either 160 or 325 mg qd. The optimal dose of aspirin has not been established.

(3) **Beta-adrenergic antagonists** have been shown to decrease the incidence of nonfatal reinfarction and recurrent ischemic events in patients treated with t-PA for acute MI (*N Engl J Med* 320:618, 1989). Although definitive criteria have not been established, their use should be considered in patients without contraindications (see sec. **III.C.1**).

(4) **Lidocaine should only be used to treat potentially life-threatening ventricular arrhythmias** (see sec. **IV.A.1.a** and Chap. 7).

Table 5-7. Doses of fibrinolytic agents for myocardial infarction

Agents without fibrin specificity

Streptokinase

1.5 million IU IV over 60 minutes (more rapid infusion can cause hypotension)

Urokinase*

3 million IU IV over 60 minutes

Anistreplase (acylated streptokinase-plasmin complex)

  30 IU IV bolus over 2 minutes

Agents with fibrin specificity

Alteplase (recombinant tissue plasminogen activator [rt-PA])

  100 mg IV over 3 hours, usually with an initial 6-mg bolus followed by continuous infusion for a total of 60 mg the first hour, and then 40 mg over the next 2 hours

  Although not approved by the FDA, a front-loaded regimen in which the dose of rt-PA is given more rapidly is preferred by many and is administered as a 15-mg IV bolus followed by 0.75 mg/kg (up to 50 mg) IV infusion over 30 minutes, then 0.5 mg/kg (up to 35 mg) IV infusion over 60 minutes (*J Am Coll Cardiol* 14:1566, 1989)

* Not approved for IV administration by the FDA.

---

  d. **Monitoring thrombolytic therapy** with coagulation assays is of value in documenting the effects of fibrinolytic agents on hemostasis and is necessary to titrate the dose of heparin (*Prog Cardiovasc Dis* 34:279, 1992). With SK, there is extensive fibrinogen degradation resulting in increased concentrations of fibrin degradation products (FDPs) and increases in the thrombin time and aPTT. Fibrinogen degradation is modest in most patients treated with rt-PA, and the aPTT is often not prolonged in the absence of heparin. Routine assessment of fibrinogen levels is not mandatory. Although fibrinogen levels less than 100 mg/dl are associated with an increased risk of bleeding, they are not predictive in an individual patient. The aPTT should be monitored in all patients to allow titration of heparin and should be maintained at 2.0–2.5 times control (see Chap. 17). In patients in whom there is systemic lytic activity, the aPTT may be markedly prolonged for 6–8 hours after administration of the fibrinolytic agents because of the effects of fibrinogen degradation and FDPs.

  e. **Complications.** Bleeding is the most common adverse effect of thrombolytic therapy. Hematomas develop at sites of vascular access in as many as 45% of patients, and transfusions are required in 10–20% of patients. Therefore venipuncture should be limited and arterial puncture avoided in patients to be treated with thrombolytic therapy. In patients who hemorrhage, fresh-frozen plasma can be given to reverse the lytic state. Cryoprecipitate can also be used to replete fibrinogen and factor VIII levels. Because platelet dysfunction often accompanies the lytic state, platelet transfusions may be useful in patients with markedly prolonged bleeding times (*Ann Intern Med* 12:1010, 1989). The incidence of intracranial hemorrhage is approximately 0.5% in patients treated with SK and 0.7% in those treated with rt-PA. SK can occasionally cause fever, chills, and anaphylaxis. No serious allergic reactions have been reported with rt-PA administration.

  2. **Primary PTCA** for MI results in a level of myocardial salvage comparable to that obtained with thrombolytic therapy, with lower rates of intracranial hemorrhage and recurrent ischemia (*N Engl J Med* 328:673, 1993). However, primary PTCA can be performed within 60–90 minutes only in specialized centers; therefore prompt administration of thrombolytic therapy remains the treatment of choice in patients without contraindications. The role of primary PTCA in MI requires further investigation, but the greatest benefit has been

observed in high-risk patients, such as those with anterior MI, age greater than 70 years, or persistent sinus tachycardia. In addition, primary PTCA has been associated with improved mortality in patients with cardiogenic shock (*J Am Coll Cardiol* 19:639, 1992). PTCA should not be performed routinely during the first 48 hours after successful thrombolytic therapy, but **salvage PTCA** may be indicated in patients in whom reperfusion has apparently failed, such as those with persistent chest pain and ST segment elevation.

3. **Coronary angiography** should be considered in patients with recurrent myocardial ischemia after MI and in those in whom ischemia is provoked during predischarge exercise testing (*N Engl J Med* 320:618, 1989). In addition, many cardiologists recommend that selected high-risk patients undergo coronary angiography to determine the extent of CAD and assess vessel patency.

4. **CABG.** Acute surgical revascularization has been performed successfully in the setting of MI (*Ann Thorac Surg* 41:119, 1986), but delays required in preparation for surgery make this approach an unacceptable alternative to thrombolysis or PTCA as primary treatment for acute MI. Patients with three-vessel CAD and impaired left ventricular function after MI should be considered for elective CABG.

C. **Other measures to reduce infarct size**

1. **Beta-adrenergic antagonists** decrease myocardial oxygen consumption by reducing the heart rate, contractility, and BP. IV beta-adrenergic antagonists have been shown to reduce infarct size and mortality in several clinical trials (*Am J Med* 74:113, 1983; *Lancet* 2:57, 1986) and are indicated in most patients with acute MI who present within the first 4–6 hours after the onset of symptoms. Patients with continued ischemic pain or evidence of sympathetic hyperactivity manifested by tachycardia and hypertension **in the absence of heart failure** may particularly benefit.

   a. **Contraindications to beta-adrenergic antagonists.** Patients with a resting heart rate below 50–55 beats/minute, systolic BP less than 95 mm Hg, significant first-degree AV block (PR >0.24 sec), second- or third-degree AV block, obstructive lung disease by history, wheezing on examination, or evidence of significant heart failure on examination or chest radiograph should not receive beta-adrenergic antagonists.

   b. **IV doses of beta-adrenergic antagonists. Metoprolol** (15 mg IV given in 5-mg doses, q5min, followed by a 50- to 100-mg PO dose q12h), **propranolol** (0.1 mg/kg divided into three doses IV q5–10min, followed in 1 hour by a 20- to 40-mg PO dose q6–8h), **atenolol** (5–10 mg IV, followed by a 100-mg PO daily dose), and **timolol** (1 mg repeated after 10 minutes and followed by a 0.6-mg/kg maintenance infusion for 24 hours and then by a 10-mg PO dose q12h) have all been used in the treatment of patients with acute MI (*Eur Heart J* 6:199, 1985; *N Engl J Med* 310:9, 1984). Although there is no evidence that **esmolol hydrochloride** reduces infarct size or decreases mortality, because of its extremely short half-life (10 minutes) it is particularly useful in patients at high risk for complications of beta-adrenergic antagonists. It is administered as an initial 250- to 500-µg/kg bolus over 1 minute, followed by a maintenance infusion beginning at 50 µg/kg/minute and titrated to a heart rate of 55–60 beats/minute (*Circulation* 72:873, 1985). Timolol for IV injection is not available in the United States.

2. **Nitroglycerin** may have a beneficial effect on infarct size in selected subgroups of patients when treatment is started early and hypotension is avoided (*Circulation* 76:906, 1989). However, in a large randomized trial, IV nitroglycerin did not reduce mortality compared to placebo (*Lancet* 343:1115, 1994). Therefore, routine use of IV nitroglycerin cannot be recommended in patients with acute MI. Nitroglycerin should be used in acute MI complicated by CHF or recurrent ischemia. IV nitroglycerin is initiated as a 10-µg/minute infusion that is increased in 10-µg/minute increments at 10- to 15-minute intervals. The BP should be monitored closely, and the dose should

Table 5-8. Doses and actions of vasoactive and inotropic agents used in patients with myocardial infarction

Agent	Dose	Action	Precautions
Dobutamine (see Appendix C)	2.5–15.0 µg/kg/ min; start at lower doses	Positive inotrope, beta-adrenergic agonist	Heart rate and oxygen consumption may increase; may exacerbate arrhythmias
Amrinone (*Am J Cardiol* 56:29B, 1985)	0.75 mg/kg initial dose, followed by 5–10 µg/kg/ min infusion	Positive inotrope, phosphodiesterase inhibitor	May exacerbate arrhythmias
Dopamine (see Appendix C)	0.5–2.0 µg/kg/min	Dilates renal and mesenteric arteries	
	2.0–6.0 µg/kg/min	Positive inotrope, beta-adrenergic agonist	Increases heart rate and increases PAOP
	>10 µg/kg/min	Vasopressor, alpha-adrenergic agonist	Similar but less potent than norepinephrine at these doses
IV nitroglycerin	10–400 µg/min; start at lower doses	Venodilator with modest arteriolar dilator effects, coronary vasodilator	Hypotension in patients with low PAOP
Nitroprusside (see Appendix C)	0.25–2.0 µg/kg/ min	Arteriolar and venodilator	Thiocyanate toxicity in patients with renal failure or with high doses

PAOP = pulmonary artery occlusive pressure.

not be increased further without invasive hemodynamic monitoring once there has been a 10–15% reduction in systolic BP. Hypotension is most likely to occur in patients with MI who have relative volume depletion (low preload) or those with inferior MI complicated by right ventricular dysfunction (see Appendix C and Table 5-8).

3. **Calcium channel antagonists** have failed to limit infarct size in large clinical trials. When administered after MI, **nifedipine** has been associated with excess mortality and an increased incidence of reinfarction (*Br Med J* 299:1187, 1989). **Verapamil** has no benefit in the acute treatment of MI but does not cause excess mortality (*Am J Cardiol* 67:1295, 1991). When started in the first week after MI, verapamil appears to decrease mortality and reduce the incidence of reinfarction in patients without heart failure who are not treated with beta-adrenergic antagonists (*Am J Cardiol* 66:779, 1990). In the subgroup of patients with non–Q-wave MI, **diltiazem** was found to have no benefit when given to patients with MI and increased mortality in patients with left ventricular ejection fractions less than 40% or with clinical evidence of heart failure (*N Engl J Med* 319:385, 1988). In contrast, in patients with non–Q-wave MI and good left ventricular function, treatment with diltiazem may help prevent recurrent infarction (*N Engl J Med* 315:423, 1986). Thus

there is **little indication for the acute use of calcium channel antagonists in patients with MI** and a significant potential for harm in those with impaired left ventricular function.

D. **Anticoagulant and antiplatelet therapy**
1. **Heparin**, administered either as a continuous IV infusion or a high dose SC (12,500 units SC q12h), appears to decrease mortality in patients with MI regardless of whether they receive thrombolytic therapy (*Lancet* 2:182, 1989) and may decrease the incidence of mural thrombi (*J Am Coll Cardiol* 8:419, 1985). However, the risk of bleeding complications due to anticoagulation are probably greater than the potential benefits in patients at low risk for complications after MI. Therefore, in the absence of contraindications, anticoagulation with IV or high-dose SC heparin should be considered in patients with large anterior MIs, patients at risk of developing mural thrombosis, and selected patients at risk for recurrent MI. In the absence of more aggressive anticoagulation, all patients admitted to the cardiac care unit should be given low-dose heparin, 5,000 units SC q8–12h, until they are fully ambulatory to prevent the development of deep venous thrombosis (*Am Heart J* 99:574, 1980).
2. **Warfarin.** Patients with documented mural thrombus or extensive anterior MI with apical involvement should be treated with warfarin for 3–6 months to minimize the risk of systemic embolism. An international normalized ratio (INR) of approximately 2.5 should be maintained. In the absence of these conditions, either **aspirin** or **warfarin** can be given for secondary prevention (see sec. **VII.B.2**).
3. **Aspirin.** It is reasonable to give most patients with MI aspirin on admission and to continue aspirin long term for secondary prevention. In patients fully anticoagulated with IV heparin or when long-term anticoagulation with warfarin is anticipated, concurrent aspirin therapy has been associated with an increase in bleeding complications. Aspirin may also increase bleeding in patients who subsequently undergo cardiac surgery.
E. **Additional pharmacologic therapy in MI patients**
1. **Prophylactic lidocaine** is generally unnecessary once the patient has been admitted to the intensive care unit, where ventricular arrhythmias can be treated promptly. However, if lidocaine has been started before admission, it can be continued for at least 24 hours (see sec. **IV.A.1**).
2. **IV magnesium sulfate**, despite earlier reports of beneficial effects (*Lancet* 339:1553, 1992), failed to reduce mortality in acute MI in a large randomized study (*Circulation* 88(Suppl):I-292, 1993). Therefore, routine use of IV magnesium in acute MI is not indicated. Patients with ventricular arrhythmias should have hypomagnesemia and hypokalemia corrected. The IV dose of magnesium sulfate is 2 g over 5–10 minutes, repeated q4–6h, with careful monitoring of serum magnesium levels. Patients with serum creatinine levels greater than 3.0 mg/dl or complete heart block should not be treated with magnesium.
3. **Angiotensin-converting enzyme inhibitors** have an established role in the long-term management of patients with depressed left ventricular function following acute MI (see sec. **VII.B.3**). Data from large randomized studies have demonstrated a modest improvement in 1- and 6-month survival in patients treated with an oral ACE inhibitor within the first 24 hours after acute MI (*Lancet* 343:1115, 1994; *Circulation* 88(Suppl):I-292, 1993). The patient groups demonstrating the greatest benefit were high-risk groups including those with CHF, anterior MI, or previous MI.
F. **Subsequent management of patients with MI**
1. **General measures.** Patients with MI should be admitted to the intensive care unit. IV access is mandatory. Continuous ECG monitoring should be established and observed by nursing personnel trained in the recognition of arrhythmias. Visitors should be limited, and visitation periods should be kept brief to allow for patient rest. Oral rather than rectal temperatures should be obtained. Patients with uncomplicated MIs generally spend 2–3 days in the

intensive care unit and can then be transferred to a "step down" unit with ambulatory monitoring capability for the remainder of their 7- to 10-day hospital stay. If complications arise during the initial post-MI period, the stay in the intensive care unit should be extended until the patient's condition stabilizes.

2. **Sedation** is beneficial during the initial days after MI and can be achieved with low doses of a benzodiazepine or other anxiolytic agent (see Chap. 1).

3. **Diet and bowel care.** For the first day after MI, the diet should be liquid or soft, followed by a 1,200- to 1,800-calorie, no added salt, low-cholesterol diet. Caffeinated beverages, as well as very hot or cold liquids, should be avoided. Since constipation is a common problem in MI patients, stool softeners or mild laxatives are routinely given.

IV. **Complications**

A. **Arrhythmias** often occur during the first 24 hours after MI. While life-threatening arrhythmias such as ventricular tachycardia (VT) or fibrillation (VF) are of most concern, any arrhythmia that results in hemodynamic compromise should be vigorously treated. Sustained arrhythmias causing hypotension, angina, or CHF should be terminated with synchronized electrical cardioversion. Potentially exacerbating conditions should be considered and corrected, including adverse effects of drugs, hypoxemia, acidosis, or electrolyte imbalances (especially potassium, calcium, and magnesium disorders). Left ventricular failure, recurrent ischemia, or hypotension may also predispose to arrhythmias and should be promptly managed.

1. **Ventricular arrhythmias**

a. **Ventricular premature depolarizations (VPDs)** occur commonly in the acute MI period and may herald VT or VF. In the majority of patients, VT and VF are not preceded by "warning arrhythmias" (*Circulation* 74:653, 1986). Routine treatment of VPDs is not recommended but should be considered if they occur more frequently than 5/minute, appear in the vulnerable period of the cardiac cycle (R-on-T phenomenon), occur in salvos of two or more with sufficient frequency to induce hemodynamic compromise, or occur in multiple forms (see Chap. 7).

(1) **Lidocaine** is the treatment of choice for suppression of VPDs. It is administered as an IV bolus of 1 mg/kg followed by one or more boluses of 0.5 mg/kg 3–5 minutes apart until ectopy resolves, or a total dose of 3 mg/kg has been given. A continuous IV infusion of 2–4 mg/minute (20–50 μg/kg/minute) should then be initiated. Since the half-life of lidocaine is prolonged with heart failure, liver disease, hypotension, and advanced age, the total dose should be decreased by 50% in these situations. Blood levels should be monitored in patients in whom lidocaine clearance may be impaired, or when high doses or prolonged infusions are used.

(2) **Procainamide** is used when lidocaine is ineffective and is started as a 500- to 1,000-mg loading dose given at a rate not exceeding 50 mg/minute, followed by a 2- to 5-mg/minute maintenance infusion (see Appendix C). During the infusion, QRS duration, QT interval, vital signs, and procainamide and *N*-acetylprocainamide (NAPA) blood levels should be carefully monitored. In patients with renal failure, accumulation of the active metabolite NAPA may occur.

b. **VT and VF.** Immediate defibrillation or cardioversion is the treatment of choice for VF or VT with hemodynamic compromise. Specific protocols are outlined in Chap. 8.

c. **Accelerated idioventricular rhythm (AIVR)** occurs frequently in patients in whom coronary reperfusion is achieved, and occasionally in other patients with MI. AIVR is a wide complex escape rhythm (rate 60–110 beats/minute) that occurs when the sinus rate slows below 60 beats/minute and is not usually accompanied by hemodynamic compromise. AIVR is usually benign, with a duration of less than 48 hours, and does not require specific therapy except for close observation. When AIVR is associated with hemodynamic deterioration or it precipitates VT or VF, administration of atropine or overdrive pacing is effective treatment. Lidocaine is generally not indicated in the treatment of AIVR, unless the AIVR appears to contribute to the development of sustained VT.

2. **Supraventricular tachycardias** (see Chap. 7)

   a. **Sinus tachycardia** is common in patients with acute MI and is frequently associated with heart failure, hypoxemia, pain, anxiety, fever, hypovolemia, or adverse drug effects. Persistent sinus tachycardia is a poor prognostic indicator and is often an indication for invasive hemodynamic evaluation. Treatment is directed at correcting underlying causes. In the absence of heart failure and after correction of contributing causes, judicious use of a beta-adrenergic antagonist is indicated, especially when hypertension accompanies sinus tachycardia. IV metoprolol, propranolol, or esmolol is usually effective treatment (see sec. **III.C.1.b**).

   b. **Paroxysmal supraventricular tachycardia (PSVT)** occurs infrequently in patients with MI but should be treated to prevent exacerbation of myocardial ischemia. Synchronized cardioversion is the treatment of choice in the presence of hypotension, ischemia, or heart failure. If the patient's condition is stable, vagotonic maneuvers such as careful carotid sinus massage can be attempted. For PSVT that is refractory to vagotonic maneuvers, IV **adenosine, diltiazem, verapamil, propranolol, or digoxin** can be given, as outlined in Chap. 7. IV adenosine is the drug of choice.

   c. **Atrial flutter** often responds poorly to pharmacologic measures. If the patient's condition is unstable, synchronized cardioversion beginning at low energy levels (50 joules) is the treatment of choice. This may convert the rhythm to sinus or atrial fibrillation. Rapid atrial pacing may also be beneficial and is the treatment of choice in patients with digitalis intoxication. For patients in stable condition, IV diltiazem, verapamil, propranolol, or digoxin can be used (see Chap. 7). These drugs will decrease the ventricular response but may convert the rhythm to atrial fibrillation. Because of the risk of atrial flutter with 1 : 1 conduction, even patients in stable condition should be electrically cardioverted when there is no response to initial pharmacologic therapy (see Chap. 7).

   d. **Atrial fibrillation** is deleterious to the ischemic myocardium because the ventricular response is usually rapid and the atrial contribution to ventricular filling is lost. Cardioversion beginning at 100 joules is the treatment of choice for atrial fibrillation with rapid ventricular response associated with hemodynamic compromise. If the ventricular rate is slow (less than 100 beats/minute) in the absence of treatment with drugs that depress AV nodal conduction, placement of a transvenous endocardial pacemaker to avoid asystole should be considered before cardioversion. For patients who are hemodynamically stable, IV diltiazem, verapamil, propranolol, or digoxin can be used to control ventricular response (see Chap. 7). Frequently, atrial fibrillation in the acute MI period may be transient and not require long-term treatment.

   e. **Accelerated junctional rhythm** is usually a benign escape rhythm in patients with sinus bradycardia and requires no specific therapy. Occasionally in patients with cardiogenic shock or digitalis toxicity, **nonparoxysmal junctional tachycardia** (70–130 beats/minute) may occur. Treatment is directed toward the underlying condition.

3. **Bradycardias**

   a. **Sinus bradycardia** may occur in patients with acute MI, particularly in those with inferior MI. Treatment is indicated only in patients with hypotension or decreased cardiac output due to the bradycardia. Atropine sulfate, 0.5–1.0 mg IV, repeated at 5-minute intervals to a maximum of 2–3 mg, is usually effective. Temporary atrial or ventricular pacing is preferred for refractory or recurrent symptomatic bradycardia.

   b. **Atrioventricular conduction disturbances**, including first-degree, second-degree, or third-degree (complete) AV block, occur frequently in patients with MI.

(1) First-degree AV block (prolonged PR interval) should be recognized because it may be a contraindication to the use of verapamil, diltiazem, or beta-adrenergic antagonists. Often, first-degree AV block is caused by treatment with digoxin or other agents that slow AV node conduction.

(2) Second-degree block is classified as either Mobitz type I (Wenckebach), manifested by gradual prolongation of the PR interval and a narrow QRS complex before the nonconducted P-wave, or Mobitz type II, in which the dropped beats are not preceded by PR prolongation and the QRS complex is wide. In Mobitz type I, the site of block is usually within the AV node. The block in Mobitz type II is located below the bundle of His. Mobitz type I (Wenckebach) block does not require specific therapy, but temporary transvenous pacing is indicated in the presence of symptomatic bradycardia. **Mobitz type II block may progress to complete AV block and requires pacemaker insertion regardless of whether the patient is symptomatic.**

(3) In third-degree heart block there is AV dissociation, often with a slow ventricular escape rhythm. In patients with anterior MI, complete AV block may develop abruptly, often preceded only by first-degree AV block or some form of intraventricular block, and is associated with a large area of infarction and high mortality. In patients with inferior MI, heart block may be preceded by first- or second-degree AV block, and often the junctional or ventricular escape rhythm is not associated with symptoms. Nonetheless, **third-degree AV block in the setting of an MI requires emergency transvenous pacing** because of the potential for progression to asystole. The consequences of third-degree AV block are the most deleterious in patients in whom maintenance of cardiac output depends on a synchronized atrial contribution to ventricular filling. Thus, when third-degree AV block occurs in those with large anterior MI or inferior MI complicated by right ventricular infarction, temporary AV pacing is indicated.

(4) Indications for transvenous pacing in patients with MI include (1) asystole, (2) third-degree heart block, (3) new right bundle branch block with left anterior or posterior hemiblock (new right bundle branch block alone is considered by many an indication for temporary pacing), (4) new left bundle branch block, (5) Mobitz type II second-degree heart block, and (6) symptomatic bradycardia not responsive to atropine. Indications for permanent pacing after MI are discussed in Chap. 7.

B. Hypertension in patients with MI is common and should be treated promptly. Increases in afterload and subsequent elevation in myocardial oxygen demand may increase infarct size or produce infarct expansion. In general, patients with MI should be treated initially with short-acting titratable IV agents. The following approach to treatment of patients with MI and hypertension is suggested:

1. Bed rest, analgesia, and sedation are frequently sufficient in controlling mild-to-moderate elevations in BP.

2. Beta-adrenergic antagonists are often appropriate and should be administered in small parenteral doses, as described in sec. **III.C.1.b.** If IV preparations are tolerated, oral therapy can be initiated (see Table 5-2).

3. Angiotensin-converting enzyme inhibitors. In view of the favorable influence of angiotensin-converting enzyme inhibitors on mortality following acute MI, these agents, in combination with a beta-adrenergic antagonist, should be the preferred approach to moderate hypertension (see Chap. 4).

4. Indications for the use of calcium channel antagonists in the treatment of hypertension in the acute MI period have not been well defined. However, these agents are effective in reducing BP and may be appropriate if angiotensin-converting enzyme inhibitors or beta-adrenergic antagonists are ineffective or contraindicated. Given concerns about the safety of dihydropyridines such as nifedipine in patients with MI, verapamil or diltiazem may be preferable. The safety of newer dihydropyridines in patients with MI has not been established (see sec. III.C.3 and Table 5-3).

5. **IV nitroprusside** is indicated in the treatment of moderate to severe hypertension and results in a prompt reduction in BP by dilation of the venous and arterial circulation. The initial dose is 10–15 μg/minute (or 0.25 μg/kg/minute) administered as a continuous IV infusion, increasing by 5- to 10-μg/minute increments q5–10min as required for control of BP (see Appendix C and Table 5-8). Doses as high as 400 μg/minute are occasionally necessary. Solutions should be prepared in 5% dextrose and water just before use and shielded from light because the drug is photosensitive. Thiocyanate, a metabolite excreted by the kidneys, may increase to toxic levels with prolonged therapy (>72 hours), high doses, or renal dysfunction. **Plasma thiocyanate levels should be monitored under these circumstances.** Cyanide toxicity may occur with even brief infusions or low infusion rates and may be manifested by confusion, delirium, or the development of lactic acidosis resulting from inhibition of aerobic metabolism. The maximum dose rate of 10 μg/kg/minute should never be used for more than 10 minutes (*Clin Pharmacokinet* 9:239, 1984).

6. **IV nitroglycerin** induces venodilation and modest arteriolar dilation. In patients with elevated left ventricular filling pressures, doses sufficient to decrease modest hypertension can often be given, but with normal left ventricular filling pressures, the antihypertensive effects are limited. This drug is often effective in the treatment of hypertension associated with heart failure, or when there are continued ischemic symptoms. The initial dose is 10 μg/minute by continuous infusion with increases in 5- to 10-μg/minute increments until BP is controlled (see Table 5-8).

C. **Hemodynamic complications**
1. **Left ventricular pump failure** in the setting of MI is associated with both decreased left ventricular systolic function and decreased compliance (e.g., stiff ventricle). The severity of pump failure is related to the extent of infarction, ranging from mild pulmonary congestion to cardiogenic shock. Acute mechanical complications of MI such as acute mitral regurgitation, ventricular septal rupture, or exacerbation of underlying chronic valvular disease may also result in pulmonary edema or shock. Thus, in patients with clinical evidence of pump failure or shock, the initial evaluation should include noninvasive imaging of ventricular function with radionuclide ventriculography or two-dimensional echocardiography and Doppler studies.
   a. **Treatment of mild heart failure.** In patients with mild pulmonary congestion or an S3 gallop:
      (1) **Diuretics** are generally appropriate but must be used cautiously, because most patients with MI are not volume overloaded. Excessive diuresis may lead to hypovolemia, hypotension, and inappropriate reduction in left ventricular filling pressures. Furosemide, 10–20 mg IV, is the treatment of choice (see Chap. 4).
      (2) **Topical nitrates or low doses of IV nitroglycerin** in patients who are hemodynamically stable will often be of benefit by decreasing left ventricular filling pressures.
      (3) **Digoxin,** 0.125–0.250 mg PO qd, is often used in the treatment of patients with mild chronic heart failure, but its effects on long-term survival are not well established. **Digoxin should not be used in the acute management of heart failure in patients with MI.**
      (4) **ACE inhibitors** improve symptoms in patients with mild-to-moderate heart failure (*JAMA* 259:539, 1988) and improve survival in patients with severe heart failure (*N Engl J Med* 316:1429, 1987). **Captopril,** 6.25–50.0 mg PO q6–8h, or **enalapril,** 2.5–20.0 mg PO bid, can be used starting with the lower doses to avoid hypotension (see Chap. 6).

In patients with significant CHF or hypotension who do not respond to initial therapy, invasive hemodynamic monitoring with a balloon-tipped pulmonary artery catheter should be considered.

b. **Indications for pulmonary artery catheterization** include the following: (1) severe or progressive CHF; (2) cardiogenic shock or hypotension unresponsive to simple conventional measures (i.e., IV fluids); (3) clinical signs suggestive of severe mitral regurgitation, ventricular septal defect, or hemodynamically significant pericardial effusion; (4) unexplained or severe cyanosis, hypoxemia, tachypnea, diaphoresis, or acidosis; (5) unexplained or refractory sinus tachycardia or other tachyarrhythmias; or (6) the need for parenteral vasoactive agents that must be closely monitored to avoid deleterious changes in heart rate or BP (*J Am Coll Cardiol* 16:249, 1990). Pulmonary arterial and systemic arterial catheters should be inserted only by trained individuals under sterile conditions (see Chap. 9). In patients with left bundle branch block, consideration should be given to placing a temporary pacemaker because pulmonary artery catheterization can induce complete heart block in such individuals. In addition, in patients undergoing pulmonary artery catheterization, systemic BP should be measured frequently, either noninvasively or by use of a radial or femoral arterial catheter. Urinary output should be closely monitored with an indwelling catheter if necessary.

c. **Management of hemodynamic subsets of patients with left ventricular dysfunction.** Pulmonary artery catheterization allows for measurement of right atrial pressure (RAP), right ventricular pressure, pulmonary artery pressure, and pulmonary artery occlusive pressure (PAOP). Pressures should be measured at end-expiration and should be determined using a strip chart recording. In addition, cardiac index (CI = cardiac output/body surface area) can be measured by the thermodilution or Fick methods, and mixed venous blood gases can be obtained. The systemic vascular resistance (SVR = [(mean arterial pressure − RAP)/cardiac output] × 80) should also be calculated (normal range 900–1,350 dynes/sec/cm^{-5}). In some circumstances, catheters that allow for continuous measurement of mixed venous oxygen saturation or right ventricular ejection fraction may be useful. Patients with MI can be categorized into several hemodynamic subsets that are useful for defining treatment strategies (*J Am Coll Cardiol* 16:249, 1990). Establishing baseline measurements and subsequent trends is more important than single absolute values. It is also important to recognize that, although guidelines for management of hemodynamic complications are useful, therapy must be based on individual responses to initial therapy. All hemodynamic data should be evaluated in terms of the clinical response and viewed critically if they fail to correlate with other physiologic parameters (such as urine output). Patients should be managed aggressively to minimize the duration of catheterization.

(1) **Decreased left filling pressure (PAOP <15–18 mm Hg)** when accompanied by hypotension, decreased cardiac index (<2.5 liters/minute/m^2), oliguria, or persistent sinus tachycardia should be treated by rapid infusion of normal saline. Because left ventricular compliance is decreased in patients with anterior MI, a PAOP of 15–18 mm Hg is generally an appropriate end point for volume resuscitation.

(2) **Elevated left ventricular filling pressure (PAOP >18 mm Hg) with normal cardiac index (>2.5 liters/minute/m^2)** is an indication of volume overload or decreased LV compliance. Often, such patients can be treated with a diuretic alone. Topical nitrates or IV nitroglycerin can also be used when increased filling pressures persist despite diuresis.

(3) **Elevated left ventricular filling pressure (PAOP >18 mm Hg), decreased cardiac index (<2.5 liters/minute/m^2), and systolic arterial pressure greater than 100 mm Hg** are indications of significant left

ventricular systolic dysfunction. Because the BP is maintained, after-load reduction with nitroglycerin or nitroprusside is the treatment of choice. Nitroglycerin is preferred early after the onset of infarction because it may also induce coronary vasodilatation and increase myocardial blood flow to ischemic regions. Nitroprusside has less favorable effects in terms of coronary blood flow (*N Engl J Med* 306:1121, 1129, 1168, 1982) but is a more potent vasodilator and is indicated when marked hypertension is present. If BP falls or cardiac index does not improve, an inotropic agent, such as dobutamine or amrinone, should be added (see Table 5-8).

(4) **Elevated left ventricular filling pressure (PAOP >18 mm Hg), decreased cardiac index (<2.5 liters/minute/m^2), and systolic arterial pressure less than 100 mm Hg** are indications of extensive left ventricular dysfunction. **Cardiogenic shock** is defined as systolic BP of less than 90 mm Hg in the presence of organ hypoperfusion (such as oliguria or confusion). Thrombolysis is contraindicated in most patients with shock because of the unpredictable pharmacokinetics of fibrinolytic agents in this setting and the need for invasive vascular procedures in these patients. However, because the mortality of patients with cardiogenic shock is nearly 80% despite aggressive intervention, once stabilized the patient should be aggressively evaluated for myocardial salvage with emergency PTCA (*Circulation* 78:1345, 1988) and for the presence of treatable mechanical complications of infarction, such as severe mitral regurgitation or ventricular septal rupture (see sec. **IV.D**). Initial support of the circulation with a vasopressor is essential; norepinephrine is preferred in markedly hypotensive patients (systolic BP <70 mm Hg), but dopamine is usually sufficient in patients with a systolic BP of 70–90 mm Hg. In patients with a systolic BP near 90 mm Hg, inotropic support with dobutamine is often sufficient (see Table 5-8). Patients who are candidates for aggressive intervention and do not respond to initial pharmacologic therapy or require high doses of vasopressors should be supported with an intraaortic balloon pump.

(5) **Right ventricular myocardial infarction (RVMI)** is characterized by a decreased cardiac index (<2.5 liters/minute/m^2), with normal or decreased left ventricular filling pressures and elevated right atrial pressure (>10 mm Hg) in patients with inferior MI (*Chest* 77:220, 1980). In some patients, elevation of right atrial pressure may not be evident until IV fluids are administered. Clinical signs may include hypotension, elevation of the jugular venous pulsation, a positive Kussmaul's sign (increase in jugular venous pressures with inspiration), and right-sided third and fourth heart sounds with clear lung fields. Right precordial ECG leads should be obtained and analyzed for ST elevation in lead V$_4$R, a specific marker of RVMI. Echocardiographic demonstration of decreased right ventricular systolic function is often useful in confirming the diagnosis of RVMI (*Am Heart J* 107:505, 1984). Hemodynamic responses to right ventricular infarction range from asymptomatic elevation of right-sided pressures to severe shock. Patients with a systolic BP of 90–100 mm Hg and a depressed cardiac index often respond to IV fluids, which should be given until the PAOP is 15–18 mm Hg; excessive fluid administration should be avoided. If the cardiac index is still decreased after fluid administration or if hypotension is more severe, dobutamine should be administered. Most often the combination of volume resuscitation and inotropic support with dobutamine will increase the systolic BP to greater than 90 mm Hg. However, patients with refractory severe hypotension should be supported with intraaortic balloon counterpulsation. In patients with heart block causing AV dysynchrony, AV sequential pacing may have marked beneficial hemodynamic effects.

D. Mechanical complications

1. **Infarct expansion.** Thinning and expansion of the infarcted myocardial wall after MI may adversely alter ventricular geometry and function. Agents that decrease afterload, particularly **ACE inhibitors**, may limit infarct expansion and ventricular dilatation after MI (*N Engl J Med* 319:80, 1988, and sec. **VII.B.3**). Use of glucocorticoids or nonsteroidal anti-inflammatory drugs should be avoided in patients with MI because they appear to augment myocardial thinning (*Circulation* 53 [Suppl I]: I-204, 1976; *Can J Cardiol* 5:211, 1989).

2. **Hemodynamically significant mitral regurgitation** may occur in patients with acute MI and is associated with a worse prognosis compared with that for patients without mitral regurgitation (*Am J Cardiol* 65:1169, 1990).

   a. **Diagnosis.** Most patients with hemodynamically significant mitral regurgitation have a typical holosystolic murmur. With moderate-to-severe mitral regurgitation, pulmonary edema is usually present. Papillary muscle rupture or severe papillary muscle dysfunction is often associated with severe mitral regurgitation and cardiogenic shock. Although the presence of a large V-wave on the pulmonary artery pressure tracing obtained at pulmonary artery catheterization suggests mitral regurgitation, it is neither sensitive nor specific and may occur in patients with ventricular septal rupture. Two-dimensional echocardiography with Doppler imaging is the diagnostic test of choice. However, in critically ill patients, technical difficulties often limit the sensitivity of conventional echocardiographic imaging; these limitations can be overcome by use of transesophageal echocardiography.

   b. **Initial management** of patients with mitral regurgitation should include pharmacologic afterload reduction with IV nitroglycerin or nitroprusside; dobutamine may be of benefit in patients with borderline hypotension. In patients with severe mitral regurgitation, intraaortic balloon counterpulsation is often necessary to stabilize the patient before coronary angiography and surgical intervention can be performed.

3. **Rupture of the interventricular septum** is suggested by the development of a systolic murmur, the concomitant onset of pulmonary edema, and, almost always, cardiogenic shock. Interventricular septal rupture complicates 1–3% of MIs and generally occurs within 7 days.

   a. **Diagnosis.** Ventricular septal rupture typically produces a holosystolic murmur that is heard best along the lower left sternal border and is most often associated with a systolic thrill. Two-dimensional echocardiography with Doppler imaging is an extremely sensitive and specific technique for detecting intracardiac shunts and valvular regurgitation and should always be part of the initial evaluation of patients with a new murmur or cardiogenic shock after MI. The presence of a ventricular septal rupture can be documented by a greater than 5% increase in hemoglobin oxygen saturation between the right atrium and right ventricle with right heart catheterization.

   b. **Management.** Initial management of patients with ventricular septal rupture is similar to that already outlined for those with cardiogenic shock and should include invasive hemodynamic monitoring. Vasodilators such as nitroglycerin or nitroprusside are indicated to reduce afterload, but the majority of patients will require intraaortic balloon counterpulsation before an attempt at surgical repair is made.

4. **Rupture of the left ventricular free wall (cardiorrhexis)** is a catastrophic complication of MI responsible for 10% of deaths associated with MI. Rupture is more frequent in female patients, patients with MI as the first indication of CAD, patients with hypertension, and those treated with glucocorticoids or nonsteroidal antiinflammatory drugs (*Am J Cardiol* 40:429, 1977). Rupture typically occurs during the first week after MI and presents as sudden hemodynamic collapse. Left ventricular rupture may be accompanied by sinus or junctional bradycardia, idioventricular rhythm, ST

segment and T-wave abnormalities, and rapid development of electromechanical dissociation. Although sudden death is usual, some instances of left ventricular rupture may be preceded by recurrent pericardial pain secondary to the accumulation of blood in the pericardial space with or without the signs of pericardial effusion, tamponade, and hypotension. Echocardiography may be useful in identifying patients with thin ventricular walls at risk for rupture or those in whom partial rupture has occurred. Prompt recognition at this stage may allow for successful surgical repair. Pericardiocentesis in the event of tamponade and the prompt institution of intraaortic balloon counterpulsation may prove life-sustaining until surgical correction can be performed.

5. **Ventricular aneurysm,** a localized outpouching of the left ventricular cavity related to a region of dyskinetic myocardium, may be suspected on the basis of persistent ST segment elevation after MI, intractable heart failure, or poorly controlled ventricular arrhythmias (*N Engl J Med* 311:1001, 1984). Patients with aneurysms are at risk for development of mural thrombi and peripheral embolization.

   a. **Diagnosis.** Echocardiography and left ventricular angiography are useful to define the extent of aneurysmal involvement of the left ventricular wall, but two-dimensional echocardiography is the test of choice for determining the presence of mural thrombus.

   b. **Management.** Patients with mural thrombi should be anticoagulated (see sec. **III.D**). Delayed surgical repair of a left ventricular aneurysm is indicated in some patients with refractory left heart failure, life-threatening ventricular arrhythmias, or recurrent systemic embolization.

6. **Ventricular pseudoaneurysm** is a form of cardiac rupture in which pericardial extravasation of blood is contained locally by the visceral pericardium. Thus, a free communication exists between the left ventricle and the pseudoaneurysm. Two-dimensional echocardiography is useful in differentiating pseudoaneurysms from true left ventricular aneurysms. Pseudoaneurysms should be repaired promptly because of the high incidence of rupture (*Thorax* 38:25, 1983).

E. **Recurrent ischemia and infarction**
   1. **Recurrent ischemia.** Patients with signs or symptoms of recurrent ischemia in the post-MI period should be aggressively managed, and prompt coronary angiography should be performed to identify those patients who will benefit from interventional therapy with PTCA or CABG.
   2. **Extension or recurrence of infarction** occurs in 10–20% of patients after MI (*Circulation* 65:918, 1982) and is often preceded by recurrent chest discomfort despite initial therapy. Patients with recurrent chest pain or ECG changes should be reevaluated for new myocardial necrosis with MB-CK isoenzyme measurements. Most infarct extensions occur within 7–10 days of infarction; therefore, discharge from the hospital before this time is not advised in high-risk patients (e.g., patients with recurrent ischemia, extensive infarction, symptomatic heart failure, or arrhythmias).

F. **Pericardial complications after MI**
   1. **Acute pericarditis** generally occurs in patients with large infarctions. Pain due to pericarditis is typically substernal, radiates to the back, is exacerbated by deep breathing or movement, and is relieved by sitting up. A pericardial friction rub may be appreciated on careful examination but is often evanescent. The classic ECG findings associated with pericarditis may be masked by the infarct (*N Engl J Med* 311:1211, 1984). Aspirin can be used to relieve the pain. **Use of glucocorticoids or non-aspirin–containing nonsteroidal anti-inflammatory drugs is contraindicated** because they retard myocardial scar formation and may increase the incidence of rupture (see sec. **IV.D.1**). In patients who are being treated with IV heparin, the presence of active pericarditis may increase the risk of hemorrhagic cardiac tamponade. In such patients, the potential risk should be balanced against the need for continued anticoagulation.

2. **Post-MI or Dressler's syndrome** is an uncommon late complication of MI characterized by pericarditis, pleuritis, pericardial or pleural effusions, fever, leukocytosis, elevated sedimentation rate, and elevated levels of antimyocardial antibodies (*Am J Cardiol* 50:1269, 1982). Patients typically have malaise, fever, and chest pain, but the syndrome may be mistaken for angina or MI, and the ECG may show diffuse, marked ST segment elevation. Onset of symptoms is usually between the second and tenth weeks after MI, and the course may be lengthy, with frequent remissions and exacerbations. Therapy is aimed at relieving symptoms and consists of **nonsteroidal antiinflammatory** agents such as aspirin (650 mg PO q6–8h) or indomethacin (25–50 mg PO q6–8h). Glucocorticoids such as **prednisone** (1 mg/kg PO qd) may be required for severe symptoms and, when used, should be tapered gradually to minimize exacerbation of symptoms. Anticoagulants should be discontinued if possible, since hemorrhagic pericarditis with tamponade can occur. Constrictive pericarditis may complicate the post-MI syndrome but is rare.

V. **Rehabilitation.** Although tissue repair may not be complete for up to 6 weeks after MI, the length of hospitalization and level of activity should be adjusted to the individual patient. In general, the length of hospitalization for patients with uncomplicated MI is 7–10 days, with ECG monitoring in a telemetry unit. Longer hospitalization is often necessary for those with complications. Patients should initially be kept at bed rest, but movement in bed and dangling the feet over the side of the bed should be encouraged. Within 24 hours after admission, patients with an uncomplicated course should begin sitting in a chair, may use a bedside commode, and should be encouraged to help themselves to shave, use the toilet, and eat. Patients should be encouraged to begin walking in the room on the third day after admission and should be fully ambulatory by 5–7 days. Instructions about activity, including sexual activity, should be provided before discharge. Generally, patients can tolerate daily walking programs but should avoid driving, heavy lifting, and vigorous climbing until completion of a maximal stress test. Depending on the extent of infarction, patients can return to work 4–8 weeks after hospital discharge. Supervised exercise rehabilitation can begin on discharge from the hospital.

VI. **Risk stratification after MI** with exercise stress testing, with or without the use of thallium perfusion imaging, radionuclide ventriculography, or echocardiography, can help identify patients with inducible ischemia and a high risk for subsequent cardiac events. Submaximal exercise testing can be performed safely 7–10 days after an uncomplicated MI, and patients with a positive test result should undergo cardiac catheterization to further assess coronary anatomy, prognosis, and the need for revascularization. Those individuals who complete the submaximal exercise protocol without evidence of ischemia are at low risk for cardiac events during the year following MI (*N Engl J Med* 314:161, 1986). Coronary angiography should also be performed in patients with non–Q-wave infarctions or post-MI courses complicated by recurrent ischemia, significant heart failure, or sustained ventricular arrhythmias. Maximal exercise testing can be performed safely 4–6 weeks after MI.

VII. **Secondary prevention**
A. **Modification of cardiac risk factors** is important after MI. Cessation of tobacco use is recommended, and information regarding hospital or American Heart Association smoking cessation programs should be provided. Patients with hypercholesterolemia, hypertension, or diabetes mellitus should be identified and treated appropriately. Regular aerobic exercise, preferably in a structured setting, is recommended for those patients who have had an uncomplicated post-MI course and are at low risk for subsequent cardiac events.

B. **Medical therapy** for secondary prevention should include drugs that have been shown in randomized trials to reduce the incidence of reinfarction and death after MI:
1. **Beta-adrenergic antagonists** (such as timolol, 10 mg bid; propranolol, 20–80 mg qid; or metoprolol, 100 mg bid) reduce mortality, sudden death, and reinfarction after MI (*N Engl J Med* 313:1055, 1985). Beta-adrenergic antagonists with ISA do not appear to be as effective (see Table 5-2). Therapy should be continued for at least 2 years following MI.

2. **Antiplatelet therapy** with **aspirin** (325 mg/day) may also be valuable in secondary prevention (*Br Med J* 296:320, 1988). Therapeutic **anticoagulation** with **warfarin** has also been shown to be effective (*N Engl J Med* 323:147, 1990), but whether it is more effective than aspirin has not been determined. Following successful thrombolytic therapy, patients treated with aspirin were found to have improved event-free survival compared with those treated with warfarin (*Circulation* 87:1524, 1993). Aspirin therapy should be continued indefinitely after MI. Patients with large anterior MI or left ventricular aneurysm should be treated initially with warfarin for 3–6 months and then can be treated with aspirin alone indefinitely. Patients with severe LV dysfunction should be treated with warfarin chronically to decrease the risk of systemic embolization.

3. **Angiotensin-converting enzyme inhibitors.** In asymptomatic patients with left ventricular ejection fraction less than 40% after MI, captopril reduced mortality, incidence of heart failure, and recurrent infarction. An improved clinical outcome with angiotensin-converting enzyme inhibitor therapy was present regardless of infarct location, use of thrombolytic therapy, or treatment with aspirin and beta-adrenergic antagonists (*N Engl J Med* 327:669, 1992). In high-risk patients with recent MI (e.g., large anterior MI, CHF, left ventricular aneurysm), therapy with an angiotensin-converting enzyme inhibitor should be continued for at least 1–2 years and continued indefinitely in those with persistent left ventricular dysfunction.

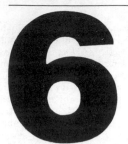

Heart Failure

Joseph G. Rogers and
Edward M. Geltman

Clinical Diagnosis

I. **Definition.** Heart failure (HF) is the inability of the heart to maintain an output adequate to meet the metabolic demands of the body. It is an increasingly common condition associated with extremely high morbidity and mortality.

II. **Pathophysiology.** The clinical syndrome of HF manifests as organ hypoperfusion and inadequate tissue oxygen delivery due to a low cardiac output and decreased cardiac reserve, as well as pulmonary and systemic venous congestion. A variety of compensatory adaptations occur, including (1) increased left ventricular volume (dilatation) and mass (hypertrophy), (2) increased systemic vascular resistance (SVR) secondary to enhanced activity of the sympathetic nervous system and elevated levels of circulating catecholamines, and (3) activation of the renin-angiotensin and vasopressin (ADH) systems. These secondary mechanisms, in conjunction with actual "pump failure," play a role in the pathophysiology of HF.

III. **The clinical manifestations** of HF vary depending on the rapidity of cardiac decompensation, underlying etiology, and age of the patient. Signs and symptoms of **low cardiac output** include fatigue, exercise intolerance, and decreased peripheral perfusion. Extreme deterioration in cardiac output and elevated SVR result in hypoperfusion of vital organs such as the kidney (decreased urine output) and brain (confusion and lethargy) and ultimately in shock. **Chronic pulmonary and systemic venous congestion** results in orthopnea, dyspnea on exertion, peripheral edema, elevated jugular venous pressure, pleural and pericardial effusions, hepatic congestion, and ascites. Acute elevations in left ventricular diastolic pressure and pulmonary venous pressure result in pulmonary edema. Associated laboratory abnormalities include elevated levels of BUN and creatinine, hyponatremia, and elevated levels of serum enzymes of hepatic origin.

IV. **The diagnosis** of HF should be suspected by clinical presentation. Radiographic evidence of cardiomegaly and pulmonary vascular redistribution is common. Depressed ventricular function may be confirmed by echocardiography, radionuclide ventriculography, or cardiac catheterization with cineangiography. Abnormalities in the ECG are common and include arrhythmias, conduction delays, and nonspecific ST-T changes.

V. **Etiology.** Hypertension and coronary artery disease are the most frequent causes of HF in the United States. Additional etiologies include primary abnormalities of myocardial muscle, abnormalities of valvular function, and pericardial disease. "High output" HF may occur with severe anemia, arteriovenous shunts, thyrotoxicosis, or beriberi. Depending on the etiology, the heart may be dilated (predominantly systolic dysfunction) or nondilated (predominantly diastolic dysfunction). Table 6-1 contains one of many schemes for classifying the etiologies of HF.

VI. **Precipitants** of HF include myocardial ischemia or infarction, hypertension, ventricular or supraventricular arrhythmias, infection, anemia, pregnancy, thyroid disease, volume overload, toxins (alcohol, doxorubicin), drugs (beta-adrenergic antagonists, nonsteroidal antiinflammatory drugs [NSAIDs], calcium channel antagonists), pulmonary embolism, and dietary or medical noncompliance.

Table 6-1. Common causes of heart failure

I. Coronary artery disease
II. Hypertensive heart disease
  A. Diastolic dysfunction
  B. Systolic dysfunction
III. Dilated cardiomyopathy
  A. Idiopathic
  B. Toxic (e.g., alcohol, doxorubicin)
  C. Infection (viral, parasitic, and others)
  D. Collagen vascular disease
IV. Valvular heart disease
V. Hypertrophic cardiomyopathy
VI. Restrictive cardiomyopathy
  A. Amyloidosis
  B. Sarcoidosis
  C. Hemochromatosis
VII. Constrictive pericarditis
VIII. High-output heart failure
  A. Chronic anemia
  B. Atrioventricular shunts
  C. Thyrotoxicosis

General Management Considerations

I. **The initial approach to the patient with HF must be individualized** according to severity, acuity of presentation, etiology, presence of coexisting illness, and precipitating factors. Identification of etiology and precipitating factors is essential since the beneficial effect of one type of treatment of HF (e.g., nitrates for ischemia) may be deleterious when applied to another (e.g., aortic stenosis). After a careful history, physical examination, and directed diagnostic evaluation, treatment should be based on clinical assessment of the degree of myocardial dysfunction, total body and intravascular volume status, and extent of peripheral vasoconstriction. General principles of treatment include correction of precipitating processes, control of fluid and sodium retention, optimization of myocardial contractile function, minimization of cardiac workload, and reduction of pulmonary and systemic venous congestion. Close attention to clinical parameters such as weight, vital signs, fluid intake, and urine output is critical to guiding treatment of HF.

II. **Nonpharmacologic** therapeutic measures are generally used in conjunction with specific pharmacologic measures.

  A. **Restriction of physical activity** and bed rest are useful acutely to reduce myocardial workload and oxygen consumption in patients with symptomatic HF. After stabilization, carefully guided cardiac rehabilitation and exercise may improve functional capacity in selected patients with HF (*Circulation* 79:324, 1989). Prophylaxis for deep venous thrombosis should be provided with heparin (5,000 IU SC bid) during periods of bed rest.

  B. **Weight loss** in obese patients reduces SVR as well as myocardial oxygen demand; however, maintenance of adequate caloric intake in patients with severe heart failure is necessary to prevent or correct cardiac cachexia.

  C. **Dietary sodium restriction** (<2 g Na^+/day) will facilitate control of signs and symptoms of HF and minimize diuretic requirements.

D. **Fluid and free water restriction** (<1.5 liters/day) is important in the setting of hyponatremia (serum sodium <130 mEq/liter) and volume overload. Fluid restriction is critical when serum sodium is <125 mEq/liter to prevent arrhythmias and neurologic abnormalities.

E. **Discontinuation of medications with negative inotropic effects** (e.g., beta-adrenergic antagonists, verapamil, diltiazem, disopyramide, flecainide), if possible, may improve signs and symptoms of HF in patients with impaired ventricular contractility. Aspirin and NSAIDs may attenuate the efficacy of or potentiate the renal toxicity of angiotensin-converting enzyme (ACE) inhibitors (*J Am Coll Cardiol* 20:1549, 1992).

F. **Administration of oxygen** may relieve dyspnea, improve oxygen delivery, reduce the work of breathing, and limit pulmonary vasoconstriction in patients with hypoxemia. **Smoking cessation** is also important to optimize oxygen-carrying capacity and to reduce the risk of coronary disease.

G. **Dialysis or ultrafiltration** may be necessary in patients with severe HF and renal dysfunction who cannot respond adequately to fluid and sodium limitation or diuretics. Other mechanical methods of fluid removal such as therapeutic thoracentesis, paracentesis, phlebotomy, and rotating tourniquets may provide temporary symptomatic relief of dyspnea and ascites, as well as edema and pulmonary congestion. Care must be taken to avoid excessively rapid fluid removal and subsequent hypotension.

Specific Pharmacologic Agents

Principles of pharmacologic therapy include vasodilator therapy, control of sodium and fluid retention, and inotropic support of depressed left ventricular function. Vasodilators are the cornerstone of therapy for patients with HF. Diuretics are reserved for patients with volume overload. Several large multicenter studies have demonstrated the importance of a multidrug regimen to prolong survival in patients with HF.

I. **Vasodilator therapy.** Arterial and venous vasoconstriction occurs in patients with HF due to compensatory activation of the adrenergic and renin-angiotensin systems, as well as increased secretion of arginine vasopressin. Arterial vasoconstriction impairs myocardial performance by increasing the impedance (**afterload**) against which the ventricle ejects blood, raising intracardiac filling pressures, increasing myocardial wall stress, and predisposing to subendocardial ischemia. Reflexive arteriolar vasoconstriction in renal, hepatic, mesenteric, cerebral, and myocardial vascular beds results in further hypoperfusion and vital organ dysfunction in patients with severe HF. Venous vasoconstriction limits venous capacitance, resulting in venous congestion and elevated diastolic ventricular filling pressures (**preload**). Pulmonary arterial vasoconstriction may occur as a result of hypoxia, in response to chronically elevated pulmonary blood flow (e.g., left-to-right intracardiac shunts), or chronically elevated left atrial pressure (e.g., mitral stenosis, mitral regurgitation, or left ventricular failure).

Vasodilators can selectively reduce afterload, preload, or both (balanced vasodilators). Agents with predominantly venodilatory properties decrease preload and ventricular filling pressures by favoring redistribution of blood from the pulmonary to the systemic venous bed. In the absence of left ventricular outflow tract obstruction, arterial dilators reduce afterload by decreasing SVR, which results in improved cardiac output, decreased ventricular filling pressure, and decreased wall stress. Patients with valvular regurgitation, severe HF with elevated SVR, or HF with associated hypertension will most likely benefit from afterload reduction with arterial vasodilators. The efficacy and toxicity of vasodilator therapy depend on intravascular volume status and preload. Hypotension, orthostasis, and prerenal azotemia may result from treatment with venous or arterial dilators in the setting of low or normal ventricular filling pressures. Particular caution is necessary in patients with a fixed cardiac output (e.g., aortic stenosis, idiopathic hypertrophic subaortic stenosis) or with predominantly diastolic dysfunction (restrictive or hypertrophic cardiomyopathy and tamponade).

A. Oral vasodilators should be considered initial therapy in patients with symptomatic chronic HF and in patients in whom parenteral agents are being discontinued. When initiating treatment with oral vasodilators, it may be prudent to use agents that have short half-lives.

   1. Angiotensin-converting enzyme (ACE) inhibitors attenuate vasoconstriction, vital organ hypoperfusion, hyponatremia, hypokalemia, and fluid retention attributable to compensatory activation of the renin-angiotensin system. Treatment with ACE inhibitors decreases ventricular filling pressures and SVR while increasing cardiac output, with little or no change in BP or heart rate. Hypotension and renal insufficiency may develop in the setting of reduced preload and may respond to a reduction in the dose of diuretics or venodilating agents or to cautious volume expansion. Absence of an initial beneficial response to treatment with an ACE inhibitor does not preclude long-term benefit. Acute renal insufficiency may occur in patients with **bilateral renal artery stenosis**. Additional adverse effects include rash, angioedema, dysgeusia, increases in serum creatinine, proteinuria, hyperkalemia, leukopenia, and cough. Levels of serum creatinine and electrolytes, urinalysis, and blood counts should be monitored periodically during treatment. Oral potassium supplements, potassium salt substitutes, and potassium-sparing diuretics should be used with caution during treatment with ACE inhibitors, and serum potassium levels should be followed closely. Most ACE inhibitors are excreted by the kidneys, necessitating careful dose titration in patients with renal insufficiency.

      a. Captopril has been shown to significantly reduce symptoms of HF, improve exercise tolerance, and increase functional capacity (*J Am Coll Cardiol* 2:755, 1983). Captopril attenuates ventricular enlargement and improves hemodynamics and survival rates in patients with left ventricular dysfunction due to myocardial infarction (*N Engl J Med* 327:669, 1992). It may also reduce mortality in patients with severe HF when compared with patients receiving hydralazine and nitrates (*J Am Coll Cardiol* 19:842, 1992). Treatment is initiated at dosages of 6.25–12.50 mg PO q6–8h. The dose of captopril can be increased at each subsequent dosage interval, with close attention to BP, urine output, and serum creatinine, and may be titrated up to 50 mg q6h as BP and renal function permit. Because captopril contains a sulfhydryl group, agranulocytosis and angioedema may be more common than with other ACE inhibitors, particularly in patients with associated collagen vascular disease or serum creatinine greater than 1.5 mg/dl.

      b. Enalapril is hepatically hydrolyzed to the active ACE inhibitor enalaprilat. Enalapril has been shown to improve survival rates in patients with mild, moderate, and severe heart failure (*N Engl J Med* 316:1429, 1987; *N Engl J Med* 325:293, 1991). Enalapril also significantly reduced the development of HF in patients with asymptomatic left ventricular dysfunction (*N Engl J Med* 327:685, 1992). The onset of action and duration of effect (12–24 hours) are significantly longer than with captopril (6–8 hours). The initial dose is 2.5–5.0 mg PO qd–bid; however, patients with severe HF, diabetes, hyponatremia (sodium <130 mEq/liter), or creatinine greater than 1.6 mg/dl should start treatment at 2.5 mg PO qd under close observation. Higher initial doses may result in prolonged hypotension, renal insufficiency, and hyperkalemia. Doses should be titrated carefully to a maximum of 20 mg PO bid. The incidence of agranulocytosis may be less with enalapril than with captopril.

      c. Lisinopril is a long-acting ACE inhibitor approved for use in hypertension and HF. The initial dose is 10 mg PO qd in patients with a creatinine clearance (Cl_{cr}) greater than 30 ml/minute. Patients with a Cl_{cr} of 10–30 ml/minute should start at 5 mg PO qd. In patients with severe renal insufficiency (CL_{cr} <10 ml/minute), the initial dose should be 2.5 mg PO qd. The hypotensive effect of lisinopril is potentiated by diuretics, and careful monitoring is suggested for patients receiving diuretics and lisinopril.

   d. Quinapril has recently been approved for use in HF. The initial dose is 10 mg PO qd with a maximum dose of 80 mg qd or 40 mg bid. The dosage should be lowered for patients with impaired renal function or those receiving diuretics.

   e. Ramipril, fosinapril, and benazepril are available and approved for use in hypertension. Although these agents are not approved for use in HF, there are data indicating their efficacy. The experience with these agents is limited compared to that with captopril, enalapril, and lisinopril (see Chap. 4).

2. **Nitrates** are predominantly venodilators and are therefore beneficial in relieving symptoms of venous and pulmonary congestion. Nitrates reduce myocardial ischemia by decreasing ventricular filling pressures and directly dilating coronary arteries. In combination with hydralazine, nitrates have been demonstrated to decrease mortality in patients with HF (*N Engl J Med* 314:1547, 1986). Nitrate therapy may induce hypotension in patients with reduced preload. Hypotension is usually responsive to volume expansion and reduction in dose. Improved hemodynamics and symptomatic relief may be seen after the first dose in the majority of patients but may be transient due to development of nitrate tolerance (see Chap. 5). Nitrates can be administered as oral short-acting or sustained-release forms as well as transdermally.

3. **Hydralazine** is an afterload-reducing agent that acts directly on arterial smooth muscle to produce vasodilation. It is particularly useful in the treatment of regurgitant valvular lesions (see Specific Management Considerations, sec. I). In combination with nitrates, hydralazine offers a survival advantage to patients with HF. Dosage requirements vary widely but average 25–100 mg PO tid or qid. Hemodynamic tolerance has been reported and may be reduced by concomitant diuretic use. Reflex tachycardia and increased myocardial oxygen consumption may occur, requiring cautious use in patients with ischemic heart disease. Other adverse effects include headache, flushing, nausea, vomiting, and fluid retention. A **drug-induced lupus-like syndrome** may develop in patients receiving daily doses of 200 mg or more for prolonged periods but is generally reversible with discontinuation of the drug. Antinuclear antibodies (ANAs) may develop in up to 50% of patients, but the drug should not be discontinued unless symptoms of lupus develop.

4. **Adrenergic receptor antagonists** theoretically may attenuate some of the adverse effects attributable to compensatory activation of the sympathetic nervous system in HF. Alpha-adrenergic blockade reduces vasoconstriction, SVR, and afterload by antagonizing the effects of norepinephrine. Beta-adrenergic blockade in the treatment of HF is controversial but may limit the adverse effects of high levels of endogenous catecholamines on the failing heart.

   a. Alpha-adrenergic receptor antagonists such as **prazosin** and **doxazosin** have vasodilatory properties and are effective antihypertensive medications, with side effects of orthostatic hypotension and reflex tachycardia. Neither has been shown to improve survival in HF patients, possibly because beneficial hemodynamic effects are short lived secondary to the development of tolerance (*N Engl J Med* 314:1547, 1986).

   b. Beta-adrenergic receptor antagonists are theoretically useful in the treatment of HF by blocking the cardiac effects of chronic adrenergic stimulation (direct myocyte toxicity, down-regulation of cardiac beta receptors). Some new beta-adrenergic antagonists have $beta_2$ receptor agonist activity and peripheral vasodilatory actions, which clinically compensate for their negative inotropy. Many HF patients experience improvement in ejection fraction, exercise tolerance, and functional class following the institution of a beta-adrenergic antagonist, but caution must be used when initiating this therapy. It has been shown that 2–3 months of therapy are required to observe significant hemodynamic improvement, but the effect may be long-lasting (*Am J Cardiol* 71:12C, 1993). Except in patients with hypertrophic cardiomyopathy and dynamic outflow tract obstruction or those with diastolic dysfunction, beta-adrenergic receptor antagonist therapy in HF is still investigational.

5. **Calcium channel antagonists** directly relax vascular smooth muscle and inhibit calcium entry into myocardial cells. These agents have a beneficial effect on diastolic relaxation and are useful in the treatment of ischemic heart disease. However, the vasodilatory effects of some of the first-generation calcium channel antagonists (**diltiazem** and **verapamil**) are counterbalanced by their negative inotropic properties and have been shown to have detrimental effects in patients with left ventricular dysfunction (*J Am Coll Cardiol* 22:139A, 1993). Nicardipine has a more favorable hemodynamic profile, but preliminary data on its efficacy in the treatment of patients with HF are contradictory and clinical deterioration in HF has been reported (*J Am Coll Cardiol* 17[Suppl. A]:274A, 1991; *J Am Coll Cardiol* 21[Suppl. A]:377A, 1993). Preliminary results suggest that the addition of amlodipine or felodipine to diuretics, digoxin, and an ACE inhibitor may result in improved exercise tolerance and symptoms compared to placebo (*J Am Coll Cardiol* 17:274A, 1991).

B. **Parenteral vasodilators** should be reserved for patients with severe HF or those unable to take oral medications. IV vasodilator therapy should be guided by continuous central hemodynamic monitoring (pulmonary artery catheterization) to assess efficacy and avoid hypotension. Parenteral agents should be started at low doses, titrated to hemodynamic effect, and discontinued slowly to avoid rebound vasoconstriction.

1. **Nitroglycerin** is a potent vasodilator with effects on venous and, to a lesser extent, arterial vascular beds. It relieves pulmonary and systemic venous congestion. It is also an effective coronary vasodilator and is the preferred vasodilator for treatment of HF in the setting of acute myocardial infarction or unstable angina. Onset of action is rapid, with a half-life of 1–3 minutes, which allows rapid titration and discontinuation if necessary. IV nitroglycerin is initiated at a dose of 10 μg/minute through adsorption-resistant tubing by infusion pump. The dose can be titrated according to hemodynamic effect and is limited by the development of hypotension. Doses greater than 300 μg/minute provide no additional benefit and may be associated with significant hypotension. In the absence of adequate preload, IV nitroglycerin may cause hypotension that is typically responsive to discontinuation of the infusion and volume expansion. Nitrate tolerance, necessitating increased dose, develops in as little as 12 hours. Conversion to intermittent oral or topical nitrate preparations should be accomplished as early as possible to reduce the probability of developing tolerance.

2. **Sodium nitroprusside** is a direct arterial vasodilator with less potent venodilatory properties. Its predominant effect is to **reduce afterload**, and it is particularly effective in patients with HF who are hypertensive or have severe valvular regurgitation. Nitroprusside should be used cautiously in patients with myocardial ischemia due to potential reduction in regional myocardial blood flow ("coronary steal"). The initial dose of 10 μg/minute can be titrated (maximum dose of 300–400 μg/minute) to the desired hemodynamic effect or until hypotension develops. The half-life of nitroprusside is 1–3 minutes, and its metabolism results in the release of cyanide, which is hepatically metabolized to thiocyanate that is renally excreted. Toxic levels of thiocyanate (>10 mg/dl) may develop in patients with renal insufficiency, necessitating close monitoring of serum levels. Thiocyanate toxicity is manifested as nausea, mental status changes, abdominal pain, seizures, and metabolic acidosis (see Chap. 4). Methemoglobinemia is a rare complication of treatment with nitroprusside.

3. **Enalaprilat** is a deesterified active metabolite of enalapril available for IV administration. Onset of action is more rapid, and pharmacologic half-life is shorter than that of enalapril. The initial dose is 1.25 mg IV q6h, which can be titrated to a maximum dosage of 5 mg IV q6h. Patients taking diuretics or those with impaired renal function (serum creatinine >3 mg/dl, Cl_{cr} <30 ml/minute) should initially receive 0.625 mg IV q6h. When converting from IV to PO administration, 0.625 mg IV q6h of enalaprilat is approximately equivalent to 2.5 mg PO qd of enalapril.

II. **Digitalis glycosides** increase myocardial contractility through reversible inhibition of sarcolemmal sodium-potassium adenosine triphosphatase (ATPase) activity. Digoxin is most efficacious in the management of HF (1) accompanied or caused by atrial fibrillation or flutter (or other supraventricular tachycardias that respond to digoxin) or (2) in patients with dilated left ventricles and impaired systolic function manifested by a third heart sound, low ejection fraction, and large cardiothoracic ratio. Several studies have shown improvement in ejection fraction and exercise tolerance in patients with chronic HF who receive digoxin (*N Engl J Med* 320:677, 1989). Discontinuation of digoxin in patients who are stable on a regimen of digoxin, diuretics, and an ACE inhibitor may result in clinical deterioration (*N Engl J Med* 329:1, 1993). The toxic-therapeutic ratio is narrow, and serum levels should be followed closely. Hypokalemia and hypoxemia may exacerbate toxicity and should be corrected prior to initiation of and during digoxin therapy.

A. **Dosage and route of administration** are dictated by the underlying condition and the severity of illness. Bioavailability is less with oral preparations (approximately 60–85% in tablet form, 90–100% in liquid-filled capsules), and onset of action is most rapid with IV therapy (15–30 minutes versus two hours with oral administration). The serum half-life is 33–44 hours with normal renal function. **Digoxin loading** is accomplished by giving 0.25–0.50 mg PO or IV initially, followed by 0.25 mg q6h to a total dose of 1.0–1.5 mg. Evidence of toxicity (see sec. **II.D**) should be sought before each successive dose. **Maintenance therapy** is affected by the patient's age, lean body weight, and renal function. The usual daily dose is 0.125–0.375 mg and should be decreased in patients with renal insufficiency. Assessment of serum digoxin levels should ultimately determine optimum dosing in patients with renal insufficiency, in those receiving drugs that may interfere with digoxin metabolism, and when noncompliance is suspected. Levels of 0.8–2.0 ng/ml are generally considered therapeutic, but toxicity can occur in this range. Some patients may require high levels to control the ventricular response in atrial fibrillation. Drug levels should not be drawn within 8 hours of administration of a dose since distribution is incomplete and the result is not interpretable.

B. **Drug interactions** with digoxin are frequent and include impaired absorption of digoxin by cholestyramine, kaolin-pectin, and antacids, which may decrease bioavailability by 25%. Oral antibiotics such as erythromycin and tetracycline may increase digoxin levels by 10–40%. **Quinidine increases serum digoxin levels up to twofold;** the maintenance dose of digoxin should therefore be reduced by 50% in patients receiving both drugs. Verapamil, flecainide, and amiodarone also increase digoxin levels significantly.

C. **Contraindications** to digoxin use are rare, but additional caution should be exercised in several settings. Since digoxin may increase myocardial oxygen demand, its use in the presence of acute myocardial infarction should be limited to the treatment of supraventricular tachyarrhythmias and overt HF due to reduced systolic performance. Atrioventricular (AV) conduction disturbances may be exacerbated by digoxin; conversely, conduction through accessory AV pathways may be potentiated. Electrolyte abnormalities, especially hypokalemia and hypomagnesemia, increase the likelihood of digoxin toxicity and should always be corrected before initiation of therapy. **Cardioversion in the presence of digoxin toxicity is contraindicated,** as potentially fatal ventricular arrhythmias may be precipitated; however, with serum levels in the therapeutic range, cardioversion can be attempted with little increased risk.

D. **Digoxin toxicity** remains an important clinical problem, occurring in 5–15% of patients at some time during therapy. The therapeutic range is narrow, and toxicity may develop despite serum levels within the usual therapeutic range. Factors that may contribute to the development of toxicity include drug interactions, electrolyte abnormalities (particularly hypokalemia), hypoxemia, hypothyroidism, renal insufficiency, and volume depletion.

1. **Clinical manifestations** of digoxin toxicity include virtually all forms of cardiac arrhythmias. Ventricular premature depolarizations (often in a bigeminal pattern), junctional tachycardia, and varying degrees of second-degree AV block are frequently present. Bidirectional ventricular tachycardia, paroxysmal atrial tachycardia with AV block, and regularization of atrial fibrillation occur almost exclusively as a result of digoxin toxicity. Noncardiac manifestations of toxicity include GI and neuropsychiatric symptoms. Anorexia, nausea, vomiting, and diarrhea may compound toxic effects by worsening hypokalemia. Altered mental status, agitation, lethargy, and visual disturbances (scotomas and color perception changes) are frequent.

2. **Treatment of digoxin toxicity** includes discontinuation of the drug, correction of precipitating factors, and continuous ECG monitoring. The serum potassium should be maintained in the high-normal range but should be repleted cautiously since rapid increases in serum potassium (even within the normal range) can precipitate complete heart block. Symptomatic bradycardia can be controlled with atropine or temporary pacing as needed; sympathomimetics should be avoided, as they may precipitate or worsen ventricular arrhythmias. Lidocaine or phenytoin should be used to control ventricular and atrial arrhythmias; **quinidine should not be used,** because it may elevate serum levels further (see Chap. 7). Cardioversion is contraindicated unless all other measures of controlling hemodynamically significant arrhythmias have been exhausted.

3. **Digoxin-specific Fab antibody fragments** are effective in rapidly reversing life-threatening digoxin intoxication (*J Am Coll Cardiol* 17:590, 1991) and should be considered when other modes of therapy are inadequate. Digoxin-Fab fragment complexes are cleared from the circulation via renal excretion. **Total serum digoxin levels are no longer meaningful following administration of Fab fragments;** free (unbound) digoxin can be measured when serum level monitoring is required. Significant adverse effects have not been reported with the use of the antibody fragments. Each 40-mg vial of Fab fragments neutralizes approximately 0.6 mg of digoxin. Dosage is based on the estimated amount of drug ingested or the steady-state serum level and can be calculated as follows:

Acute digoxin ingestion:

Dose (no. of vials) = [ingested digoxin dose (mg) × 0.8]/0.6

Chronic digoxin intoxication:

Dose (no. of vials) = [serum level (ng/ml) × weight (kg)]/100

The Fab fragments should be reconstituted in **sterile water** (4 ml/vial). The reconstituted solution may then be diluted in 0.9% sodium chloride solution to a convenient volume for infusion. The solution should be infused over 15–30 minutes through a 0.22-μm filter to remove remaining protein aggregates. The dosage should be repeated if toxicity is not adequately reversed with the initial administration.

III. **Diuretics** (Table 6-2; see Chap. 4) in conjunction with restriction of dietary sodium and fluids often lead to clinical improvement in patients with mild to moderate HF. Frequent assessment of the patient's weight along with careful observation of fluid intake and output are essential during initiation and maintenance of therapy. When diuretics are initiated for an acute exacerbation of HF, the goal of therapy should be a maximum net loss of 0.5–1.0 liter of fluid/day (0.5–1.0 kg body weight) to prevent intravascular volume depletion. Frequent complications of therapy

Table 6-2. Diuretic agents used in heart failure

Agent	Site of action	Relative potency	Route of administration[a]	Average daily dose (mg)[b]	Onset of action	Duration of action
Thiazides						
Chlorothiazide	Distal tubule	++	PO	250–500	2 hr	6–12 hr
			IV	500	15 min	1 hr
Hydrochlorothiazide	Distal tubule	++	PO	25–100	2 hr	12 hr
Chlorthalidone	Distal tubule	++	PO	25–100	2 hr	48 hr
Metolazone	Proximal, distal tubules	+++	PO	2.5–20.0	1 hr	24–48 hr
Indapamide	Distal tubule	++	PO	2.5–5.0	2 hr	24 hr
Loop diuretics						
Furosemide	Loop of Henle	++++	PO	20–80[c]	1 hr	6–8 hr
			IV, IM	10–80[c]	5 min	2–4 hr
Ethacrynic acid			PO	25–100	30 min	6–8 hr
			IV	50	5 min	3 hr
Bumetanide			PO	0.5–2.0	30 min	2 hr
			IV, IM	0.5–2.0 (10 max)	5 min	30 min
Torsemide			PO	5–10	2 hr	8–12 hr
			IV	5–10	5 min	6–8 hr
Potassium-sparing diuretics	Distal tubule, collecting duct	+				
Spironolactone			PO	50–200	1–2 days	2–3 days
Triamterene			PO	100–200	2–4 days	7–9 days
Amiloride			PO	5–10	2 hr	24 hr

[a] IV doses should be given slowly over 1–2 minutes.
[b] Dose and dosing intervals should be determined by the patient's clinical response.
[c] Larger doses may be required in patients with renal insufficiency.

include hypokalemia, hyponatremia, hypomagnesemia, volume contraction alkalosis, and intravascular volume depletion. Serum electrolytes, BUN, and creatinine should be followed closely after institution of diuretic therapy. Hypokalemia may be life-threatening in patients receiving digoxin or in those who have severe left ventricular dysfunction predisposing to ventricular arrhythmias. Potassium supplementation or a potassium-sparing diuretic should be considered in addition to careful monitoring of serum potassium levels.

A. Thiazide diuretics (hydrochlorothiazide, chlorthalidone) can be used as initial agents in patients with normal renal function in whom only a mild diuresis is desired. Metolazone, unlike other thiazides, exerts its action at the proximal as well as the distal tubule and may be useful in combination with a loop diuretic in patients with a low glomerular filtration rate (GFR). Use of thiazides may be complicated by hypercalcemia, hyperuricemia, rash, pancreatitis, vasculitis, and increased low-density lipoprotein levels. Indapamide is a long-acting agent with a potency equal to other thiazide diuretics but appears to have fewer adverse effects on serum lipids.

B. Loop diuretics (furosemide, bumetanide, ethacrynic acid) should be used in patients who require significant diuresis and in patients with markedly decreased renal function. Furosemide reduces preload acutely by causing direct venodilatation when administered intravenously. This property renders furosemide particularly useful for the management of severe HF or acute pulmonary edema. Patients with chronic HF may become refractory to oral diuretics as a result of diminished GI absorption secondary to bowel edema but respond readily when given an equivalent dose of IV diuretic. Use of loop diuretics may be complicated by hyperuricemia, hypocalcemia, ototoxicity, rash, and vasculitis. Furosemide and bumetanide are sulfa derivatives and may cause drug reactions in sulfa-sensitive patients. Ethacrynic acid can generally be used safely in such patients; however, ototoxicity may be more common with this agent.

C. Potassium-sparing diuretics (spironolactone, triamterene, amiloride) are minimally effective for the management of HF when used alone. However, when combined with a thiazide or loop diuretic they are often effective in maintaining normal serum potassium levels. The potential for development of life-threatening hyperkalemia exists with the use of these agents. Serum potassium must be monitored closely following their administration; concomitant use of ACE inhibitors and NSAIDs and diabetes increase the risk of hyperkalemia.

IV. Inotropic agents

A. Sympathomimetic agents (see Appendix C) are potent inotropes primarily used to treat severe HF. Beneficial and adverse effects are mediated by stimulation of myocardial beta adrenoreceptors. The most important adverse effects are related to the arrhythmogenic nature of these agents and the potential for exacerbation of myocardial ischemia; tachycardia and ventricular arrhythmias may be decreased by lower dosage. Treatment should be guided by careful hemodynamic and electrocardiographic monitoring.

1. Dopamine is an endogenous catecholamine that exerts selective renal and mesenteric vasodilatation at doses of 1–3 µg/kg/minute via dopaminergic-receptor stimulation, resulting in improved renal blood flow and urine output. Positive inotropic effects are produced with doses of 2–5 µg/kg/minute and are secondary to **beta$_1$-adrenoreceptor stimulation.** At doses of 5–10 µg/kg/minute, **alpha-adrenoreceptor** stimulation occurs; the resulting peripheral vasoconstriction increases SVR and may be deleterious in patients with low cardiac output and HF. Dopamine should be used primarily for stabilization of the hypotensive patient.

2. Dobutamine is a synthetic agent that selectively stimulates beta$_1$-adrenoreceptors; beta$_2$ and alpha receptors are activated to a much lesser degree. Its predominant hemodynamic effect is direct inotropic stimulation with reflex arterial vasodilatation, resulting in afterload reduction and augmentation of cardiac output. BP generally remains constant and heart rate may increase minimally. Tachycardia may result from excessive doses or if left ventricular filling pressure falls in response to improved ventricular performance. Dobutamine is administered as a constant infusion that is initiated at a rate of 1–2 µg/kg/minute and is titrated to obtain the desired hemodynamic effect or until excessive tachycardia or ventricular arrhythmias occur. In the absence of tachycardia, dobutamine does not increase myocardial oxygen requirements excessively. Patients with refractory chronic HF may benefit symptomatically from intermittent dobutamine infusion for 2–4 days or from continuous ambulatory administration via a portable infusion device. The latter usually requires placement of a central venous catheter. Dobutamine tolerance has been described, and some studies have indicated an increased mortality for patients treated with continuous dobutamine. Patients undergoing continuous therapy should be closely monitored, and infusion rates of 10 µg/kg/minute or less should be used. Dobutamine has no significant role in the treatment of HF resulting from diastolic dysfunction (e.g., hypertrophic cardiomyopathy) or a high-output state.

B. Phosphodiesterase inhibitors (see Appendix C) increase myocardial contractility and produce vasodilation by increasing intracellular cyclic adenosine monophosphate (cAMP). **Amrinone** and **milrinone** are currently available for clinical use and are indicated for short-term treatment of refractory HF. Amrinone has hemodynamic effects similar to dobutamine but with more vasodilatory properties. Thus, hypotension may develop in patients receiving vasodilator therapy or who have intravascular volume contraction. Amrinone may improve hemodynamics in patients treated concurrently with digoxin, dobutamine, or dopamine. IV administration of a 750-µg/kg bolus over 2–3 minutes followed by a continuous infusion of 2.5–10.0 µg/kg/minute is recommended. Milrinone is structurally similar to amrinone and has comparable hemodynamic effects. A loading dose of 50 µg/kg is administered over 10 minutes, followed by a continuous infusion of 0.375–0.750 µg/kg/minute to achieve the desired clinical response. The principal side effects of the phosphodiesterase inhibitors include atrial and ventricular arrhythmias and thrombocytopenia.

C. Vesnarinone is a quinoline derivative with positive inotropic properties that is currently investigational but has demonstrated efficacy for long-term oral use. When added to digoxin and ACE inhibitors in patients with HF, vesnarinone, 60 mg/day, has been demonstrated to reduce mortality rates by 50% and improve quality of life (*N Engl J Med* 329:149, 1993). However, higher doses (120 mg/day) should be avoided due to potential deleterious effects. The primary side effect appears to be neutropenia that is reversible with discontinuation of the drug.

V. Mechanical circulatory support may be considered for patients in whom other therapeutic modalities have failed, who have transient myocardial dysfunction, or in whom a more definitive procedure is planned.

A. The **intraaortic balloon pump** can be placed percutaneously through the femoral artery and is positioned in the aorta with its tip distal to the left subclavian artery. Balloon inflation is synchronous with the cardiac cycle and occurs during diastole. The hemodynamic consequences of balloon counterpulsation are decreased myocardial oxygen demand and improved coronary blood flow. Additionally, significant preload and afterload reduction occurs, resulting in improved cardiac output.

B. Ventricular assist devices (VADs) require surgical implantation and are indicated for patients with severe HF following cardiac surgery, in patients who have intractable cardiogenic shock following acute MI, and in patients who deteriorate while awaiting cardiac transplantation. Currently available devices vary with regard to degree of mechanical hemolysis, intensity of anticoagulation required, and the difficulty of implantation. Therefore the decision to institute VAD circulatory support must be made in consultation with a cardiac surgeon experienced in this procedure.

VI. Cardiac transplantation is an effective therapeutic option for selected patients with severe end-stage heart disease that has become refractory to aggressive medical therapy and for whom there are no other conventional treatment options.

A. Candidates considered for transplantation should be less than 60 years old (although selected older patients derive significant benefits), have advanced HF (New York Heart Association functional class III–IV), have a strong psychosocial support system, have exhausted all other therapeutic options, and be free of irreversible extracardiac organ dysfunction that would limit functional recovery or predispose to posttransplant complications (*J Am Coll Cardiol* 22:1, 1993).

B. Survival rates of 90% at 1 year and 65–70% at 5 years have been reported since the introduction of cyclosporine. In general, functional capacity and quality of life improve significantly after transplantation.

C. Immunosuppressive therapy typically includes glucocorticoids, cyclosporine, and azathioprine. Several new immunosuppressive agents are under investigation and may offer benefits in selected patients.

D. Posttransplant complications include acute rejection, infection due to immunosuppression (see Chap. 14), and adverse effects of immunosuppressive agents. Aggressive posttransplant coronary artery disease is the leading cause of death after the first posttransplant year.

Specific Management Considerations

I. Valvular heart disease

A. Mitral stenosis (MS) impedes blood flow from the lungs and left atrium into the left ventricle. Rheumatic heart disease is the most common etiology; much less commonly, it may result from calcium deposition in the mitral annulus and leaflets, a congenital valvular malformation, or in association with connective tissue disorders. Left atrial myxoma and cor triatriatum may mimic MS clinically. Prosthetic mitral valves (particularly bioprosthetic valves) may become stenotic late after implantation.

 1. Pathophysiology. Significant MS results in elevation of left atrial, pulmonary venous, and pulmonary capillary pressures with resultant pulmonary congestion. The degree of pressure elevation depends on the severity of the pressure gradient across the mitral valve, which depends on the severity of obstruction, flow across the valve, time allowed for diastolic filling, and presence of effective atrial contraction. Therefore, factors that augment flow across the stenotic mitral valve, such as tachycardia, exercise, fever, and pregnancy, cause a marked increase in left atrial pressure and may exacerbate symptoms of HF. Left atrial enlargement and fibrillation may result in atrial thrombus formation, which is primarily responsible for the high incidence of systemic embolization in patients with MS who are not anticoagulated (approximately 20% of patients).

 2. Diagnosis. Symptoms of dyspnea and pulmonary congestion are prominent. Physical signs of pulmonary venous congestion and right heart volume and pressure overload are often present. A prominent first heart sound, early diastolic "opening snap," and rumbling diastolic murmur are present on auscultation. The diagnosis and severity of MS can be confirmed by two-dimensional and Doppler echocardiography. Cardiac catheterization is indicated in patients with (1) a likelihood of concomitant coronary artery disease, (2) technically suboptimal or nondiagnostic echocardiographic studies, and (3) other suspected valvular lesions such as mitral regurgitation. Transesophageal echocardiography (TEE) may be used to confirm the diagnosis, define the anatomy more fully, or provide diagnostic information in patients in whom transthoracic echocardiography is suboptimal.

 3. Medical management

 a. Factors that increase left atrial pressure, including tachycardia and fever, should be identified and alleviated. Vigorous physical activity should be avoided in patients with moderate to severe MS.

 b. Diuretics (see Table 6-2) are the mainstay of therapy for pulmonary congestion and edema.

     c. Anticoagulant therapy is indicated for patients with MS and atrial fibrillation, since they are at high risk for thromboembolic events. Heparin therapy should be instituted at the onset of atrial fibrillation, followed by long-term warfarin therapy (see Chap. 17). In the absence of prior embolic events, marked left atrial enlargement, or demonstrable atrial thrombi, patients with sinus rhythm do not require anticoagulation.

     d. Atrial fibrillation may not be tolerated. Synchronized DC cardioversion should be performed if hemodynamic compromise (hypotension, pulmonary edema, and angina) accompanies the onset of atrial fibrillation. In less urgent situations, the ventricular response rate to atrial fibrillation can be controlled with IV diltiazem, 0.25 mg/kg bolus over 2 minutes (an additional 0.35 mg/kg bolus may be given 10 minutes after the first bolus if the desired clinical response is not achieved), followed by an infusion of 5–15 mg/hour or 60 mg PO tid. **Digoxin** is another effective agent for ventricular rate control in atrial fibrillation (see sec. II.A). **Verapamil,** 5–10 mg IV or 80 mg PO tid, or **propranolol,** 20 mg PO q6h, can also be used to slow the ventricular response and provide greater diastolic filling time. An attempt to restore and maintain sinus rhythm is indicated except in the presence of marked left atrial enlargement (i.e., >6 cm). Following institution of rate control measures, elective cardioversion should be attempted with administration of a type I_A antiarrhythmic agent (quinidine or procainamide) (see Chap. 7). **Elective attempts at chemical or electrical cardioversion should be preceded by anticoagulation therapy for at least 3 weeks** to minimize the risk of systemic embolization on resumption of normal sinus rhythm. If chemical cardioversion fails to restore sinus rhythm, elective synchronized DC cardioversion should be performed. Following conversion to sinus rhythm, type I_A antiarrhythmics can be continued in an effort to maintain sinus rhythm.

     e. Infective endocarditis prophylaxis is indicated (see Chap. 13).

     f. Continuous prophylaxis against recurrent rheumatic fever is indicated in young patients, patients at high risk for streptococcal infection (parents of young children, school teachers, medical and military personnel, and those in crowded living conditions), and those with acute rheumatic fever within the previous 5 years. Continuous antibiotic prophylaxis may be administered through various regimens (see Chap. 13).

  4. Surgical considerations

     a. Patients with severe symptoms and significant MS (mitral valve area <1 cm^2/m^2 body surface area) should undergo commissurotomy or mitral valve replacement (MVR). Those with pulmonary hypertension, even if minimally symptomatic, should also be treated surgically.

     b. Patients with **mild to moderate symptoms** generally show improvement with diuretic therapy and can be followed clinically with serial echocardiograms.

     c. A **single systemic thromboembolic** event does not mandate MVR. However, the recurrence rate of systemic thromboembolism in patients with MS is high and MVR should be strongly considered.

     d. Percutaneous balloon mitral valvuloplasty has been shown to reduce the mitral valve pressure gradient and improve cardiac output in patients with MS. This procedure may be considered an alternative to surgery with acceptable morbidity and mortality rates in select patients without significant mitral regurgitation or a severely calcified valve. Mitral valvuloplasty is usually reserved for patients in whom the surgical risk is high.

B. Aortic stenosis (AS) in the adult population may result from (1) calcification and degeneration of a normal valve, (2) calcification and fibrosis of a congenitally bicuspid aortic valve, or (3) rheumatic valvular disease.

  1. Pathophysiology. Aortic stenosis produces a pressure gradient from the left ventricle to the aorta, causing pressure overload of the left ventricle, which leads to concentric hypertrophy. As a result, left ventricular compliance is reduced, left ventricular end-diastolic pressure rises, and myocardial oxygen demand is increased as left ventricular mass and wall stress are increased. Elevated left ventricular end-diastolic pressure decreases the perfusion pressure across the myocardium, leading to subendocardial ischemia.

2. **The diagnosis** of significant aortic stenosis may be difficult, as the condition may be asymptomatic for a number of years. Clinical suspicion is often raised by the presence of one or more of the classic symptom triad of **angina, syncope, and HF.** The physical findings of AS include a slowly rising carotid pulse that is sustained (pulsus parvus et tardus), and a mid- to late-peaking systolic murmur, which is usually harsh in quality. The pressure gradient across the stenotic aortic valve is directly related to the severity of obstruction and cardiac output. Therefore, the intensity of the systolic murmur may diminish as the cardiac output decreases with increasingly severe AS. In general, murmurs of long duration that peak late in systole indicate severe AS. Doppler echocardiography provides a noninvasive estimation of the aortic valve gradient and aortic valve area that correlate well with those found at cardiac catheterization. Most patients being considered for aortic valve replacement require preoperative cardiac catheterization with coronary arteriography to determine the presence and extent of concomitant CAD.

3. **Medical management**
   a. **Infective endocarditis** occurs with increased frequency, and prophylaxis is indicated (see Chap. 13).
   b. **Vigorous exercise and physical activity should be avoided** in patients with moderate to severe AS.
   c. **Atrial (and ventricular) arrhythmias** are poorly tolerated and should be treated aggressively.
   d. **Digoxin** may be useful in patients with HF in the presence of left ventricular dilatation and impaired systolic function. However, in severe AS due to the fixed obstruction of left ventricular outflow, inotropic therapy is of little benefit.
   e. **Diuretics** may be useful in treating congestive symptoms but must be **used with extreme caution.** Reduction of left ventricular filling pressure in patients with AS may decrease cardiac output and systemic BP.
   f. **Nitrates and other vasodilators should be avoided** in patients with severe AS if possible. These agents reduce left ventricular filling pressure and may lower systemic BP, resulting in hemodynamic collapse. Patients with AS in whom angina develops may occasionally require treatment with nitroglycerin. Such therapy should be initiated only under strict supervision by a physician at the bedside. Volume expansion with saline may be necessary to avoid excessive preload reduction. If nitroglycerin results in hypotension that does not respond to aggressive volume expansion, parenteral inotropic agents (e.g., dobutamine), vasopressors, or both should be given.
   g. **Asymptomatic patients** with mild to moderate AS can be followed closely with clinical assessment and Doppler echocardiography performed at 6- to 12-month intervals.

4. **Surgical considerations**
   a. **Symptomatic patients** should undergo evaluation for aortic valve replacement (AVR), including two-dimensional and Doppler echocardiography. In patients with suboptimal transthoracic echocardiograms, TEE may be diagnostic. Coronary arteriography should be performed in men older than 40 years and women older than 50 years, as well as in all patients with anginal symptoms; left ventriculography is indicated in patients with coexistent mitral regurgitation (although a high-quality transthoracic or TEE may provide adequate information and limit the total amount of contrast material administered). Patients with severe AS (aortic valve area <0.75 cm^2) should undergo valve replacement unless comorbid conditions preclude surgery. Asymptomatic patients with severe AS are rare and should be considered for valve replacement if left

ventricular dilatation or decreased systolic function is present. Patients with significant **concomitant coronary disease** should undergo surgical revascularization at the time of AVR, because the operative morbidity and mortality for the combined procedure are no greater than for AVR alone.

   b. Intraaortic balloon counterpulsation may stabilize patients with critical AS and hemodynamic decompensation until AVR can be accomplished. It should not be used when significant aortic insufficiency coexists with AS.

   c. Percutaneous balloon aortic valvuloplasty can reduce the aortic valve gradient and improve symptoms and left ventricular function with relatively low morbidity and mortality in select patients. Unfortunately, restenosis occurs in approximately 50% of patients within 6 months. At present, its use should be limited to patients who refuse surgery or who are poor surgical candidates due to comorbid conditions.

C. Mitral regurgitation (MR)

   1. Chronic MR, as an isolated lesion, is most commonly caused by myxomatous degeneration of the mitral valve. Other etiologies include rheumatic heart disease, calcification of the mitral valve annulus, coronary artery disease with associated papillary muscle dysfunction, infective endocarditis, and connective tissue diseases (e.g., Marfan's syndrome, Ehlers-Danlos syndrome). MR may occur as a secondary phenomenon in any patient with left ventricular dilatation.

   a. Pathophysiology. Chronic MR imposes volume overload on the left ventricle as a result of regurgitation of a fraction of the left ventricular blood flow into the left atrium. Normal forward cardiac output is maintained early in the course of the disease, but with progressive MR, compensatory mechanisms no longer accommodate increasing left ventricular end-diastolic volume. Accordingly, ejection fraction falls and symptoms of right and left HF develop.

   b. The diagnosis is suggested by characteristic physical findings of well-preserved carotid pulsations, an enlarged point of maximal impulse (PMI), and an apical holosystolic murmur. Doppler and two-dimensional echocardiography may confirm the diagnosis, estimate the severity of MR, and provide clues to its etiology. TEE is particularly useful for the evaluation of the mitral valve and is used instead of left ventriculography in some institutions. Cardiac catheterization and contrast left ventriculography remain the standard for determining the severity of MR and are required for assessing the need for mitral valve replacement in most patients.

   c. Medical management

   (1) Infective endocarditis prophylaxis should be given (see Chap. 13).

   (2) Anticoagulant therapy should be considered, particularly in the presence of atrial fibrillation, an enlarged left atrium, or a previous embolic event; however, the incidence of thromboembolic events is lower than in MS.

   (3) Atrial fibrillation should be anticipated in the later stages of MR as the left atrium dilates and should be treated as outlined in sec. **I.A.3.c–d.**

   (4) Vasodilators provide hemodynamic improvement in MR by reducing SVR, thus decreasing the mitral regurgitant fraction and augmenting forward cardiac output. Beneficial effects have been demonstrated with **nitroprusside, captopril, enalapril, and hydralazine.**

   (5) Digoxin may be useful in the presence of impaired left ventricular systolic function.

   (6) Diuretics are useful for treating congestive symptoms (see Table 6-2). **Nitrates** can also be used to reduce preload and ventricular size, which may decrease the severity of MR (*Am J Cardiol* 43:773, 1979).

   d. Surgical considerations

   (1) Moderate to severe symptoms despite medical therapy should prompt consideration of mitral valve repair or replacement, provided that left ventricular function is adequate (left ventricular ejection fraction >40%).

(2) **Patients with minimal or no symptoms** should be followed closely with noninvasive assessment of left ventricular size and systolic function (by echocardiography or radionuclide ventriculography) every 6–12 months. Generally, by the time a significant decrease in ejection fraction is noted, marked left ventricular dysfunction has occurred and MVR with its attendant increase in left ventricular afterload may be poorly tolerated or may fail to improve the patient's symptoms. Patients should be considered for mitral valve repair or replacement when the ejection fraction approaches 50–55%.

2. **Acute MR** can result from papillary muscle dysfunction or rupture due to myocardial ischemia or infarction, infective endocarditis with flail or perforated leaflets, severe myxomatous disease with rupture of a chorda resulting in a flail leaflet, or trauma.

   a. **The pathophysiology** of acute MR differs from that of chronic MR in that compensatory increases in left atrial and left ventricular compliance do not occur. The result is a sudden increase in pulmonary venous pressure leading to acute pulmonary edema. Acute MR frequently results in cardiogenic shock necessitating urgent diagnostic evaluation and treatment.

   b. **Medical management**

      (1) **Afterload reduction** should be initiated emergently with **sodium nitroprusside** guided by systemic BP and central hemodynamics. Approximately 50% of patients with acute MR can be stabilized in this manner allowing MVR to proceed under more controlled conditions. The usual starting dose is 0.25 µg/kg/minute.

      (2) **Furosemide,** with or without nitrates, can be used as systemic BP tolerates to relieve pulmonary congestion. However, the direct venodilating effect of nitroprusside may render other preload-reducing maneuvers unnecessary.

      (3) **Intraaortic balloon counterpulsation** is indicated in cases of severe hemodynamic instability to reduce SVR and improve forward cardiac output.

   c. **Surgical therapy** is indicated urgently in patients with acute MR and hemodynamic compromise whose condition cannot be stabilized medically. In those with infective endocarditis who are hemodynamically stable, MVR should be delayed for several days while antibiotic therapy is initiated. If refractory hemodynamic deterioration develops, surgery should not be delayed.

D. **Aortic insufficiency (AI)** may occur as a result of an abnormality of the aortic valve itself, dilatation and distortion of the aortic root, or both. Causes of valvular aortic insufficiency include rheumatic fever, endocarditis, trauma, connective tissue diseases, and congenital bicuspid aortic valve. Dilatation or distortion of the aortic root producing AI may be due to systemic hypertension, ascending aortic dissection, syphilis, cystic medionecrosis, Marfan's syndrome, ankylosing spondylitis, and osteogenesis imperfecta. Chronic AI typically presents insidiously, while acute AI usually is manifested as severe HF and impending cardiogenic shock.

   1. **Pathophysiology.** The diastolic regurgitant flow from the aorta into the left ventricle causes increased left ventricular end-diastolic volume (LVEDV) and pressure (LVEDP). In turn, the left ventricle becomes dilated and hypertrophied, which maintains stroke volume and prevents further increase in LVEDP. In acute AI, the chronic compensatory mechanisms are not active and therefore the increase in LVEDP is marked. In chronic AI, increases in peripheral resistance (e.g., hypertension) lead to increased regurgitant flow and raise diastolic filling pressure and volume.

   2. **Diagnosis** of AI may be suspected based on clinical findings including a wide pulse pressure, bounding pulses, and an aortic diastolic murmur. The presence of AI can be confirmed by two-dimensional and Doppler echocardiography or cardiac catheterization with ascending aortography.

3. **Medical management** is reserved for patients with chronic, stable AI or for stabilization of patients with severe or acute AI before definitive surgical treatment.
   a. **Treatment of underlying or precipitating causes** such as endocarditis, syphilis, and connective tissue diseases should occur concomitantly with treatment of HF.
   b. Patients with AI should receive **prophylaxis for endocarditis** (see Chap. 13).
   c. **Strenuous physical activity** should be restricted in patients with AI and associated left ventricular dysfunction with limited cardiac reserve. Activities involving increases in isometric work (lifting heavy objects) are more detrimental than activities such as walking or swimming.
   d. **Fluid and salt restriction,** diuretics, and digoxin are the cornerstones of therapy for patients with chronic AI who have evidence of LV dysfunction.
   e. **Vasodilators** are beneficial in symptomatic patients with **chronic AI.** In patients with **acute AI,** afterload reduction with sodium nitroprusside and/or positive inotropes should be employed to stabilize the patient's condition prior to valve replacement.
4. **Surgical treatment**
   a. **Aortic valve replacement (AVR)** and repair of associated aortic root abnormalities should be performed urgently in patients with **acute AI.** In patients with infective endocarditis who are hemodynamically stable with medical therapy, AVR can be deferred for several days while treatment with antibiotics is initiated. Patients in whom hemodynamic instability develops require urgent surgery.
   b. AVR should be recommended in patients with severe **chronic AI** in whom signs or symptoms of moderate HF (New York Heart Association functional class II–III) or left ventricular dysfunction develop. Echocardiography should be performed serially and AVR considered when left ventricular dilatation or left ventricular systolic dysfunction becomes significant. The clinical outcome and extent of reversibility of left ventricular dysfunction following AVR depend on the duration of dysfunction, dilatation of the left ventricle (end-systolic diameter and volume), and degree of systolic dysfunction.

II. **Cardiogenic pulmonary edema (CPE)**
   A. **Pathophysiology.** CPE occurs when the pulmonary capillary pressure (PCP) exceeds the forces (serum oncotic pressure and interstitial hydrostatic pressure) that maintain fluid within the vascular space. Accumulation of fluid in the pulmonary interstitium is followed by alveolar flooding and disturbance of gas exchange. Increased PCP may be caused by left ventricular failure of any cause, obstruction to transmitral flow (e.g., mitral stenosis, atrial myxoma), or, rarely, by pulmonary veno-occlusive disease.
   B. **Diagnosis**
      1. **Clinical manifestations** of CPE usually occur rapidly and include dyspnea, air hunger, anxiety, and restlessness. Physical signs of decreased peripheral perfusion, pulmonary congestion, use of accessory respiratory muscles, and wheezing are often present. The patient may expectorate a pink frothy fluid.
      2. **Radiographic abnormalities** include cardiomegaly, interstitial and perihilar vascular engorgement, Kerley B lines, and pleural effusions. The radiographic abnormalities may lag several hours behind the development of symptoms, and their resolution may be out of phase with clinical improvement.
   C. **Management**
      1. **Initial supportive treatment** of CPE includes administration of oxygen via nasal cannula or mask in a concentration sufficient to raise PO_2 to greater than 60 mm Hg. Mechanical ventilation is indicated if hypercapnia coexists or if oxygenation is inadequate while using a high-flow, tight-fitting mask at 100% FIO_2 concentration. **A sitting position** improves pulmonary function and assists in venous pooling. Cardiac workload should be decreased by placing the patient on strict bed rest and by reducing pain and anxiety.

2. Pharmacologic treatment

a. **Morphine sulfate** reduces anxiety and dilates pulmonary and systemic veins. Morphine, 2–5 mg IV, can be given safely over several minutes and can be repeated q10–25min until an effect is seen. An opioid antagonist (naloxone, 0.4–0.8 mg IV) must be available in case respiratory depression results from morphine therapy (see Chaps. 1 and 9).

b. **Furosemide** is a potent venodilator and decreases pulmonary congestion within minutes of IV infusion, well before its diuretic action begins. An initial dose of 20–40 mg should be given IV over several minutes and can be increased, based on response, to a maximum of 200 mg on subsequent doses.

c. **Nitroglycerin** (TNG) is a venodilator that can potentiate the effect of furosemide but should be used cautiously. IV TNG titrated from an initial dose of 5 μg/minute is preferable to oral and topical forms since it offers the advantage of rapid titration to the desired effect and eliminates prolonged or delayed absorption from subcutaneous tissues should hypotension develop.

d. **Nitroprusside** is often an effective adjunct in the treatment of acute CPE secondary to its balanced vasodilatory properties. It is particularly useful in CPE resulting from acute valvular regurgitation and/or hypertension. Direct pulmonary and systemic arterial catheterization should be considered to guide titration of nitroprusside therapy.

e. **Inotropic agents** such as dobutamine or phosphodiesterase inhibitors may be helpful after initial treatment of CPE in patients with concomitant hypotension or shock (see secs. **IV.A** and **B**).

3. Mechanical reduction of pulmonary congestion

may be of temporizing benefit in cases of severe pulmonary edema. **Soft rubber tourniquets** or sphygmomanometer cuffs can be applied to all but one extremity, allowing arterial perfusion but restricting venous flow (i.e., inflate cuff to a pressure greater than diastolic, but less than systolic), and should be rotated every 15–20 minutes to the free extremity. **Phlebotomy** and removal of 250–500 ml blood is occasionally helpful in patients with relatively fixed intravascular volume (e.g., those with renal failure) or when pharmacologic therapy is inadequate. These procedures are only rarely used since aggressive pharmacologic therapy with nitrates, diuretics, vasodilators, and inotropes is usually successful. Acute hemodialysis and ultrafiltration are preferable to phlebotomy if they are available.

4. Right heart catheterization

and placement of an indwelling pulmonary artery catheter (e.g., **Swan-Ganz catheter**) may be helpful in cases in which a prompt response to therapy does not occur. The Swan-Ganz catheter will allow differentiation between cardiogenic and noncardiogenic causes of pulmonary edema via measurement of the PCP and will allow hemodynamic monitoring during therapy (see Chaps. 5 and 9).

5. Precipitating factors

should be identified if possible because several causes are correctable. Common precipitants of pulmonary edema include severe hypertension, myocardial infarction or ischemia (particularly if associated with MR), acute valvular regurgitation, new onset tachyarrhythmias or bradyarrhythmias, and volume overload in the setting of severe LV dysfunction. Successful resolution of pulmonary edema can often only be accomplished by correction of the underlying process.

III. Dilated cardiomyopathy is a disease of heart muscle characterized by dilatation of the cardiac chambers and reduction in ventricular contractile function. Dilatation may be secondary to progression of any process that causes HF, although certain etiologies appear to primarily cause an isolated myopathic process (see Table 6-1). The majority of cases, however, are idiopathic.

A. Pathophysiology and clinical features. Dilatation of the cardiac chambers and varying degrees of hypertrophy are anatomic hallmarks. Symptomatic HF is often present. Tricuspid and mitral regurgitation are common due to the effect of chamber dilatation on the valvular apparatus. Atrial and ventricular arrhythmias are seen in as many as half of these patients and are probably responsible for the high incidence of sudden death in this population.

B. Diagnosis can be confirmed with echocardiography or radionuclide ventriculography. Two-dimensional and Doppler echocardiography are helpful in differentiating this condition from hypertrophic or restrictive cardiomyopathy, pericardial disease, and valvular disorders. The ECG is almost always abnormal, but changes are typically nonspecific. Endomyocardial biopsy is of very limited value in providing information that is clinically useful in patients with dilated cardiomyopathies (*Am Heart J* 124:1251, 1992).

C. Medical management of symptomatic patients is similar to that for HF from any cause. The therapeutic strategies include control of total body sodium and volume as well as appropriate **preload and afterload reduction** using vasodilator therapy. Immunizations against influenza and pneumococcal pneumonia are recommended. Additional therapeutic considerations are as follows.

1. **Complex ventricular ectopy,** including nonsustained ventricular tachycardia, is frequently seen during ambulatory monitoring of these patients. Patients with complex ventricular ectopy and HF have a high incidence of sudden death. However, the empiric use of antiarrhythmic agents to suppress nonsustained asymptomatic ventricular ectopy has not been shown to improve survival and could result in drug-induced depression of ventricular function, proarrhythmic effects, or both. The value of signal-averaged ECGs and electrophysiologic studies for the prediction of sudden death in patients with dilated cardiomyopathy is controversial. Patients with dilated cardiomyopathy and asymptomatic nonsustained ventricular tachycardia should be treated aggressively to improve their HF and myocardial ischemia, if present; electrolyte imbalance should be identified and corrected, and proarrhythmic drugs should be discontinued. The treatment of patients with symptomatic nonsustained ventricular tachycardia, sustained ventricular tachycardia, or history of sudden death is evolving and consultation with an electrophysiologist is warranted (see Chap. 7).

2. **Chronic oral anticoagulation** should be considered because of the high incidence of **mural thrombi** found by echocardiography or autopsy (*Circulation* 78:1388, 1988). Patients with severe left ventricular dysfunction (LVEF <25%) due to myocardial infarction or dilated cardiomyopathy, a prior history of thromboembolic events, or atrial fibrillation are at highest risk for a thromboembolic event. The level of anticoagulation recommended varies but is generally a prothrombin time 1.3–1.5 times control or an international normalized ratio (INR) of 2.0–3.0 (see Chap. 17).

3. **Immunosuppressive therapy** with agents such as prednisone, azathioprine, and cyclosporine for biopsy-proven **active myocarditis** has been advocated by some, but the efficacy has not been definitely established. Large-scale randomized trials designed to determine the efficacy of these agents in patients with myocarditis are ongoing.

D. Surgical management. Primary valvular disease and coronary disease should be evaluated and surgically corrected as indicated (see sec. I and Chap. 5). Revascularization with percutaneous transluminal coronary angioplasty (PTCA) or coronary artery bypass surgery reduces ischemia, resulting in improved or stabilized left ventricular function in selected patients with coronary artery disease. Intraaortic balloon counterpulsation and VADs may be necessary for stabilization of patients in whom cardiac transplantation is an option or before other definitive surgical therapies.

IV. Hypertrophic cardiomyopathy (HCM) is a myocardial disorder characterized by ventricular hypertrophy, diminished left ventricular cavity dimensions, normal or enhanced contractile function, and impaired ventricular relaxation (diastolic dysfunction). The idiopathic form of HCM has an early onset (as early as the first decade of life) without associated hypertension. Many cases have a **genetic component** with mutations in the myosin heavy-chain gene that follow an autosomal dominant transmission with variable phenotypic expressivity and penetrance. An **acquired form** also occurs in elderly patients with a long history of hypertension.

A. **Pathophysiology.** Myocardial hypertrophy is typically predominant in the ventricular septum (asymmetric hypertrophy) but may involve all ventricular segments equally. The disease can be classified according to the presence or absence of **left ventricular outflow tract obstruction.** Left ventricular outflow obstruction may occur at rest but is enhanced by factors that increase left ventricular contractility or decrease ventricular volume. **Ventricular diastolic abnormalities** of delayed ventricular relaxation and decreased compliance are common and may lead to pulmonary congestion. Myocardial ischemia occurs and is likely secondary to a myocardial supply-demand mismatch. Systolic anterior motion of the anterior leaflet of the mitral valve is often associated with MR and may play a role in left ventricular outflow tract obstruction.

B. **Clinical presentation** varies considerably but may include dyspnea, angina, arrhythmias, syncope, cardiac failure, or sudden death. Patients of all ages may be affected, but **sudden death** is most common in children and young adults between 10 and 35 years of age and often occurs during periods of strenuous exertion. Physical findings include a bisferiens carotid pulse (in the presence of obstruction); a forceful, double or triple apical impulse; and a coarse systolic outflow murmur localized along the left sternal border that is accentuated by maneuvers that decrease preload (e.g., Valsalva maneuver).

C. **The diagnosis** is suspected on the basis of clinical presentation and/or a family history suggestive of familial HCM and is confirmed by two-dimensional echocardiography. Doppler flow studies may be useful in establishing the presence of a significant left ventricular outflow gradient at rest or with provocation.

D. **Management** is directed toward relief of symptoms and prevention of endocarditis, arrhythmias, and sudden death. The treatment of asymptomatic individuals is controversial, and there is no conclusive evidence that medical therapy is beneficial to them. All individuals with HCM should avoid participation in strenuous physical activities including most competitive sports.

1. **Medical therapy**

   a. **Beta-adrenergic antagonists** may reduce symptoms of HCM by reducing myocardial contractility and heart rate. Unfortunately, symptoms may recur during long-term therapy. Many patients will show improvement with oral doses of propranolol in the range of 160–320 mg/day (or an equivalent dose of another beta-adrenergic antagonist). Higher doses of beta-adrenergic antagonist therapy may be necessary in patients with refractory or recurrent symptoms, although dosages over 480 mg/day are associated with a higher incidence of side effects.

   b. **Calcium channel antagonists,** particularly verapamil and diltiazem, often improve the symptoms of HCM, primarily through their action on augmentation of diastolic ventricular filling. Because of their vasodilatory properties, the **dihydropyridines should be avoided in patients with left ventricular outflow tract obstruction.** Therapy should be initiated at low doses, with careful hemodynamic monitoring in those patients with outflow obstruction. The dose should be increased gradually over several days to weeks if symptoms persist.

   c. **Diuretics** may improve pulmonary congestive symptoms in those patients with elevated pulmonary venous pressures (particularly in the small subset of patients in whom a congestive form of cardiomyopathy develops). **These agents should be used cautiously** in patients with severe left ventricular outflow obstruction because excessive preload reduction may worsen the obstruction.

   d. **Nitrates and vasodilators should be avoided** because of the risk of increasing the left ventricular outflow gradient.

2. **Atrial and ventricular arrhythmias** occur commonly in patients with HCM. Supraventricular tachyarrhythmias are tolerated poorly and should be

aggressively treated; DC cardioversion is indicated if hemodynamic compromise develops. Digoxin is relatively contraindicated because of its positive inotropic properties and potential for exacerbating ventricular outflow obstruction. **Atrial fibrillation** is poorly tolerated and should be converted to sinus rhythm when possible. Diltiazem, verapamil, or beta-adrenergic antagonists can be used to control the ventricular response before cardioversion. Procainamide or disopyramide (see Chap. 7) may be efficacious in the chronic suppression of atrial fibrillation. Patients with nonsustained ventricular tachycardia detected on ambulatory monitoring are at increased risk for sudden death. However, the benefit of suppression of these arrhythmias with medical therapy has not been established, and the risk of a proarrhythmic effect of antiarrhythmic therapy exists. Invasive electrophysiologic testing should be considered in these patients. Symptomatic ventricular arrhythmias should be treated as outlined in Chap. 7.

3. **Dual-chamber pacing** has been used successfully in treating patients with HCM (*Circulation* 85:2149, 1992). Alteration of the ventricular activation sequence via right ventricular pacing is a useful way to minimize left ventricular outflow tract obstruction secondary to asymmetric septal hypertrophy.

4. **Prophylaxis for endocarditis** is indicated (see Chap. 13).

5. **Anticoagulation** is recommended if paroxysmal or chronic atrial fibrillation develops.

6. **Surgical therapy** is useful in the treatment of symptoms but has not been shown to alter the natural history of HCM. The most frequently used operative procedure involves septal myotomy or myectomy or MVR.

V. Restrictive cardiomyopathy results from pathologic infiltration of the myocardium by a variety of processes such as amyloidosis and sarcoidosis. Less common causes include glycogen storage diseases, hemochromatosis, endomyocardial fibrosis, and hypereosinophilic syndromes.

A. **Pathophysiology and diagnosis.** Myocardial infiltration results in abnormal diastolic ventricular filling and varying degrees of systolic dysfunction depending on the duration and nature of the underlying disease. It is often difficult to differentiate between restrictive cardiomyopathy and constrictive pericarditis because of similar clinical presentations and hemodynamics, but this distinction is critical as surgical therapy is an effective treatment for constrictive pericarditis. Echocardiography may reveal thickening of the myocardium and varying degrees of systolic ventricular dysfunction. Doppler echocardiographic analysis may demonstrate evidence of abnormal diastolic filling patterns and elevated venous pressure. The ECG may show conduction system disease or low voltage, in contrast to the increased voltage seen with ventricular hypertrophy. Cardiac catheterization reveals elevated right and left ventricular filling pressures and a classic dip-and-plateau pattern in the right and left ventricular pressure tracing. Right ventricular endomyocardial biopsy may be diagnostic and should be considered in patients in whom a diagnosis is not established.

B. **Management**

1. **General measures** include judicious use of diuretics for pulmonary and systemic congestion and digoxin if left ventricular systolic dysfunction is present. Digoxin should be avoided in patients with cardiac amyloidosis because they appear to be more susceptible to the development of digoxin toxicity. In some cases, vasodilator therapy may be beneficial, but these agents should be used with caution to avoid excessive reduction in preload; elevated filling pressures may be required to maintain adequate cardiac output.

2. **Specific therapy** aimed at amelioration of the underlying cause should be instituted. Cardiac hemochromatosis may respond to reduction of total body iron stores via phlebotomy or chelation therapy with deferoxamine. Cardiac sarcoidosis may respond to glucocorticoid therapy, but prolongation of survival with this approach has not been established. There is no known effective therapy to reverse the progression of cardiac amyloidosis.

VI. Pericardial disease
  A. Cardiac tamponade results from increased intrapericardial pressure secondary to fluid accumulation within the pericardial space. Pericarditis of any cause may lead to cardiac tamponade. Idiopathic (or viral) and neoplastic forms are the most frequent etiologies.

1. **The diagnosis** should be suspected in patients with elevated jugular venous pressure, hypotension, pulsus paradoxus, tachycardia, evidence of poor peripheral perfusion, and distant heart sounds. The 12-lead electrocardiogram often reveals a tachycardia with low-voltage and electrical alternans. Echocardiography can confirm the diagnosis of pericardial effusion and demonstrate the hemodynamic significance by revealing right atrial and ventricular diastolic collapse, increased right-sided flows during inspiration, and respiratory variation of the transmitral flow. Right heart catheterization is also helpful in determining the hemodynamic significance of a pericardial effusion, especially in patients with a subacute or chronic presentation. Hemodynamic findings of elevated, equalized, diastolic pressures are present in the patient with cardiac tamponade.

2. **Definitive treatment** consists of drainage of the pericardial space via **pericardiocentesis or surgical pericardiotomy.** Urgent pericardiocentesis should be performed with echocardiographic guidance if possible. If pericardial drainage cannot be performed, stabilization with parenteral inotropic support and aggressive administration of IV saline to maintain adequate ventricular filling are indicated. **Diuretics, nitrates, or any other preload-reducing agents are absolutely contraindicated.**

  B. Constrictive pericarditis may develop as a late complication of pericardial inflammation. The majority of cases are of unknown etiology, but postpericardiotomy syndrome following cardiac surgery and mediastinal irradiation are important identifiable causes. Tuberculous pericarditis is a leading cause in some underdeveloped countries.

1. **Pathophysiology and diagnosis.** The noncompliant pericardium causes impairment of ventricular filling and progressive elevation of venous pressure. In contrast to cardiac tamponade, the clinical presentation is characteristically insidious, with gradual development of fatigue, exercise intolerance, and venous congestion. Physical findings include jugular venous distention with prominent X and Y descents, inspiratory elevation of the jugular venous pressure (Kussmaul's sign), peripheral edema, ascites, and a pericardial knock during diastole. Echocardiography may reveal pericardial thickening and diminished diastolic filling. In addition, a chest CT scan or MRI may detect pericardial thickening. Cardiac catheterization is usually necessary to demonstrate elevated and equalized diastolic pressures in all four cardiac chambers. The diagnosis of constrictive pericarditis is often difficult to distinguish from restrictive cardiomyopathy (see sec. **V**).

2. **Definitive treatment requires complete pericardiectomy,** which is accompanied by significant perioperative mortality (5–10%), but results in clinical improvement in 90% of patients. Patients who are minimally symptomatic can be managed with judicious sodium and fluid restriction and diuretic therapy but must be followed closely to detect hemodynamic deterioration.

VII. Shock is a clinical syndrome of systemic hypotension, acidemia, and impairment of vital organ function resulting from tissue hypoperfusion. Although typically acute, its onset may be gradual and insidious. Shock can be classified based on characteristic pathophysiologic and hemodynamic changes (Table 6-3). Treatment of shock requires hemodynamic stabilization with IV fluids and vasopressors to maintain vital organ perfusion, with concomitant identification and treatment of underlying pathologic processes.
  A. Classification

1. **Cardiogenic shock** occurs as a result of inadequate cardiac output, impaired oxygen delivery, and reduced tissue perfusion caused by loss of effective contractile function of myocardium (acute myocardial infarction, hemodynamically significant tachyarrhythmias or bradyarrhythmias, cardiomyop-

Table 6-3. Classification of shock

Type of shock	Hemodynamics			Potential etiologies
	Filling pressures	CO	SVR	
Cardiogenic	↑	↓	↑	Myocardial infarction
				Cardiomyopathy
				Valvular heart disease
				Arrhythmias
				Acute VSD, MR
Distributive (septic)	↓	↑	↓	Sepsis
				Anaphylaxis
				Toxic shock syndrome
Hypovolemic	↓	↑↓	↑	Hemorrhage
				Volume depletion
				Hypoadrenal crisis
Obstructive	↑ (proximal)	↓	↑	Pulmonary embolism
	↓ (distal)			Tamponade
				Tension pneumothorax

CO = cardiac output; SVR = systemic vascular resistance; VSD = ventricular septal defect; MR = mitral regurgitation.

athy), or from mechanical processes reducing adequate forward output (acute valvular regurgitation, acute ventricular septal defect, critical aortic stenosis, HCM). Intracardiac pressures are elevated (pulmonary artery wedge pressure >18 mm Hg), cardiac output is depressed (index <2.0 liters/minute/m^2), peripheral vascular resistance is increased, and mean arterial blood pressure is low (<60 mm Hg).

    a. Initial treatment is directed toward maintaining adequate systemic BP, cardiac output, and myocardial perfusion with volume expansion in combination with vasopressors or inotropes. Initial treatment is guided by hemodynamic monitoring while the precipitating cause is identified and treated. Prompt diagnosis is mandatory and may require urgent echocardiography or cardiac catheterization.

    b. Mechanical support with intraaortic balloon counterpulsation may be necessary during the acute phase of cardiogenic shock.

2. Distributive shock (septic shock) is characterized by vasodilation, low central filling pressures, decreased intravascular volume, reduction in peripheral vascular resistance, loss of capillary integrity with transudation of intravascular fluid (capillary leak), and an initially increased cardiac output.

    a. Treatment includes hemodynamic support with IV fluids (saline, colloid) and vasopressors (dopamine, epinephrine, norepinephrine [Levophed], phenylephrine [Neo-Synephrine]) as identification of underlying processes is initiated. Adjunctive treatment includes antibiotics, surgical drainage of abscesses, and removal of potential sources of infection (e.g., urethral and IV catheters, wound packing, tampons).

    b. Treatment of **anaphylaxis** is discussed in Chap. 9.

    c. Use of **steroids** in the treatment of septic shock is not recommended in the absence of adrenal suppression.

3. Hypovolemic shock results from loss of greater than 20% of the circulating blood volume due to acute hemorrhage, fluid depletion, or dehydration. In the absence of obvious trauma or hemorrhage, occult sources of bleeding and volume loss should be considered (GI, intra- or retroperitoneal, femoral compartment, intrathoracic, aortic dissection). Intracardiac filling pressures are decreased, cardiac output is normal or increased, and systemic vascular resistance is elevated due to compensatory vasoconstriction.

    a. Rapid volume expansion with fluids, colloid, and blood products is paramount. Coexisting problems such as congestive heart failure, valvular heart disease, myocardial ischemia, or renal insufficiency must be carefully monitored, and invasive hemodynamic monitoring should be considered during acute management.

b. **Correction of coagulopathy and electrolyte imbalance** as well as use of invasive diagnostic and therapeutic procedures (surgery, endoscopy, interventional radiologic procedures) need to be addressed urgently.

c. **Hypoadrenal (Addisonian) crisis** is a form of hypovolemic shock due to inadequate release of mineralocorticoids and glucocorticoids from the adrenal gland. In addition to hypotension, patients may manifest hyponatremia, hyperkalemia, acidosis, and hypoglycemia. Adrenal insufficiency may occur acutely (adrenal hemorrhage) or insidiously (metastatic cancer, tuberculosis). In patients whose adrenal function has been suppressed by chronic steroid therapy, hypoadrenal crisis may develop if glucocorticoid replacement is discontinued abruptly or if metabolic or physical stress (i.e., infection, surgery) develops. Once the diagnosis is suspected on clinical grounds, treatment should be initiated immediately by volume expansion with IV saline and glucocorticoid replacement with hydrocortisone, 100 mg IV q8h (see Chap. 21).

4. **Obstructive shock** may result from massive pulmonary embolism, cardiac tamponade, atrial myxoma, acute valvular stenosis (e.g., prosthetic valve thrombosis), or tension pneumothorax. Cardiac output is severely reduced due to impairment of ventricular filling or obstruction to blood flow, despite adequate intravascular volume, contractility, and vascular tone.

a. **Initial treatment** is supportive, with volume expansion and vasopressors. However, since the precipitating factors are mechanical, rapid diagnosis is essential to identify the obstructive process and guide therapy.

b. **Specific treatment** of mechanical problems may include pericardiocentesis, chest tube placement, thrombolytic therapy (for massive pulmonary embolus or valve thrombosis), embolectomy, or cardiac surgery.

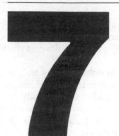

Cardiac Arrhythmias

Joseph M. Smith

Recognition and Management

I. **Clinical diagnosis of arrhythmias.** Accurate diagnosis and selection of appropriate therapy for cardiac arrhythmias requires interpretation of data directly pertaining to the arrhythmia as well as assessment of other patient-specific information. The frequency, duration, mode of onset and offset (gradual vs. abrupt), response to vagal maneuvers, and presence or absence of associated symptoms (e.g., chest pain, near-syncope, syncope) should be determined. A history of symptoms of organic heart disease and noncardiac diseases that potentiate rhythm abnormalities (e.g., inflammatory diseases, endocrinopathies, infiltrative diseases, infectious processes [e.g., Chagas' disease, Lyme disease], or familial or congenital causes of arrhythmias [e.g., hypertrophic heart disease, Wolff-Parkinson-White syndrome, congenital long QT syndrome]) should be sought. Physical examination should emphasize pulse rate and regularity, BP (both supine and standing), evidence of atrioventricular (AV) synchrony as manifested by the pattern of jugular venous pulsation and the regularity of the first heart sound, signs of organic heart disease as manifested by right- or left-sided heart failure (HF), or evidence of relevant systemic diseases. Serum electrolytes (K^+, Ca^{2+}, and Mg^{2+}), antiarrhythmic drug levels, and thyroid function studies should be performed in all patients under investigation for an unknown arrhythmia.

II. **Electrocardiographic data** should focus on identification of atrial activity and its relation to ventricular activity during the rhythm disturbance. Diagnostic tests useful for interpreting a rhythm disturbance include the following:

   A. **A 12-lead ECG** should be performed both at rest and during the arrhythmia.

   B. **A rhythm strip** should document the response to interventions (e.g., vagal maneuvers, bolus administration of antiarrhythmic agents, attempted cardioversion). If atrial activity is not readily apparent in the recorded rhythm strip, additional tests may be performed to enhance detection of atrial activity.

   1. **Lewis leads** are bipolar exploring leads that facilitate recording of atrial activation during an arrhythmia (*Cardiol Clin* 5:349, 1987). The recording electrodes can be positioned on the precordium to maximize the electrical signal corresponding to atrial activation. The largest atrial deflections are recorded with the negative electrode positioned high and to the right of the sternum and the positive electrode positioned low and to the left of the sternum.

   2. **Transesophageal electrograms** are obtained by placing a recording electrode within the esophagus near the left atrium. Using either a bipolar configuration similar to that used for Lewis leads or a unipolar electrode connected as V_1 of the standard 12-lead ECG, atrial activity and its relationship to ventricular activity can be determined. Special esophageal electrodes are available for this purpose.

   3. **Direct atrial electrograms** are obtained either by placing a transvenous temporary pacing electrode into the right atrium or by recording from temporary pacing wires left in place immediately after cardiac surgery. Recordings may be made in either unipolar or bipolar configuration.

III. Bradyarrhythmias. A bradyarrhythmia is defined as any rhythm resulting in a ventricular rate of less than 60 beats/minute.

   A. Sinus bradycardia occurs when the sinus mechanism is slowed and the pattern of atrial and ventricular activation is normal. Increased vagal tone, antiarrhythmic drug effect, myocardial ischemia, and primary sinus node disease are typical etiologies. The patient may be asymptomatic or may experience light-headedness, breathlessness, angina, near-syncope, and syncope. The **ECG** reveals an atrial rate of less than 60, P waves with a normal configuration and axis, a normal or prolonged PR interval, and a normal QRS pattern. **Asymptomatic patients** require no therapy. In **symptomatic** patients, therapy is directed toward the specific etiology and includes treatment with atropine, 0.5–2.0 mg IV, or cardiac pacing (see Chap. 8). If bradycardia is refractory to atropine and a transcutaneous pacemaker is unavailable, dopamine, 5–20 μg/kg/minute, epinephrine, 2–20 μg/minute, or isoproterenol, 2–10 μg/minute, can be used.

   B. AV block occurs when an atrial impulse is conducted with delay or fails to conduct to the ventricle at a time when the AV node is not physiologically refractory.

   1. First-degree AV block usually results from the delay of impulse propagation within the AV node. Rarely, intraatrial delay or delay within the His-Purkinje system is responsible, in which case conduction system disease is usually manifested by a bundle branch block pattern. **Etiologies** include increased vagal tone, antiarrhythmic drug effects, electrolyte abnormalities, myocardial ischemia, and conduction system disease. First-degree block is usually asymptomatic but may exacerbate HF if marked conduction delay affects AV synchrony. The **ECG** characteristically shows a PR interval greater than 200 ms. **Therapy** is not indicated in the asymptomatic patient. In the symptomatic patient, electrolyte abnormalities should be corrected and drugs that affect AV conduction should be withdrawn. In symptomatic patients, therapy should be instituted as outlined in sec. **III.A.**

   2. Second-degree AV block occurs when some of the atrial impulses are not conducted to the ventricle at times when the AV node is not physiologically refractory. Two types of second-degree AV block are recognized. Clinically, the distinctions between type I and type II are important, as they carry different prognostic implications.

   a. Mobitz type I (Wenckebach block) is characterized by a delay that progressively prolongs AV conduction prior to conduction block. The site of conduction block is almost always within the AV node. **Etiologies** include increased vagal tone, antiarrhythmic drug effects, electrolyte abnormalities, myocardial ischemia, acute inferior myocardial infarction (MI), and conduction system disease. Type I AV block, especially in the setting of a normal QRS, is a benign rhythm disturbance and usually does not portend an increased likelihood of developing complete heart block. The **ECG** reveals gradual PR prolongation preceding a nonconducted P wave on a rhythm strip such that QRS complexes occur in regular groupings (**grouped beating**). The shortest PR interval occurs with the first conducted P wave following a blocked P wave, and the RR interval shortens prior to a blocked P wave. **Symptomatic** type I AV block is **initially managed** with atropine, 0.5–2.0 mg IV. Persistent symptoms refractory to this regimen require temporary pacing, if available. Alternative therapy includes dopamine, epinephrine, or isoproterenol (see sec. **III.A**).

   b. Mobitz type II is characterized by conduction block without preceding conduction delay. The site of block is most often localized to the His-Purkinje system, particularly in the setting of a bundle branch block pattern. **Etiologies** include conduction system disease, antiarrhythmic drug effects, acute anterior MI, and increased vagal effects on the AV node. Type II AV block, especially in the setting of a bundle branch block pattern, **often antedates the development of transient complete heart block.** Symptoms may include feelings of a "skipped beat," lightheadedness, near-syncope, and syncope. The **ECG** reveals no change in PR interval duration preceding a blocked P wave. Symptomatic patients should be treated as outlined in sec. **III.A**. Permanent pacemaker insertion must also be considered in patients with Mobitz type II block. The development of heart block in the setting of an acute MI requires special consideration (see Cardiac Pacing).

3. **Third-degree (complete) AV block** occurs when there is an absence of transmission of atrial impulses to the ventricles. The site of complete conduction block may be the AV node (as occurs in congenital heart block), within the His bundle or the distal Purkinje system (as occurs with acquired heart block). **Acquired complete AV block** is usually the result of drug toxicity, MI with scarring, or degenerative processes involving the conduction system. Other etiologies include infiltrative diseases (amyloidosis, sarcoidosis), rheumatologic disorders (polymyositis, scleroderma, rheumatoid nodules), infectious diseases (Chagas' disease, Lyme disease), inadvertent surgical interruption, calcific aortic stenosis, endocarditis, or metastatic disease.

The extent of **symptoms** largely depends on the underlying escape rhythm and rate and include light-headedness, breathlessness, angina, near-syncope, and syncope. In complete heart block, the **atrial rate exceeds the ventricular rate**, there is no fixed relation between atrial and ventricular activity (AV dissociation), and the ventricular rate is usually regular, due to the regularity of the escape rhythm focus. Complete heart block should be distinguished from competitive AV dissociation. The latter results from the increased rate of an AV nodal or ventricular focus exceeding the sinus or atrial rate and is usually benign. Symptomatic bradycardia can be **treated** with atropine, 0.5–2.0 mg IV, epinephrine, 2–20 μg/minute, dopamine, 5–20 μg/kg/minute, or isoproterenol, 2–10 μg/minute IV. Persistent symptoms despite medical therapy, an underlying etiology likely to recur, or the failure to identify a readily reversible cause necessitates pacemaker therapy (see Cardiac Pacing).

IV. Premature complexes represent the most common interruption of normal sinus rhythm, most frequently arising from the ventricles. They occur with diminishing likelihood from the atria, the AV node, and the atrial region of the sinus node.

A. **Premature atrial complexes (PACs)** are atrial depolarizations that occur prior to the onset of the next atrial depolarization from the sinus node. They most often result from abnormal automaticity but may also occur as a manifestation of intraatrial reentry. They often occur in the absence of structural heart disease but may occur de novo in a variety of clinical settings including infection, inflammation, myocardial ischemia, drug toxicities, catecholamine excess, electrolyte imbalance, or excessive use of tobacco, alcohol, or caffeine. Symptoms range from none to feelings of "skipped" beats. The P wave of a PAC is early with respect to the next anticipated sinus P wave and is typically different in contour and axis from the sinus P wave. Depending on the degree of prematurity, the PR interval following the PAC may be slightly prolonged. There is usually a compensatory pause between the PAC and the next sinus P wave, reflecting the resetting of the sinus mechanism by the PAC. PACs typically require no therapy. When patients are symptomatic, therapy should be directed toward correction of underlying abnormalities (e.g., removing offending drugs or toxins, correcting electrolyte abnormalities). Beta-adrenergic antagonists or calcium channel antagonists may be useful.

B. **Premature AV junctional complexes (JPCs)** are premature depolarizations with their site of origin in the AV node or the proximal portion of the His-Purkinje system, and may result from increased automaticity. JPCs most often occur in the absence of structural heart disease but may occur de novo in a variety of clinical settings including MI, drug toxicity, catecholamine excess, electrolyte imbalance, or excessive use of tobacco, alcohol, or caffeine. The patient may be asymptomatic or have feelings of "skipped" beats. JPCs typically result in a premature, normally conducted QRS. With intact retrograde AV nodal conduction, an inverted P wave will occur during or just after the inscription of the QRS. With retrograde AV block, the retrograde (inverted) P wave is absent, and the next, normally timed sinus P wave may experience delay or block in the AV node. JPCs typically require no therapy.

C. Premature ventricular complexes (PVCs) are depolarizations originating from the ventricles and begin prematurely with respect to the scheduled arrival of the next normally conducted sinus beat. They may result from abnormal automaticity within the ventricles or from reentry. PVCs most often occur in the absence of structural heart disease, with an increasing frequency with age. Increasing frequency, increased number of morphologies, and the occurrence of complex forms (couplets, triplets) may accompany infection, inflammation, myocardial ischemia, drug toxicities, catecholamine excess, electrolyte imbalance, or excessive use of tobacco, alcohol, or caffeine. The patient may be asymptomatic or have feelings of "skipped" beats. The frequency of occurrence, the number of morphologies, and the occurrence of complex forms has limited prognostic significance. The **ECG** reveals a premature QRS complex with a bizarre morphology, typically greater than 120 ms in duration, with a T wave that is larger in amplitude than normal and a polarity opposite to that of the QRS complex. PVCs typically require no therapy. When patients are **symptomatic, therapy** should be directed toward correction of underlying abnormalities. Specific antiarrhythmic agents may be effective in suppressing PVCs, but adverse effects (e.g., arrhythmia aggravation, proarrhythmia, death) preclude their widespread use (*N Engl J Med* 321:406, 1989). In the setting of acute myocardial ischemia or infarction, IV lidocaine (1–4 mg/minute with initial boluses of 1 mg/kg and 0.5 mg/kg 10 minutes apart) may suppress PVCs, but toxic effects (e.g., increased risk of asystole and CNS effects) appear to outweigh potential benefits in most cases.

V. Tachycardia is defined as a heart rate in excess of 100 beats/minute. Tachycardias are distinguished as being supraventricular (SVT) or ventricular (VT), depending on the site of origin. **Distinction between SVT and VT is critical** as they are associated with vastly different clinical outcomes, require different levels of evaluation, and respond to different therapeutic interventions. Many ECG criteria have been proposed to distinguish between SVT and VT (see sec. **V.B.4.c**). While the underlying mechanism of the tachycardia critically determines both prognosis and therapy, initial investigation may only allow for characterization of the tachycardia as either a narrow complex tachycardia (QRS duration ≤120 ms) or a wide complex tachycardia (QRS duration >120 ms).

A. Narrow complex tachycardias are almost exclusively supraventricular in origin and, in the absence of organic heart disease, are associated with an excellent prognosis.

   1. Sinus tachycardia occurs when the sinus mechanism is accelerated and the pattern of atrial and ventricular activation is normal. Increased sympathetic or diminished vagal tone, increased levels of circulating catecholamines, pain, hypovolemia, hypoxemia, myocardial ischemia or infarction, pulmonary embolism, fever, and inflammation are common etiologies. The atrial rate is typically between 100 and 160 beats/minute, the P waves have a normal configuration and axis, the PR interval is normal or slightly shortened, and the QRS pattern is usually normal. Occasionally, aberrant conduction in a bundle branch or fascicle of the His-Purkinje system may occur secondary to the increased rate. Therapeutic interventions should be targeted at the underlying pathophysiologic process. In the setting of myocardial ischemia or infarction, beta-adrenergic antagonists (see Table 4-3) may be used to slow the sinus rate.

   2. Atrial tachycardia is typically automatic or, infrequently, due to reentry and occurs in the setting of coronary artery disease with or without MI, chronic lung disease, acute alcohol ingestion, or digitalis intoxication. Rarely, automatic atrial tachycardias may occur in patients with otherwise normal hearts.

      a. Paroxysmal atrial tachycardia, especially with second-degree AV block **(PAT with block)** is typically associated with digitalis toxicity.

      b. Multifocal atrial tachycardia (MAT) is often associated with chronic obstructive pulmonary disease (COPD) and HF and may be potentiated by concomitant therapy with theophylline.

  c. The **ECG** reveals an atrial rate of 130–200 beats/minute. The P waves have an abnormal configuration and axis, the PR interval depends on the atrial rate, and the QRS pattern is either normal or reflects aberrant conduction in a bundle branch or fascicle of the His-Purkinje system secondary to the increased rate. Atrial tachycardia secondary to digitalis toxicity is typically associated with second-degree AV block. MAT is present when at least 3 distinct P wave morphologies are noted.

  d. **Therapy** is targeted at the underlying pathophysiologic process. PAT with block in the setting of digitalis therapy should be treated by discontinuing digitalis and maintaining normal serum potassium levels; if refractory and symptomatic, lidocaine, propranolol, or phenytoin may also be used. In clinical situations not associated with digitalis toxicity, calcium channel antagonists, beta-adrenergic antagonists, or digitalis may be used to slow the ventricular response rate. If atrial tachycardia persists, class Ia, Ic, or III agents can be added. Automatic atrial tachycardia can often be permanently prevented with surgical ablation (*J Am Coll Cardiol* 22:85, 1993), but the advent of radio frequency catheter ablation has largely supplanted the need for surgical intervention.

3. **AV junctional tachycardia** is thought to be automatic and occurs in the setting of MI, myocarditis, catecholamine excess states, and digitalis toxicity, and following heart surgery. The atrial rate is typically 60–130 beats/minute. With intact retrograde conduction from the site of the junctional tachycardia and the atria, the P waves are inverted and occur during or immediately after the inscription of the QRS complex. With retrograde conduction block from the site of the tachycardia, there is competitive AV dissociation, with normal-appearing, nonconducted P waves occurring at a rate slower than the ventricular rate. The ventricular rate is 60–130 beats/minute, and the QRS pattern is either normal or reflects aberrant conduction in a bundle branch or fascicle of the His-Purkinje system secondary to the increased rate. **Therapy** consists of discontinuing potentially offending agents (e.g., exogenous catecholamines, digitalis preparations) and correcting the underlying pathophysiologic process. With these measures, the arrhythmia typically abates spontaneously. Phenytoin, lidocaine, or propranolol may also be effective. Atrial overdrive pacing may restore AV synchrony in patients with hemodynamic compromise secondary to competitive AV dissociation.

4. **AV nodal reentrant tachycardia (AVNRT)** occurs when there is a reentrant circuit involving two anatomically and physiologically distinct pathways (fast and slow pathways) that link the right atrium to the distal part of the AV node (Fig. 7-1). AVNRT is one of the most common forms of narrow complex tachycardia and is the most common of the paroxysmal supraventricular tachycardias (PSVTs). Occurrence of AVNRT may be potentiated by physiologic or emotional stress, increased levels of circulating catecholamines, pain, fever, inflammation, or myocardial ischemia or infarction. Symptoms include palpitations, nervousness, light-headedness, near-syncope, angina, and syncope.

  a. In **typical (slow-fast)** AVNRT, the heart rate is 150–250 beats/minute, the P wave is not usually apparent because atrial and ventricular depolarization are nearly synchronous, and the QRS complex is normal or may show rate-related aberrant conduction. The onset of AVNRT is abrupt, usually initiated by a PAC that conducts with a long PR interval (typical of slow-pathway conduction).

  b. In **atypical (fast-slow)** AVNRT, the heart rate is similar to that for typical AVNRT, but an inverted P wave is usually readily apparent in the T wave. The PR interval is normal or minimally prolonged. The onset of atypical AVNRT is abrupt, usually initiated by a PVC that conducts with a long RP (R wave of QRS to the next P wave) interval.

  c. **Initial therapy** of acute episodes of narrow complex tachycardias, particu-

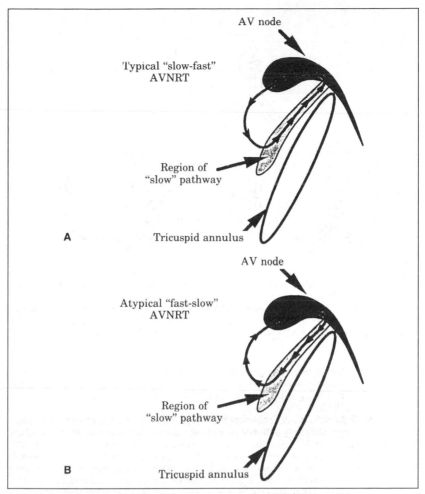

Fig. 7-1. The anatomic substrate for AV nodal reentrant tachycardia (AVNRT) is a region of slow conduction residing within the atrium nearly adjacent to the tricuspid annulus. A. In typical AVNRT, a premature atrial depolarization may experience antegrade block in the AV node (fast pathway), with conduction proceeding via the slow pathway and with sufficient delay to allow for retrograde activation of the fast pathway, giving rise to sustained slow-fast AVNRT. B. In atypical AVNRT, a premature ventricular depolarization may experience retrograde block in the AV node (fast pathway), with retrograde conduction proceeding via the slow pathway and with sufficient delay to allow for antegrade activation of the fast pathway, giving rise to sustained fast-slow AVNRT.

larly AVNRT, includes vagal maneuvers (e.g., carotid massage, Valsalva maneuver), and, if unsuccessful, bolus administration of short-acting agents that slow or block AV nodal conduction, such as adenosine (6–12 mg IV), verapamil (5 mg IV q5min for a maximum of 3 doses), or diltiazem (15- to 20-mg bolus over 2 minutes for a maximum of 2 doses). Chronic therapy for recurrent AVNRT may include calcium channel antagonists,

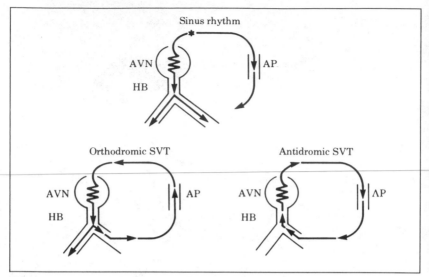

Fig. 7-2. Atrioventricular conduction in the WPW syndrome. During normal sinus rhythm, antegrade conduction occurs over both the AV node (AVN) and the accessory pathway (AP). During orthodromic SVT, there is antegrade conduction in the AVN and retrograde conduction via the AP. During antidromic SVT, there is antegrade conduction in the AP and retrograde conduction via the AVN. (HB = His bundle.)

beta-adrenergic antagonists, or digoxin. The advent of radio frequency catheter ablation of the slow pathway often cures this tachyarrhythmia and has greatly limited the need for empiric drug trials (*N Engl J Med* 327:313, 1992).

5. **Orthodromic AV reciprocating tachycardia using a concealed (retrograde only) accessory pathway** consists of a macro-reentrant circuit involving the atria, the AV node, the ventricles, and an accessory bypass tract (Fig. 7-2). Electrical activation conducts (orthodromically) down the AV node, speeds throughout the ventricles, and then travels retrograde in the accessory bypass tract to excite the atria. Concealed accessory bypass tracts account for up to 30% of clinical SVTs. The accessory bypass tract is congenital in origin and is independent of other forms of heart disease.

a. **Symptoms** include palpitations, nervousness, light-headedness, near-syncope, angina, and syncope. Bypass tract–mediated orthodromic tachycardias typically occur at rates of 150–250 beats/minute. Unlike typical AVNRT, atrial and ventricular activation are not synchronous but occur in sequence, with atrial activation typically occurring near the end or shortly after ventricular depolarization is complete. A retrograde P wave is typically appreciated at the end of the normal or aberrant QRS complex or in the early part of the ST segment. The onset of orthodromic tachycardia is typically abrupt, initiated by a premature atrial or ventricular complex. Acute episodes of tachycardia are managed in the same fashion as AVNRT (see sec. **V.A.4.c**).

b. **Chronic therapy** may include calcium channel antagonists, beta-adrenergic antagonists, and specific antiarrhythmic therapy targeted at slowing conduction and prolonging refractory periods of the accessory bypass tract (see sec. **V.A.6.b**). Radio frequency catheter ablation of accessory bypass tract conduction is often the treatment of choice (*N Engl J Med* 324:1605, 1991).

6. **Wolff-Parkinson-White syndrome (WPW)** is characterized by **preexcitation** (a **short PR** interval and the presence of a **delta wave** slurring the upstroke of the QRS complex) and paroxysmal SVT. Depending on the conduction characteristics of the accessory bypass tract, WPW may present as orthodromic tachycardia (see sec. **V.A.5**) or antidromic tachycardia when excitation conducts down the accessory pathway, throughout the ventricles, and then retrogradely through the AV node to the atria (see Fig. 7-2). The accessory AV connection (bypass tract), which mediates both orthodromic and antidromic tachycardia, represents a congenital defect with an incidence of 3 in 1,000 in the general population. The typical orthodromic SVT in these patients uses the accessory pathway as a retrograde limb, and thus the QRS complex during the tachycardia is normal (not preexcited). The most common wide complex tachycardia seen in patients with WPW is orthodromic SVT with rate-related aberration (right bundle branch block, left bundle branch block). The combination of ventricular preexcitation and atrial fibrillation may, in a small number of patients, predispose to very frequent conduction of the atrial impulses to the ventricle, initiating ventricular fibrillation.
   a. The **diagnosis** of WPW requires the presence of ventricular preexcitation on a routine ECG, as well as paroxysmal SVT. While enhanced conduction through the AV node or slow or intermittent conduction in the accessory pathway may obscure ventricular preexcitation in the resting ECG, a delta wave is usually apparent. Carotid sinus massage, vagal maneuvers, bolus administration of short-acting AV nodal–blocking agents, or spontaneous PACs can enhance the degree of preexcitation by effectively slowing conduction through the AV node.
   b. **Therapy.** Acute episodes of tachycardia are managed in the same fashion as AVNRT (see sec. **V.A.4.c**). Bolus administration of adenosine may infrequently potentiate brief bouts of atrial fibrillation, and it is prudent to have a DC cardioverter present when administering adenosine to patients with WPW. The choice of chronic therapy must be made with recognition that AV nodal–blocking agents (including calcium channel antagonists, beta-adrenergic antagonists, and digoxin) will not prevent and may occasionally precipitate a very rapid ventricular response to atrial fibrillation, which may trigger ventricular fibrillation in this patient group. Pharmacologic therapy targeted at slowing conduction and prolonging refractoriness in the accessory bypass tract (class Ia, Ic, and III agents) may be used to prevent recurrence of bypass tract–mediated tachycardia, but the proven efficacy of radio-frequency catheter ablation has limited the need for lifelong drug therapy.
7. **Atrial fibrillation (AF)** is the most common sustained arrhythmia patients seek treatment for and afflicts as many as 10% of Americans over age 75. The majority of strokes and peripheral thromboembolic events of cardiac origin occur in association with AF. AF occurs when multiple wandering wave fronts of activation simultaneously occur within the atria. Any disease process that increases atrial size and/or focally or globally decreases conduction velocity or refractory period duration may result in AF.
   a. **Etiologies** that are potentially treatable include hypertension, acute alcohol ingestion, toxic effects of theophylline or other stimulants, endocrinopathies (hypothyroidism, hyperthyroidism, pheochromocytoma), pericarditis, and MI.
   b. **Symptoms** are related to the loss of coordinated AV synchrony and the irregular and frequently rapid pulse rate, and may include palpitations, "skipped" beats, anxiety, light-headedness, breathlessness, angina, near-syncope, and syncope.
   c. **The ECG** reveals an irregularly fluctuating baseline without well-defined P waves, irregular spacing between R waves, and frequently a rate greater than 100 beats/minute in the untreated patient.
   d. **Therapy.** AF with a rapid ventricular response in the setting of myocardial ischemia, MI, hypotension, or worsening heart failure should be

managed with **prompt DC cardioversion** (see Chap. 8). For well-tolerated AF, **control of ventricular rate** is the initial treatment goal, with a target rate of 60–100 beats/minute. This is typically accomplished by treatment with AV nodal–blocking agents. Calcium channel antagonists and beta-adrenergic antagonists afford more rapid control of ventricular response than digoxin therapy, but digoxin is preferable in the setting of severe left ventricular dysfunction or HF. **Anticoagulation** for stroke prophylaxis is achieved with heparin administration in the short term, followed by subsequent warfarin therapy for long-term anticoagulation (see Chap. 17). **Sinus rhythm** can be restored with either short-term administration of antiarrhythmic agents (chemical cardioversion) or electrical (DC) cardioversion, but any attempt to restore normal sinus rhythm should be made in consideration of the potential for thromboembolism associated with cardioversion. In general, prior to cardioversion, **patients should be anticoagulated** for at least 3 weeks, and anticoagulation should be continued for at least 3 weeks following cardioversion. In circumstances where the episode of AF is known to be of less than 48 hours' duration, cardioversion has been conducted without apparent increase in the incidence of thromboembolic events. Long-term antiarrhythmic therapy to prevent the recurrence of AF is controversial, with a variety of agents showing only modest efficacy in suppression of symptomatic arrhythmia, no clear beneficial impact on stroke risk, and a modest rate of proarrhythmic effects. Interruption of AV nodal conduction via radio frequency catheter ablation with concomitant implantation of a permanent pacemaker affords nonpharmacologic rate control but does not restore AV synchrony or alter stroke risk and must be considered a palliative procedure. **Chronic warfarin anticoagulation is the most effective therapy for attenuating the risk of stroke associated with AF** (see Chap. 17).

8. **Atrial flutter** results from a single macro-reentrant circuit involving only atrial tissue around functional or structural barriers to conduction. Typical atrial flutter may occur in otherwise healthy patients but also occurs in any of those conditions that predispose to the development of atrial fibrillation (see sec. **V.A.7.a**). Atypical atrial flutter occurs in patients with organic heart disease, in patients receiving drug therapy for AF, and in patients with prior cardiac surgery involving the atria.

a. **The ECG** reveals a regular undulation (sawtooth pattern) in the baseline, most notable in V_1 and the inferior leads (II, III, avF), with an effective atrial rate of 280–350 beats/minute). The RR intervals may be regular, reflecting a fixed-ratio AV block (2:1, 3:1), or may be variable, reflecting a Wenckebach periodicity. In the presence of class Ia or Ic antiarrhythmic drugs, atrial rates may be substantially slowed.

b. **Therapy** is similar to that for AF, except that the role of anticoagulation is not clear. DC cardioversion should be performed if evidence of clinical instability is noted. Restoration of normal sinus rhythm is often preferable to attempted control of the ventricular rate, as the ventricular response to atrial flutter may vary greatly with very modest changes in autonomic influences on AV nodal conduction characteristics. In addition to pharmacologic therapy and DC cardioversion, overdrive pace termination of atrial flutter may be attempted, particularly in patients with temporary pacemaker leads or newer models of permanent pacemakers capable of atrial overdrive pacing. Chronic therapy for preventing recurrent arrhythmia is controversial, and the advent of radio frequency catheter ablation for the cure of typical atrial flutter may limit the need for empiric drug therapy in these patients (*Circulation* 86:1233, 1992). For those patients with drug-refractory atrial flutter not amenable to catheter ablation, interruption of AV nodal conduction via radio frequency catheter ablation with concomitant implantation of a permanent pacemaker is a palliative procedure.

B. **Wide complex tachycardias** may be either supraventricular or ventricular in origin, and correct identification of the origin and mechanism of the tachycardia is critical to the selection of appropriate treatment. Demographic and ECG criteria are helpful in distinguishing between SVT and VT (see sec. **V.B.4.c**).

1. **SVTs with aberration** can present as wide complex tachycardias due to rate-dependent aberration of conduction (right bundle branch block, left bundle branch block) or to the presence of a fixed intraventricular conduction defect.

2. **In the setting of WPW**, the most common wide complex tachycardia is an **aberrantly conducted orthodromic tachycardia** (see sec. **V.A.6.a**), but it must be distinguished from **antidromic tachycardia** and **atrial fibrillation** with conduction down the bypass tract.

   a. **Antidromic tachycardia** occurs when electrical activation propagates down the accessory pathway, throughout the ventricle, with retrograde (antidromic) activation up the AV node to the atria, completing the macro-reentrant circuit. It is characterized by the presence of an inverted P wave prior to every QRS, a short but constant PR interval with the absence of an isoelectric PR segment, and a wide and bizarre QRS morphology.

   b. **Preexcited atrial fibrillation** occurs when ventricular activation during atrial fibrillation occurs via the accessory bypass tract as opposed to via the AV node. Patients with WPW have an increased propensity to develop atrial fibrillation. Preexcited atrial fibrillation is characterized by an irregularly undulating baseline without recognizable P waves, an irregular and typically rapid ventricular rate (180–300 beats/minute), and QRS complexes demonstrating variable fusion between normal complexes and fully preexcited (wide, bizarre) complexes. **For preexcited AF, AV nodal–blocking agents (adenosine, calcium channel antagonists, digoxin) should be avoided**, and hemodynamic compromise or clinical instability should be treated with prompt DC cardioversion. Otherwise, class Ia, Ic, or III antiarrhythmic drugs may be used to prolong the pathway refractory period, which slows the ventricular response rate and may chemically cardiovert AF to normal sinus rhythm. Interruption of accessory pathway function, in addition to removing the mechanism for the associated AV reentrant tachycardias, prevents recurrence of AF in up to 90% of patients (*Am J Cardiol* 69:493, 1992).

3. **Accelerated idioventricular rhythm (AIVR)** is an automatic ectopic rhythm, with its origin in the terminal Purkinje system or in ventricular myocardium. The abnormal automaticity responsible for AIVR occurs with acute MI or with drug toxicities (e.g., digitalis). When associated with acute MI or digitalis toxicity, AIVR is a transient and intermittent arrhythmia, without additional adverse prognostic implications. It is usually asymptomatic but may be a cause of hemodynamic deterioration in patients who require AV synchrony. The **ECG** reveals a ventricular rate of 60–110 beats/minute, usually exceeding the spontaneous atrial rate. The QRS complex in AIVR is wide (typically >120 ms) and bizarre. With intact ventriculo-atrial conduction, retrograde P waves are seen after each wide QRS. With ventriculo-atrial block, there is interruption of the sequence of wide QRS complexes by a narrow QRS preceded by a normal P wave (atrial capture). AIVR is suppressed when the atrial rate exceeds the ventricular rate. AIVR is typically a self-limited arrhythmia and does not routinely require aggressive management. In symptomatic patients, therapy is directed at increasing the sinus rate (e.g., with atropine, isoproterenol, overdrive atrial pacing).

4. **Ventricular tachycardia (VT)** is the most frequently encountered life-threatening arrhythmia. Its prompt recognition and acute treatment are often critical to preventing adverse clinical outcomes.

   a. **Etiology.** VT may be caused by abnormalities of impulse conduction (reentry) or abnormalities of impulse initiation (abnormal automaticity or triggered activation). Coronary artery disease with MI is the most common form of organic heart disease that predisposes to VT. The nonconductive scar from the MI, together with the abnormal conduction characteristics of the peri-infarct region, provide the substrate for reentry. Drug and electrolyte abnormalities may alter myocardial membrane characteristics and promote VT. Nonischemic cardiomyopathies (idiopathic, hypertrophic, valvular), infiltrative diseases (amyloidosis, sarcoidosis), infectious diseases (viral myocarditis or cardiomyopathy, Chagas' disease, Lyme disease), congenital diseases (inborn errors of metabolism, long QT syndrome), inflammatory diseases that affect the myocardium (systemic lupus erythematosus, rheumatoid arthritis), and primary and metastatic malignancies that involve the heart may all provide the substrate for the evolution of VT. Finally, a variety of distinct forms of VT have been described in otherwise normal patients without evidence of structural heart disease.

    b. Symptoms. VT may be asymptomatic, particularly when the rate of the tachycardia is relatively slow, the patient is supine, and baseline hemodynamic function is well-preserved. Symptoms include palpitations, neck pounding (associated with AV dissociation), breathlessness, lightheadedness, near-syncope, angina, and syncope. Untreated, VT may degenerate to ventricular fibrillation, resulting in hemodynamic collapse and death. VT is defined as a series of three or more ventricular complexes occurring at a rate of 100–250 beats/minute, where the origin of activation is within the ventricle. Typically, the QRS is wide (usually >120 ms) with a bizarre morphology, accompanied by T waves with a polarity opposite to that of the major QRS deflection.

    c. Classification. Sustained VT is defined as lasting longer than 30 seconds or associated with hemodynamic collapse. **Monomorphic VT** is defined as VT in which the QRS complexes maintain a single morphology throughout the arrhythmia. **Polymorphic VT** is characterized by an ever-changing QRS morphology. **Differentiation of VT from SVT with aberrancy** is critical in determining appropriate therapy, the need for further clinical investigation, as well as the need for and type of long-term arrhythmia management. Distinguishing between SVT with aberrancy and VT based on analysis of the surface ECG can be challenging (*Am J Med* 64:27, 1978; *Circulation* 83:1649, 1991). Features that favor VT include (1) AV dissociation, (2) the presence of capture or fusion beats, (3) left axis deviation, (4) QRS duration greater than 0.14 seconds, and (5) precordial concordance of the dominant QRS deflection. For **right bundle branch block morphology tachycardias**, monophasic or biphasic QRS complexes in V_1, left axis deviation, and an R/S ratio of less than 1 in V_6 favors VT. For **left bundle branch block morphology tachycardias**, R in V_1 or V_2 greater than 30 ms in duration, any Q in V_6, onset of QRS to nadir of S in V_1 or V_6 greater than 60 ms, and notching of the downstroke of the S in V_1 or V_2 favor VT (*Am J Cardiol* 61:1279, 1988).

    d. Therapy. Immediate synchronized DC cardioversion is indicated for sustained VT associated with hemodynamic compromise (hypotension, altered consciousness, heart failure, dyspnea, or angina). **Pharmacologic cardioversion** with IV lidocaine (and/or procainamide and/or bretylium) may be attempted in the patient with clinically stable VT (see Chap. 8). Recurrent sustained VT should be managed with continuous infusion of IV lidocaine (alternate therapy includes procainamide or bretylium) until such time as the acute alteration in the arrhythmogenic substrate has been modified. Selection of a specific therapeutic alternative is determined by the combination of the response to programmed electrical stimulation during cardiac electrophysiology studies, the response of the arrhythmia to antiarrhythmic drug therapy, and the response to exercise testing.

5. Ventricular fibrillation (VF) is the simultaneous presence of multiple activation wave fronts within the ventricle producing uncoordinated electrical activity and ineffective mechanical contraction, leading to hemodynamic collapse and death. Any structural, toxic, or metabolic derangement that

Table 7-1. Drugs associated with torsades de pointes

Amiodarone	Haloperidol	Probucol
Arsenic	Indapamide	Procainamide
Astemizole	Itraconazole	Propafenone
Bepridil	Ketoconazole	Quinidine
Cocaine	Ketanserin	Quinine
Disopyramide	Maprotiline	Sotalol
Droperidol	Moricizine	Sultopride
Encainide	Pentamidine	Terfenadine
Erythromycin	Perhexiline	Terodiline
FK506	Prenylamine	Thioridazine
Flecainide		

adversely affects the homogeneity of electrical recovery and repolarization characteristics of ventricular myocardium can precipitate VF. VF is invariably associated with hemodynamic collapse and death unless prompt cardioversion is successful. The **ECG** reveals rapid (250–400 beats/minute) and irregular oscillations in the baseline, without uniquely identifiable P waves, QRS complexes, or T waves. **Immediate unsynchronized DC cardioversion is primary therapy**. Cardiopulmonary resuscitation should be initiated and continued until cardioversion is successful and hemodynamic stability is restored (see Chap. 8). If DC cardioversion is initially unsuccessful, repeated attempts at cardioversion should be attempted following bolus infusion of first epinephrine and then lidocaine. Following successful cardioversion, continuous IV infusion of lidocaine (procainamide and bretylium are alternates) should be maintained until the acute alterations in the electrophysiologic substrate (myocardial ischemia or infarction, hypoxemia, acidosis, electrolyte abnormalities, drug toxicities) have been corrected. The choice of chronic antiarrhythmic therapy depends on the nature of the conditions responsible for the initial VF episode. Primary VF occurring within the first 72 hours of an acute MI is not associated with an elevated risk of postdischarge recurrence and does not require antiarrhythmic therapy. VF without an identifiable and reversible cause (such as MI, hyperkalemia, drug toxicity, coronary artery spasm) requires chronic therapy in the form of either prophylactic antiarrhythmic drug therapy (e.g., amiodarone) or implantation of an automatic defibrillator (see Antitachycardia Devices).

6. **Torsades de pointes** (twisting of the points) describes a polymorphic VT characterized by successive QRS complexes that gradually migrate from one polarity to another, giving the appearance of a twisting axis of depolarization. The exact electrophysiologic mechanism responsible for torsades de pointes is incompletely understood. Both intraventricular reentry and triggered activity secondary to early after-depolarizations have been implicated as playing important roles in initiating and sustaining this arrhythmia. Torsades de pointes typically occurs in the setting of congenital **long QT syndromes** (Romano-Ward syndrome and Jervell and Lange-Nielsen syndrome), drug-induced prolongation of the QT interval, and end-stage cardiomyopathies. A variety of pharmacologic agents have been associated with QT prolongation and torsades de pointes (Table 7-1). Torsades de pointes is most often an intermittent and recurrent arrhythmia associated with transient hemodynamic compromise (light-headedness, near-syncope, or syncope), although complete hemodynamic collapse may occur. Torsades de pointes is characterized by a variety of **ECG** features. There is prolongation of the QT interval during normal sinus rhythm prior to the onset of the arrhythmia. The initiation of the arrhythmia is triggered by a long-short sequence (e.g., closely coupled premature ventricular complexes during sinus bradycardia or following a sinus pause, ventricular bigeminy). During the arrhythmia, the

QRS complexes appear to undergo a gradual modulation in amplitude and axis. **Sustained arrhythmia in the presence of hemodynamic compromise should be treated with DC cardioversion.** All potentially offending agents should be discontinued. **Magnesium sulfate**, 1–2 g administered by IV bolus, is highly effective in the treatment and prevention of drug-induced torsades de pointes and should be considered primary therapy. Elimination of the triggering (long-short) RR interval sequences and shortening of the QT interval can be achieved by increasing the heart rate to 90–120 beats/minute by either isoproterenol infusion or temporary pacing. Torsades de pointes in the setting of congenital long QT syndromes most often responds to beta-adrenergic antagonists. **Class Ia and class III antiarrhythmic agents should be avoided** because of their propensity to further prolong the QT interval.

Antiarrhythmic Agents

The task of identifying safe and effective antiarrhythmic drug therapy remains complex because our ability to uniquely ascribe a single mechanism to each clinical arrhythmia is imperfect, and the actions of antiarrhythmic agents are modulated by intercurrent disease states and concurrent drug therapies. Antiarrhythmic agents are classified according to the Vaughan-Williams classification (*J Clin Pharmacol* 24:129, 1984; *Am J Cardiol* 52(Suppl):1C, 1983). Class I agents are those that predominantly inhibit the fast sodium channel, class II agents are beta-adrenergic antagonists, class III agents prolong repolarization, and class IV agents are calcium channel antagonists. It is important to remember that a specific antiarrhythmic agent may have actions that span multiple classes of action, and that active metabolites of a given antiarrhythmic agent may have electrophysiologic actions substantially different from the parent compound.

I. **Class I agents** (Table 7-2) possess **local anesthetic** and **membrane stabilizing** effects, and their predominant action is to bind to sodium channels and impede sodium influx during phase 0 of the action potential, resulting in depression of intracardiac conduction. Class I drugs can be further classified into Ia, Ib, and Ic based on additional aspects of their actions in conduction and refractoriness. Class Ia agents prolong ventricular refractoriness and QT interval. Class Ib agents are less potent sodium channel blockers and at high tissue concentrations shorten action potential duration and refractoriness. Class Ic agents are potent sodium channel blocking agents, markedly slowing conduction with little effect on repolarization.

A. **Class Ia agents** (see Table 7-2)
   1. **Quinidine** is effective in suppressing symptomatic atrial premature depolarizations and complex ventricular ectopy, converting atrial fibrillation to sinus rhythm, terminating and preventing recurrence of paroxysmal SVTs, and preventing recurrence of atrial fibrillation. In a highly select minority of patients, quinidine may be useful in preventing recurrence of sustained VT or VF.
      a. **Dosages. Quinidine sulfate** is available in tablets or capsules of 200 and 300 mg. The usual initial dosage is 200 mg PO q6h, with a maximum dosage of 2.4 g/day. Extended-release tablets (300 mg) are given q8–12h. Loading regimens range from 600 mg to 1,000 mg in divided doses over 6–10 hours. **Quinidine polygalacturonate** is available in 275-mg tablets. This form reduces gastric irritation and can be given q8–12h. **Quinidine gluconate** is available in sustained-release tablets of 324 mg. The drug can be administered q8–12h.
      b. **IV administration** should be avoided when possible because of quinidine's propensity to cause hypotension. The ECG and BP must be monitored continuously. Maintenance therapy with IV infusion is not recommended.
      c. **Absorption** of an oral dose of quinidine sulfate or quinidine gluconate is virtually complete, with peak serum levels achieved 90 minutes following

a dose of quinidine sulfate and 3–4 hours after a dose of quinidine gluconate. The serum half-life is 5–8 hours. The serum half-life increases significantly with age and in the presence of hepatic dysfunction, and modestly with CHF and renal failure. Serum levels of 1.3–5.0 µg/ml correlate with clinical efficacy.

d. **Drug toxicity** includes **GI side effects**, which are the most common adverse effects and include nausea, vomiting, diarrhea, abdominal pain, and anorexia. **Cinchonism** is the term used to describe the CNS toxicities of quinidine, which include tinnitus, hearing loss, visual disturbances, confusion, delirium, and psychosis. **Allergic reactions** including rash, fever, immune-mediated thrombocytopenia, and hemolytic anemia may occur. **Proarrhythmic effects** are associated with quinidine therapy in 1–3% of patients and is most often manifest as "quinidine syncope," the result of recurrent episodes of torsades de pointes associated with QT interval prolongation. It is recommended that quinidine and all class Ia agents be avoided in patients with a history of torsades de pointes and that these agents be discontinued if the QT_c exceeds 500 ms or prolongs by more than 25% on therapy [QT_c = measured QT ÷ $\sqrt{(RR)}$]. Hypokalemia, hypomagnesemia, and severe left ventricular dysfunction identify patients at increased risk for development of quinidine-induced torsades. **Cardiac conduction abnormalities** may occur, either in the form of accentuating existing AV block or causing new sinoatrial exit block, intraventricular conduction block, or asystole. Quinidine should be avoided in patients with high-degree AV block and/or evidence of extensive conduction system disease. **An increase in ventricular rate** in patients with atrial flutter and AF can occur with quinidine therapy due to slowing of the atrial rate and vagolytic effects that increase AV nodal conduction. It is recommended that ventricular rate control of atrial fibrillation and flutter first be achieved with AV nodal–blocking agents before initiation of quinidine therapy. **Serum digoxin levels increase approximately twofold with therapeutic doses of quinidine.** Warfarin effects may be potentiated by quinidine. Phenobarbital and phenytoin reduce the serum half-life significantly. Other agents that prolong the QT interval (other class Ia or class III antiarrhythmics, phenothiazines, tricyclic antidepressants, erythromycin, terfenidine, astemizole) should be avoided in patients taking quinidine.

2. **Procainamide** shares quinidine's effects on automaticity, conduction, and refractoriness. Its major metabolite, **N-acetylprocainamide** (NAPA), exerts an action typical of class III agents. The clinical utility of procainamide parallels that of quinidine. Additionally, IV procainamide is more effective than lidocaine in the acute termination of sustained VT (*Circulation* 80:652, 1989).

a. **Dosages.** Capsules of 250, 375, and 500 mg are available. A sustained-release preparation is available with tablets of 250, 500, and 750 mg. A total **oral daily dosage** of 50 mg/kg body weight administered in divided doses results in therapeutic serum levels (4–12 µg/ml). To rapidly obtain therapeutic levels, an oral loading dose of 750–1,000 mg is frequently necessary. The suggested maintenance dosage is 0.5–1.0 g q4–6h.

b. **IV administration** should be given at a rate not exceeding 50 mg/minute (to avoid hypotension) until the arrhythmia is suppressed, the QRS widens by 50%, or a maximum loading dose of 15 mg/kg has been administered. Vital signs should be observed continuously during the initial infusion. A maintenance infusion of 2–5 mg/minute can then be used (see Appendix C).

c. The **peak serum concentration** is reached 1 hour after an oral dose and almost immediately with IV administration. Elimination is by both hepatic metabolism and renal excretion. The major metabolic pathway is hepatic acetylation to NAPA, the metabolite that accounts for the prolongation of repolarization (class III action). The serum half-life of procainamide is approximately 3 hours and may be significantly prolonged by HF

Table 7-2. Dosages of class I and III antiarrhythmic agents[a]

Drug	Normal half-life	Half-life in ESRD (hr)	Elimination	Oral dosage	IV dosage
Ia					
Procainamide	3–6 hr	6–59	Renal 76–93%; hepatic 7–24%	250–1,000 mg q3–4h; sustained release q6h	100 mg q5min or 50 mg/min up to 15 mg/kg; maintenance infusion 2–6 mg/min
Quinidine	5–7 hr	5–14	Hepatic 80–90%; renal 10–20%	Sulfate 200–400 mg q6h; polygalacturonate 275–550 mg q8–12h; glucuronate 324–648 mg q8–12h	Gluconate 16 mg/min to therapeutic plasma concentration (300–700 mg)[b]
Disopyramide	4–10 hr	10–18	Renal 90%; hepatic 10%	100–200 mg q6–8h	—
Ib					
Lidocaine	1–2 hr	1–3	Hepatic 90%; renal 10%	—	1 mg/kg; repeat 0.5 mg/kg q8–10 min, if needed, to total of 3 mg/kg; maintenance infusion of 2 mg/kg
Mexiletine	8–10 hr	9–13	Hepatic 85–95%; renal 10–15%	200–400 mg q8h	—
Moricizine	2–4 hr	?	Renal 40% (metabolites); hepatic 99%	100–300 mg q8h	—
Tocainide	10–14 hr	27	Hepatic 60%; renal 20–40%	300–800 mg q8h	—

Ic

Flecainide	12–27 hr	26	Renal 35%; hepatic 65%	100–200 mg q12h	—
Propafenone[c]	2–32 hr	?	Hepatic, renal	150–300 mg q8h	—
III					
Amiodarone	18–40 days	—	Hepatic	800–1,600 mg qd for 7–14 days; then maintenance dose of 200–400 mg qd	5 mg/kg IV over 2–3 min; then 10 mg/kg/day; use central IV line
Bretylium	4–17 hr	36	Renal 80%; hepatic 20%	—	VF: 5–10 mg/kg bolus; VT: 5–10 mg/kg diluted 1:4 over 8 min; then 1–2 mg/min IV
Sotalol	12 hr	36	Renal 90%	80–160 mg q12h[d]	—

ESRD = end-stage renal disease.
[a] Dosage reductions are often indicated in the presence of renal or hepatic dysfunction.
[b] May cause significant hypotension.
[c] Moderate beta-adrenergic antagonist at usual doses. Long half-life in patients who are poor metabolizers (7% of population).
[d] Significant dose reduction and increased dosing interval in patients with renal insufficiency (see text).

or renal dysfunction. NAPA has a serum half-life of 6–8 hours, but it may be as long as 70 hours in patients with severe renal dysfunction. **Serum procainamide levels** of 4–12 µg/ml correlate with clinical efficacy. Combined procainamide and NAPA levels greater than 30 µg/ml are associated with increased toxicity.

d. **Toxicity and side effects** of procainamide include a **lupus-like syndrome** (fever, pleuropericarditis, hepatomegaly, arthralgias), which may be seen in up to one-third of patients during chronic therapy and may be more likely in the slow acetylator phenotype. This syndrome usually spares the kidneys and resolves when the drug is discontinued. **Antinuclear antibodies**, frequently in high titer, develop in 75% of patients during chronic administration but do not mandate discontinuation of the drug in the absence of other signs or symptoms. **Proarrhythmic effects**, particularly torsades de pointes, has been associated with procainamide use. Class Ia effects (procainamide) and class III effects (NAPA) cause prolongation of the QT_c interval (see sec. **I.A.d**), and the rhythm and QT_c interval should be monitored during initiation of therapy. QT_c prolongation of more than 25% on therapy or a QT_c interval of greater than 500 ms may require discontinuation of the drug. **Agranulocytosis** may result from a hypersensitivity reaction to procainamide. Fever, rash, and constitutional symptoms are manifestations of typical allergic reactions. **Other agents** that prolong the QT interval (other class Ia or class III antiarrhythmics, phenothiazines, tricyclic antidepressants, erythromycin, terfenidine, astemizole) should be avoided in patients taking procainamide.

3. **Disopyramide's** electrophysiologic effects in slowing conduction and prolonging refractoriness are similar to those of procainamide and quinidine. The clinical utility of disopyramide is similar to that of quinidine. Additionally, disopyramide has been shown effective for preventing inducible and spontaneous neurally mediated syncope (*Am J Cardiol* 65:1339, 1990).

a. **Dosages.** Available formulations include 100- and 150-mg capsules. The usual maintenance dosage is 100–300 mg PO q6–8h. In patients with hepatic dysfunction, heart failure, or moderate renal insufficiency (creatinine clearance >40 ml/minute), the dosage should not exceed 100 mg q6h. In patients with marked renal impairment, the recommended dosage regimen is a 200-mg loading dose, followed by 100 mg q12h for creatinine clearances of 15–40 ml/minute, or 100 mg q24h for creatinine clearances less than 15 ml/minute. A sustained-release preparation is available and permits a q12h dosing interval.

b. Oral doses of disopyramide reach a **peak plasma concentration** in approximately 2 hours. In healthy subjects, the serum half-life ranges from 4–10 hours, with a mean of 7 hours. The half-life increases in patients with renal impairment and acute MI. Serum levels of 2–4 µg/ml correlate with clinical efficacy.

c. **Toxicity and side effects** include the following: **Depression of myocardial contractility** may occur and is more marked in patients with preexisting ventricular dysfunction. Disopyramide should not be used in patients with overt heart failure or shock. **Anticholinergic effects** include dry mouth, urinary retention, constipation, blurred vision, abdominal pain, exacerbation of glaucoma, and drying of bronchial secretions. It should be used with caution in patients with myasthenia gravis because its anticholinergic properties may precipitate a myasthenic crisis. **Proarrhythmic effects**, particularly torsades de pointes, may occur. Recommendations regarding monitoring of rhythm and QT_c interval during initiation of therapy are similar to those for the other class Ia agents. **Hypoglycemia,** as well as masking of hypoglycemic symptoms, may accompany disopyramide therapy, particularly in patients with renal dysfunction. **Other agents** that prolong the QT interval (other class Ia or class III antiarrhythmics, phenothiazines, tricyclic antidepressants, erythromycin, terfenidine, astemizole) should be avoided in patients taking disopyramide.

B. **Class Ib agents** (see Table 7-2) are similar to type Ia agents with regard to their effect on fast sodium channels and intracardiac conduction but differ in their effect on repolarization. Type Ib agents shorten repolarization time, in contrast to type Ia agents, which prolong repolarization and refractoriness.

1. **Lidocaine** is effective in the management of ventricular tachyarrhythmias, particularly in the setting of acute MI; however, the routine prophylactic administration of lidocaine in patients with acute MI is not indicated (*Arch Intern Med* 149:2694, 1989).

   a. **Dosages. Initial therapy** should consist of an IV bolus of 1 mg/kg, with subsequent bolus injections of 0.5 mg/kg every 8–10 minutes, if necessary, to a total of 3 mg/kg. At the time of the initial bolus, **maintenance therapy** should also begin with an IV infusion at a rate of 2–4 mg/minute (see Appendix C). The initial bolus and maintenance dose should be reduced by 50% in patients with heart failure, shock, or hepatic dysfunction, and in patients over 70 years of age. In such instances plasma levels should be monitored during prolonged infusions. Endotracheal or IM administration should only be used when IV administration is not possible. The recommended dose is 300 mg, although in the early hours of acute MI, higher doses may be necessary.

   b. **The onset of action** is immediate following IV administration. Serum half-life is prolonged in patients with hepatic dysfunction, in patients over 70 years of age, and in the setting of prolonged administration. Therapeutic serum levels are 2–6 μg/ml, but adverse reactions have been observed at even lower levels.

   c. **Toxicities** of lidocaine include **CNS effects** (convulsions, confusion, stupor, and, rarely, respiratory arrest), all of which resolve with discontinuation of therapy. **Negative inotropic effects** are seen only with high levels of drug. **Induction of arrhythmias** may occur occasionally, including sinus arrest, AV block, and augmentation in AV conduction or atrial rate in patients with atrial flutter or fibrillation. The serum half-life of lidocaine is prolonged when administered with propranolol and cimetidine.

2. **Mexiletine** is similar to lidocaine in its chemical structure, electrophysiologic properties, antiarrhythmic activity, and toxicities. Mexiletine can be used alone or in combination with a class Ia drug for treatment of ventricular arrhythmias. It is not effective in the management of supraventricular arrhythmias and has not proved effective in preventing recurrence of sustained life-threatening ventricular arrhythmias.

   a. **Dosages.** When it is used in combination with type Ia, type II, or type III agents, a synergistic interaction may allow a lower dose of each agent to be used. Mexiletine is available as 150-, 200-, and 250-mg capsules. A loading dose of 400 mg can be administered when rapid control of ventricular arrhythmias is essential. The usual maintenance dosage is 200 mg PO q8h. Patients may have fewer GI-related side effects if mexiletine is taken with food. A minimum of 2–3 days between dosage adjustments is recommended.

   b. **Peak plasma concentrations** are observed within 2–4 hours; however, absorption may be delayed and less complete in patients with acute MI. It is eliminated primarily by the liver, but 10% is excreted unchanged by the kidneys. Hepatic dysfunction and MI may prolong elimination half-life (>20 hours). The margin between therapeutic (0.75–2.00 μg/ml) and toxic (>2 μg/ml) concentrations is narrow.

   c. **Toxicities. CNS toxicity** includes fine tremor, dizziness, and blurred vision. Higher levels of mexiletine may result in dysarthria, diplopia, nystagmus, and an impaired level of consciousness. **GI side effects,** such as nausea and vomiting, are common and may be reduced by administering mexiletine with food. **Proarrhythmic effects,** particularly torsades de pointes, are less common with mexiletine and the other type Ib agents than with type Ia and III agents. **Drug interactions** may be observed with concomitant use of mexiletine and lidocaine. Rifampin and phenytoin reduce plasma levels of mexiletine by enhancing hepatic metabolism. Mexiletine can increase theophylline plasma levels.

3. **Tocainide** can be used alone or in combination with class Ia drugs for treatment of ventricular arrhythmias. It is not effective for the management of SVTs and has not proved to be effective in preventing recurrence of sustained life-threatening ventricular arrhythmias.

   a. **Dosages.** Tocainide is available as 400- and 600-mg tablets. The usual daily dose is 1,200–1,800 mg PO in divided doses q8–12h.

   b. **Peak plasma concentrations** occur within 2 hours. The half-life ranges from 10–14 hours and appears to be prolonged in patients with acute MI. Therapeutic serum levels are 4–10 µg/ml. Increased toxicity is observed with levels exceeding 10 µg/ml.

   c. **Toxicities and side effects** include **neurologic** symptoms, such as dizziness, tremor, paresthesias, and confusion (the most commonly reported adverse reactions), and **GI side effects,** including nausea and vomiting, which are relatively common and may be reduced by administering tocainide with food. **Pulmonary** complications including pulmonary fibrosis, interstitial pneumonitis, and fibrosing alveolitis have been reported in 0.1% of patients. **Hematologic** complications including agranulocytosis, leukopenia, hypoplastic anemia, and thrombocytopenia have been reported in 0.1–0.2% of patients. CBCs should be monitored during long-term therapy. Tocainide may decrease theophylline metabolism.

4. **Phenytoin** is used primarily in the treatment of digitalis-induced ventricular and supraventricular arrhythmias. It may have a limited role in the treatment of ventricular arrhythmias associated with congenital long QT syndromes.

   a. **Dosages.** The **IV loading dose** is 250 mg diluted in normal saline (crystallization occurs in dextrose-containing solutions), given slowly over 10 minutes. Subsequent doses of 100 mg can be given q5min as needed to a total of 1,000 mg. Frequent monitoring of the ECG and BP and examination for signs of nystagmus are required. A **continuous infusion should not be used**.

   b. **The onset of action** after IV administration is prompt. The serum half-life is 22–25 hours and is prolonged with concomitant administration of any drug that competes with phenytoin for hepatic degradation. Therapeutic serum levels are 10–20 µg/ml, and levels exceeding 20 µg/ml are associated with toxicity.

   c. **Toxicities** of phenytoin include **hypotension, sinus bradycardia,** and **respiratory depression,** which may occur with rapid IV administration and may be minimized by slow administration (maximum 50 mg/minute). **Neurologic** manifestations of toxicity such as nystagmus, nausea, vertigo, ataxia, stupor, and coma may occur. The risk of **thrombophlebitis,** which occurs as a result of the vehicle in which phenytoin is dissolved, may be minimized by administration via a large central vein. Phenytoin levels are increased by amiodarone, fluconazole, isoniazid, and cimetidine. Carbemazepine, folic acid, and rifampin decrease phenytoin levels. Serum quinidine levels or effects of warfarin may be diminished by phenytoin.

5. **Moricizine** is structurally similar to the phenothiazines and has electrophysiologic effects that represent a combination of class Ia and Ib actions. Moricizine can be used to treat ventricular arrhythmias. It is not effective for the management of SVTs and has not proved to be effective in preventing recurrence of sustained life-threatening ventricular arrhythmias.

   a. **Dosages.** Moricizine is available in 200-, 250-, and 300-mg tablets. The initial dosage is 200 mg PO q8h, which can be increased every 3 days by 150 mg/day to a maximum of 900 mg/day. Twice-daily dosing may provide effective therapy but may increase side effects, due to increased peak plasma levels.

   b. **Toxicities** of moricizine include **proarrhythmic effects,** which occur in approximately 3% of treated patients, with greater frequency in those with prior history of potentially lethal arrhythmias or severe left ventricular dysfunction. The potential for serious proarrhythmia limits the widespread use of moricizine (*N Engl J Med* 327:227, 1992). **GI side effects** include nausea, vomiting, and diarrhea. **CNS** toxicities include tremor, mood changes, headache, vertigo, dizziness, and nystagmus. Moricizine may decrease serum levels of theophylline.

C. **Class Ic agents** (see Table 7-2) profoundly depress the maximum rate of rise of phase 0 of the action potential and markedly slow conduction, with less prolongation of refractoriness than with class Ia agents. **Flecainide and propafenone** have pronounced effects on conduction in the AV node, the His-Purkinje system, and ventricular myocardium. Automaticity is decreased in the sinus node, Purkinje fibers, and ventricular tissue. The ECG characteristically shows a widening of the QRS and lengthening of the QT_c interval (see sec. **I.A.d**), attributable to QRS prolongation.

1. **Flecainide** is effective in the management of a variety of supraventricular arrhythmias including AF, atrial flutter, and the PSVTs, and can effect chemical cardioversion of AF to normal sinus rhythm. Flecainide prevents induction of ventricular tachyarrhythmias in less than 30% of patients, yet it does not appear to favorably affect survival or incidence of sudden cardiac death. It is more effective than quinidine in suppressing complex ventricular ectopy and nonsustained ventricular tachycardia, although routine use is not recommended because of the risk of proarrhythmia and sudden death (*N Engl J Med* 324:781, 1991).

   a. **Dosages.** Flecainide is available in 100-mg tablets. The initial dosage is 100 mg PO bid and can be increased cautiously by an increment of 50 mg bid every fourth day until clinical efficacy is obtained or a total dose of 400 mg/day is reached. Dosages exceeding 400 mg/day should be avoided in patients with heart or renal failure.

   b. **Therapeutic serum levels** range from 0.4–0.9 µg/ml. The mean plasma elimination half-life is approximately 20 hours and is prolonged in the setting of renal impairment or HF.

   c. **Toxicities** of flecainide include **conduction abnormalities**, which may occur or worsen. A 20% increase in the PR and QRS intervals is commonly observed and is not cause for concern. Patients who have an increase of more than 50% in the PR and QRS intervals should be closely monitored. The dose should be reduced or the drug discontinued if the PR interval exceeds 0.3 seconds, the QRS duration exceeds 0.2 seconds, or bifascicular block, second-degree AV block, or third-degree AV block occurs. **Proarrhythmic effects** manifested as exacerbation of ventricular arrhythmias have been reported in up to 5% of patients. This risk may be higher in patients with underlying heart disease or malignant ventricular arrhythmias (*N Engl J Med* 324:781, 1991). Flecainide serum levels above 1 µg/ml appear to be associated with a higher risk of sustained ventricular arrhythmias. When used in the treatment of AF (particularly in the absence of AV nodal–blocking agents), flecainide may result in conversion to atrial flutter with 1 : 1 AV conduction. **Negative inotropic effects** may exacerbate HF, and flecainide should be used very cautiously in patients with left ventricular dysfunction. **Pacing thresholds** of the atria and ventricles may increase by as much as 200%. Flecainide should be used cautiously in pacemaker-dependent patients and in patients with implanted defibrillators. **Noncardiac effects** include confusion, irritability, blurred vision, dizziness, nausea, and headache. Modest increases in plasma digoxin levels will occur when flecainide is administered. Plasma levels of both flecainide and propranolol are increased when these agents are used concurrently. **Amiodarone increases flecainide levels**, requiring a one-third reduction in the dosage of flecainide. Concomitant use of beta-adrenergic antagonists or calcium channel antagonists may precipitate symptomatic bradycardia or high-degree AV block.

2. **Propafenone** is structurally related to flecainide and to some beta-adrenergic

antagonists. At therapeutic levels it has both type Ic actions and moderate beta-adrenergic antagonist actions. It is effective in the management of atrial fibrillation, atrial flutter, AV nodal reentrant tachycardia, and bypass tract–mediated tachycardias, and can effect chemical cardioversion of AF to normal sinus rhythm. Propafenone is effective in suppressing complex nonsustained ventricular ectopy and, in highly select patients, SVT.

a. **Dosages.** Propafenone is available in 150- and 300-mg tablets. The initial dosage is 150 mg PO tid, which can be increased at 3- to 4-day intervals to 225 mg tid, and then 300 mg tid. The dosage should be increased cautiously in patients with hepatic or renal insufficiency.

b. **Plasma concentration.** The relationship between serum level and therapeutic effect is poor. Propafenone reaches peak plasma concentration in 2–3 hours, and metabolism occurs in the liver. Bioavailability increases with dose, such that a threefold increase in dose (300–900 mg/day) may result in a tenfold increase in plasma concentration. Caution is advised in patients with renal insufficiency, as the parent drug and the metabolites are eliminated in the urine. **Therapeutic serum concentrations** range from 0.2–1.5 μg/ml. The dose for patients with hepatic insufficiency is 20–30% of the usual dose.

c. **Toxicities** of propafenone include **conduction abnormalities,** similar to those seen with flecainide, which may occur or worsen in conjunction with propafenone therapy (see sec. **I.C.1.c**). **Proarrhythmic effects** in the form of exacerbation of ventricular arrhythmias have been reported in up to 5% of patients. This risk may be higher in patients with underlying heart disease or malignant ventricular arrhythmias. **Bronchospasm** may occur as a result of the beta-adrenergic antagonistic actions of propafenone. **Negative inotropic effects** may precipitate or worsen CHF. **Noncardiac effects** include dizziness, disturbances in taste, blurred vision, and nausea. Drugs that inhibit the cytochrome P_{450} system in the liver may inhibit propafenone metabolism. Plasma digoxin concentration, effects of beta-adrenergic antagonists, and effects of warfarin are all increased by propafenone.

II. Class II agents (see Table 4-3) are beta-adrenergic antagonists that exert their antiarrhythmic actions by attenuating the binding of circulating catecholamines to beta-adrenergic receptor sites on myocytes and diminishing increases in automaticity. Beta-adrenergic antagonists are effective in decreasing automaticity and abolishing reentrant arrhythmias involving the AV node. In ventricular tissue, beta-adrenergic antagonists have little direct effect on action potential characteristics of ventricular muscle but can favorably influence arrhythmias by their effects on myocardial oxygen supply and demand. Class II agents are clinically useful in the following situations:

A. **After MI,** beta-adrenergic antagonists reduce both overall death rate and sudden death rate (*Am J Cardiol* 70:21, 1992; *Circulation* 85:1107, 1992).

B. In **thyrotoxicosis, pheochromocytoma,** and states of clear **catecholamine excess** (exercise, postoperative state, extreme emotional stress), the associated arrhythmias often respond to beta-adrenergic antagonist therapy.

C. In **atrial fibrillation** and **atrial flutter,** beta-adrenergic antagonists reduce the ventricular response rate and reduce the incidence of postoperative atrial fibrillation in cardiac surgery patients (*Circulation* 84:236, 1991).

D. **SVTs** may respond to therapy with beta-adrenergic antagonists.

E. **Sinus tachycardia,** while rarely requiring specific treatment, responds to beta-adrenergic blockade.

F. In **congenital long QT syndromes** complicated by recurrent episodes of torsades de pointes, beta-adrenergic antagonists may be effective in preventing recurrent episodes of torsades de pointes (*Ann NY Academy Sciences* 644:112, 1992).

G. **Neurocardiogenic syncope** may be effectively managed with beta-adrenergic antagonists.

Toxicities and side effects of class II agents include **negative inotropic** effects that can precipitate or exacerbate left ventricular dysfunction and HF, particularly when administered by the IV route. Their use should be avoided in patients with severe heart failure or shock. **Negative chronotropic effects** may cause symptomatic sinus bradycardia and may exacerbate AV nodal conduction abnormalities. **Abrupt withdrawal** of beta-adrenergic antagonists may precipitate cardiac arrhythmias or angina. After chronic administration, discontinuation of drug therapy should be tapered over several days. In **insulin-dependent diabetics**, beta-adrenergic antagonists may mask the symptoms of hypoglycemia. **Coronary artery spasm** may be potentiated or exacerbated by beta-adrenergic antagonists due to unopposed alpha-adrenergic stimulation. **Bronchospasm** may be exacerbated in patients with asthma, chronic obstructive pulmonary disease, or allergic rhinitis; it may be partially averted by using lower doses of beta$_1$-selective agents. Other side effects include lethargy, confusion, diminished concentration, mental depression, impotence, potentiation of Raynaud's phenomenon, nightmares, and insomnia.

III. **Class III agents** (see Table 7-2) prolong action potential duration and repolarization to a greater extent than they depress conduction velocity.

   A. **Amiodarone** prolongs action potential duration, repolarization, and refractoriness in atrial and ventricular tissue. It slows the sinus rate and recovery time and prolongs AV nodal conduction. Amiodarone blocks the peripheral conversion of thyroxine (T_4) to triiodothyronine (T_3). It is a noncompetitive alpha- and beta-adrenergic antagonist and a relatively potent antianginal agent. It reduces systemic vascular resistance and mean arterial BP without a significant change in left ventricular function; however, hemodynamic deterioration has been reported in patients with severe underlying left ventricular failure. Amiodarone is a potent antiarrhythmic agent effective for a variety of arrhythmias but in high doses is associated with significant toxicities (*Am Heart J* 125:109, 1993). Amiodarone is effective in the management of **supraventricular arrhythmias,** but the emergence of other definitive therapies and amiodarone's potential toxicities limit its use in these settings. Amiodarone prevents recurrence of **AF** and **atrial flutter** and can effect chemical conversion of AF to normal sinus rhythm. In chronic AF, it slows the ventricular response, but the onset of this effect is slow in comparison to that of conventional agents (calcium channel antagonists, beta-adrenergic antagonists, digoxin). Amiodarone prevents the recurrence of sustained **spontaneous VT or VF** in up to 60% of patients. A therapeutic latency of 5–15 days exists before beneficial antiarrhythmic effects are observed, and full suppression of arrhythmias may not be obtained for 4–6 weeks after initiating therapy.

   1. **Dosages.** Amiodarone is available as a 200-mg scored tablet. The initial loading schedules are empiric and vary between 800 and 1,600 mg PO qd for 1–2 weeks. The usual maintenance dose rarely exceeds 400 mg qd, and the minimum effective dose should be used to avoid the potential toxicities. Approximately 50% of an oral dose is absorbed, and a peak plasma concentration occurs 3–8 hours after ingestion. Achieving steady state without an initial high-dose loading period may take more than 6 months.

   2. **Elimination** is via hepatic excretion into bile. The slow uptake and release from reservoir tissues contribute to a multiphasic elimination half-life in which plasma levels fall to 50% within the first 3–5 days after discontinuation of therapy, with a subsequent half-life of 26–107 days. **Therapeutic serum levels** range from 1.0–2.5 µg/ml. Measurements of serum concentrations of amiodarone are of only limited value but may be helpful in documenting compliance and absorption.

   3. **Adverse effects** are partially dose-dependent and may occur in up to 75% of patients treated with amiodarone at high doses for 5 years, but in fewer than 20% of cases do these adverse effects require discontinuation of therapy. The incidence of **pulmonary toxicity** has been reported as 5–15%. It may occur early or late in the course of therapy at a wide range of doses but is unlikely to occur in patients receiving less than 300 mg/day (*Circulation* 82:51, 1990). Patients characteristically have dry cough and dyspnea associated with

pulmonary infiltrates and rales. The process appears to be reversible if detected early, but undetected cases may result in a mortality rate of up to 10%. A **chest x-ray** should be obtained every 3–6 months to detect interstitial changes. Changes in pulmonary function tests, especially a decrease in diffusing capacity, are of value in the diagnosis of amiodarone pulmonary toxicity. **Photosensitivity** is a common adverse reaction, and in some patients a violaceous skin discoloration develops in sun-exposed areas. The blue-gray discoloration may not completely resolve with discontinuation of therapy (*Mayo Clin Proceed* 66:721, 1991). **Corneal microdeposits,** detectable on slit-lamp examination, develop in virtually all patients. Their occurrence is dose-dependent and reversible with discontinuation of the drug. These deposits rarely interfere with vision, although a small number of patients may notice halos around lights at night. **Hypothyroidism** and **hyperthyroidism** have been reported, with an incidence of approximately 3%. Thyroid function should be monitored annually. The diagnosis of hyperthyroidism may be obscured by elevation of T_4 (observed routinely during chronic amiodarone therapy) but clinical hyperthyroidism is confirmed by suppression of the TSH level to less than 0.1 μU/ml together with an elevated plasma T_4. Hypothyroidism is typically associated with a markedly increased TSH level. **Cardiovascular effects** include asymptomatic sinus bradycardia and prolonged AV node conduction; however, severe bradycardia or high-grade AV block may occur, more often in patients with preexisting conduction abnormalities. Exacerbation of ventricular arrhythmias has been reported but occurs less commonly than with class I agents. The ECG effects of amiodarone are a lengthened PR interval, QRS duration, and QT interval. Torsades de pointes is a rare complication of amiodarone therapy. Other agents that prolong the QT interval (other class Ia or class III antiarrhythmics, phenothiazines, tricyclic antidepressants, erythromycin, terfenidine, astemizole) should be avoided in patients taking amiodarone. **GI side effects** including nausea, anorexia, and constipation may occur, especially during the initial high-dose loading phase. A transient rise in **hepatic transaminases** is commonly observed early in the course of therapy but is usually asymptomatic. If the increase exceeds 3 times normal or doubles in a patient with an elevated baseline level, amiodarone should be discontinued or the dose reduced. Amiodarone has been reported to markedly potentiate the effects of warfarin and to increase flecainide and digoxin levels. **Maintenance doses of digoxin should be routinely reduced by one-half** when amiodarone is started.

B. **Sotalol** decreases the frequency and duration of nonsustained VT in up to 40% of patients, prevents inducibility of sustained VT via programmed electrical stimulation (PES) in 35% of patients, and prevents recurrence of sustained VT and VF in 70% of patients (*N Engl J Med* 329:452, 1993). Sotalol may be effective in preventing recurrence of symptomatic AF and atrial flutter, but concern about proarrhythmia limits widespread use.

   1. **Dosages.** Sotalol is available as 80-, 160-, and 240-mg tablets. Initial dosage is 80 mg bid, with dosage increments every 2–3 days until the desired dose is attained. A therapeutic response is obtained at a daily dose of 240–360 mg/day in most patients.

   2. **Peak plasma concentrations** occur in 2.5–4.0 hours, with an elimination half-life of approximately 12 hours. Steady-state plasma concentrations occur in 2–3 days. Sotalol is predominantly excreted unchanged in the urine. The dosing interval should be 24 hours for a creatinine clearance of 30–60 ml/minute, with extension to 36–48 hours for a creatinine clearance of 10–30 ml/minute.

   3. **Toxicities** of sotalol include **proarrhythmic effects,** typically torsades de pointes, the risk of which appears to be dose dependent and related to the QT interval. Hypokalemia should be avoided, as it has been associated with an increased risk of torsades de pointes in patients receiving sotalol. Other agents that prolong the QT interval (other class Ia or class III antiarrhythmics,

phenothiazines, tricyclic antidepressants, erythromycin, terfenidine, astemizole) should be avoided in patients taking sotalol. **Bradyarrhythmias** (e.g., sinus bradycardia or advanced AV block) may occur with sotalol therapy, particularly when sotalol is used in combination with other agents that suppress sinus node function or AV nodal conduction. It is contraindicated in patients with sinus bradycardia or second- or third-degree AV block. **Bronchospasm** may be precipitated by sotalol therapy, particularly in patients with asthma. **HF** may be precipitated or exacerbated by sotalol therapy. New-onset HF occurs in approximately 3% of patients. **Hypoglycemic** symptoms may be attenuated and recovery may be impaired by sotalol therapy. Effects on sinus nodal conduction, AV nodal conduction, left ventricular dysfunction, and BP are additive with **calcium channel antagonists**. Concomitant use of reserpine, guanethidine, and bretylium may produce excessive reduction in resting sympathetic tone.

C. **Bretylium tosylate** is a quaternary ammonium compound that has direct electrophysiologic effects as well as important interactions with the autonomic nervous system. Bretylium markedly prolongs action potential duration and refractoriness in Purkinje fibers and ventricular muscle. Automaticity transiently increases after drug exposure due to the initial release of norepinephrine from adrenergic nerve terminals. Efficacy in terminating reentrant arrhythmias is probably related to marked alterations in refractoriness and stabilization of sympathetic tone. Bretylium's chief clinical utility is in the treatment of **VT and VF**. It may be effective in cardiac arrest, even after protracted episodes of ventricular fibrillation refractory to conventional maneuvers (see Chap. 8).

1. **Dosages.** In the treatment of **VF**, a 5-mg/kg undiluted bolus is given rapidly IV, and defibrillation is attempted after CPR-assisted circulation. If VF recurs or persists, a second bolus of 10 mg/kg can be administered at intervals of 15 minutes to a maximum dose of 30 mg/kg. For patients with hemodynamically stable refractory or recurrent **VT**, rapid injections of bretylium should be avoided as they may cause hypotension, nausea, and vomiting. In those patients who do not require immediate cardioversion, 5–10 mg/kg bretylium should be injected over 10 minutes, followed by an infusion of 2 mg/minute (see Appendix C).

2. The **onset of action** is prompt with IV administration, although maximum efficacy may require 15–20 minutes. The serum half-life varies from 4–17 hours.

3. **Toxicities** include **proarrhythmic effects,** which may occur as a result of initial elaboration of catecholamines. **Orthostatic hypotension** may occur. Transient **hypertension** and increased sinus rate may accompany initiation of therapy. Other side effects include nausea, vomiting, parotid pain and swelling, light-headedness, rash, emotional lability, and renal dysfunction. Bretylium may potentiate the response to infused catecholamines. The hypotensive effects of diuretics or vasodilator drugs may also be augmented during bretylium administration.

IV. **Class IV agents** are calcium channel antagonists (see Table 4-3). These agents selectively block the slow inward current carried primarily by calcium ions. In tissues dependent on slow-channel activity (sinoatrial and AV nodes and some areas of diseased atrial and ventricular tissue), verapamil induces a concentration-dependent depression in phase 4 depolarization and a prolongation in refractoriness, resulting in depressed automaticity and slowed conduction.

A. **Verapamil** is effective in slowing the ventricular response rate of atrial fibrillation and flutter and in slowing or abolishing the SVTs that use the AV node as their reentrant circuit. IV formulations are useful for termination of paroxysmal reentrant SVTs, though bolus administration of adenosine appears equally effective, with a diminished incidence of prolonged hypotension. Verapamil is effective in preventing recurrence of SVTs and in achieving a well-controlled ventricular response in primary atrial arrhythmias.

1. **Dosages.** For **IV administration,** verapamil is supplied in 5-mg vials. An initial dose of 5–10 mg should be administered as a slow IV bolus over 2–3

minutes. This dose can be repeated after 15–30 minutes if the initial response is unsatisfactory. A continuous infusion of verapamil is seldom required but can be administered as a rapid loading infusion (in isotonic saline) of 0.375 mg/minute for 30 minutes, followed by a maintenance infusion of 0.125 mg/minute. The cardiac rhythm and vital signs should be monitored closely during administration. For **oral administration**, verapamil is available in 40-, 80-, and 120-mg tablets. The usual initial dosage is 80 mg q6–8h. The total daily dose ranges from 240–480 mg. Sustained-release tablets (120-, 180-, 240-mg) may permit a once daily dosing interval.

2. The **onset of action is within 1–2 minutes** following IV administration, with a peak effect occurring in 10–15 minutes. Depression of AV node conduction is detectable up to 6 hours after drug administration. Hemodynamic effects occur 3–5 minutes after bolus injection and usually dissipate within 20 minutes. After oral ingestion, peak plasma concentrations are reached in 1–2 hours. The elimination half-life is 4–12 hours, with up to 70% of the drug excreted by the kidneys.

3. **Toxicities** of verapamil include **bradycardia, high-degree AV block, and asystole.** Verapamil should not be used in patients with preexisting second- or third-degree AV block or patients with sinus node dysfunction. **Hypotension** may occur after IV administration. Therapy with IV fluids and pressor agents is generally effective, and pretreatment with IV calcium salts (1 g calcium gluconate) may blunt verapamil-induced hypotension (*Ann Intern Med* 107:623, 1987). Verapamil should be used cautiously in patients with mild to moderate HF and in the elderly, and it is contraindicated in the presence of severe heart failure or hypotension. **Verapamil is contraindicated in patients with WPW syndrome and atrial fibrillation,** as it may increase the ventricular response rate by enhancing anterograde conduction over the accessory pathway, potentially initiating VF. **Transient ventricular ectopy** may be observed after verapamil-induced termination of reentrant SVTs and is generally self-limited. In **hepatic dysfunction,** toxic levels may be reached quickly. Verapamil's **negative inotropic and chronotropic effects are additive** with those of other antiarrhythmic agents, and combination therapy should be used with caution in patients with heart failure or preexisting conduction system disease. Serious adverse effects have been reported with concomitant use of verapamil and IV beta-adrenergic antagonists in patients with impaired ventricular function or impaired AV nodal conduction. Verapamil may be used with digoxin, but caution should be exercised as both drugs impair AV conduction.

B. **Diltiazem** also slows conduction within the AV node. Continuous infusion allows titration of effect in critical care settings (*Am J Cardiol* 69:36B, 1992). IV bolus of diltiazem is effective in terminating nearly 90% of PSVTs within 3 minutes of a first or second bolus but is not as effective in preventing recurrence.

1. **Dosages.** The recommended dose for **IV bolus** administration is 0.25 mg/kg of body weight over 2 minutes, with a repeat bolus of 0.35 mg/kg if the desired effect is not obtained. After bolus administration, a continuous infusion may be initiated at 10 mg/hr, with the infusion rate titrated to desired effect. Continuous administration for longer than 24 hours is not recommended. **Oral** preparations include 30-, 60-, 90-, and 120-mg tablets for tid or qid dosing, with longer-acting preparations available in 60-, 90-, 120-, 180-, 240-, and 300-mg preparations for qd or bid dosing. Oral administration should begin at 120–180 mg/day, initially in divided doses.

2. The **plasma elimination half-life** is 3–4 hours following a single IV injection and prolongs by as much as 50% with continuous IV administration. For conversion from IV to PO dosing, the approximate PO daily dose is 150% of the 24-hour cumulative IV infusion.

3. **Toxicity and side effects** of diltiazem include **bradyarrhythmias;** diltiazem is contraindicated in patients with sick sinus syndrome and second- or third-degree AV block. The concomitant use of other agents that slow sinus rate or block AV nodal conduction (beta-adrenergic antagonists, calcium

channel antagonists, type I or type III antiarrhythmics, or digoxin) may precipitate symptomatic bradycardia or high-degree AV block. In patients with **WPW**, diltiazem is contraindicated for treatment of AF or atrial flutter, as paradoxical enhancement of conduction in the accessory bypass tract may precipitate VF. Symptomatic **hypotension** may be observed in up to 3% of patients treated with IV bolus infusion. Diltiazem should be used with caution in patients with HF. Hepatic dysfunction may allow for accumulation of drug to toxic levels. Acute hepatic injury has rarely been reported following oral diltiazem. Diltiazem has been shown to increase propranolol levels, increasing the possibility of bradycardia and AV block.

C. **Adenosine** is an endogenous nucleoside with significant electrophysiologic effects, including inhibition of sinus node automaticity, depression of AV node conduction, and prolongation of AV nodal refractoriness. Adenosine is indicated for the treatment of reentrant SVT that can be terminated by blocking AV node conduction. Adenosine and verapamil have comparable efficacy for termination of AV nodal reentry and orthodromic SVT (WPW) (*Ann Intern Med* 113:104, 1990). Adenosine is not effective in converting atrial flutter, AF, or VT to sinus rhythm, but adenosine-induced AV nodal blockade may facilitate the diagnosis of these arrhythmias by causing transient AV dissociation.

1. **Dosages.** The recommended initial dose is 6 mg given IV as a rapid bolus via an antecubital vein, followed by a 10- to 30-ml saline flush. If SVT is not terminated within 1–2 minutes, 12 mg should be given and can be repeated if necessary. A lower initial dose (1–3 mg) should be used if the drug is injected through a central venous line.

2. **The serum half-life** of adenosine—approximately 10 seconds—is not affected by hepatic or renal failure. A **continuous infusion of adenosine is not effective** and should not be used for control of supraventricular arrhythmias.

3. **Toxicities.** Adenosine may precipitate prolonged asystole in patients with sick sinus syndrome or second- or third-degree AV block. Facial flushing, dyspnea, and chest pressure are common adverse side effects but are usually of brief duration. The effects of adenosine are antagonized by **methylxanthines** such as caffeine or theophylline. Accordingly, adenosine may be ineffective or larger doses may be required in patients who have taken methylxanthines. The effects of adenosine are potentiated by **dipyridamole**, which blocks cellular uptake of adenosine and delays its metabolism. Carbamazepine also potentiates the effects of adenosine.

D. **Digitalis glycosides** are useful in the control of the ventricular rate response to AF or atrial flutter in the setting of left ventricular dysfunction and heart failure. It may also be useful as adjunctive therapy in combination with calcium channel antagonists or beta-adrenergic antagonists for optimum rate control of chronic AF (*Am J Cardiol* 69:78G, 1992).

1. **Dosages.** Digoxin, the most commonly used digitalis glycoside, is available as digoxin solution in capsules (0.05-, 0.1-, and 0.2-mg), as tablets (0.125-, 0.25-, and 0.5-mg), as a solution for injection (0.25 mg/ml and 0.1 mg/ml), and as an elixir (0.05 mg/ml). The bioavailability varies with preparation. **Loading regimens** for digoxin vary widely, with as much as 0.5 mg given as a single IV dose and loading accomplished after 1.0–1.5 mg has been administered in divided doses over 8–24 hours. Maintenance doses of 0.125–0.500 mg qd are common.

2. **Therapeutic digoxin levels** are not well defined, but a range of 0.8–2.0 ng/ml correlates with effect in most patients. Levels >2 ng/ml should raise concern of digitalis toxicity. Digoxin levels should not be drawn within 6 hours after an IV dose or 8 hours after a PO dose as distribution will be incomplete. Most of an oral dose is absorbed, with peak effect occurring in 90 minutes to 5 hours. Following IV injection, peak effect is observed in 1–4 hours. The average serum half-life is 36–48 hours. The excretion pathway is predominantly renal, and serum half-life is prolonged in patients with renal insufficiency.

3. **Digitalis toxicity** is not well correlated with serum levels and is potentiated by

hypomagnesemia, hypokalemia, hypercalcemia, and renal impairment (see Chaps. 6 and 9). Manifestations of digitalis toxicity include **constitutional** symptoms such as fatigue and malaise. **GI** side effects include anorexia, nausea, and vomiting. **Neurologic** symptoms such as headache, confusion, delirium, seizures, visual aberrations (scotomas, halos, changes in color perception) may occur. **Cardiac arrhythmias** including MAT or PAT with block, bidirectional VT, and VF may occur. Increases in **outflow obstruction** in patients with hypertrophic obstructive cardiomyopathy may be precipitated by treatment with digitalis glycosides. Digitalis may increase the duration of episodes of **paroxysmal AF** without slowing the ventricular response rate (*Br Heart J* 64:409, 1990). **In patients with WPW,** digitalis, like all AV nodal–blocking agents, is contraindicated as it may facilitate conduction down the accessory pathway during AF, potentially resulting in VF. Concomitant therapy with calcium channel antagonists and beta-adrenergic antagonists may result in complete heart block. Quinidine, verapamil, amiodarone, and propafenone increase serum digoxin concentration. **Quinidine administration will increase the serum digoxin level twofold** and requires decreasing the maintenance dose of digoxin accordingly. IV calcium may produce serious arrhythmias in patients receiving digitalis.

V. General principles of antiarrhythmic drug therapy

A. Initiation. Antiarrhythmic drugs constitute a diverse set of agents with a wide range of potential adverse effects and toxicities, chief among them the potential for **proarrhythmia**, defined as aggravation of the rhythm under treatment or initiation of a different, potentially life-threatening arrhythmia. In general, class Ia, Ic, and III agents appear to have a greater propensity for proarrhythmia, with the likelihood of proarrhythmic complications being highest in the setting of ischemic heart disease, left ventricular dysfunction, and high drug doses. While it is recommended that the initiation and titration of antiarrhythmic drug therapy be performed in a monitored setting in a hospital, it must be noted that drug initiation is not the only time proarrhythmia may develop. These observations underscore the importance of exercising caution in the selection of antiarrhythmic drug therapy.

B. Assessment of efficacy of drug therapy. Appropriate strategies for assessing antiarrhythmic drug efficacy depend on the goals of therapy (e.g., relieving symptoms, diminishing recurrence rate, or complete prevention), the specific arrhythmia under treatment, and the arrhythmia-induced physiologic manifestations.

1. Continuous ECG monitoring in a coronary care unit (CCU) or telemetry unit is advisable for patients with incessant arrhythmias or recurrent arrhythmias with adverse sequellae (particularly sustained VT or VF). For patients whose arrhythmias are nonsustained and well tolerated, **Holter monitoring** may be useful. **Event recorders,** patient-activated ECG recording devices, are useful in patients with infrequent symptoms potentially related to transient rhythm abnormalities. However, using quantitative measures of transient arrhythmia as markers of drug efficacy remains controversial due to the day-to-day variability in arrhythmia frequency. For assessment of the efficacy of antiarrhythmic therapy in completely preventing recurrence of sustained VT or VF, surrogate markers such as the frequency and duration of nonsustained VT have shown only limited value (*N Engl J Med* 329:445, 1993), and in some studies, the demonstrated ability to reduce transient ectopy has been associated with increased overall mortality (*N Engl J Med* 321:406, 1989; *N Engl J Med* 327:227, 1992).

2. Provocative tests

a. Exercise testing may be useful in the evaluation of antiarrhythmic drug efficacy, particularly in the small subset of patients with arrhythmias triggered by exertion or changes in sympathetic tone. However, exercise testing is less sensitive than 24-hour ECG recording for detecting atrial or ventricular arrhythmias. In a minority of patients with sustained ventricular arrhythmias and frequent ventricular ectopy, exercise testing in combination with ambulatory monitoring may be useful in identifying antiarrhythmic therapy that prevents recurrence of sustained ventricular arrhythmias (N Engl J Med 329:445, 1993).

b. In **electrophysiology studies,** percutaneously placed endocardial catheter electrodes are used to record intracardiac electrograms and provide **programmed electrical stimulation (PES)** for the evaluation of complex supraventricular and ventricular arrhythmias. In the evaluation of **supraventricular arrhythmias,** PES is useful in replicating the clinical arrhythmia, determining the arrhythmia mechanism, and, when appropriate, ablating the arrhythmia mechanism. **Ablation procedures** using radio frequency energy to induce highly localized thermal injury may yield success rates in excess of 95% for permanently ablating the mechanisms responsible for bypass tract–mediated tachycardias, AVNRT, atrial tachycardias, and typical atrial flutter. In the evaluation and management of **ventricular arrhythmias,** PES reproducibly induces sustained VT or VF in 75% of survivors of sudden cardiac death and 95% of patients with sustained monomorphic VT (Circulation 72:1, 1985). In patients in whom PES induces VT, subsequent studies may be performed to guide antiarrhythmic drug therapy based on efficacy in preventing induction of ventricular arrhythmias (N Engl J Med 317:1681, 1987). Patients treated with antiarrhythmic therapy based on suppression of inducibility of VT experience significantly lower arrhythmia recurrence rates than those treated with therapy that fails to prevent induction of VT (N Engl J Med 303:1073, 1980). This management scheme is limited by (1) the imperfect reproducibility of individual responses to PES, (2) the appreciation that the arrhythmia substrate continues to evolve over time, potentially rendering once-effective therapy ineffective, and (3) the complications of long-term antiarrhythmic drug therapy. The advent of implantable antitachycardia devices with antitachycardia pacing algorithms, back-up DC cardioversion, and bradycardia pacing capabilities provides an effective alternative to chronic antiarrhythmic drug therapy for patients with sustained VT or VF (see Antitachycardia Devices).

Cardioversion

Cardioversion is the term used to describe delivery of an electrical impulse across the myocardium to terminate a sustained arrhythmia. All modern cardioverter-defibrillator units can be synchronized to the QRS complex to enable energy delivery during or immediately after ventricular depolarization, avoiding discharge during the period of partial ventricular recovery (the "vulnerable period" during which external electrical stimulation might initiate ventricular fibrillation). Cardioversion should be accomplished at the lowest effective energy level to reduce the incidence of complications and the degree of discomfort. Successful conversion to sinus rhythm occurs in more than 90% of patients with recent-onset atrial flutter, AF, reentrant SVTs, and VT. Following successful cardioversion, the need for antiarrhythmic drugs to prevent arrhythmia recurrence should be assessed.

I. **Indications.** Immediate cardioversion is indicated for any potentially responsive arrhythmia (AF, atrial flutter, AV reentrant SVTs resistant to adenosine, VT, and VF) when accompanied by **hemodynamic compromise.** Elective cardioversion is indicated for AF, atrial flutter, AV reentrant SVTs, and VT when chemical cardioversion has been ineffective.

A. **Atrial fibrillation** is one of the most common indications for cardioversion. A transthoracic discharge of at least 100 joules is typically required for successful reversion to normal sinus rhythm, with many clinical situations requiring 200–360 joules. When possible, patients in AF for 2 days or longer (or an unknown duration) should undergo systemic anticoagulation for at least 3 weeks prior to elective cardioversion and should remain on anticoagulation therapy for at least 3 weeks following cardioversion (see Chap. 17). Chronic anticoagulation therapy should be considered in patients with organic heart disease in whom a recurrence of AF is likely. Patients are less likely to maintain sinus rhythm if AF is of longstanding duration or the echocardiographically determined left atrial dimension exceeds 4.5 cm.

B. **Atrial flutter** often requires cardioversion with less than 50 joules, but low energy discharges (5–10 joules) may convert atrial flutter to AF. The need for pre- and postcardioversion anticoagulation in patients with atrial flutter remains controversial, with limited data suggesting that the risk of thromboembolism in atrial flutter, while smaller than that seen with AF, may be greater than that of the general population (*Pace Pacing Clin Electrophysiol* 15:2308, 1992), suggesting a need for individual patient recommendations.

C. **Reentrant SVTs.** Cardioversion of reentrant SVTs due to dual AV nodal pathways or accessory pathways generally requires 25–100 joules. Chemical cardioversion with IV adenosine or verapamil (in hemodynamically stable patients) should be attempted before electrical cardioversion is pursued.

D. **Ventricular tachycardia** may respond to synchronized cardioversion with as little as 20–50 joules. However, in patients with evidence of hemodynamic deterioration, the initial shock energy should be 200 joules, with a repeat cardioversion attempt with 360 joules if the initial shock is unsuccessful. Recurrence of arrhythmia suggests a need for pharmacologic intervention in addition to repeat cardioversion (see Chap. 8).

E. **Ventricular fibrillation** should be treated with prompt defibrillation, initially with 200 joules, with increasing energy levels if initially unsuccessful (see Chap. 8).

II. **Contraindications.** Cardioversion is relatively contraindicated in the following circumstances:

A. **Digitalis toxicity.** A therapeutic level of digoxin is not a contraindication to cardioversion. If digitalis toxicity is suspected, elective cardioversion for AF or atrial flutter should be deferred. Digitalis toxicity associated with ventricular tachycardia should be treated (see Chaps. 6 and 9), and prophylactic lidocaine therapy should be administered.

B. **Repetitive, short-lived tachycardias** should not be treated with electrical cardioversion, as their recurrence demonstrates an abnormal substrate requiring pharmacologic manipulation.

C. **Multifocal atrial tachycardia** or other automatic arrhythmias.

D. **Hyperthyroidism** patients should be functionally euthyroid before elective cardioversion to limit the likelihood of recurrence.

III. **Caution** should be exercised when initiating cardioversion in (1) elderly patients with coronary artery disease and conduction system disease, (2) patients with AF and a slow ventricular response in the absence of digitalis or verapamil, and (3) those with evidence of sick sinus syndrome. In such patients either a transcutaneous pacemaker should be available or a temporary pacemaker should be placed before cardioversion.

IV. **Technique.** Prior to cardioversion, all antiarrhythmic **drug levels** should be titrated to their therapeutic ranges, and digoxin levels should be determined to exclude digoxin toxicity. Concerns about **anticoagulation**, particularly for AF and atrial flutter, should be addressed (see Chap. 17). Informed consent should be obtained, reliable **IV access** should be established, and continuous monitoring of the **ECG** should be initiated, with a final 12-lead ECG being done to confirm persistence of the index arrhythmia. Supplemental oxygen and equipment necessary for intubation and manual ventilation should be available. Adhesive defibrillation pads should then be positioned, with consideration given to the arrhythmia being treated. For ventricular arrhythmias, the anterior electrode should be placed just right of the sternum at the level of the third or fourth intercostal space, with the second electrode being positioned lateral to the cardiac apex or more posteriorly in the left infrascapular region. For atrial arrhythmias the anterior electrode should be positioned just right or left of the sternum at the level of the third or fourth intercostal space, with the second electrode positioned just below the left scapula. In all cases, care should be taken to position electrodes at least 6 cm from permanent pacemaker or defibrillator generators. **Amnesia** should be induced with midazolam (1–2 mg IV q2min to a maximum of 5 mg) or methohexital (25–75 mg IV). The BP and respiratory rate should be carefully monitored. If possible, an anesthetist should be present for optimal airway management. **Synchronization** of the cardioverter should be evaluated by visual confirmation of the presence of a synchronization artifact superimposed on the QRS complex. If electrode paddles are being used, firm pressure should be applied to minimize contact impedance. Direct contact with the patient or the bed should be avoided. The cardioversion pulse should be provided at end-expiration to minimize transthoracic impedance. As a result of synchronization, the discharge may be delayed a short time, and the electrodes should be maintained in place until discharge occurs.

V. **Adverse effects** with DC cardioversion are rare but include **arrhythmias,** which may occur because of the release of catecholamines, acetylcholine, and potassium, or the interaction of these substances with cardioactive drugs. Sinus pauses, as well as atrial, junctional, or ventricular ectopic beats, may occur transiently after restoration of sinus rhythm, especially in patients with longstanding AF and a slow ventricular response. Reports of serious arrhythmias, such as VT, VF, or asystole, are rare and are more likely in the setting of improperly synchronized cardioversion or digitalis toxicity. **Systemic or pulmonary embolic events,** while uncommon, appear to be more likely in patients with AF and atrial flutter of more than 3 days' duration who have not been anticoagulated (3 weeks) prior to cardioversion. An increased likelihood of embolic events may extend for weeks after the cardioversion, perhaps due to the gradual return of atrial mechanical function following cardioversion. **Muscle pain,** with a concomitant rise in lactate dehydrogenase (LDH), SGOT, and creatine kinase (CK), and irritation of the skin at the paddle site may occur. Elevation of MB-CK is related to the total amount of energy delivered to the patient and generally does not occur until a cumulative discharge greater than 425 joules has been given.

Cardiac Pacing

Technical advances since the mid-1980s have greatly improved the performance of cardiac pacemakers. The most recent designs maintain AV synchrony and adapt the rate of pacing to optimize the physiologic response to exertion. When cardiac pacemakers are used appropriately, they enhance the quality of life in patients with symptomatic bradyarrhythmias. Before the decision is made to implant a pacemaker, the indications, appropriate mode of pacing, and arrangements for follow-up study should be carefully considered.

I. **Pacing modalities.** An alphabetical code has been devised to identify the various pacing modalities available for the treatment of bradyarrhythmias, which comprise the major indications for cardiac pacing. The first initial defines the chamber paced (**V**entricle, **A**trial, **D**ouble), the second identifies the sensing chamber, and the third indicates the response to a sensed event (**I**nhibited, **T**riggered, and **D**ouble). The letter D in the response position indicates that atrial sensing will inhibit the atrial stimulus and trigger a ventricular response after an appointed interval, and ventricular sensing will inhibit both ventricular and atrial outputs. The VVI, DVI, and DDD modes are most commonly used. VVI units pace and sense in the ventricle; a sensed event inhibits the ventricular stimulus. DVI units pace both chambers. Atrial sensing does not occur, but an event sensed in the ventricle inhibits both the atrial and ventricular stimuli. DDD units pace and sense in both chambers and respond in the manner previously described. In addition, rate-adaptive pacemakers may integrate inputs from various sensors (e.g., acceleration, QT interval, ventricular impedance, thoracic impedance, and temperature) to modulate heart rate in response to physiologic demands. These are indicated by the letter R (rate adaptive) in the pacemaker code.

II. **Indications**

A. **Temporary pacing** may be achieved by either external transthoracic pacing

(**Zoll** pacemaker) or, preferably, insertion of a temporary transvenous pacemaker. Symptomatic second- or third-degree heart block due to transient drug intoxication or electrolyte imbalance as well as complete heart block, Mobitz II, or bifascicular block in the setting of acute MI (*Circulation* 58:689, 1978) require temporary pacing. A temporary pacemaker is often required when new right or left bundle branch block occurs in the setting of acute MI and is indicated for treatment of Mobitz I AV block if the arrhythmia causes hemodynamic compromise or angina. Symptomatic sinus bradycardia, AF with a slow ventricular response, or other bradycardic manifestations of conduction system disease may necessitate temporary pacing until a permanent pacemaker can be inserted.

B. **Permanent pacing.** Indications for which there is a general consensus that placement of a permanent pacemaker is necessary are designated class I (*J Am Coll Cardiol* 18:1, 1991). There are other indications for permanent pacing on which opinion is divided (class II), as well as indications for which there is general agreement that permanent pacing is not indicated (class III). The following are class I indications for pacemaker placement:

1. **Acquired AV block**
   a. Acquired permanent or intermittent AV block resulting in symptomatic bradycardia, HF, asystolic pauses of longer than 3 seconds, or an escape rate less than 40 beats/minute; confusional states that clear with temporary pacing; and AV block following AV junction ablation or occurring in the setting of myotonic dystrophy.
   b. Permanent or intermittent second-degree AV block with symptomatic bradycardia.
   c. AF, atrial flutter, or other SVTs with advanced or complete AV block that are symptomatic.

2. **AV block associated with myocardial infarction**
   a. Persistent advanced second- or third-degree AV block after acute MI **with block in the His-Purkinje system** (bilateral bundle branch block).
   b. Transient advanced AV block and associated bundle branch block.

3. **Bifascicular and trifascicular block (chronic)**
   a. Bifascicular block with intermittent complete AV block associated with symptomatic bradycardia.
   b. Bifascicular or trifascicular block with intermittent type II second-degree AV block.

4. **Sinus node dysfunction** with documented symptomatic bradycardia (in the absence of nonessential medications that depress sinus node function).

5. **Neurocardiogenic abnormalities**
   a. Recurrent syncope associated with clear spontaneous events provoked by carotid sinus stimulation.
   b. Carotid sinus hypersensitivity as manifested by induced asystole of longer than 3 seconds' duration with minimal carotid sinus pressure (in the absence of nonessential medications that depress sinus or AV nodal function).

6. **Permanent pacing in children**
   a. Second- or third-degree AV block with symptomatic bradycardia or marked exercise intolerance.
   b. External ophthalmoplegia with bifascicular block.
   c. Sinus node dysfunction with symptomatic bradycardia.
   d. Congenital AV block with a wide QRS escape rhythm or infra-His block.
   e. Advanced second- or third-degree AV block persisting 14 days after cardiac surgery.

III. **Complications associated with permanent pacing**
   A. **Failure of pacemaker system function** may result from battery depletion, intermittent or nonsecure contact between electrode lead and generator, elevation in pacing threshold secondary to local tissue reaction or drug effects, electrode lead fracture, lead insulation fracture, electrode dislodgment, erosion or perforation of the myocardium with the electrode, or myopotential sensing with or without lead or insulation failure. Investigation of potential pacemaker

system malfunction should include prolonged ECG monitoring (with temporary pacing facilities available until the nature of the failure has been discerned), pacemaker interrogation with reconfirmation of pacing and sensing function, and radiographic examination of the generator/lead system.

B. **Pacemaker-mediated tachycardia (PMT)** occurs in dual-chamber pacemakers programmed to the DDD mode when a ventricular depolarization (usually a VPC) results in retrograde atrial activation that is then sensed by the atrial lead, resulting in a paced ventricular depolarization. The paced ventricular beat then reinitiates the same sequence, resulting in an incessant A-sensed, V-paced rhythm at or near the upper rate limit of the pacemaker. Diagnostic features include (1) a V-paced rhythm at or near the upper rate limit of the pacemaker, and (2) retrograde P waves without atrial pacing. PMT may be terminated by vagal maneuvers (which transiently interrupt retrograde AV nodal conduction), applying a magnet (which transiently disables pacemaker tracking), or programming to a different mode (DVI, VVI). Adjustment of other pacing parameters generally allows the DDD mode to be resumed.

C. **Pacemaker syndrome** is the name given a variety of symptomatic manifestations (e.g., dizziness, syncope) referable to either the loss of atrioventricular synchrony during single-chamber ventricular pacing or the abnormal atrioventricular synchrony associated with retrograde atrial conduction. The mainstay of therapy is revision of pacing modality to a dual-chamber mode to restore normal AV synchrony.

Antitachycardia Devices

Long-term management of patients with life-threatening ventricular arrhythmias includes consideration of implantation of antitachycardia devices capable of automatic recognition and treatment of ventricular arrhythmias. These devices include tiered therapy (e.g., paced arrhythmia termination and/or low-energy cardioversion strategies for stable VT, DC cardioversion for unstable VT or VF, and back-up pacing for bradycardia).

I. **Class I indications**, for which there is general agreement, include at least one documented episode of hemodynamically significant VT or VF in a patient in whom (1) PES and ambulatory monitoring cannot be used to accurately predict efficacy of pharmacologic therapy, (2) no tolerable drug therapy is effective, or (3) PES reveals persistently inducible, hemodynamically significant ventricular arrhythmia despite the best available drug therapy, surgery, or catheter ablation (*J Am Coll Cardiol* 18:1, 1991).

II. **Class II indications**, for which there is a divergence of opinion, include (1) at least one documented episode of hemodynamically significant VT or VF in a patient in whom drug efficacy testing is impossible and (2) recurrent syncope of undetermined origin in a patient with hemodynamically significant VT or VF induced via PES in whom no tolerable and effective drug therapy can be identified.

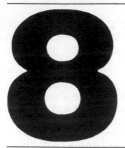

Cardiopulmonary Resuscitation and Advanced Cardiac Life Support

Dino Recchia

The development of cardiopulmonary resuscitation (CPR) and external defibrillation in the late 1950s made possible the rescue of patients with acute cardiopulmonary arrest. Resuscitation guidelines have been established and updated by the American Heart Association (*JAMA* 268:2171, 1992). All therapeutic interventions are classified as follows: **Class I** interventions are always acceptable and considered useful and effective. **Class II** interventions are acceptable but of uncertain efficacy, and are further classified as: **class IIa** when the weight of evidence is in favor of its usefulness and **class IIb** when the evidence of its usefulness is not well established and the intervention is probably not harmful. **Class III** interventions are not appropriate and may be harmful.

CPR alone is of limited benefit without the prompt initiation of advanced cardiac life support (ACLS). Emphasis should be placed on achieving the following sequence of events as soon as possible: (1) recognition of cardiopulmonary arrest, (2) activation of the emergency medical system (EMS), (3) basic CPR, (4) defibrillation, (5) intubation, and (6) IV administration of appropriate medications. Ventricular arrhythmias are responsible for a majority of sudden cardiac arrests in adults; therefore, it is imperative that activation of the EMS occur immediately after unresponsiveness is determined to facilitate rapid initiation of ACLS. The specific clinical circumstances regarding any particular patient may require deviation from these guidelines.

Basic Life Support

The ABCs of basic life support (BLS) include **A**irway, **B**reathing, and **C**irculation. The goal of BLS is to provide oxygen to the brain and heart until definitive treatment (i.e., ACLS) can be delivered. Without proper BLS, ACLS is futile. When one encounters an unconscious patient, the following procedures are recommended.

I. **Determine responsiveness** by gently shaking the patient. **Do not shake the patient's head or neck if trauma to this area is suspected.**

II. **Activate the EMS system.**

III. **Position the patient** on a firm, flat surface. If the victim must be moved from the facedown position, roll him or her as a unit so the head, neck, and torso move simultaneously.

IV. **Open the patient's mouth,** leaving dentures in place as they facilitate a good mouth-to-mouth seal.

V. **Open the patient's airway.** If neck injury is not suspected, the **head tilt–chin lift** is the maneuver of choice. Place the palm of one hand on the patient's forehead and apply firm pressure to tilt the head backward. At the same time, place the index and middle fingers of your other hand under the patient's chin and displace the mandible anteriorly; this movement raises the tongue away from the posterior pharynx and opens the airway. If a neck injury is suspected, avoid the head tilt and use the **jaw thrust maneuver** to limit the potential for spinal cord injury in the setting of a cervical fracture. This maneuver is performed by grasping the angles of the patient's mandible with the fingers of both hands, one on each side, and moving the mandible anteriorly.

VI. Assess for the presence of respiration with the airway open. Place your ear above the patient's mouth to listen and feel for airflow while observing for chest movement. Maintenance of an open airway may be all that is necessary for spontaneous respiration to resume and continue.

VII. If spontaneous respiration is not present, gently pinch the patient's nose closed with the index finger and thumb of the hand that is on the forehead. Make a tight seal over the patient's mouth and give 2 slow breaths (1.5–2.0 seconds/breath) followed by 10–12 breaths/minute. Avoid rapid and high-pressure breaths as they may result in gastric distention. Take a breath after each ventilation. Each ventilation should be performed with sufficient volume to make the patient's chest rise and followed by a 2-second pause. Indicators of adequate ventilation are the rise and fall of the chest and detection of escaping air during the patient's exhalation. **Improper chin or head position is the most common cause of difficult ventilation.** If the patient cannot be ventilated, reposition the head and attempt ventilation again. If ventilation is still unsuccessful, use obstructed airway maneuvers (see sec. **XI**).

VIII. Palpate the patient's carotid pulse for at least 5 seconds. If a carotid pulse is present, continue rescue breathing at a rate of 10–12 slow breaths/minute.

IX. In the absence of a carotid pulse, initiate chest compressions. There should be a firm surface under the patient. Perform chest compressions by placing the heel of one hand on the back of the other positioned 1 in. above (cephalad to) the patient's xiphoid process, with your shoulders directly above your hands and your elbows in a locked position. Compress the patient's sternum 1.5–2.0 in., thrusting straight down toward the spine. Compressions should be smooth and regular, with an equal amount of time allowed for compression and release. Pressure must be completely released from the patient's chest after each compression, but your hands should remain in contact with the chest to maintain proper hand position. The recommended compression rate is 80–100/minute. Assess the adequacy of compressions by periodically palpating the carotid pulse (two-rescuer BLS). During one-rescuer BLS, 15 chest compressions should be performed followed by 2 ventilations. For two-rescuer BLS, the compression-ventilation ratio is 5 : 1, with a 1.0–1.5 second pause for ventilation after every 5 compressions. Once the patient is intubated, ventilations can be given at a rate of 12–15/minute, without pausing for compressions.

X. Stop BLS for 5 seconds at the end of the first minute, and every 2–3 minutes thereafter, to determine whether the patient has resumed spontaneous breathing or circulation. If a spontaneous pulse has returned, continue ventilation as needed. BLS should otherwise not be withheld for more than 5 seconds except to intubate or defibrillate the patient. Attempts at intubation should not exceed 30 seconds before resuming CPR.

XI. If an unconscious patient cannot be ventilated after two attempts at positioning the head and chin, perform abdominal thrusts (the Heimlich maneuver). Use careful technique to avoid an improper hand position that may damage internal organs. Straddle the patient's thighs and place the heel of one hand against the patient's abdomen slightly above the umbilicus and well below the tip of the xiphoid. Place the second hand directly on top of the first. Then press posteriorly and cephalad with 6–10 quick upward thrusts. Follow this maneuver by sweeping debris from the patient's mouth with your finger, and repeat attempts at ventilation. When removing debris from the mouth, grasp the tongue and lower jaw as a unit with the thumb and fingers of one hand and lift them anteriorly and caudad. Place the index finger of the opposite hand down along the inside of the person's cheek deeply into the throat to the base of the tongue. Then use a hooking action to dislodge a foreign body and move it into the mouth, where it can be grasped and removed. If attempts are unsuccessful in relieving the obstruction, repeat this sequence. Cricothyrotomy and transtracheal ventilation are rarely necessary (see Chap. 9).

Advanced Cardiac
Life Support

I. **Proper leadership of the resuscitative effort is essential to optimize patient survival.** Supervision is the responsibility of the **team leader**, who must ensure that (1) **BLS** is performed adequately, (2) **early defibrillation** is used when appropriate, (3) **intubation** occurs as early as possible without excessive (>30 seconds) interruption of BLS, (4) **adequate IV access** is maintained, and (5) **pharmacologic treatment** is initiated in the proper sequence and at the proper dose. The team leader also has the responsibility of deciding when resuscitative efforts should be terminated.

II. **General considerations**
   A. **Arrhythmia recognition and defibrillation should be performed as quickly as possible.** Quick-look paddles on defibrillators can be used to avoid delay prior to establishing ECG monitoring. It is critical that the presence of a palpable pulse, obtainable blood pressure, and the patient's level of consciousness be considered in the overall treatment plan.
      1. **If pulseless ventricular tachycardia (VT) or ventricular fibrillation (VF) is present, perform defibrillation immediately.** Patients with an automatic implantable cardioverter/defibrillator (AICD) or a pacemaker can be externally defibrillated without damage to the device, provided a defibrillation paddle is not placed over the device. Higher energy levels (>200 joules) and anterior-posterior paddle positions may be necessary for defibrillation in patients with an AICD.
      2. **If a "flat line" appears on the monitor**, the differential diagnosis includes loose leads, a lack of connection between the patient and monitor, isoelectrical VF masquerading as asystole, or true asystole. Operator mistakes are the most frequent cause of false asystole. Determining the rhythm in two or more leads should clarify the underlying rhythm.
      3. **Blind defibrillation** in the absence of a rhythm diagnosis is rarely necessary because of the monitoring capabilities on most modern defibrillators. It should be considered only when monitoring is unavailable.
      4. **Proper technique** is essential to the success of defibrillation. Place one paddle along the upper right sternal border below the clavicle and the other lateral to the nipple centered in the midaxillary line. Use conductive gel or pads if available, and apply firm paddle pressure to reduce transthoracic resistance. **Individuals using the paddles must ensure that no one is touching the bed or the patient during a defibrillation attempt.**
   B. **Internal cardiac compression along with defibrillation** is rarely useful but can be considered in the following situations: (1) penetrating chest trauma, (2) anatomic deformity of the chest that precludes adequate chest compressions, (3) severe hypothermia, (4) ruptured aortic aneurysm or pericardial tamponade unresponsive to pericardiocentesis, (5) during or shortly after procedures requiring open thoracotomy, and (6) when VF is refractory to standard techniques. This procedure is successful only if implemented early during the arrest sequence by experienced personnel rather than as a last resort.
   C. **A solitary precordial "thump"** may convert VT or VF to a more stable rhythm if delivered quickly. It should be considered an optional technique (class IIb) for a witnessed arrest in a pulseless patient when a defibrillator is not immediately available. It should never delay defibrillation attempts.
   D. **Airway management and oxygen therapy** are essential to any resuscitative effort. Oxygen (100%) should be administered, and endotracheal intubation should be accomplished by a qualified individual as soon as possible. Endotracheal tube position must be assessed immediately after placement. Equal bilateral breath sounds during ventilation should be present to ensure that a mainstem bronchus has not been intubated. Auscultation over the stomach should be performed to exclude accidental esophageal intubation. BLS should not be interrupted for more than 30 seconds for intubation. Ventilation with a

well-fitting pocket mask and protection of the airway by suctioning is preferable to making repeated unsuccessful attempts at intubation. Because of difficulty in maintaining a seal, a bag-valve device with a mask should only be used by experienced personnel. If airway obstruction is present and cannot be relieved by abdominal thrusts, transtracheal catheter ventilation or cricothyrotomy is indicated (see Chap. 9).

E. **Route of drug administration.** If an internal jugular or subclavian central venous line is in place before the arrest, it should be used for drug administration. If central access is not available, an antecubital vein should be cannulated so that BLS is not interrupted. The femoral venous route is not adequate unless a long catheter is used that reaches above the diaphragm. When an antecubital vein is used, rapid entry of drugs into the central circulation can be facilitated by using a long IV catheter, elevating the extremity, and flushing with a 20- to 30-ml bolus of IV fluid. If there is a delay in gaining venous access, isotonic agents such as epinephrine, atropine, and lidocaine may be diluted in 10 ml saline and injected into the endotracheal tube and distributed into the bronchi by several forceful lung inflations. The dosage for drugs used in this manner should be 2.0–2.5 times the recommended IV dose. If circulation is not rapidly restored after initial drug administration via a peripheral IV line, a subclavian or internal jugular IV line should be placed with minimal interruption of BLS. Intracardiac injections are not recommended.

F. **IV fluids** for volume expansion are indicated in patients with cardiac arrest and evidence of acute blood loss, hypovolemia, or hypotension. Patients with acute myocardial infarction (MI), especially right ventricular infarction, may also benefit from volume expansion with normal saline. Routine IV fluid administration in patients with cardiac arrest and no evidence of volume depletion is not recommended because it may diminish blood flow to the cerebral and coronary circulations.

III. **Common drugs**

A. **Epinephrine** produces beneficial effects during CPR by increasing myocardial and cerebral blood flow. It is presently the catecholamine of choice for resuscitative efforts (class I). The recommended dose is 1 mg (10 ml of a 1 : 10,000 solution) repeated at 3- to 5-minute intervals. The benefits of higher doses of epinephrine during resuscitation have not been proved in randomized studies. High-dose epinephrine (5.0 mg or 0.1 mg/kg) is considered a class IIb recommendation and should only be considered after the standard dose has failed. Epinephrine is well absorbed via the endotracheal route.

B. **Atropine sulfate** is the treatment of choice for symptomatic bradycardia (class I). It may be beneficial (class IIa) for treatment of atrioventricular (AV) block at the nodal level, ventricular asystole, and pulseless electrical activity (PEA). The recommended dose for symptomatic bradycardia is 0.5–1.0 mg IV, repeated every 3–5 minutes if necessary, to a total dose of 0.4 mg/kg. For asystole or PEA, the dose is 1 mg repeated every 3–5 minutes. **A total dose of 3 mg results in full vagal blockade in humans.** Atropine should be used cautiously in the setting of acute myocardial ischemia or MI since excessive increases in heart rate may worsen ischemia or increase the zone of infarction. Atropine is well absorbed via the endotracheal route.

C. **Lidocaine** is the antiarrhythmic of choice for treatment of VT or VF that persists following defibrillation and administration of epinephrine. It is also beneficial in stable VT and wide-complex tachycardias of uncertain type. An initial bolus of 1.0–1.5 mg/kg is required to rapidly achieve therapeutic levels. Additional boluses of 0.5–1.0 mg/kg can be administered every 5–10 minutes as needed to a total of 3 mg/kg. Only bolus dosing should be used in cardiac arrest. With the return of perfusion, a maintenance infusion of 2–4 mg/min is recommended. Toxicity is more likely with decreased cardiac output (i.e., acute MI, shock, and heart failure), a patient older than 70 years, and hepatic dysfunction. In these situations, the bolus dose remains unchanged but the maintenance infusion should be decreased by one-half.

D. **Procainamide hydrochloride** is recommended for the treatment of patients with recurrent VT when lidocaine is contraindicated or has failed. It is acceptable (class IIa) for treatment of wide-complex tachycardias associated with a pulse that cannot be distinguished from VT. Procainamide is administered by infusion of 20–30 mg/minute until the arrhythmia is suppressed, hypotension ensues, the QRS is widened by 50%, or a total dose of 17 mg/kg is reached. The maintenance infusion rate is 1–4 mg/minute. This drug should be avoided in patients with preexisting QT prolongation or torsades de pointes. Hypotension may occur if the drug is injected too rapidly.

E. **Bretylium tosylate** is used for treatment of refractory VT and VF when defibrillation, epinephrine, and lidocaine have failed. It is also indicated when lidocaine and procainamide have failed to control VT associated with a pulse, or adenosine, lidocaine, and procainamide have failed to control wide-complex tachycardias of unknown type. The dosage is 5 mg/kg given as an IV bolus for refractory VT and VF. If cardiac arrest persists, the dosage is increased to 10 mg/kg and repeated every 5 minutes to a total dosage of 30–35 mg/kg. For recurrent VT associated with a pulse, 5–10 mg/kg of the drug is diluted in 50 ml of D5W and delivered over 10 minutes, followed by a maintenance infusion of 1–2 mg/minute.

F. **Magnesium sulfate** is of probable benefit (class IIa) in treating torsades de pointes, VT, and VF associated with a hypomagnesemic state, and severe refractory VF. The dose is 1–2 g IV administered over 1–2 minutes.

G. **Adenosine** is the agent of choice (class I) for paroxysmal supraventricular tachycardia (PSVT) and can be used following lidocaine for treatment of wide-complex tachycardia of unknown type in a patient who is hemodynamically stable. The initial dose is 6 mg delivered as a rapid IV bolus over 1–3 seconds followed by a 20-ml saline flush. If there is no response in 1–2 minutes, the dose should be increased to 12 mg and delivered in the same fashion. The 12-mg dose can be repeated if necessary. Theophylline antagonizes the actions of adenosine, and patients taking this drug may require larger doses of adenosine to achieve the desired effect. Dipyridamole interferes with adenosine metabolism and potentiates its effects; therefore, adenosine should be used with caution in patients taking dipyridamole.

H. **Diltiazem**, given IV, is useful in the management of atrial fibrillation or flutter and multifocal atrial tachycardia. It also can be administered for treatment of PSVT if adenosine has failed in patients who are not hypotensive and have a narrow QRS complex. The initial dose is 15–20 mg (0.25 mg/kg) IV. A second dose of 20–25 mg (0.35 mg/kg) can be administered in 15 minutes if necessary, followed by a maintenance infusion of 5–15 mg/hour to control the ventricular rate.

I. **Isoproterenol** is not indicated (class III) in most patients with cardiac arrest. It may be useful (class IIa) for refractory torsades de pointes (after magnesium has failed) and hemodynamically significant bradycardia in the denervated heart of a transplant patient.

J. **Sodium bicarbonate** is not recommended for routine use during the resuscitative effort. Its use should be based on a clearly defined diagnosis. Bicarbonate administration is indicated (class I) for hyperkalemia. It may also be beneficial (class IIa) for a known preexisting acidosis, overdose with tricyclic antidepressants, and to alkalinize the urine in patients with drug overdose. The initial dosage is 1.0 mEq/kg given IV followed by 0.5 mEq/kg given every 10 minutes. In most patients with cardiac arrest, acidosis is uncommon if BLS is adequately performed. When acidosis is present, it is usually due to inadequate ventilation, and treatment should be directed to increasing minute ventilation. There is no convincing evidence that acidosis adversely affects the ability to defibrillate the patient, the effectiveness of adrenergic agents, or survival. The use of bicarbonate is poorly defined for patients with a prolonged arrest interval (class IIb). It is not useful in hypoxic lactic acidosis (class III).

K. **Calcium** has not been shown to improve survival in patients with cardiac arrest. Its use should be limited to situations in which definite indications exist (class IIa), including **hyperkalemia, hypocalcemia, and calcium channel blocker** toxicity. When indicated, **10% calcium chloride** is the preferred preparation and is given as an IV bolus of 5–10 ml (500–1,000 mg); **caution should be used in patients taking digitalis,** because its toxic effects may be potentiated by calcium administration.

IV. **Transcutaneous cardiac pacing** has resulted in improved survival in patients with hemodynamically unstable bradycardia defined as (1) systolic blood pressure less than 80 mm Hg, (2) altered mental status, (3) myocardial ischemia, or (4) pulmonary edema. Transcutaneous pacing can be used following atropine administration in these patients. Effectiveness of cardiac pacing should be evaluated by palpation of the femoral, radial, or brachial pulses. Transvenous pacing should be considered if transcutaneous pacing is not available. In the postresuscitation period, transvenous pacing is more effective and can be placed more safely than during active resuscitation.

Specific Arrest Sequences

The following sequences are useful in treating a broad range of patients with cardiac arrhythmias but should be modified as the clinical situation warrants (*JAMA* 268:2171, 1992). **The emphasis should be to consider the overall condition of the patient, not only the arrhythmia displayed on the cardiac monitor.** Figures 8-1 through 8-5 outline the algorithms recommended by the American Heart Association; however, some patients may require care not specified in these algorithms.

I. **Ventricular fibrillation and pulseless ventricular tachycardia** (see Fig. 8-1). VF and VT are responsible for a majority of nontraumatic adult cardiac arrests. Definitive treatment with immediate defibrillation improves the likelihood of success. Correction of underlying etiologic abnormalities (e.g., hypokalemia, MI, hypoxia) should be performed promptly after successful defibrillation.

   A. **Early defibrillation is critical** and should be performed before intubation or IV access. The patient's rhythm on the monitor should be assessed after each defibrillation attempt, and shocks should be delivered in sequence with minimal delay (other than to assess for a rhythm and pulse). Defibrillation should be attempted with 360 joules after each subsequent dose of antiarrhythmic medication.

   B. **Epinephrine is critical for patients with cardiac arrest** and should be repeated every 3–5 minutes until a pulse is established.

   C. **If VF or pulseless VT is refractory** to defibrillation and epinephrine, medications of probable benefit (class IIa) in persistent or recurrent VF should be administered (lidocaine, bretylium, magnesium, and procainamide).

   D. **If VF or pulseless VT recurs** during the arrest sequence, defibrillation should be performed at previously successful energy levels.

   E. **Torsades de pointes** is a characteristic form of VT that displays a gradual alteration in the amplitude and direction of electrical activity and commonly occurs with a prolonged QT interval (see Chap. 7). It should be considered when VT is refractory to the treatment outlined above. Defibrillation should always be attempted if the arrhythmia is sustained or associated with hemodynamic instability. For nonsustained or recurrent torsades de pointes, immediate therapy consists of **magnesium sulfate.** The initial dose is 2 g IV followed by an infusion of 2–20 mg/minute. If magnesium is ineffective, electrical pacing or isoproterenol infusion should be considered. Electrical pacing is initiated at rates of 80–120 beats/minute and produces an immediate decrease in the QT interval (secondary to increased heart rate). A transcutaneous pacemaker can be used until a transvenous pacemaker can be placed. Isoproterenol can be infused at a rate of 2–10 μg/minute, titrated to a target heart rate. Isoproterenol should be avoided in patients with severe coronary artery disease or myocardial ischemia. Some patients may respond to treatment with lidocaine, phenytoin, or bretylium. Class Ia and class III antiarrhythmic agents should be avoided in patients with torsades de pointes.

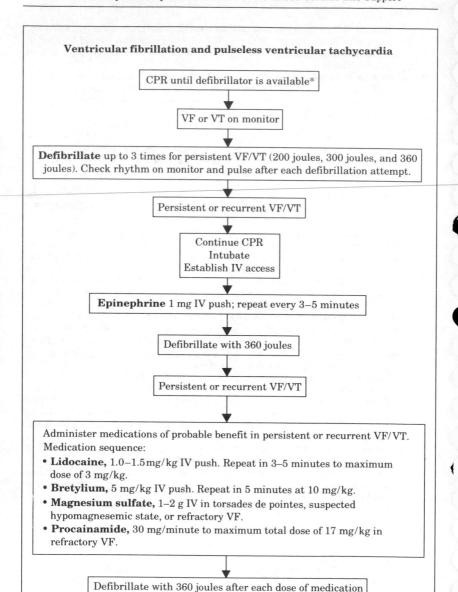

Ventricular fibrillation and pulseless ventricular tachycardia

CPR until defibrillator is available*

↓

VF or VT on monitor

↓

Defibrillate up to 3 times for persistent VF/VT (200 joules, 300 joules, and 360 joules). Check rhythm on monitor and pulse after each defibrillation attempt.

↓

Persistent or recurrent VF/VT

↓

Continue CPR
Intubate
Establish IV access

↓

Epinephrine 1 mg IV push; repeat every 3–5 minutes

↓

Defibrillate with 360 joules

↓

Persistent or recurrent VF/VT

↓

Administer medications of probable benefit in persistent or recurrent VF/VT. Medication sequence:
- **Lidocaine,** 1.0–1.5 mg/kg IV push. Repeat in 3–5 minutes to maximum dose of 3 mg/kg.
- **Bretylium,** 5 mg/kg IV push. Repeat in 5 minutes at 10 mg/kg.
- **Magnesium sulfate,** 1–2 g IV in torsades de pointes, suspected hypomagnesemic state, or refractory VF.
- **Procainamide,** 30 mg/minute to maximum total dose of 17 mg/kg in refractory VF.

↓

Defibrillate with 360 joules after each dose of medication

* A solitary precordial "thump" may convert VT or VF to a stable rhythm if delivered quickly and should be considered an optional technique (class IIb) for a witnessed arrest in a pulseless patient. It should never delay defibrillation attempts. In patients who have a pulse, a defibrillator must be available before a precordial thump is administered as it may induce VF.

Fig. 8-1. Ventricular fibrillation and pulseless ventricular tachycardia. Flow of the algorithm presumes that VF is continuing. (VF = ventricular fibrillation; VT = ventricular tachycardia.) (Adapted from Part III. Adult advanced cardiac life support. *JAMA* 268:2172, 1992.)

II. **Asystole** is usually associated with severe underlying cardiac disease and often occurs in the hospitalized patient. This rhythm often constitutes a terminal condition, and the likelihood of resuscitation is poor. An algorithm for the management of asystole is outlined in Fig. 8-2.

   A. **Asystole should be confirmed** in more than one lead, as fine VF can sometimes masquerade as asystole (see General Considerations, sec. **II.A**). If the diagnosis is unclear, the presence of fine VF should be assumed and defibrillation attempted, but routine defibrillation for asystole may be detrimental and is not recommended.

   B. **The possible causes of asystole should be considered** and appropriate therapy instituted if identified. Causes include hypoxia, hyperkalemia, hypokalemia, preexisting acidosis, drug overdose, and hypothermia.

   C. **Transcutaneous pacing** may be beneficial in a patient with asystole if it is instituted early and is considered a class IIb recommendation. This modality is seldom of benefit in patients with prehospital cardiac arrest, and **routine transcutaneous pacing in patients with asystolic cardiac arrest should not be performed**.

   D. **Asystole is often a confirmation of death;** termination of resuscitative efforts should be considered if asystole persists despite adequate CPR, intubation, and administration of appropriate medications.

III. **Bradycardia** is treated according to the patient's hemodynamic stability and type of arrhythmia. **The focus should be on the patient's clinical status and not the absolute heart rate.** The manifestations of hemodynamic instability include hypotension, congestive heart failure, altered mentation, ischemic chest pain, or acute MI. An algorithm for the management of bradycardia is outlined in Fig. 8-3.

   A. **Sinus bradycardia, junctional rhythm, and type I second-degree AV block** should be observed in asymptomatic patients.

   B. **Type II second-degree and complete AV block** are unstable rhythms and may progress to asystole or ventricular fibrillation. **A pacemaker is required even in the absence of symptoms.** Atropine or transcutaneous pacing should be used in the symptomatic patient until a transvenous pacemaker can be placed. Atropine may exacerbate ischemia or induce VT and VF when used to treat bradycardia associated with acute MI.

   C. **If the bradycardia is a ventricular escape rhythm, the use of lidocaine may be lethal** as it will suppress ventricular escape.

   D. **Transcutaneous pacing** is a class I intervention for all symptomatic bradycardias and should be considered early in the resuscitative effort if it is available.

IV. **Pulseless electrical activity (PEA)** includes electromechanical dissociation (EMD); idioventricular ventricular escape; and postdefibrillation idioventricular, bradycardic, and asystolic rhythms all characterized by electrical activity (other than VT and VF) in the absence of a pulse. These arrhythmias are associated with a very poor outcome, especially in the prehospital setting. They are frequently associated with an underlying clinical condition that, if identified early and appropriately treated, increases the chance of survival. An algorithm for management of PEA is outlined in Fig. 8-4.

   A. **It is critical that potential reversible causes be considered in all patients with PEA.** These include hypovolemia, hypoxia, cardiac tamponade, tension pneumothorax, hypothermia, massive pulmonary embolism, drug overdose, hyperkalemia, severe acidosis, and massive MI. If a reversible cause is identified, appropriate therapy should be instituted.

   B. **Immediate use of Doppler ultrasound** may reveal blood flow not detected by arterial palpation. These patients should be aggressively treated for severe hypotension (see Chap. 9).

V. **Tachycardias** are treated in a similar fashion to bradycardias. The manifestations of hemodynamic instability (hypotension, congestive heart failure, altered mentation, ischemic chest pain, or acute MI) should be sought before deciding on appropriate therapy. An algorithm for the approach to these patients is outlined in Fig. 8-5.

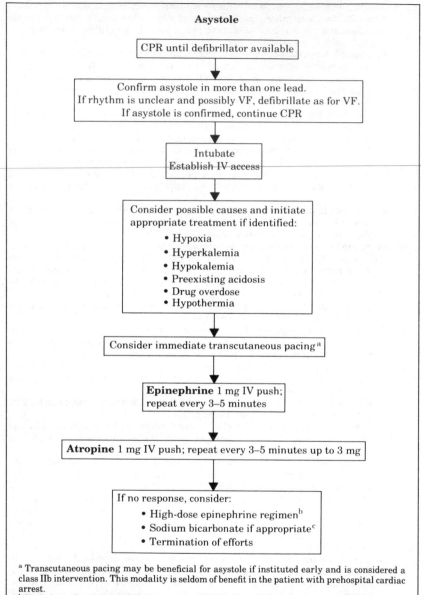

Asystole

CPR until defibrillator available

Confirm asystole in more than one lead.
If rhythm is unclear and possibly VF, defibrillate as for VF.
If asystole is confirmed, continue CPR

Intubate
Establish IV access

Consider possible causes and initiate
appropriate treatment if identified:
 • Hypoxia
 • Hyperkalemia
 • Hypokalemia
 • Preexisting acidosis
 • Drug overdose
 • Hypothermia

Consider immediate transcutaneous pacing[a]

Epinephrine 1 mg IV push;
repeat every 3–5 minutes

Atropine 1 mg IV push; repeat every 3–5 minutes up to 3 mg

If no response, consider:
 • High-dose epinephrine regimen[b]
 • Sodium bicarbonate if appropriate[c]
 • Termination of efforts

[a] Transcutaneous pacing may be beneficial for asystole if instituted early and is considered a class IIb intervention. This modality is seldom of benefit in the patient with prehospital cardiac arrest.
[b] High-dose alternative epinephrine regimens include: 2–5 mg IV push every 3–5 minutes; 1 mg–3 mg–5 mg IV push (3 minutes apart); 0.1 mg/kg IV push every 3–5 minutes.
[c] Sodium bicarbonate is not recommended for routine use early during the resuscitative effort. When acidosis is present, it is usually due to inadequate ventilation, and treatment should be directed at increasing minute ventilation. If bicarbonate is indicated, the initial dosage is 1 mEq/kg given IV followed by 0.5 mEq/kg every 10 minutes.

Fig. 8-2. Asystole treatment algorithm. (Adapted from Part III. Adult advanced cardiac life support. *JAMA* 268:2172, 1992.)

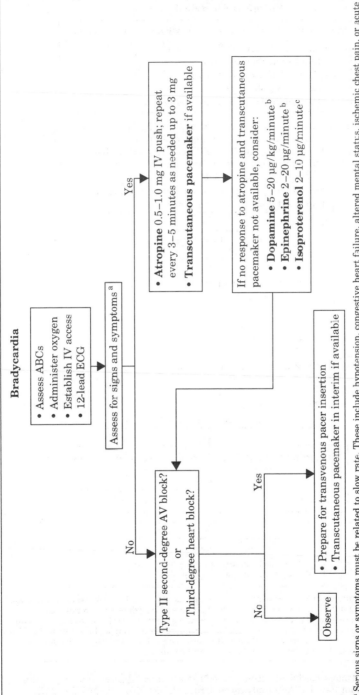

Bradycardia

- Assess ABCs
- Administer oxygen
- Establish IV access
- 12-lead ECG

Assess for signs and symptoms [a]

Yes

- **Atropine** 0.5–1.0 mg IV push; repeat every 3–5 minutes as needed up to 3 mg
- **Transcutaneous pacemaker** if available

If no response to atropine and transcutaneous pacemaker not available, consider:

- **Dopamine** 5–20 µg/kg/minute [b]
- **Epinephrine** 2–20 µg/minute [b]
- **Isoproterenol** 2–10 µg/minute [c]

No

Type II second-degree AV block?
or
Third-degree heart block?

Yes

- Prepare for transvenous pacer insertion
- Transcutaneous pacemaker in interim if available

No

Observe

[a] Serious signs or symptoms must be related to slow rate. These include hypotension, congestive heart failure, altered mental status, ischemic chest pain, or acute myocardial infarction.
[b] These drugs are considered class IIb interventions and should be considered temporizing measures until preparations for a transvenous pacemaker can be made.
[c] Isoproterenol is not indicated in most patients with cardiac arrest.

Fig. 8-3. Bradycardia treatment algorithm. This algorithm assumes the patient is not in cardiac arrest. (Adapted from Part III. Adult advanced cardiac life support. *JAMA* 268:2172, 1992.)

Pulseless Electrical Activity

Electrical activity other than VF/VT on monitor includes:

- Electromechanical dissociation
- Idioventricular rhythms
- Ventricular escape rhythms
- Bradyasystolic rhythms
- Postdefibrillation idioventricular rhythms

↓

Assess for presence of a pulse.
Use Doppler ultrasound if available to assess for blood flow.

↓

If blood flow present, treat for severe hypotension.
If no blood flow present, continue CPR.

↓

Intubate
Establish IV access

↓

Consider possible causes and treat if identified:

- Hypovolemia
- Hypoxia
- Cardiac tamponade
- Tension pneumothorax
- Hypothermia
- Massive pulmonary embolus
- Drug overdose
- Hyperkalemia
- Severe acidosis
- Massive acute myocardial infarction

↓

Epinephrine 1 mg IV push; repeat every 3–5 minutes

↓

If absolute (<60 beats/minute) or relative bradycardia,
atropine 1 mg IV push; repeat every 3–5 minutes up to 3 mg

↓

If no response, consider:

- High-dose epinephrine regimen[a]
- Sodium bicarbonate if appropriate[b]

[a] High-dose alternative epinephrine regimens include: 2–5 mg IV push every 3–5 minutes; 1 mg–3 mg–5 mg IV push (3 minutes apart); 0.1 mg/kg IV push every 3–5 minutes.
[b] Sodium bicarbonate is not recommended for routine use early during the resuscitative effort. When acidosis is present, it is usually due to inadequate ventilation, and treatment should be directed at increasing minute ventilation. If bicarbonate is indicated, the initial dosage is 1 mEq/kg given IV followed by 0.5 mEq/kg every 10 minutes.

Fig. 8-4. Pulseless electrical activity (electromechanical dissociation) algorithm. (Adapted from Part III. Adult advanced cardiac life support. *JAMA* 268:2172, 1992.)

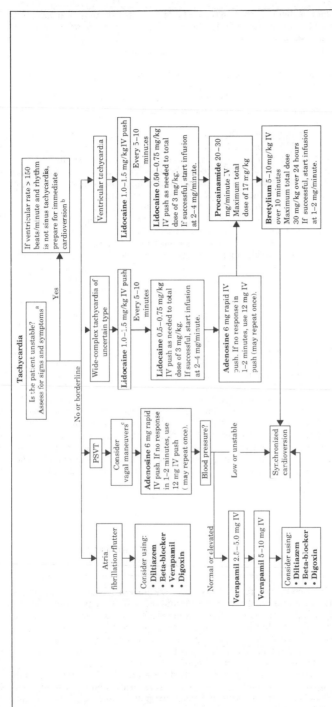

Fig. 8-5. Tachycardia treatment algorithm. Algorithm assumes patient has a pulse. If patient becomes unstable at any point, move to immediate cardioversion. If delays in synchronization occur and the patient is unstable, go to immediate unsynchronized cardioversion. (Adapted from Part III. Adult advanced cardiac life support. *JAMA* 268:2172, 1992.)

[a] Serious signs or symptoms must be related to the tachycardia. These include hypotension, congestive heart failure, altered mental status, ischemic chest pain, or acute myocardial infarction.

[b] A brief trial of appropriate medication can be used while preparations for cardioversion are under way, but the delay should be minimal. Immediate cardioversion is seldom necessary for rates less than 150 beats/minute.

[c] Carotid sinus pressure is the most commonly used vagal maneuver. It should be performed carefully and is contraindicated in the elderly and patients with carotid bruits. Bilateral carotid sinus massage should never be performed.

A. **If the patient is hemodynamically unstable and the rhythm is a nonsinus tachycardia at a rate greater than 150 beats/minute, preparations for immediate cardioversion should be made.** A brief trial of appropriate medication can be used while preparations for cardioversion are under way, but the delay should be minimal.
   1. **IV access and supplemental oxygen** should be in place. Equipment necessary to support the airway should also be readily available. If possible, a short-acting sedative should be administered. Assistance from trained anesthesia personnel is optimal if they are available and the patient's condition permits.
   2. **Synchronized cardioversion** should be performed starting at 100 joules and increasing to 200, 300, and 360 joules if the tachycardia does not respond. Atrial flutter and PSVT will often respond to an initial shock of 50 joules. Polymorphic VT should initially be cardioverted with 200 joules. **If delays in synchronization occur and the patient's condition is critical, unsynchronized cardioversion should be performed immediately.**
   3. **Immediate cardioversion** is seldom necessary for rates less than 150/minute. In the case of sinus tachycardia, cardioversion is not appropriate, and a search for the underlying cause should be performed.
B. **If the patient is stable,** treatment is based on the underlying cardiac rhythm.
   1. **Hemodynamically stable VT** is initially treated with lidocaine. If this fails, procainamide followed by bretylium may be used. If there is no response to pharmacologic therapy, synchronized cardioversion is indicated.
   2. **Wide-complex tachycardia of unknown type** should initially be treated with lidocaine (class I). If this fails, adenosine may be administered (class IIa) for possible PSVT with aberrant conduction. Procainamide can also be considered (class I). **Verapamil should not be used** (class III) because it may worsen the arrhythmia if it is due to an underlying accessory pathway (e.g., Wolff-Parkinson-White syndrome). If a wide-complex tachycardia is **known** to be PSVT, and the patient has a normal blood pressure, verapamil may be used.
   3. **Paroxysmal supraventricular tachycardia** should initially be treated with vagal maneuvers if they are not contraindicated. Various vagal maneuvers are possible, but the most commonly used is carotid sinus massage. This should be performed carefully. It should be avoided in elderly patients and those with carotid bruits. Bilateral carotid sinus pressure should never be applied. If vagal maneuvers are contraindicated or unsuccessful, adenosine is the drug of choice (class I). Verapamil is acceptable, but it may cause hypotension. If patients do not respond to adenosine or verapamil, other drugs (digoxin, beta blockers, diltiazem) or elective synchronized cardioversion may be used.
   4. **Treatment of atrial fibrillation and flutter** is outlined in Chap. 7.

Postresuscitation Management

Management of successfully resuscitated patients depends on treatment of the underlying disease process and continued maintenance of electrical and hemodynamic stability. All patients require careful and repeated assessment and should be monitored in an ICU. Evaluation and management of electrolytes, volume status, and previously initiated therapies (e.g., antiarrhythmics or pacing) are essential to successful long-term survival. Hypotension is frequently encountered in the postresuscitation period, and successful management depends on rapid determination of its etiology. Hypotension following cardiac arrest is frequently due to derangements in a patient's intravascular volume, heart rate, cardiac performance, or a combination of these etiologies, and making an exact diagnosis often requires invasive hemodynamic monitoring.

Discontinuation of CPR

The decision to discontinue CPR is the responsibility of the team leader. No guidelines for terminating resuscitative efforts are available, and the outcome of resuscitative efforts is heavily influenced by pre-arrest conditions. The duration of arrest before CPR-ACLS is initiated is a critical factor in determining survival. Patients with asystole or EMD as the initial rhythm have a very poor survival rate, and prolonged resuscitative efforts are probably not warranted. The following conditions should be met before discontinuing resuscitative efforts: (1) countershocks for ventricular fibrillation (if present) have been delivered; (2) the patient has been oxygenated and ventilated via properly performed endotracheal intubation; (3) IV access has been achieved and appropriate medications according to ACLS protocols have been administered; and (4) asystole or an agonal rhythm persists despite continued resuscitative efforts and an appropriate search for reversible causes. The duration of the resuscitative effort should be considered, as studies have shown that resuscitation attempts persisting for 30 minutes are usually unsuccessful. Neither the presence nor absence of any neurologic signs short of regaining consciousness provides a reliable end point for resuscitative efforts. The decision to terminate resuscitative efforts should be individualized and based on the lack of cardiovascular responsiveness to acceptable resuscitative techniques.

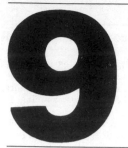

Critical Care and Medical Emergencies

Marin Kollef and
Daniel Goodenberger

Medical emergencies may not allow time for orderly information gathering and formulation of a differential diagnosis prior to initiation of therapy. **The first responsibility** of the physician is to provide basic life support (i.e., maintain an intact airway, adequate ventilation, and circulation).

Acute Upper Airway Obstruction

In the **conscious patient,** manifestations of airway obstruction may include stridor, impaired or absent phonation, sternal or suprasternal retractions, display of the universal choking sign, and respiratory distress. Urticaria, angioedema, fever, or evidence of trauma may be present. The **unconscious patient** may have labored breathing or apnea. Airway obstruction should always be suspected in a nonbreathing patient whom rescuers find difficult to ventilate. The **differential diagnosis** includes trauma to the face and neck, foreign body, infection (croup, epiglottitis, Ludwig's angina, retropharyngeal abscess, and diphtheria), tumor, angioedema, laryngospasm, anaphylaxis, retained secretions, or blockage of the upper airway by the tongue in the unconscious patient. **Therapy** is directed at rapid relief of obstruction to prevent cardiopulmonary arrest and anoxic brain damage.

I. **Partial obstruction in the awake patient with adequate ventilation** requires rapid history taking. A directed physical examination should include examination for airway swelling, trismus, pharyngeal obstruction, respiratory retractions, angioedema, stridor, wheezing, and grossly swollen lymph nodes and masses in the neck. Indirect laryngoscopy or fiberoptic nasopharyngolaryngoscopy may be performed if the patient is stable. A careful examination is unlikely to cause acute airway obstruction in an adult. Soft-tissue **radiographs of the neck** (posteroanterior and lateral view) are less sensitive and specific than direct examination but may be a valuable adjunct. It should be performed in the emergency department as a portable study, as the patient should not be left unattended. **Treatment** is aimed at the underlying disease process; the patient should be carefully observed, and the physician must be prepared to intervene to maintain an airway.

II. **Airway obstruction in the awake patient without ventilation** is usually caused by a foreign body (usually food) or angioedema. Other causes include infection or posttraumatic hematoma. History is usually unavailable. The **Heimlich maneuver** (subdiaphragmatic abdominal thrust) should be performed repeatedly until the object is expelled from the airway or the patient becomes unconscious (*JAMA* 268:2193, 1992) (see Chap. 8, Basic Life Support, sec. **XI**).

III. **Airway obstruction in an unconscious patient without intact ventilation** may be due to coma (in which the upper airway is obstructed by the tongue). It may also be caused by a foreign body, trauma, infection, or angioedema. A history is often unavailable except from paramedics or relatives. Examination reveals an unresponsive patient with no air movement or paradoxical respiratory efforts. **The first maneuver** should be head tilt-chin lift if cervical spine trauma is not suspected. If cervical spine trauma is suspected, the best maneuver is a jaw thrust (see Chap. 8). If these maneuvers are effective, an oral or nasal airway may be placed. If they are ineffective, an attempt should be made to ventilate the patient with a bag-valve-mask apparatus. If this is unsuccessful, the oropharynx and hypopharynx should be rapidly examined. A blind finger sweep should be avoided if **direct examination** using a laryngoscope and McGill forceps can be performed. The supine Heimlich maneuver (straddling the supine patient and applying repeated subdiaphragmatic thrusts) may be attempted (*JAMA* 268:2193, 1992) if laryngoscopy cannot be performed immediately or a foreign body is suspected. If this maneuver fails, direct laryngoscopy and endotracheal intubation should be attempted. If the patient cannot be intubated, establishing a surgical airway becomes crucial. If a surgeon is not immediately available, needle cricothyrotomy using a 12- to 16-gauge over-the-needle catheter may be performed with high-flow oxygen to provide adequate oxygenation (15 liters/minute). However, inappropriate catheter placement or high airway pressures may result in pneumomediastinum and tension pneumothorax. Surgical cricothyrotomy is rapid and simple and is the procedure of choice when it can be performed by physicians with appropriate training (*JAMA* 268:2203, 1992) (see Airway Management and Tracheal Intubation, sec. **III.B**). An endotracheal tube may then be placed through the incision.

Airway Management and Tracheal Intubation

Establishment of a patent airway and ventilatory support are required by many ICU patients. Specific indications for airway support in the form of endotracheal intubation include (1) initiation of mechanical ventilation, (2) airway protection, (3) inadequate oxygenation using less invasive methods, (4) prevention of aspiration and allowing for the suctioning of pulmonary secretions, and (5) hyperventilation for the treatment of increased intracranial pressure. In an emergency situation, simple maneuvers like a jaw thrust with mask-to-face ventilation may assist the patient in clearing an obstructed airway and in maintaining adequate ventilation until endotracheal intubation can be performed.

I. Airway management
- **A. Head and jaw positioning.** The oropharynx should be inspected and all foreign bodies removed. For patients with inadequate respirations the jaw thrust or head-tilt–chin-lift maneuvers should be performed (see Chap. 8, Basic Life Support, sec. **V**).
- **B. Oral and nasopharyngeal airways.** When head and jaw positioning fail to establish a patent airway or when more permanent airway maintenance is desired, an oral or nasopharyngeal airway can be used. Oral airways are initially positioned with the concave curve of the airway facing up into the roof of the mouth. The oral airway is then turned 180 degrees so that the concave curve of the airway follows the natural curve of the tongue. Alternatively a tongue depressor can be used to displace the tongue inferiorly and laterally to allow direct positioning of the oral airway. Oral airways can be taped in place to create a passageway for ventilation and suctioning of secretions. Careful monitoring of airway patency is required since malpositioning of oral airways can push the tongue posteriorly and result in obstruction of the oropharynx. Nasopharyngeal airways are made of soft plastic. These airways are easily passed down one of the nasal passages to the posterior pharynx following topical nasal lubrication and anesthesia with viscous lidocaine jelly.
- **C. Mask-to-face ventilation.** After establishing an airway, respiratory efforts should be evaluated and closely monitored. Ineffective respiratory efforts can be augmented with simple mask-to-face ventilation. Proper fitting and positioning of the mask will ensure a tight seal around the mouth and nose, optimizing ventilation. The patient's mandible is lifted into the mask to produce a tight seal. Significant leaks may develop between the mask and the patient's face, which may result in less effective ventilation. Additionally, proper head positioning (see sec. **II.A**) and the use of airway adjuncts (e.g., oral or nasopharyngeal airways) will further optimize ventilation with a mask-to-face system.

Table 9-1. Procedure for direct orotracheal intubation

1. Administer oxygen by face mask.
2. Ensure basic equipment is present and easily accessible (oxygen source, bag-valve device, suctioning device, ET tube, blunt stylet, laryngoscope, 20-ml syringe).
3. Place patient on nonmobile rigid surface.
4. If patient is in hospital bed, remove backboard and adjust bed height.
5. Depress patient's tongue with tongue depressor and administer topical anesthesia to patient's pharynx.
6. Position patient's head in "sniffing position" (see sec. **II.A**).
7. Administer IV sedation and neuromuscular blocker if necessary.*
8. Have assistant apply Sellick maneuver (compressing cricothyroid cartilage posteriorly against vertebral bodies) to prevent regurgitation and aspiration of stomach contents from esophagus.
9. Grasp laryngoscope handle in left hand while opening patient's mouth with gloved right hand.
10. Insert laryngoscope blade on right side of patient's mouth and advance to base of tongue, displacing tongue to the left.
11. Lift laryngoscope **away** from patient at a 45-degree angle using arm and shoulder strength. Avoid using patient's teeth as a fulcrum.
12. Suction oropharynx and hypopharynx if necessary.
13. Grasp ET tube with inserted stylet in right hand and insert it into right corner of patient's mouth, avoiding obscuration of epiglottis and vocal cords.
14. Advance ET tube through vocal cords until cuff no longer visible and remove stylet.
15. Inflate cuff with enough air to prevent significant air leakage.
16. Verify correct ET tube positioning by auscultation of both lungs and the abdomen.
17. Obtain a chest radiograph to verify correct position of the ET tube.

ET = endotracheal.

* Neuromuscular blockade can result in complete airway collapse and airway obstruction. Personnel skillful in establishment of an emergency surgical airway should be available if paralysis is used.

II. Endotracheal intubation (*Clin Chest Med* 12:449, 1991)

   A. Technique. Depending on the skill of the operator and the urgency of the situation, one of several techniques can be selected for intubation of the trachea. These techniques include (1) direct laryngoscopic orotracheal intubation, (2) blind nasotracheal intubation, and (3) flexible fiberoptic guided orotracheal or nasotracheal intubation. In emergency situations, the direct laryngoscopic technique allows for the most rapid intubation of the trachea with the largest endotracheal tube. Nasotracheal intubation often requires smaller endotracheal tubes that are more susceptible to kinking and obstruction and is associated with a higher incidence of otitis media and sinusitis compared to orotracheal intubation. Prior to attempted endotracheal intubation a systematic evaluation of the patient's head and neck positioning must be performed. The oral, pharyngeal, and tracheal axis should be aligned prior to any intubation attempts. This "sniffing" position is achieved by flexing the patient's neck and extending the head. A small pillow or several towels placed under the occiput will assist in maintaining this position. Table 9-1 offers a step-by-step approach to performing successful orotracheal intubation.

   B. Verification of correct endotracheal tube positioning may include (1) direct view of the endotracheal tube entering the trachea through the vocal cords, (2) fiberoptic inspection of the airways through the endotracheal tube, and (3) use of an end-tidal carbon dioxide monitor.

   C. Complications. Improper endotracheal tube positioning is the most important immediate complication to be recognized and corrected. Ideally, the tip of the endotracheal tube should be 3–7 cm above the carina depending on head and neck positioning. Esophageal or right mainstem intubation should be suspected if hypoxemia, hypoventilation, barotrauma, or cardiac decompensation occur. Abdominal distention, lack of breath sounds over the thorax, and regurgitation of food contents through the endotracheal tube indicate an esophageal intubation. If there is any uncertainty regarding the possibility of an esophageal intubation, tube positioning should be immediately verified or the patient should be reintubated with direct confirmation of endotracheal tube positioning. Although chest radiographs usually indicate the presence of an esophageal intubation, they should not be routinely used as a means of verifying suspected esophageal positioning due to delays associated with their acquisition (*South Med J* 87:248, 1994). Other complications associated with endotracheal intubation include dislodgement of teeth, trauma to the upper airway, and increased intracranial pressure.

III. Surgical airways

    A. Tracheostomy (*Persp Critical Care* 3:105, 1990). The main indications for surgical tracheostomy are (1) the need for prolonged respiratory support, (2) potentially life-threatening upper airway obstruction (due to epiglottitis, facial burns, or worsening laryngeal edema), (3) obstructive sleep apnea unresponsive to less invasive therapies, and (4) congenital abnormalities (e.g., Pierre-Robin syndrome). Tracheostomy sites usually require at least 72 hours to mature. Tube dislodgement before their maturation, followed by blind attempts at tube reinsertion, can lead to tube malpositioning within a false channel in the pretracheal space; this can result in complete loss of the airway followed by progressive hypoxemia and hypotension. If a tracheostomy tube cannot be easily reinserted, standard direct orotracheal intubation should be performed (see Table 9-1). Surgical tracheostomy to manage respiratory failure should be considered after 11–14 days of mechanical ventilation but can be performed earlier if prolonged ventilation is anticipated (*Am Rev Respir Dis* 147:768, 1993). Tracheostomy tube placement can facilitate liberation from mechanical ventilation in the difficult-to-wean patient by (1) decreasing dead space, (2) allowing patients to eat, and (3) increasing patient mobility. Various types of cuffed tracheostomy tubes are available. Metal uncuffed tracheostomy tubes can keep a tracheostomy patent in spontaneously breathing patients until it is no longer needed. Tracheal tube cuff pressures should be monitored every 4–6 hours with a manometer and maintained below capillary-filling pressure (i.e., <25 mm Hg) to prevent ischemic mucosal injury.

    B. Cricothyrotomy is indicated for the establishment of an emergency airway when direct tracheal intubation cannot be performed due to upper airway obstruction (Table 9-2). A pillow or towel roll should be placed under the patient's shoulders to extend the neck. The thyroid cartilage superiorly and the cricoid cartilage inferiorly should be located where they border the cricothyroid membrane. The thumb and second finger of the nondominant hand should grasp and stabilize the lateral aspects of the cricothyroid membrane. With a scalpel, a transverse skin incision is made over the entire distance of the membrane. The incision is then deepened down to the cricothyroid membrane, avoiding injury to surrounding structures. The incision can be dilated with the handle of the scalpel to facilitate cannulation with an airway. Standard tracheostomy tubes or endotracheal tubes can be inserted into the stoma to ventilate the patient. Appropriate surgical consultation should be obtained after the patient is stabilized.

    C. Cricothyroid needle cannulation. In emergency settings when standard endotracheal intubation cannot be performed and placement of a surgical airway is not immediately possible, needle cannulation of the cricothyroid membrane may be performed as an intermediate procedure until a more definitive airway can be established. After grasping the ends of the cricothyroid membrane with the nondominant hand, a 22-gauge needle is inserted into the airway, aspirating air to confirm positioning. Lidocaine is then injected into the trachea to blunt the patient's cough reflex before withdrawal of the needle. Using the same technique,

Table 9-2. Causes of upper airway obstruction

I. Inhalational injury
  A. Primarily upper airway injury due to water-soluble substances
    1. Anhydrous ammonia
    2. Hydrogen chloride
  B. Both upper airway and lower airway injury due to water-insoluble substances
    1. Chlorine
    2. Cadmium
    3. Zinc chloride
    4. Osmium tetroxide
    5. Paraquat
II. Traumatic injury
  A. Facial
  B. Laryngeal
  C. Hemorrhage
  D. Airway burns
III. Foreign body
IV. Laryngospasm
V. Infection
  A. Epiglottitis
  B. Retropharyngeal abscess
  C. Diphtheria
  D. Ludwig's angina
VI. Angioedema
VII. Tumor
  A. Primary
  B. Metastatic
VIII. Vocal cord paralysis/dysfunction

a 14-gauge (or larger) needle-through-cannula device can be passed through the cricothyroid membrane at a 45-degree angle to the skin. When air is freely aspirated the outer cannula is passed into the airway caudally and the needle is removed. A 3-ml syringe barrel can then be attached to the catheter and a 7-mm inner-diameter endotracheal tube adapter attached to the syringe will allow bag-valve ventilation. Additionally the cannula can be directly attached to high-flow oxygen (i.e., 10–15 liters/minute).

Oxygen Therapy

The goal of oxygen administration is to facilitate adequate uptake of oxygen into the blood to meet the needs of peripheral tissues. When this goal cannot be accomplished with the methods outlined below, endotracheal intubation may be necessary.
I. **Methods of delivery**
  A. **Nasal prongs** allow patients to eat, drink, and speak when the prongs are in place. Their disadvantage is that the exact concentration of inspired oxygen (i.e., FiO_2) delivered is not known as it is influenced by the patient's peak inspiratory flow demand. As an approximation the following guide can be used: 1 liter/minute of nasal prong oxygen flow is approximately equivalent to an FiO_2 of 24% with each additional liter of flow increasing the FiO_2 by approximately 4%. Flow rates should be limited to less than 5 liters/minute.
  B. **A Venturi mask** allows the precise administration of oxygen. Usual FiO_2 values delivered with these masks are 24, 28, 31, 35, 40, and 50%. Venturi masks are often useful in patients with chronic obstructive pulmonary disease (COPD) and

hypercapnia because they titrate the arterial oxygen tension (PaO_2) as to minimize carbon dioxide retention.

C. **A nonrebreathing mask** achieves higher oxygen concentrations (approximately 90%) compared to partial rebreathing systems. A one-way valve prevents exhaled gases from entering the reservoir bag in a nonrebreathing system to optimize the FiO_2

D. **Continuous positive airway pressure (CPAP)** (*N Engl J Med* 325:1825, 1991). If the PaO_2 is less than 60–65 mm Hg while using a nonrebreathing mask (i.e., FiO_2 >90%) and the patient is conscious and cooperative, able to protect the lower airway, and hemodynamically stable, then a CPAP mask can be used. CPAP is delivered by a tight-fitting mask equipped with pressure-limiting valves. Many patients will not tolerate a CPAP mask due to feelings of claustrophobia, aerophagia, persistent hypoxemia, or hemodynamic instability. In these patients, endotracheal intubation should be performed. Initially 3–5 cm H_2O of CPAP should be applied while monitoring the PaO_2 or hemoglobin saturation (SaO_2). If the PaO_2 is still less than 60 mm Hg (SaO_2 <90%), then the level of CPAP should be incremented in steps of 3–5 cm H_2O up to a level of 10–15 cm H_2O.

E. **Bilevel positive airway pressure (BiPAP)** (*Am Rev Respir Dis* 147:1050, 1993) is a method whereby inspiratory and expiratory pressure can be applied by a mask during the patient's respiratory cycle (i.e., noninvasive ventilation). The inspiratory support decreases the patient's work of breathing. The expiratory support (CPAP) improves gas exchange by preventing alveolar collapse. Noninvasive ventilation using face or nasal masks has been successfully used in patients with neuromuscular disease, COPD, and postoperative respiratory insufficiency as a means of decreasing the need for endotracheal intubation and mechanical ventilation (*N Engl J Med* 323:1523, 1990). When using BiPAP, a pressure-supported ventilation (PSV) level of 5–10 cm H_2O and a CPAP level of 3–5 cm H_2O are reasonable starting points. The PSV level can be increased in increments of 3–5 cm H_2O using the patient's respiratory rate as a guide of effectiveness (less labored breathing at a rate less than 30 breaths/minute).

Blood Gas Analysis

I. **Clinical approach to acid-base disorders**
  A. Determine if acidemia (pH <7.36) or alkalemia (pH >7.44) is present.
  B. Determine the source of the primary acid-base disturbance:

  $[HCO_3^-]$ <20 mEq/liter for a metabolic acidosis.

  $PaCO_2$ >44 mm Hg for a respiratory acidosis.

  $[HCO_3^-]$ >28 mEq/liter for a metabolic alkalosis.

  $PaCO_2$ <36 mm Hg for a respiratory alkalosis.

  C. Determine if appropriate compensation has occurred using the appropriate formula (see Table 3-2). If an appropriate compensation has not occurred, then a mixed acid-base disorder may be present or compensation may not yet be complete.
  D. Determine the anion gap:

  $$[Na^+] - [Cl^-] - [HCO_3^-] = 12 \pm 2 \text{ mEq/liter}$$

  E. Start appropriate treatment (see Chap. 3, Acid-Base Disturbances).
II. **Evaluation of PaO_2.** Arterial hypoxemia can be caused by hypoventilation, pulmonary diffusion abnormalities, right-to-left shunt, ventilation-perfusion mismatch, and alveolar hypoxia. Alveolar hypoxia usually occurs at high altitude or because of gaseous inhalation. Both hypoventilation and alveolar hypoxia are usually associ-

Table 9-3. Hemodynamic patterns associated with specific shock states

Type of shock	CI	SVR	PVR	SVO$_2$	RAP	RVP	PAP	PAOP
Cardiogenic (e.g., MI, cardiac tamponade*)	D	I	N	D	I	I	I	I
Hypovolemic (e.g., hemorrhage)	D	I	N	D	D	D	D	D
Distributive (e.g., septic)	I	D	N	N/I	N/D	N/D	N/D	N/D
Obstructive (e.g., massive pulmonary embolism)	D	I/N	I	D	I	I	I	N/D

CI = cardiac index; SVR = systemic vascular resistance; PVR = pulmonary vascular resistance; SVO$_2$ = mixed venous oxygen saturation; RAP = right atrial pressure; RVP = right ventricular pressure; PAP = pulmonary artery pressure; PAOP = pulmonary artery occlusion pressure; D = decreased; I = increased; N = normal.
* Equalization of RAP, PAOP, diastolic PAP, and diastolic RVP establishes a diagnosis of cardiac tamponade.

ated with normal lung function, which is manifested by a normal alveolar oxygen tension to arterial blood oxygen tension gradient (P[A-a]O$_2$ gradient). Diffusion abnormalities, right-to-left shunt, and ventilation-perfusion mismatch are the usual pathophysiologic processes responsible for a widened P(A-a)O$_2$ gradient. Supplemental oxygen will usually improve the PaO$_2$ in patients with ventilation-perfusion abnormalities (e.g., COPD) and diffusion mismatch (e.g., interstitial lung disease). Patients with a significant right-to-left shunt (e.g., adult respiratory distress syndrome [ARDS]) will be resistant to the effects of supplemental oxygen and will often require the addition of positive end-expiratory pressure (PEEP) or CPAP to improve arterial oxygenation.

Shock

Circulatory shock is a process in which blood flow and oxygen delivery to tissues is disturbed; this leads to tissue hypoxia with resultant compromise of cellular metabolic activity and organ function. Altered tissue perfusion that results in oliguria, decreased mental status, decreased peripheral pulses, and diaphoresis represents the major clinical manifestation of circulatory shock. Survival from shock is related to both the adequacy of the initial resuscitation and the degree of subsequent organ system dysfunction. Rapid cardiovascular resuscitation with the reestablishment of tissue perfusion using fluid therapy and vasoactive drugs is the main goal of therapy.

Circulatory shock can be classified into four broad categories based on the primary defect that results in the shock state. These categories include hypovolemic shock (e.g., hemorrhage, dehydration), cardiogenic shock (e.g., acute myocardial infarction [MI], cardiac tamponade), obstructive shock (e.g., acute pulmonary embolism), and distributive shock (septic shock and anaphylactic shock). Table 9-3 gives the main hemodynamic patterns seen with each of these shock states.

I. **Individual shock states**
   A. **Hypovolemic shock** results from a decrease in effective intravascular volume that decreases venous return to the right ventricle. Significant hypovolemic shock (i.e., >40% loss of intravascular volume) lasting more than several hours is often associated with a fatal outcome despite resuscitative efforts. Therapy of hypovolemic shock is usually aimed at reestablishing the adequacy of the intravascular compartment. At the same time ongoing sources of volume loss such as a

bleeding vessel may require surgical intervention. Table 9-4 lists crystalloid and colloid solutions generally used for the resuscitation of patients in shock states. Blood products are an important part of the resuscitative effort, especially when hypovolemic shock is secondary to hemorrhage. In general, resuscitation with colloid solutions results in more rapid correction of the intravascular volume deficits using smaller total volumes of infusate compared to crystalloid solutions (*Crit Care Clin* 9:239, 1993). However, because of ease of use and availability, in most circumstances isotonic crystalloid solutions represent the fluid of choice for the resuscitation of patients in shock. **Fluid resuscitation** must be prompt and should be given through large-bore catheters placed in large peripheral veins. In the absence of overt signs of congestive heart failure, the patient should receive a 500-ml initial bolus of normal saline, with further infusions adjusted to achieve adequate blood pressure and tissue perfusion. When shock is due to hemorrhage, packed red blood cells should be given as soon as feasible. When hemorrhage is massive, type-specific unmatched blood can be given safely. Rarely, type O blood may be needed (see Chap. 18).

    The pneumatic antishock garment (PASG), with sequential inflation of legs and abdominal compartments to 15–40 mm Hg, may temporarily stabilize patients in hypovolemic, obstructive, distributive, and mixed states of shock. **PASG is contraindicated in cardiogenic shock**. Its beneficial effects are due to an increase in peripheral systemic vascular resistance (*Ann Emerg Med* 15:886, 1986). Patients with severe noncardiogenic shock may benefit from PASG until adequate fluid or pressor therapy, or both, can be established. **Trendelenburg's position** increases venous return and cardiac index.

B. Cardiogenic shock is most commonly seen following acute MI (see Chap. 5). Other causes of cardiogenic shock include septal wall rupture, acute mitral regurgitation, myocarditis, dilated cardiomyopathy, arrhythmias, and pericardial tamponade. Cardiogenic shock secondary to MI is usually associated with a depressed cardiac output and elevated PAOP (see Table 9-3). See Chap. 5 for management strategies.

C. Obstructive shock is usually caused by massive pulmonary embolism. Occasionally air embolism, amniotic fluid embolism, or tumor embolism may also cause obstructive shock. When shock complicates pulmonary embolism, therapy is directed toward preserving peripheral organ perfusion and removing the vascular obstruction. Fluid administration and the use of vasoconstrictors (e.g., norepinephrine, dopamine) may preserve BP while more definitive measures such as thrombolytic therapy (e.g., streptokinase, urokinase, tissue plasminogen activator) or surgical embolectomy are considered.

D. Distributive shock. Septic shock and anaphylactic shock are the two main forms of distributive shock associated with significant decreases in vascular tone.

    1. Septic shock is caused by the systemic release of mediators that are usually triggered by circulating gram-negative bacteria or their products, although septic shock can be seen without evidence of infection (e.g., pancreatitis, crush injuries) (*Chest* 101:1644, 1992). Septic shock is primarily characterized by hypotension due to decreased vascular tone. Cardiac output is also increased due to increased heart rate and end-diastolic volumes despite overall myocardial depression (*N Engl J Med* 328:1471, 1993). The main goals of **treatment** of septic shock include initial fluid resuscitation, adequate treatment of the underlying infection, and interruption of the mediator-associated systemic inflammatory response. Initial resuscitation includes appropriate large-volume fluid administration due to the decrease in vascular tone and dilated ventricular capacity. Pulmonary artery (PA) catheter–directed therapy is most important in such patients to determine the adequacy of preload and the need for inotropic or vasoconstrictor agents.

    2. Anaphylactic shock. Anaphylaxis is the result of an IgE-mediated acute allergic reaction in a sensitized individual. Death may occur from anaphylaxis; Hymenoptera stings and penicillin (parenteral) are the most common causes. Other causes include local anesthetics, other antimicrobials, serum, and food products. **Anaphylactoid reactions** result from the direct release of

Table 9-4. Fluids available for intravascular volume resuscitation

	Sodium (mEq/liter)	Chloride (mEq/liter)	Osmolarity (mOsm/liter)	Oncotic pressure (mm Hg)	Lactate (mEq/liter)	Cost per unit[a] (dollars)
0.9% sodium chloride	154	154	310	0	0	0.75 (1 liter)
Ringer's lactate	130	109	275	0	28	0.90 (1 liter)
3% saline solution	513	513	1,025	0	0	8.35 (0.50 liter)
5% albumin	145	145	290	20	0	55.00 (0.25 liter)
25% albumin	145	145	290	70	0	55.00 (0.05 liter)
6% hetastarch	154	154	310	30	0	72.50 (0.5 liter)
Dextran 40	154	154	310	40	0	37.50[b] (0.5 liter)
Dextran 70	154	154	310	70	0	25.00[b] (0.5 liter)

[a] These represent 1993 average wholesale prices for these solutions at Barnes Hospital, St. Louis, MO.
[b] Costs for generic products.

mediators, including histamine and leukotrienes. IV radiographic contrast reagents are the most common cause; reactions occur in 5.0–7.5% of those exposed (*Invest Radiol* 23:S88, 1988; *Am J Cardiol* 66:34F, 1990). Other agents include salicylates and other nonsteroidal antiinflammatory drugs.

a. **Clinical manifestations** are the same for both anaphylaxis and anaphylactoid reactions. Onset may be immediate or delayed. Manifestations include pruritus, urticaria, angioedema, respiratory distress (due to laryngeal edema, laryngospasm, or bronchospasm), hypotension, and abdominal pain. Hypotension and shock may be due to hypoxemia, vasodilation, and capillary leak. The most common cause of death is airway obstruction, followed closely by hypotension.

b. **Treatment**

(1) **Management of the airway** is the first priority. If the patient cannot be ventilated, an endotracheal tube should be placed and ventilation begun with 100% oxygen. If laryngeal edema is not rapidly responsive to epinephrine and endotracheal intubation is unsuccessful, surgical airway management may be necessary (see Airway Management and Tracheal Intubation, sec. **III**).

(2) **Epinephrine** is the cornerstone of therapy and is given in a dose of 0.3–0.5 mg (0.3–0.5 ml of 1 : 1,000 solution) SC and repeated twice at 20-minute intervals if necessary. Patients with major airway compromise or hypotension may be given epinephrine SL (0.5 ml of 1 : 1,000 solution), in a femoral or internal jugular vein (3–5 ml of 1 : 10,000 solution), or via endotracheal tube (3–5 ml of 1 : 10,000 solution). For severe reactions not immediately responsive to these measures, an epinephrine drip may be useful. One milligram is diluted in 250 ml 5% dextrose in water, and the infusion is begun at 0.1 µg/kg/minute, titrating to BP. Patients taking beta-adrenergic antagonists may require glucagon (see sec. **I.D.2.b.(8)**).

(3) **Volume expansion** with 500–1,000 ml of crystalloid or colloid, followed by titration to BP and urine output, may be used in addition to epinephrine and glucagon to treat hypotension. The PASG may also be useful when the BP is persistently less than 80 mm Hg (*Ann Emerg Med* 13:189, 1989; *J Emerg Med* 2:349, 1985).

(4) **Inhaled beta-agonists.** Metaproterenol, 0.3 ml, or albuterol, 0.5 ml in 2.5 ml normal saline, should be used to treat resistant bronchospasm. **Aminophylline** may be used as a second-line drug (see Appendix C).

(5) **General measures include delay of absorption of the offending antigen.** When the allergen has been injected, slight constriction (constricting pressure less than arterial pressure) and local epinephrine injection at the affected site may be useful. The patient should be carefully examined; honeybee stingers are removed by gentle scraping, not squeezing. For orally ingested antigens, activated **charcoal** (50–100 g) with 1–2 g/kg (maximum 150 g) of sorbitol or 300 ml of magnesium citrate may decrease absorption of the antigen from the GI tract. **Emesis is not indicated.**

(6) **Antihistamines** (e.g., diphenhydramine, 25–50 mg PO or IM q6h) do not have an immediate effect, but they may shorten the duration of the reaction. For persistent or recurrent symptoms, addition of an H_2-antagonist (e.g., cimetidine, 300 mg q6h IV) may be useful (*Ann Allergy* 63:235, 1989).

(7) **Glucocorticoids** have no significant effect for 6–12 hours. However, they may prevent recurrence or relapse of severe reactions. Either hydrocortisone, 500 mg IV q6h, or methylprednisolone, 125 mg IV q6h, is adequate.

(8) **Glucagon,** given as a 10-mg bolus followed by a drip of 2–8 mg/hour, provides direct inotropic support for patients taking beta-adrenergic antagonists (*Ann Intern Med* 105:65, 1986). **Beta-adrenergic antagonist** therapy increases the risk of anaphylaxis and anaphylac-

toid reactions and makes the anaphylactic state more resistant to beta-adrenergic therapy (*Ann Intern Med* 115:270, 1991). Alpha-agonist vasopressors should be avoided, as they may prolong the anaphylactic state.

II. **Observation.** Patients with mild to moderate reactions (urticaria or very mild bronchospasm) should be observed for a minimum of 6 hours. Patients with moderate to severe reactions (especially with orally ingested antigens) may relapse and **should be admitted to the hospital** (with close monitoring if there has been severe bronchospasm, laryngeal edema, hypotension, or rhythm disturbances).

III. **Prevention of recurrence.** If the allergen is identified, it should be avoided in the future. Low–ionic strength contrast should be used in those patients with a history of prior reaction (*Invest Radiol* 23:S88, 1988; *Radiology* 183:105, 1992). In addition, the patient should receive prednisone, 50 mg PO q6h for 3–4 doses (the last dose taken 1 hour before the procedure), and hydroxyzine, 100 mg PO 1 hour before the procedure (*Radiology* 184:383, 1992). Advanced cardiac life support capability must be present in the radiology suite. Those patients who have had severe Hymenoptera reactions should receive epinephrine self-injection kits with adequate instructions and should be referred to an allergist for evaluation and potential desensitization.

Establishment of Vascular Access

I. **Arterial access.** A fixed arterial line can be established in a number of sites including the radial, ulnar, brachial, axillary, femoral, dorsalis pedis, and posterior tibial arteries. The radial artery is frequently used due to its accessibility and the presence of collateral circulation from the ulnar artery. The femoral artery is also frequently used in hemodynamically unstable patients. Indications for fixed arterial access include the need for continuous arterial pressure monitoring and the need for repeated arterial blood sampling. Radial artery cannulation should only be performed after determining the presence of collateral arterial blood flow by ultrasound or by Allen's test, which is performed by simultaneously occluding the radial and ulnar arteries with the thumbs of the examiner's right and left hands. The patient's hand clenching will exsanguinate the hand and produce a blanched appearance. The artery that is not being cannulated is then released and normal color should return in 4–6 seconds. If normal color does not appear for more than 10–15 seconds, an alternative site should be selected for arterial cannulation.

For radial artery cannulation the patient's wrist is usually dorsiflexed with a towel roll placed underneath it and the fingers are taped to an armboard to prevent inadvertent movements. The skin is anesthetized with about 1 ml of 1% lidocaine. Using sterile technique, the examiner advances a 20- or 22-gauge catheter-over-needle device at a 30- to 45-degree angle through the patient's skin until blood return is demonstrated. The catheter is then advanced with a twisting motion into the artery, the needle is removed, and the catheter is sutured to the skin to prevent accidental dislodgement. Complications associated with arterial line placement include bleeding, infection, atherosclerotic plaque embolization with distal limb ischemia, peripheral nerve injury, arteriovenous fistula formation, and pseudo-aneurysm formation.

II. **Central venous access.** The Seldinger technique is used for cannulation of central veins. The internal jugular, subclavian, femoral, and external jugular veins are the most common access sites used. The skin over the access site is anesthetized with 1% lidocaine. A 16- or 18-gauge needle attached to a syringe is advanced through the patient's skin at a 45-degree angle until blood is easily aspirated. Persistent blood return usually confirms intravascular access. Following needle cannulation of a central vein, a guidewire is advanced through the needle 5 to 10 cm into the vessel. When resistance to advancement is encountered the wire should be withdrawn and blood should be reaspirated through the needle to reconfirm intravascular positioning. When resistance is encountered with withdrawal of the wire, the needle and wire should be withdrawn as a single unit to prevent wire embolization. After successful wire advancement the needle is removed and a small skin incision is made over the skin entrance site to facilitate catheter entry. A firm twisting motion with the examiner's dominant hand and wrist is used to advance the dilator-catheter assembly into position over the guidewire, and the wire and dilator are removed. If at any time resistance is met, the dilator-catheter assembly should be removed. Successfully placed catheters should be sutured in place and have an appropriate dressing placed over the skin entrance site.

A. **Complications**
   1. **Air embolism.** Needles and catheters should never be left uncovered once access to a central vein has been gained. Syringes should be attached to needles, and catheter openings should be covered with caps or a gloved finger to prevent pulmonary and systemic air embolization. If significant air embolism is suspected, the patient should be immediately placed in the headdown left lateral decubitus position. This position will allow air to pool in the right ventricle away from the pulmonary outflow tract. Air can then be aspirated from the right ventricle with a large-bore catheter, or hyperbaric therapy may be used if available. In any patient with central venous access, air embolism should be considered in the differential diagnosis of sudden pulmonary or hemodynamic deterioration.
   2. **Arrhythmias.** Wires or catheters should be immediately pulled back from the right ventricle if significant arrhythmias occur with their placement. Persistent arrhythmias occurring during subsequent attempts to pass a catheter (e.g., a PA catheter) through the right ventricle may be treated with IV lidocaine (1 mg/kg). Correction of electrolyte disorders (e.g., hypokalemia, hypomagnesemia) may also help correct the arrhythmias.
   3. **Pneumothorax.** Catheter placement should always be ipsilateral following unsuccessful attempts in the subclavian or internal jugular veins to prevent bilateral pneumothoraces. If contralateral attempts are being considered, a chest radiograph should first be obtained to exclude a complicating pneumothorax.
   4. **Vascular injury.** Vascular perforation or laceration represents a medical emergency that can result in hemothorax (subclavian or internal jugular approaches) or hemoperitoneum (femoral approach). After removal of the catheter, direct pressure should be applied if the vessel is accessible. Fistulas, aneurysms, and pseudoaneurysms can also result from attempted catheter placements. Surgical consultation should be immediately obtained when significant vascular injury is suspected.
   5. **Infection.** Local infection at the skin insertion site is an indication for catheter removal. Catheter-related infection can be defined using quantitative cultures of catheter segments (*N Engl J Med* 296:1305, 1977). As a general rule, if a central vein-catheter site is without evidence of infection and the patient is without signs of sepsis, then the catheter can remain in place for continued use beyond 48–72 hours (*N Engl J Med* 327:1062, 1992).

Hemodynamic Monitoring

I. **Pulmonary artery catheterization** (*Chest* 85:537, 1984)
   A. **Indications.** Placement of a PA catheter is usually done to differentiate between cardiogenic and noncardiogenic forms of pulmonary edema, to identify the etiology of shock (see Table 9-3), for the evaluation of acute renal failure or unexplained acidosis, for the evaluation of cardiac disorders, or to monitor high-risk surgical patients in the perioperative setting. The PA catheter allows measurement of intravascular and intracardiac pressures, cardiac output determinations, and measurement of mixed-venous oxygen tension and saturation.
   B. **Preparation and catheter insertion.** All ports of the PA catheter should be

attached to separate infusion systems and flushed with normal saline to remove all air bubbles. The balloon of the PA catheter should be inflated with 1.5 cc of air to test its integrity. The catheter should then be inserted 15 cm into the introducer to ensure it is within the vessel before inflating the balloon. The monitoring system should next be zeroed at the level of the left atrium prior to the recording of any pressure waveforms. The left atrium is usually approximated as being at the level of the fourth intercostal space in the midaxillary line.

C. **Obtaining a pulmonary capillary wedge tracing.** From the 15-cm point the PA catheter is advanced forward after the balloon is inflated. Bedside waveform analysis is used to determine successful passage of the catheter through the right atrium, right ventricle, and PA, into a PA wedge position (PA occlusive pressure [PAOP]). Fluoroscopy should be used when difficulty is encountered in positioning the PA catheter.

If at any time after passage into the PA the tracing is found to move off the scale of the graph during measurement of the PAOP, then overwedging of the catheter has occurred. An overwedged catheter should be immediately withdrawn 2–3 cm after balloon deflation, and catheter positioning should be rechecked with reinflation of the balloon. The catheter should continue to be withdrawn until the overwedge pattern has resolved and a normal PAOP tracing is obtained with balloon inflation. Overwedging of a PA catheter may increase the likelihood of serious complications.

D. **Acceptance of PAOP readings.** Respiratory variation on the waveform, atrial pressure characteristics including "a" and "v" waves, mean value of the PAOP tracing obtained at end-expiration being less than the mean value of the PA pressure measurement, and the aspiration of highly oxygenated blood with the catheter in the wedge position all indicate an accurate reading. Additionally, interpretation of the PAOP can be affected by large "v" waves reflecting mitral regurgitation or severe left ventricular dysfunction.

E. **Transmural pressure.** When PEEP is present (applied or auto-PEEP), the positive intraalveolar pressure at end-expiration is transmitted through the lung to the pleural space. In these circumstances the measured "wedge" pressure reflects the summation of the hydrostatic pressure within the vessel and the juxtacardiac pressure (P_{JC}). When significant levels of total PEEP are present (applied and auto-PEEP levels >10 cm H_2O), it is more appropriate to use the transmural pressure (P_{TM}) as a measure of left ventricular filling ($P_{TM} = PAOP - P_{JC}$). For patients with normal lung compliance, one-half of the total PEEP can be used as an estimate of P_{JC}. When lung compliance is significantly depressed (e.g., in ARDS), one-third of the total PEEP can be used as an estimate for P_{JC}.

F. **Cardiac output.** PA catheters are equipped with a thermistor to measure cardiac output. At least two measurements that differ by less than 10–15% should be obtained. Injections should be synchronized with the respiratory cycle to minimize variability between results. Thermodilution measurements of cardiac output (CO) are often inaccurate at extremely low (e.g., <1.5 liter/minute) or extremely high (e.g., >7.0 liter/minute) COs. Calculation of the CO using the Fick formula (see Appendix G) may be more accurate in these circumstances.

G. **Interpretation of hemodynamic readings.** PAOP can be used both as an index of left ventricular filling (preload) and as an index of the patient's propensity for developing pulmonary edema.

Improvements in cardiac function due to adequate preload administration are more efficient in terms of myocardial oxygen consumption compared to similar increases in cardiac output achieved by inotropes in the face of an inadequate preload. As a general rule, **preload should be optimized prior to the utilization of inotropic agents and vasodilators** that can increase myocardial oxygen consumption or cause hypotension when preload is inadequate. Fluid boluses should be administered and followed by repeat measurements of PAOP, CO, heart rate (HR), and stroke volume (SV). In low CO states, if the PAOP increases by less than 5 mm Hg without significant changes in HR, CO, and SV, then additional fluid boluses may need to be given. An increase in the PAOP by more than 5 mm Hg usually signals that adequate ventricular filling is being achieved. Once the patient's preload has been optimized, cardiac performance can be reassessed and if necessary further therapy with inotropes (e.g., dobutamine, amrinone), or vasodilators (e.g., nitroprusside, hydralazine, angiotensin-converting enzyme inhibitors) can be administered to achieve further improvements in cardiac performance.

PAOP is also a reflection of the tendency to develop pulmonary edema. Decreased left ventricular compliance will result in this "critical pressure" being reached sooner for similar volume changes compared to a normally compliant left ventricle. This difference is due to the increased stiffness of the noncompliant ventricle that causes higher pressures to be achieved for similar changes in volume. To optimize cardiac performance and to minimize the tendency for pulmonary edema formation, PAOP should be kept at the lowest point at which cardiac performance is acceptable.

Closed Tube Thoracostomy

The development of a tension pneumothorax requires immediate therapeutic intervention. Tension pneumothorax should be suspected on clinical grounds whenever agitation, progressive hypoxemia, hypotension, or electromechanical dissociation (EMD) occur. When tension pneumothorax is suspected in a hemodynamically unstable patient, emergency needle aspiration should be performed prior to thoracostomy tube placement. A 14-gauge catheter-over-needle device can be inserted into the second or third intercostal space in the midclavicular line to acutely decompress a tension pneumothorax. Once it is inserted into the pleural space a rush of air signals correct positioning. Chest tube placement in the fifth or sixth intercostal space of the midaxillary line avoids the breast in women and the pectoralis muscle in muscular patients. After infiltrating the skin, intercostal muscles, and the pleura with 1% lidocaine, an incision is made 2 cm below the desired costal interspace to facilitate an airtight seal around the chest tube. The incision should be parallel to the patient's ribs and long enough to easily admit one finger through the chest cavity. A Kelly clamp is used to create a tunnel to the pleura by spreading the clamp as it is inserted through the soft tissues. To enter the pleural space, the Kelly clamp is gripped along its shaft to prevent plunging too deeply into the chest and is used to puncture the pleura immediately over the rib, thus preventing trauma to the overlying intercostal structures. The Kelly clamp is then removed and a gloved finger is introduced into the pleural space to ensure that the tract is large enough for tube insertion and to confirm intrapleural location. Palpation of the diaphragm caudally and the lung medially will confirm intrapleural positioning after removal of the catheter. The tip of the chest tube is grasped with the Kelly clamp and guided into the pleural space. For a pneumothorax, the tube should be guided toward the apex of the thorax, whereas for evacuation of fluid a posterior location may assist in more complete drainage. The chest tube should be attached to a collection system and the skin site around the tube should be sutured using a purse-string suture.

Respiratory Failure

I. **General considerations.** Two general types of respiratory failure can occur depending on which subunits of the respiratory system are primarily involved in the disease process. **Hypercapnic respiratory failure** occurs with acute carbon dioxide retention ($PaCO_2$ >45–55 mm Hg) and the development of a respiratory acidosis (pH <7.35). **Hypoxic respiratory failure** occurs when normal gas exchange is seriously impaired, resulting in hypoxemia (PaO_2 <60 mm Hg or SaO_2 <90%). This

Table 9-5. Causes of shunts and hypoxic respiratory failure

Symptoms	Causes
Cardiogenic pulmonary edema (low permeability, high hydrostatic pressure)	Acute myocardial infarction Left ventricular failure Mitral regurgitation Mitral stenosis Diastolic dysfunction
Noncardiogenic pulmonary edema (high permeability, low hydrostatic pressure)	Sepsis Aspiration Multiple trauma Pancreatitis Drug reaction (aspirin, narcotics, interleukin-2) Near-drowning Pneumonia Reperfusion injury Inhalational injury
Mixed pulmonary edema (high permeability, high hydrostatic pressure)	Myocardial ischemia/volume overload associated with sepsis, aspiration, etc.
Pulmonary edema of unclear etiology	High-altitude exposure Upper airway obstruction Neurogenic cause Lung reexpansion

type of respiratory failure is usually associated with tachypnea and hypocapnia; however, its progression can lead to hypercapnia as well.

II. Pathophysiology

A. Hypoxic respiratory failure is usually the result of the lung's reduced ability to take up oxygen into the bloodstream due to one of the following processes: (1) shunt, (2) ventilation-perfusion mismatch, (3) low inspired oxygen tension, (4) hypoventilation, (5) diffusion impairment, and (6) low mixed-venous oxygenation (see also Blood Gas Analysis).

1. **Shunt** refers to the fraction of mixed venous blood that passes into the systemic arterial circulation after bypassing functioning gas exchange lung units. Congenital shunts are due to developmental anomalies of the heart and great vessels. Acquired shunts usually result from diseases affecting lung units, although acquired cardiac and peripheral vascular shunts can also occur. Table 9-5 lists some of the more common disease processes that produce clinically significant pulmonary shunts. Shunts are associated with a widened $P(A-a)O_2$ gradient, and the resultant hypoxemia is resistant to correction with supplemental oxygen alone when the shunt fraction of the CO is greater than 30%.

2. **Ventilation-perfusion mismatch.** Diseases associated with airflow obstruction (e.g., COPD, asthma), interstitial inflammation (e.g., pneumonia, sarcoidosis), or vascular obstruction (e.g., pulmonary embolism) often produce lung regions with abnormal ventilation-to-perfusion relationships. Ventilation-perfusion mismatch, unlike shunt physiology, responds to increases in F_IO_2 with increases in PaO_2. However, if a patient with a ventilation-perfusion abnormality is given 100% oxygen, nitrogen can be washed out of the alveoli, resulting in alveolar collapse and atelectasis; this may convert a ventilation-perfusion mismatch disorder into a shunt disorder.

3. **Low inspired oxygenation.** Usually F_IO_2 is reduced at high altitudes or due to the inhalation of toxic gases. In patients with other cardiopulmonary disease processes, an inappropriately low F_IO_2 can also contribute to hypoxic respiratory failure.

4. **Hypoventilation** is associated with elevated $PaCO_2$ values, and the resultant hypoxemia is due to increased alveolar carbon dioxide, which displaces oxygen. Oxygen therapy will usually improve hypoxemia due to hypoventilation but may worsen the overall degree of hypoventilation, especially in patients with chronic airflow obstruction. Primary treatment is directed at correcting the cause of the hypoventilation.

5. **Diffusion impairment.** Hypoxemia due to diffusion impairments usually responds to supplemental oxygen therapy.

6. **Low mixed-venous oxygenation.** Normally, the lungs fully oxygenate pulmonary arterial blood, and mixed-venous oxygen tension does not significantly affect arterial oxygen tension. However, a decreased mixed-venous oxygen tension can significantly lower the PaO_2 when either intrapulmonary shunting or ventilation-perfusion mismatch is present. Factors that can contribute to low mixed-venous oxygenation include anemia, hypoxemia, inadequate CO, and increased oxygen consumption. Improving oxygen delivery to tissues by increasing hemoglobin or CO will usually decrease oxygen extraction ($C_{a-v}O_2$) and improve both mixed-venous oxygen saturation (SvO_2) and PaO_2.

B. **Hypercapnic respiratory failure.** Three general processes are associated with significant hypercapnia leading to respiratory failure. These include: (1) increased carbon dioxide production, (2) increased dead-space ventilation, and (3) decreased total-minute ventilation.

1. **Increased carbon dioxide production.** Fever, sepsis, seizures, and excessive carbohydrate loads can precipitate respiratory acidosis in patients with underlying lung disease. The oxidation of carbohydrate fuels is associated with more carbon dioxide production per molecule of oxygen consumed compared to the utilization of fat.

2. **Increased dead space** occurs when areas of the lung are ventilated but not perfused or decreases in regional perfusion exceed decreases in ventilation. Examples include intrinsic lung diseases (e.g., COPD, asthma, cystic fibrosis, pulmonary fibrosis) and chest-wall disorders associated with parenchymal abnormalities (e.g., scoliosis). These disorders are usually associated with widened $P(A-a)O_2$ gradients.

3. **Decreased minute ventilation** can result from CNS disorders (e.g., spinal cord lesions); peripheral nerve diseases (e.g., Guillain-Barré syndrome, botulism, myasthenia gravis, amyotrophic lateral sclerosis, multiple sclerosis); muscle disorders (e.g., polymyositis, muscular dystrophy); chest-wall abnormalities (e.g., thoracoplasty, scoliosis); drug overdoses; metabolic abnormalities (e.g., myxedema, hypokalemia); and upper airway obstruction. These disorders are normally associated with a normal $P(A-a)O_2$ gradient unless accompanying lung disease is also present (see sec. II.B.2).

Mechanical Ventilation

I. **Indications.** The decision to begin mechanical ventilation is a clinical judgment that should take into account the reversibility of the underlying disease process as well as the patient's overall medical condition (*Am J Med* 88:268, 1990). Usual indications include severely impaired gas exchange, rapid onset of respiratory failure, an inadequate response to less invasive medical treatments, and increased work of breathing with evidence of respiratory muscle fatigue. Parameters that can help guide the decision about whether mechanical ventilation is needed include: respiratory rate (>35); inspiratory force (< −25 cm H_2O); vital capacity (<10–15 ml/kg); PaO_2 (<60 mm Hg with FIO_2 >60%); $PaCO_2$ (>50 mm Hg, with pH <7.35 or $\Delta[pH]/PaCO_2$ >0.008); and an absent gag or cough reflex.

II. **Initiation of mechanical ventilation.** The following variables should be considered when initiating mechanical ventilation:

A. **Ventilator type.** Ventilator selection is often dictated by what is available at a particular hospital. A volume-cycled ventilator is used in most clinical circumstances.

B. **Mode of ventilation.** Several modes of mechanical ventilation are available. Clear guidelines for the use of these modes based on scientific data are limited. General guidelines for the use of the more commonly administered or referred to modes are given below.

1. **Assist-control ventilation (ACV)** should be the initial mode of ventilation used in most patients with respiratory failure. It delivers a ventilator-delivered breath for every patient-initiated inspiratory effort. Controlled ventilator-initiated breaths are automatically delivered when the patient's spontaneous rate falls below the selected backup rate. Respiratory alkalosis is a potential concern when using ACV for patients with tachypnea.

2. **Intermittent mandatory ventilation (IMV)** allows patients to breathe at a spontaneous rate and tidal volume without triggering the ventilator, while the ventilator adds additional mechanical breaths at a preset rate and tidal volume. Synchronized IMV (SIMV) allows the ventilator to become sensitized to the patient's respiratory efforts at intervals determined by the SIMV frequency setting. The SIMV allows coordination of the delivery of the ventilator-driven breath with the respiratory cycle of the patient to prevent inadvertent stacking of a mechanical breath on top of a spontaneous inspiration. Potential advantages of the IMV include less respiratory alkalosis; fewer adverse cardiovascular effects due to lower intrathoracic pressures; less requirement for sedation and paralysis; maintenance of respiratory muscle function; and facilitation of weaning. However, considerable patient-initiated respiratory muscle work can contribute to respiratory muscle fatigue and failure to wean from mechanical ventilation in patients with compromised respiratory muscles. This added work of breathing can be alleviated by the addition of low levels of pressure support (4–8 cm H_2O) to the spontaneous ventilatory efforts.

3. **Pressure support ventilation (PSV)** augments each patient-triggered respiratory effort by an operator-specified amount of pressure that is usually between 5 and 50 cm H_2O. PSV is primarily used to augment spontaneous respiratory efforts during IMV modes of ventilation or during weaning trials (see sec. III). PSV can also be used as a primary form of ventilation in patients who can spontaneously trigger the ventilator. Increased airway resistance, decreased lung compliance, and decreased patient efforts will result in diminished tidal volumes and frequently in decreased minute ventilation. PSV is not recommended as a primary ventilatory mode in patients in whom any of the aforementioned parameters are expected to flux widely. Additionally, patients must be able to trigger the ventilator to obtain pressure-supported breaths.

4. **Inverse ratio ventilation (IRV)** (*Chest* 100:494, 1991) uses an inspiratory-to-expiratory (I:E) ratio greater than the standard 1:2 to 1:3 ratio (i.e., ≥1:1) to stabilize terminal respiratory units (i.e., alveolar recruitment) and to improve gas exchange primarily for acute lung injury (i.e., ARDS). The goals of IRV are to decrease peak airway pressures, maintain adequate alveolar ventilation, and improve oxygenation. The use of IRV should be considered with a PaO_2 that is less than 60 mm Hg despite an FiO_2 that is greater than 60%. Additionally, peak airway pressures that are greater than 40–45 cm H_2O or the need for PEEP that is greater than 15 cm H_2O may be other indications for the use of IRV. Most patients will need heavy sedation and often muscle relaxation during the implementation of IRV.

5. **Pressure targeted ventilation** (i.e., permissive hypercapnia) (*Chest* 104:578, 1993) is a method where controlled hypoventilation is allowed to occur with elevation of the $PaCO_2$ to minimize the detrimental effects of excessive peak airway pressures. This form of ventilation has been used in patients with respiratory failure due to asthma as well as in patients with ARDS. If significant respiratory acidosis occurs (pH <7.35), supplemental bicarbonate can be administered to maintain the pH.

6. **Independent lung ventilation (ILV)** uses two independent ventilators and a double-lumen endotracheal tube. This modality is usually employed for

severe unilateral lung disease such as unilateral pneumonia or respiratory failure associated with hemoptysis.

7. **High-frequency ventilation (HFV)** uses rates substantially faster (60–3,000 breaths/minute) than conventional ventilation with small tidal volumes (2–4 ml/kg). The use of HFV is controversial except during the performance of upper airway surgery.

C. **FiO_2.** Hypoxemia is more dangerous than brief exposure to high inspired levels of oxygen. The initial FiO_2 should be 100%. Adjustments in the FiO_2 can be made to achieve a PaO_2 greater than 60 mm Hg or an SaO_2 greater than 90%.

D. **Minute ventilation** is determined by the respiratory rate and the tidal volume. In general a respiratory rate of 10–15 breaths/minute is an appropriate rate to begin with. Close monitoring of minute ventilation is especially important when ventilating patients with COPD and carbon dioxide retention. In these patients, the minute ventilation should be adjusted to achieve the patient's baseline $PaCO_2$ and not necessarily a normal $PaCO_2$. Inadvertent hyperventilation with resultant metabolic alkalosis in these patients may be associated with serious serum electrolyte shifts and arrhythmias. Initial tidal volumes can usually be set at 10–12 ml/kg. Patients with decreased lung compliance (e.g., ARDS) may need smaller lung volumes (6–8 ml/kg) to minimize peak airway pressures and their associated adverse effects.

E. **PEEP** is defined as the maintenance of positive airway pressure at the end of expiration. It can be applied to the spontaneously breathing patient in the form of CPAP or to the patient receiving mechanical breaths in the form of continuous positive pressure ventilation (CPPV). The appropriate application of PEEP usually results in improved lung compliance, oxygenation, and shunt fraction and decreased work of breathing. PEEP increases peak and mean airway pressures, which can increase the likelihood of barotrauma and cardiovascular compromise. PEEP is primarily used in patients with hypoxic respiratory failure (e.g., ARDS, cardiogenic pulmonary edema). Low levels of PEEP (3–5 cm H_2O) may be useful in patients with COPD to prevent dynamic airway collapse from occurring during expiration. The use of PEEP in asthmatic patients is controversial and potentially hazardous and in most circumstances should be avoided. The main goal of PEEP is to achieve a PaO_2 greater than 55–60 mm Hg with an FiO_2 less than 60% while avoiding significant cardiovascular sequelae. PEEP is usually applied in 3- to 5-cm H_2O increments while monitoring oxygenation, organ perfusion, and hemodynamic parameters.

Levels of PEEP greater than 10–15 cm H_2O can be associated with cardiovascular dysfunction and hemodynamic compromise. Use of a PA catheter to guide medical therapy should be considered in most of these circumstances, especially when end-organ hypoperfusion is present. Patients receiving significant levels of PEEP should not have their PEEP abruptly removed, because removal can result in collapse of distal lung units, worsening shunt, and potentially life-threatening hypoxemia. The hypoxemia that results from the abrupt discontinuation of PEEP is often resistant to correction and requires hours to days for oxygenation to return to baseline. PEEP should be weaned in 3- to 5-cm H_2O increments while closely monitoring oxygenation.

F. **Inspiratory flow rate.** Flow rates set inappropriately low can be associated with prolonged inspiratory times that can lead to the development of auto-PEEP. The resultant lung hyperinflation (i.e., auto-PEEP) can adversely affect patient hemodynamics by impairing venous return to the heart. Patients with severe airflow obstruction are at the greatest risk for developing intrathoracic gas-trapping and lung hyperinflation when improper flow rates are used. Increasing the inspiratory flow rate will usually allow for longer expiratory times that help to reverse this process.

III. **Weaning from mechanical ventilation** (*J Intensive Care Med* 3:109, 1988). **Weaning** is the gradual withdrawal of mechanical ventilatory support. Successful weaning depends on the condition of the patient and the status of the cardiovascular and respiratory systems. In patients who have had brief periods of mechanical ventilation, the manner in which ventilatory support is discontinued is often not crucial. In patients with marginal respiratory function, chronic underlying lung disease, or incompletely resolved respiratory impairment, the weaning method may be critical to obtaining a favorable outcome. Decreasing mechanical ventilation too early during an illness may induce a state of chronic respiratory muscle fatigue. Prolonged mechanical ventilation may induce respiratory muscle disuse atrophy and prolong ventilator dependence. These iatrogenic problems associated with the weaning process have been termed nosocomial respiratory failure or iatrogenic ventilator dependency (*Crit Care Med* 21:171, 1993).

A. **Weaning strategies.** In general the level of supported ventilation (minute ventilation) is gradually decreased and the patient assumes more of the work of ventilation with each of the techniques described.

   1. **IMV technique** allows a change from mechanical ventilation to spontaneous breathing by gradually decreasing the ventilator rate. However, the weaning process may be prolonged if ventilator changes are not made often enough. Prolonged periods at low rates (<6 breaths/minute) may promote a state of respiratory muscle fatigue because of the imposed work of breathing through a high-resistance ventilator circuit. The addition of pressure support (see sec. **II.B.3.**) may alleviate this fatigue but can prolong the weaning process if not appropriately titrated. Very often tachypnea occurring during weaning of the IMV rate may represent a problem related to the imposed work from both the ventilator circuit and the endotracheal tube, and not a diagnosis of persistent respiratory failure. In circumstances in which this is suspected, a trial of extubation may be appropriate.

   2. **T-tube technique** intersperses periods of unassisted spontaneous breathing through a T-tube (or other continuous flow circuit) with periods of ventilator support. Short daytime periods (5–15 minutes 2–6 times/day) are used initially and are then progressively increased in duration and frequency. Small amounts of CPAP (3–5 cm H_2O) during these periods may prevent distal airway closure and atelectasis, although its effects on weaning success appear to be negligible (*Chest* 100:1655, 1991). Similar to IMV weaning, small amounts of pressure support (4–8 cm H_2O) can be used to decrease inspiratory resistance imposed by the ventilator circuit and the endotracheal tube. Extubation may be appropriate when the patient is comfortably tolerating greater than 30–90 minutes of T-tube ventilation. More prolonged periods of T-tube breathing may produce fatigue, especially when small endotracheal tubes (i.e., <8-mm internal diameter) are used.

   3. **Pressure support ventilation (PSV)** is preferred by some practitioners when respiratory muscle weakness appears to be compromising weaning success. PSV can reduce the patient's work of breathing through the endotracheal tube and the ventilator circuit. The optimal level of PSV (PSV_{max}) is selected by increasing the PSV level from a baseline of 15–20 cm H_2O in increments of 3–5 cm H_2O. A decrease in respiratory rate with achieved tidal volumes of 10–12 ml/kg signals that the optimal PSV level has been reached. When the patient is ready for weaning, the level of PSV is gradually reduced by 3- to 5-cm H_2O increments. Once a PSV level of 5–8 cm H_2O is reached, the patient can be extubated without further decreases in PSV.

B. **Failure to wean.** Patients who fail to wean from mechanical ventilation after 48–72 hours of the resolution of their underlying disease process need further investigation. Table 9-6 lists the factors that should be considered when weaning failure occurs. The acronym WEANS NOW has been developed to aid in addressing each of these factors (*J Respir Dis* 6:80, 1985). Table 9-7 lists commonly used parameters that can be assessed in predicting weaning success. Additionally, these parameters can be longitudinally followed to objectively document changes in patient respiratory status.

C. **Extubation** should be performed early in the day when full ancillary staff are available. The patient should be clearly educated about the procedure, the need to cough, and the possible need for reintubation. Elevation of the head and trunk to more than 30–45 degrees will improve diaphragmatic function. Equipment for reintubation should be available and a high-humidity, oxygen-enriched gas

Table 9-6. Factors to be considered in the weaning process

Weaning parameters
  See Table 9-7

Endotracheal tube
  Use largest tube possible
  Consider use of pressure support
  Suction secretions

Arterial blood gases
  Avoid or treat metabolic alkalosis
  Maintain PaO_2 at 60–65 mm Hg to avoid blunting of respiratory drive
  For patients with carbon dioxide retention, keep carbon dioxide at or above
    the baseline level

Nutrition
  Ensure adequate nutritional support
  Avoid electrolyte deficiencies
  Avoid excessive calories

Secretions
  Clear regularly
  Avoid excessive dehydration

Neuromuscular factors
  Avoid neuromuscular-depressing drugs

Obstruction of airways
  Use bronchodilators when appropriate
  Exclude foreign bodies within the airway

Wakefulness
  Avoid oversedation
  Wean in A.M. or when patient is most awake

source with a higher than current FiO_2 setting should be available at the bedside. The patient's airway and the oropharynx above the cuff should be suctioned. After the cuff is completely deflated, the patient should be extubated and high-humidity oxygen should be administered by a face mask. Coughing and deep breathing should be encouraged while the examiner monitors the patient's vital signs and upper airway for stridor. Inspiratory stridor may result from glottic and subglottic edema. If clinical status permits, treatment with nebulized 2.5% racemic epinephrine (0.5 ml in 3 ml normal saline) should be administered. If upper airway obstruction persists or worsens, reintubation should be performed. Extubation should not be reattempted for 24–72 hours following reintubation for upper airway obstruction. Otolaryngology consultation may be beneficial to exclude other causes of upper airway obstruction and to perform tracheostomy if upper airway obstruction persists.

IV. **Drugs commonly used** during endotracheal intubation and mechanical ventilation. Table 9-8 lists medications commonly used in the ICU to facilitate tracheal intubation and mechanical ventilation. Nondepolarizing muscle relaxants have been implicated in muscle dysfunction and prolonged paralysis after their use in ICU patients (*Am Rev Respir Dis* 147:234, 1993). Some reports suggest a drug interaction between muscle relaxants and glucocorticoids, potentiating this effect. To minimize the chances of this complication, the continuous use of muscle relaxants should be limited to as brief a period as possible. Use of muscle relaxants for more than 24–48 hours should be accompanied by daily periods of drug withdrawal when the patient is allowed to recover from the paralysis. Additionally, peripheral nerve stimulators should be used to titrate the dose of the muscle relaxant to the lowest effective dose. Finally, glucocorticoids should be avoided in patients receiving muscle relaxants unless their use is clearly indicated (e.g., for status asthmaticus, anaphylactic shock).

Table 9-7. Guidelines for assessing withdrawal of mechanical ventilation

1. Patient's mental status: awake, alert, cooperative
2. PaO_2 >60 mm Hg with an FiO_2 <50%
3. PEEP ≤5 cm H_2O
4. $PaCO_2$ and pH acceptable
5. Spontaneous tidal volume >5 ml/kg
6. Vital capacity >10 ml/kg
7. Minute ventilation (MV) <10 liters/min
8. Maximum voluntary ventilation double of MV
9. Maximum negative inspiratory pressure (MIP) > – 25 cm H_2O
10. Respiratory rate (RR) <30 breaths/min
11. Static compliance (Cst, rs) >30 ml/cm H_2O
12. Rapid shallow breathing index <100*

* Source: KL Yang et al. A prospective study of indexes predicting the outcome of trials of weaning from mechanical ventilation. *N Engl J Med* 324:1,445, 1991.

Environmental Illness

I. **Heat illness** is due to exposure to increased ambient temperature under conditions in which the body is unable to maintain appropriate homeostasis. The milder syndromes are exertional; the most severe may occur without exercise.

   A. **Heat cramps** occur in unacclimatized individuals who vigorously exercise in the heat. They are caused by salt depletion with hypotonic fluid replacement. Cramps occur in large muscle groups that have been in use, most often in the legs. Examination of the patient reveals moist, cool skin, a normal body temperature, and minimal distress. **Treatment** includes rest in a cool environment and salt replacement with 1 teaspoon of salt or a 650-mg sodium chloride tablet in 500 ml of water PO or a commercially available oral balanced electrolyte replacement solution. IV therapy is rarely required, but 2 liters of normal saline administered over several hours will cure the syndrome.

   B. **Heat exhaustion** occurs in an unacclimatized individual who exercises in the heat. It results from loss of both salt and water. The patient complains of headache, nausea, vomiting, dizziness, weakness, irritability, cramps, or diaphoresis, and has normal or minimally increased core temperature. **Therapy** consists of rest in a cool environment, acceleration of heat loss by fan evaporation, and fluid repletion with salt-containing solutions. If the patient is not vomiting and his or her blood pressure is stable, an oral commercial balanced salt solution is adequate. If vomiting occurs or hemodynamic status is unstable, electrolytes should be checked and 1–2 liters of IV normal saline given. The patient should avoid exercise in a hot environment for 2–3 additional days.

   C. **Heat stroke** causes 4,000 deaths/year in the United States; 80% occur in persons older than age 50. High core temperature causes direct thermal tissue injury; secondary effects include acute renal failure from rhabdomyolysis. Even with rapid therapy, mortality may be as high as 76% for body temperatures greater than or equal to 106°F (41.1°C) (*Dis Month* 35:301, 1989).

      1. **Classic heat stroke** occurs after several days of heat exposure in individuals at risk because of chronic illness, old age, high humidity, obesity, chronic cardiovascular disease, poverty, urban upper-story residence, lack of air-conditioning, dehydration, alcohol abuse, and use of sedatives, hypnotics, anticholinergics, or antipsychotics. Typically, such patients have core temperatures greater than 105°F (40.5°C) and are comatose and anhydrotic.

      2. **Exertional heat stroke** occurs rapidly in unacclimatized individuals who exercise in conditions of high ambient temperature and humidity. Those at risk include athletes (especially long-distance runners and football players), soldiers, and laborers without adequate access to water. Some of the risks

Table 9-8. ICU drugs to facilitate endotracheal intubation and mechanical ventilation

Drug	Bolus dosages (IV)	Continuous infusion dosages[a]	Onset	Duration after single dose
Succinylcholine	1.0–1.5 mg/kg	—	45–60 sec	2–10 min
Pancuronium	0.05–0.08 mg/kg	0.2–0.6 μg/kg/min	2–4 min	40–60 min
Vecuronium	0.08–0.10 mg/kg	0.3–1.0 μg/kg/min	2–4 min	30–45 min
Atracurium	0.4–0.5 mg/kg	5–10 μg/kg/min	2–4 min	20–45 min
Diazepam	2.5–5.0 mg up to 20–30 mg	1–10 mg/hr or titrate to effect	1–5 min	30–90 min[b]
Midazolam	1–4 mg	1–10 mg/hr or titrate to effect	1–5 min	30–60 min[b]
Morphine	2–5 mg	1–10 mg/hr or titrate to effect	2–10 min	2–4 hr[b]
Fentanyl	0.5–1.0 μg/kg	1–2μg/kg/hr or titrate to effect	30–60 sec	30–60 min[b]
Thiopental	50–100 mg; repeat up to 20 mg/kg	—	20 sec	10–20 min[b]
Methohexital	1–2 mg/kg	—	15–45 sec	5–20 min[b]
Propofol	0.25–1.00 mg/kg	50–100 μg/kg/min	15–60 sec	3–10 min[b]

[a] A continuous infusion should be started or titrated upward only after desired level of sedation is achieved with bolus administration.
[b] Duration is prolonged with continued use. Frequent titration to the minimum effective dose is required to prevent accumulation of drug.

associated with classic heat stroke may also be present, and certain congenital diseases that impair sweating may contribute. The core temperature may be less than 40.5°C; 50% of patients are still sweating at presentation. Individuals with exertional heat stroke are more likely to have **disseminated intravascular coagulation, lactic acidosis, and rhabdomyolysis** than those with classic heat stroke.

3. **Diagnosis** is based on the history of exposure, a core temperature usually 105°F (40.5°C) or above, and changes in mental status ranging from confusion to delirium and coma. Differential diagnosis includes malignant hyperthermia, neuroleptic malignant syndrome, severe hyperthyroidism, sepsis, meningitis, and Rocky Mountain spotted fever.

4. **Therapy**
   a. **Immediate cooling.** Constant misting of the patient with tepid water at 20–25°C is very effective if the patient is continuously cooled by a large electric fan, especially with maximum body surface exposure. Ice packs at points of major heat transfer, such as the groin, axilla, and chest, may speed cooling. Ice-water immersion is difficult to arrange, results in inappropriate vasoconstriction, and interferes with other resuscitative maneuvers and therefore should not be used. For a severely elevated core temperature not responsive to the above maneuvers, gastric lavage with ice water may be helpful (*Ann Emerg Med* 14:429, 1985), although this treatment is controversial (*Crit Care Med* 15:748, 1987). Cold peritoneal lavage is no more effective than evaporative cooling (*Am J Emerg Med* 11:1, 1993). **Dantrolene sodium does not appear to be effective** (*Crit Care Med* 19:176, 1991). Shivering and vasoconstriction impair cooling and may be prevented by administration of **chlorpromazine,** 10–25 mg IM, or **diazepam,** 5–10 mg IV. Core temperatures should be constantly monitored by rectal probe or tympanic membrane thermistor. Cooling measures should be discontinued when the patient's core temperature reaches 39°C (102.2°F).
   b. **Baseline laboratory studies** should include CBC, platelets, partial thromboplastin time (PTT), prothrombin time (PT), fibrin degradation products (FDP), electrolytes, BUN, creatinine, glucose, calcium, creatine kinase (CK), liver function tests (LFTs), arterial blood gases (ABGs), urinalysis, and ECG.
   c. **Hypotension** that is unresponsive to crystalloids may require vasopressors and hemodynamic monitoring (avoiding alpha-adrenergic agents as they cause vasoconstriction and impair cooling). Crystalloids should be administered cautiously to normotensive patients.
   d. **Rhabdomyolysis** or urine output less than 30 ml/hour should be treated with adequate volume replacement, mannitol (12.5–25.0 g), and bicarbonate (44 mEq/liter in 0.45% normal saline) to promote osmotic diuresis and urine alkalinization. **Renal failure** may still occur in 5% of patients with classic heat stroke and in 25% with exertional heat stroke.
   e. **Hypoxemia and ARDS** may require administration of oxygen, mechanical ventilation, and PEEP.
   f. **Other complications.** Seizures are treated with diazepam and phenytoin. Hepatic injury, congestive heart failure, and coagulopathy may occur.

II. **Cold injury.** Exposure to the cold may result in several different forms of injury. An important risk factor is accelerated heat loss, which may be promoted by exposure to high wind or by immersion. Extended cold exposure may result from alcohol or drug abuse, injury or immobilization, and mental impairment.
   A. **Chilblains** are among the mildest forms of cold injury and result from exposure of bare skin to a cold, windy environment (33–60°F). The ears, fingers, and tip of the nose are typically injured, with itchy, painful erythema on rewarming. Treatment consists of rapid rewarming, analgesics, and avoidance of recurrence.
   B. **Immersion injury** (trench foot) is caused by prolonged immersion in cold water (>10–12 hours at <50°F). Treatment includes removal from exposure, rewarming, dry dressings, and treatment of secondary infections.

C. **Frostnip** is the mildest form of frostbite and occurs most frequently on the distal extremities, the nose, or the ears. It is marked by tissue blanching and decreased sensitivity. **Rapid rewarming in a water bath at 104–108°F (40–42°C)** is the treatment of choice of all forms of frostbite. The water temperature should never be hotter than 112°F.

D. **Superficial frostbite** involves the skin and subcutaneous tissues, which are white, waxy, and anesthetic, have poor capillary refill, and are painful on thawing. No deep injury occurs and healing occurs in 3–4 weeks.

E. **Deep frostbite** involves death of skin, subcutaneous tissue, and muscle (third-degree) or deep tendons and bones (fourth-degree). The tissue appears frozen and hard. On rewarming there is no capillary filling. Healing is very slow, and demarcation of tissue with autoamputation may occur. Diabetes mellitus, peripheral vascular disease, outdoor life-style, high altitude, and nonwhite race are all additional risk factors. More than 90% of deep frostbite occurs at temperatures below 6.7°C (44°F) with exposures longer than 7–10 hours. **Initial treatment** consists of rapid rewarming with avoidance of refreezing. Analgesics (IV opioids) are given as needed. The patient should be admitted to a surgical service, with elevation of the affected extremity, non–weight-bearing positioning, separation of affected digits by cotton-wool, prevention of tissue maceration with a blanket cradle, and avoidance of smoking. Tetanus immunization should be updated if necessary. Intraarterial vasodilators, heparin, dextran, prostaglandin inhibitors, thrombolytics, and sympathectomy are not routinely justified. Antibiotics are used only for documented infection. Amputation is undertaken only after full demarcation has occurred.

F. **Hypothermia** is defined as a core temperature less than 35°C (95°F). Hypothermia is defined as mild at 34–35°C, moderate at 30–34°C, and severe at less than 30°C. The most common cause of hypothermia in the United States is cold exposure due to alcohol intoxication. Another common cause is cold-water immersion. Differential diagnosis and other risk factors include extremes of age, cerebrovascular accident, subdural hematoma, drug use, diabetic ketoacidosis, uremia, adrenal insufficiency, and myxedema.

1. **Diagnosis.** A standard oral thermometer registers only to a lower limit of 35°C. Therefore, the patient should be continuously monitored with either a rectal probe with a full range of 20–40°C or with an ear thermistor.

2. **Signs and symptoms** vary with the temperature of the patient at presentation.

   a. **All organ systems** are involved. At temperatures 35°C or below, mental processes are slowed and the affect is flattened. At temperatures below 32.2°C (90°F), the ability to shiver is lost, and deep tendon reflexes are diminished. At 28°C, coma often supervenes. At 18°C or below, the EEG is flat. On rewarming from severe hypothermia, central pontine myelinolysis may develop.

   b. **Cardiovascular effects.** After an initial increased release of catecholamines, there is a decrease in CO and HR with relatively preserved mean arterial pressure. ECG changes, manifest initially as sinus bradycardia with T-wave inversion and QT-interval prolongation, may progress to atrial fibrillation at temperatures below 32°C. Osborne waves (J-point elevation) may be visible, particularly in leads II and V6. There is an increased susceptibility to ventricular arrhythmias at temperatures below 32°C. At about 28–30°C, the susceptibility to ventricular fibrillation is significantly increased, and unnecessary manipulation, jostling, and esophageal and tracheal manipulation should be avoided. At 29°C or less, a decrease in mean arterial pressure may occur. At temperatures below 28°C, progressive bradycardia supervenes. At about 22°C, maximum ventricular fibrillation susceptibility occurs, and at temperatures below 18°C, asystole may supervene.

   c. **Respiratory complications.** After an initial increase in minute ventilation, respiratory rate and tidal volume decrease progressively with decreasing temperature. **Arterial blood gases measured with the machine**

set at 37°C should serve as the basis for therapy. Supplemental oxygen should be supplied (*Ann Emerg Med* 18:72, 1989).

   d. Renal manifestations include cold-induced diuresis as well as tubular concentrating defects.

3. **Laboratory evaluation** includes CBC, electrolytes, BUN, creatinine, glucose, coagulation studies, CK, LFTs, calcium, magnesium, amylase, urinalysis, ABGs, and ECG. All patients with a history of trauma or immersion injury should be evaluated with chest, abdominal, and cervical spine radiographs. Electrolyte abnormalities are common. Serum potassium is often increased. Elevated serum amylase may reflect underlying pancreatitis. Hyperglycemia may be noted but should not be treated, as there may be rebound hypoglycemia with rewarming. Disseminated intravascular coagulation (DIC) may be present.

4. **Therapy.** Attention should be directed toward maintaining airway patency and providing adequate ventilation and oxygenation. Intubation, when indicated, should be done by the most experienced operator in the most gentle fashion possible (see Airway Management and Tracheal Intubation).

   a. Cardiopulmonary resuscitation (CPR) is carried out in standard fashion with simultaneous vigorous core rewarming, as the patient should not be considered unresuscitatable as long as his or her core temperature is severely decreased. Reliable defibrillation requires a core temperature greater than or equal to 32°C. CPR should not be undertaken if an organized electrocardiographic rhythm is present because inability to detect peripheral pulses may be due to vasoconstriction and CPR may precipitate ventricular fibrillation. When ventricular fibrillation is present, bretylium (5 mg/kg IV) is the agent of choice; lidocaine is an alternative. Procainamide should be avoided because it may precipitate ventricular fibrillation and increase the temperature necessary to defibrillate the patient successfully. Patients with an intact circulation should have electrocardiographic rhythm, urine output, and possibly central venous pressure monitoring. Swan-Ganz catheterization should not be performed because it may precipitate ventricular fibrillation.

   b. Rewarming should be done with the goal of increasing the patient's temperature by 0.5–2.0°C/hour.

      (1) Passive external rewarming depends on the patient's ability to shiver and thus generate heat. It is effective only at core temperatures greater than or equal to 32°C. The patient is covered with blankets, placed in a warm environment, and monitored.

      (2) Active external rewarming includes application of heating blankets (40–45°C) or warm bath immersion. This type of therapy may cause paradoxical core acidosis, hyperkalemia, and decreased core temperature as cold stagnant blood returns to the central vasculature. Therefore, active rewarming should be used only on the trunk of a young, previously healthy patient with acute hypothermia and minimal pathophysiologic derangement.

      (3) Active core rewarming is preferred for treatment of severe hypothermia. Heated oxygen is the initial therapy of choice for the patient whose cardiovascular status is stable. It can be expected to raise core temperatures by 1–2°C/hour (*Am J Emerg Med* 2:533, 1984). Heated oxygen is administered through a cascade humidifier at a temperature less than or equal to 45°C. IV fluids may be heated in a microwave oven (*Am J Emerg Med* 3:316, 1985) or delivered through a blood warmer and should be given only through peripheral IV lines. Heated nasogastric or bladder lavage should be reserved for the patient with cardiovascular collapse. Heated peritoneal lavage is more effective than heated aerosol inhalation (*Am J Emerg Med* 2:210, 1984) but should be performed only for patients with cardiovascular collapse, by those experienced in its use, and in combination with other modes of rewarming. Extracorporeal circulation (cardiac bypass) is reserved for hypothermic individuals with cardiac arrest, in whom it may be dramatically effective (*Arch Surg* 127:525, 1992). It may raise the temperature as rapidly as 10–12°C/hour but must be performed in an ICU or operating room.

c. **Medications.** Most patients with exposure should receive thiamine because cold exposure due to alcohol intoxication is common. Administration of antibiotics is a controversial issue; many authorities recommend antibiotic administration for 72 hours, pending cultures. In general, those patients with hypothermia due to exposure and alcohol intoxication are less likely to have a seriously underlying infection than those who are elderly or have an underlying medical illness (*Arch Intern Med* 149:1521, 1989).

d. **Observation.** Patients with an underlying disease, physiologic derangement, or core temperature below 32°C should be admitted, preferably to an ICU. Those with mild hypothermia (32–35°C) and no predisposing medical conditions or complications may be discharged when they are normothermic if an adequate home environment can be ensured.

Near-Drowning

Drowning accounts for approximately 8,000 deaths/year, 40% of which occur in children younger than 4 years of age. **Predisposing factors** include youth, inability to swim, alcohol and drug use, barotrauma (in scuba diving), head and neck trauma, and loss of consciousness associated with epilepsy, diabetes, syncope, or dysrhythmias. **Near-drowning,** defined as survival for at least 24 hours after submersion in liquid, is more common.

I. **Pathophysiology.** Electrolyte abnormalities, hemoglobin concentration, volume status, and frequency of lung injury are similar for freshwater and saltwater drownings (*Chest* 70:231, 1976). **Major insults** (i.e., hypoxemia and tissue hypoxia, acidosis, and hypoxic brain injury with cerebral edema) are common to both. Hypothermia, pneumonia, and, rarely, DIC, acute renal failure, and hemolysis may also occur.

II. **Treatment** begins with resuscitation, focusing on airway management and ventilation with 100% oxygen. An IV line should be established with normal saline or Ringer's lactate. The Heimlich maneuver is not indicated unless upper airway obstruction is present.

A. **The cervical spine should be immobilized,** since trauma may be present.

B. **Hypothermia** should be vigorously treated (see Environmental Illness).

C. **Management of pulmonary complications** includes initial administration of 100% oxygen, with subsequent decreased titration by ABGs. Endotracheal intubation and mechanical ventilation, PEEP, and bronchodilators should be used if needed.

D. **Antibiotics should be reserved for documented infection.** Prophylactic glucocorticoids have no role (*Heart Lung* 16:474, 1987).

E. **Metabolic acidosis** is managed with mechanical ventilation, sodium bicarbonate (for a persistent pH <7.2), and BP support.

F. **Cerebral edema** may occur suddenly within the first 24 hours and is a major cause of death. Although treatment of cerebral edema does not appear to increase survival (*Crit Care Med* 14:529, 1986), intracranial pressure monitoring is recommended if there is CT evidence of cerebral edema or if the Glasgow coma scale is 7 or below (see Chap. 25). Standard management includes hyperventilation (PCO_2 approximately 25 mm Hg) and mannitol, 1–2 g/kg q3–4h, or furosemide, 1 mg/kg IV q4–6h. There is no evidence supporting use of glucocorticoids, and their routine administration is not recommended.

III. **Observation.** Patients who have survived severe episodes of near-drowning should be admitted to an ICU. Those with less severe initial immersions may still develop noncardiogenic pulmonary edema. Any pulmonary signs or symptoms mandate admission, including cough, bronchospasm, abnormal ABGs, or abnormal chest x-ray. The asymptomatic patient with a questionable or brief episode may be observed for 4–6 hours and discharged if the chest x-ray and ABGs are normal (*Ann Emerg Med* 15:1084, 1986). However, if there is a long submersion, initial cyanosis or apnea, or even brief requirement for resuscitation, **the patient must be admitted for at least 24 hours.**

High-Altitude Illness

Acute high-altitude illness typically occurs in individuals unacclimatized to altitude who ascend to more than 2,000 meters (6,500 feet) in less than 1–2 days. Symptoms usually occur within 48 hours of ascent. **Risk factors** include a prior history of altitude illness, lack of acclimatization, rapid ascent, drugs that diminish ventilatory response to hypoxia, young age, vigorous exercise, preexisting history of pulmonary disease, and alcohol use.

I. **Acute mountain sickness** is the most common manifestation. Symptoms include headache, nausea, vomiting, anorexia, dyspnea, lethargy, sleep disturbance, vertigo, palpitations, and difficulty concentrating. It typically is worst on the second to third day. **Treatment** consists of liberal fluids, mild analgesics for headache, prochlorperazine, 10 mg IM q6h, for nausea, and, for severe symptoms, oxygen at 2–3 liters/minute and descent of 1,000–1,500 meters (3,000–5,000 feet). **Acetazolamide**, 250 mg PO bid, appears to abort the illness and speed acclimatization (*Ann Intern Med* 116:461, 1992). **Dexamethasone**, 4 mg PO or IM q6h, is effective for severe headaches, vomiting, and neurologic symptoms (*N Engl J Med* 321:1707, 1989).

II. **High-altitude pulmonary edema** is most common in the young, vigorously active individual and may be fatal. Symptoms include dyspnea, cough, weakness, lethargy, tachycardia, and frothy, bloody sputum. Rales are heard on chest examination, and chest x-ray shows pulmonary edema. **Treatment is urgent descent** of at least 1,000–1,500 meters (3,000–5,000 feet). **Oxygen** is administered at high flow rates. For the severely ill, CPAP by mask or mechanical ventilation with PEEP may be lifesaving. Furosemide and morphine sulfate (in the absence of CNS manifestations) may be used but are unlikely to be effective. Early evidence suggests that nifedipine may be of use in therapy (*Int J Sports Med* 13:S65, 1992). Nifedipine, 10 mg SL and 20 mg extended-release PO are recommended (*Poisindex,* 1994). If systolic BP decreases less than or equal to 10 mm Hg, 10 mg SL is repeated, and 20 mg extended-release is given q6h, if evacuation is delayed or impossible.

III. **High-altitude cerebral edema** is rare and ordinarily occurs only at very high altitudes, usually greater than 3,500 meters (14,400 feet). Its symptoms include severe headache, ataxia, confusion, emotional lability, and hallucinations. Papilledema may be present. Untreated, it progresses to coma and death. The **primary treatment is emergency descent, with oxygen** administration at 2–4 liters/minute. If possible, endotracheal intubation with hyperventilation is indicated. Furosemide, 20–40 mg IV, and dexamethasone, 10 mg IV followed by 4 mg IV q6h, are recommended.

IV. **Prevention of high-altitude illness** depends on slow ascent and graded exercise. Travelers should not go from 0–2,300 meters (0–7,500 feet) in 1 day. At least 1 night should be spent at an intermediate altitude. **Acetazolamide,** 125–250 mg PO bid or tid or 500 mg sustained-release PO q12–24h, may be useful in prophylaxis. **Dexamethasone,** 4 mg PO q6h for 48 hours prior to ascent and during altitude exposure, is also effective (*N Engl J Med* 310:683, 1984). Preliminary results suggest a role for nifedipine, 20 mg PO q8h, in prevention of high-altitude pulmonary edema (*Int J Sports Med* 13:S65, 1992).

Overdosage

Recognition of poisoning and medication overdose requires a high index of suspicion and careful clinical evaluation. Up to 50% of all initial poisoning histories may be incorrect. The ingestion of 2 or more drugs is common. Identification of the drug or drugs ingested and their dosages should be sought from the patient's family or friends, private physician, pharmacist, and paramedical personnel. Supporting materials (e.g., pill bottles) should be sought, as should clues regarding timing of ingestion. Recognition of specific toxic syndromes is often helpful in directing initial management (Table 9-9). Vital signs, neurologic status, pupillary reactions, cardiovascular response, abdominal findings, and unusual odors and excreta, as well as evaluation of ABGs, serum electrolytes, and acid-base abnormalities, may suggest a particular toxin. Baseline screening of liver and kidney function may be helpful. Screening of blood, urine, or gastric aspirate for specific agents is important, but in most cases, therapy must proceed before such results are available. Abdominal radiography may be useful in detecting retained pills (such as iron). ECG and continuous cardiac monitoring should be performed until the ingestion is identified and thereafter as appropriate. A pregnancy test is appropriate in women of childbearing years. Although a computerized *Poisindex* system is helpful, specific advice should be sought from the regional poison control center.

I. **Supportive care** is crucial. A patent airway and adequate ventilation must be maintained. Endotracheal intubation may be required to protect the airway. Hypotension usually responds to IV fluid therapy, although vasopressors may be required in refractory cases or for pulmonary edema. Dopamine is used in most situations; norepinephrine is preferred in overdoses with alpha-adrenergic antagonists (phenothiazines) and tricyclic antidepressants (due to the proarrhythmic effect of dopamine). **Arrhythmias** may be related to cardiac or autonomic effects; treatment may vary depending on the toxin. CNS depression or coma occurs frequently and should prompt the administration of naloxone (2 mg IV) for possible narcotic overdose, 50% dextrose (50 ml IV) or immediate fingerstick glucose determination, thiamine (100 mg IV) for Wernicke-Korsakoff syndrome, and oxygen for carbon monoxide intoxication. Flumazenil may be given for known or suspected benzodiazepine overdose (see sec. **VI.L.2.b**). However, to avoid precipitating seizures it should not be given for unknown overdoses as a diagnostic trial. It also should not be given to patients who have ingested drugs known to cause seizures (e.g., cocaine, lithium, theophylline, isoniazid, cyclosporine) or who are known to have a preexisting seizure disorder (*Clin Ther* 14:292, 1992).

II. **Prevention of further drug absorption** may be facilitated by **gastric emptying** (gastric lavage, induced emesis) or administration of **activated charcoal**. Gastric emptying procedures should be initiated within 1 hour of the ingestion (*Ann Emerg Med* 14:562, 1985). Because most adult overdose patients present several hours after toxic ingestion and because the use of syrup of ipecac may delay subsequent therapy, the use of activated charcoal is recommended as the primary GI decontamination procedure for most patients (*Ann Emerg Med* 16:838, 1987).

A. **Activated charcoal** adsorbs most drugs, preventing further absorption from the GI tract. Exceptions include alkalis, cyanide, lithium, ferrous sulfate, insecticides, and mineral acids. It may also promote efflux of selected drugs (theophylline, phenobarbital, and carbamazepine) from the blood into the bowel lumen. **Activated charcoal should not be given in conjunction with an oral antidote, as it may bind and inactivate these agents**; however, it may be given 2 hours later. It is preferable not to give it simultaneously with ipecac, as it obscures gastric contents, and it should not be used when endoscopy is contemplated. Activated charcoal, 50–100 g diluted in water or sorbitol, should be given as soon as possible after the toxic ingestion; prehospital administration further enhances drug recovery. Repeated dosing (without sorbitol) also improves efficacy.

B. **Gastric emptying** may be used in obtunded patients presenting soon (within 1 hour) after ingestion and for phenothiazine overdose and ingestion of rapidly absorbed agents such as strychnine and cyanide. **The airway must be protected;** an endotracheal tube may be necessary. If the patient is awake and alert, **ipecac**, 30 ml, repeated once in 20 minutes if necessary, is a useful emetic. Additional ingestion of water is not needed and may prompt inappropriate antegrade gastric emptying. Contraindications to ipecac include decreased level of consciousness, absent gag reflex, caustic ingestion, convulsions or exposure to a substance likely to cause convulsions, and medical conditions that make

Table 9-9. Toxic syndromes and possible causes

Syndrome	Manifestations	Possible causes
Acquired hemoglobinopathies	Dyspnea, cyanosis, confusion or lethargy, headache	Carbon monoxide Methemoglobinemia (nitrites, phenazopyridine) Sulfhemoglobinemia
Anion gap metabolic acidosis	Variable	Methanol Ethanol Ethylene glycol Paraldehyde Iron Isoniazid Salicylate Vacor Cyanide
Anticholinergic	Dry mouth and skin, blurred vision; mydriasis; tachycardia; generalized sunburn-like rash or flushing of skin; hyperthermia; abdominal distention; urinary urgency/retention; confusion, hallucinations, delusions, excitation, or coma	Atropine and other belladonna alkaloids Antihistamines Tricyclics Phenothiazines Jimson seeds
Cholinergic	Hypersalivation, bronchorrhea, bronchospasm, urination/defecation, neuromuscular failure, lacrimation	Acetylcholine Organophosphate insecticides Bethanechol Methacholine Wild mushrooms
Cyanide	Nausea, vomiting, collapse, coma, bradycardia, no cyanosis, decreased AV O_2 difference with severe metabolic acidosis	Cyanide Amygdalin

Extrapyramidal	Dysphoria and dysphagia, trismus, oculogyric crisis, rigidity, torticollis, laryngospasm	Prochlorperazine Haloperidol Chlorpromazine and other antipsychotics Other phenothiazines
Narcotic	CNS depression, respiratory depression, miosis, hypotension	Morphine and heroin Codeine Propoxyphene Other synthetic and semisynthetic opiates
Salicylism	Fever, hyperpnea, respiratory alkalosis or mixed acid-base disturbance, hypokalemia, tinnitus	Aspirin Other salicylate products
Sympathomimetic	Excitation, hypertension, cardiac arrhythmias, seizures	Amphetamines Cocaine Caffeine Aminophylline Beta-agonists, inhaled or injected

Source: Modified from G Quick, P J Crocker. Toxic emergency: Agent unknown. *Emerg Decisions* 7:44, 1986.

emesis unsafe. If no response is achieved after the second ipecac dose, the patient should undergo gastric lavage. Use of a large orogastric tube (>28 French, preferably >36 French) is the preferred method for patients with a decreased gag reflex **after endotracheal intubation.** Lavage with 200-ml boluses of warm saline, repeated until the effluent is clear, is followed by instillation of activated charcoal and a single dose of cathartic. The added efficacy of a **cathartic** is not clear, but it does decrease transit time through the intestine. Acceptable forms include magnesium citrate, 4 ml/kg (300 ml maximum), sorbitol, 1–2 g/kg (150 g maximum), and magnesium or sodium sulfate, 25–30 g. Magnesium salts should not be given in renal failure. Sorbitol premixed with charcoal is available commercially. Intestinal lavage with commercially available bowel preparation materials is not routinely recommended (*Ann Emerg Med* 17:681, 1988); iron ingestion with radiographically persistent tablets in the GI tract may be an exception (*Clin Toxicol* 23:177, 1985), as may cocaine body packing (*J Clin Pharmacol* 33:497, 1993).

III. **Removal of absorbed drugs.** Enhancement of renal excretion and extracorporeal methods (e.g., dialysis) may be used. Increased urinary pH may increase elimination of weak acids.

  A. Forced diuresis should be used only when specifically indicated because of the risk of causing acid-base disturbances, electrolyte abnormalities, and cerebral or pulmonary edema. It should not be attempted in patients with renal insufficiency, cardiac disease, or existing electrolyte abnormalities. Little data exist about its efficacy in improving survival.

    1. Forced alkaline diuresis, achieving a urinary pH of 7.5–9.0, promotes excretion of drugs that are weak acids, such as salicylates, barbital, and phenobarbital. A solution of sodium bicarbonate, 50–100 mEq, added to 1 liter of 0.45% saline, may be administered at 250–500 ml/hour for the first 1–2 hours. Great care must be exercised to avoid excessive volume expansion, especially in the elderly. Alkaline solution and diuretics should be administered to maintain a urinary output of 2–3 ml/kg/hour. In salicylate poisoning, potassium supplementation will almost always be required.

    2. Forced acid diuresis is no longer recommended for any agent.

  B. Extracorporeal removal of specific toxins by dialysis or hemoperfusion is used when (1) there is clinical deterioration despite intensive supportive therapy, (2) blood levels reach potentially lethal concentrations, (3) there is a risk of lethal delayed effects, and (4) renal or hepatic failure impairs clearance of toxin.

    1. Peritoneal or hemodialysis is most useful for low-molecular-weight, water-soluble toxins that are minimally bound to plasma proteins (e.g., ethanol, ethylene glycol, lithium, methanol, and salicylates). It is also used for heavy-metal intoxication in patients with renal failure. Dialysis also corrects electrolyte, acid-base, and osmolar derangements that may accompany toxic ingestions.

    2. Hemoperfusion removes toxins by direct adsorption and is generally more effective than either peritoneal or hemodialysis. It is useful in overdoses with barbiturates, sedative-hypnotics, and lipid-soluble drugs. It may be helpful in theophylline intoxications but is of marginal value in cyclic antidepressants.

IV. **Specific antidotes** are available that neutralize or prevent the toxic effect of certain drugs (Table 9-10). The regional poison control center should be contacted immediately if it is known what drug was ingested; information on specific treatment and the pharmacokinetics of the drug can often be provided.

V. **Disposition.** Patients with apparently trivial overdoses of potentially toxic agents should be observed for at least 4 hours before contemplation of discharge. No patient who has taken an intentional overdose should be discharged from the emergency department without formal psychiatric consultation and disposition. Individuals suffering inadvertent recreational drug overdose require referral for counseling and possibly detoxification. All symptomatic (and some asymptomatic) patients require admission. Patients considered to be potentially suicidal require one-to-one constant supervision while on the medical service.

VI. Specific agents

A. Acetaminophen is a common ingredient in many analgesic and antipyretic preparations. Hepatic toxicity is due to depletion of hepatic glutathione and subsequent accumulation of a toxic intermediate metabolite, N-acetyl-p-benzoquinonimine. Toxicity usually occurs after ingestion of more than 140 mg/kg. Precise determination of probable toxicity can be obtained by plotting on a nomogram (Fig. 9-1) plasma acetaminophen level (drawn at least 4 hours after ingestion) versus time since ingestion.

1. **Symptoms** over the first 24 hours include anorexia, vomiting, and diaphoresis. Hepatic enzymes begin to rise 24–36 hours after ingestion and peak (aspartate aminotransferase [AST] earliest) 72–96 hours after ingestion. Recovery starts after approximately 4 days unless hepatic failure develops.

2. **Treatment** includes supportive measures and induced emesis or gastric lavage. **Acetylcysteine (Mucomyst)**, a specific antidote that acts as a sulfhydryl donor for glutathione synthesis, should be given within 8 hours of ingestion to prevent hepatic toxicity but may be effective when administered up to 36 hours after ingestion (*Lancet* 335:1572, 1990). The initial dosage is 140 mg/kg PO or by gastric tube; subsequent administration (70 mg/kg q4h for a total of 17 doses) is directed by the initial plasma acetaminophen levels. Administration of the first dose should not be delayed awaiting return of the blood level when history suggests a toxic dose has been ingested. **If toxic levels are detected, the full 17 doses are given;** if not, no further antidote is indicated. If vomiting occurs less than 1 hour after administration of antidote, the dose should be repeated. If vomiting is repetitive and interferes with acetylcysteine administration, metoclopramide or droperidol may be used, or acetylcysteine may be administered via a fluoroscopically placed nasoduodenal tube over a period of 30–60 minutes. Baseline AST, alanine aminotransaminase, bilirubin, BUN, and PT should be drawn and repeated at least daily for 3 days (see Chap. 16). Biochemical evidence of hepatic failure should prompt GI consultation for consideration of orthotopic liver transplantation.

   Oral charcoal should be given if the patient presents less than 4 hours after ingestion, while awaiting performance of the blood level. If activated charcoal is administered less than 1 hour before acetylcysteine, any residual charcoal should be removed by gastric lavage. If a mixed overdose requires multidose charcoal for another agent, it should be given 2 hours after each dose of acetylcysteine with lavage before each subsequent acetylcysteine dose. **IV acetylcysteine** is available at a limited number of participating centers for those who cannot or will not take oral acetylcysteine (Rocky Mountain Poison Center, 1-800-525-6115). Side effects include bronchospasm, rash, flushing, and anaphylactoid reaction.

B. Caustic ingestions

1. **Alkaline ingestions** may be either accidental or suicidal. Liquid and crystalline lye, automatic dishwater detergents, Clinitest tablets, and some toilet bowl cleaners are alkaline. Strong alkali solutions, such as liquid drain cleaner, are the agents most commonly associated with injury.

   a. **Deep tissue injury in the aerodigestive tract is common.** Oral burns are common; drooling may be a manifestation of this. Studies of whether oral burns correlate with esophageal injuries are conflicting (*Am J Surg* 157:116, 1980; *Arch Intern Med* 140:501, 1980). The overall rate of esophageal injury for all alkali ingestions is 30–40% and is suggested by vomiting, drooling, or stridor. Subsequent esophageal stricture may occur, especially with liquid lye (*Am J Surg* 157:116, 1989). Gastric injury with perforation may occur and is much more likely with liquid lye ingestions, since they pass rapidly into the stomach. Alkaline ingestions may cause severe upper airway injury, with stridor and airway obstruction requiring rapid intervention. Symptoms include oral pain, odynophagia, stridor, chest pain, abdominal pain, nausea, and vomiting.

Table 9-10. Antidotes

Poison/toxic sign	Antidote	Adult dosage
Acetaminophen	N-acetylcysteine	140 mg/kg PO, followed by 70 mg/kg q4h × 17 doses
Anticholinergics	Physostigmine sulfate	0.5–2.0 mg IV (IM) over 2 min q30–60min prn
Anticholinesterases	Atropine sulfate	1–5 mg IV (IM, SC) q15min prn to drying of secretions
	Pralidoxime (2-PAM) chloride[a]	1 g IV (PO) over 15–30 min q8–12h × 3 doses prn
Carbon monoxide	Oxygen	100%, hyperbaric
Cyanide	Amyl nitrite[b]	Inhalation pearls for 15–30 sec qmin
	Followed by Sodium nitrite[b]	300 mg (10 ml of 3% solution) IV over 3 min, repeated in half dosage in 2 hr if persistent or recurrent signs of toxicity
	Followed by Sodium thiosulfate	12.5 g (50 ml of 25% solution) IV over 10 min, repeated in half dosage in 2 hr if persistent or recurrent signs of toxicity
Digoxin	Antidigoxin Fab fragments	**Acute ingestion:** Dose (vials) = [ingested digoxin (mg)] × 0.8l/0.6 **Chronic ingestion:** Dose (vials) = [serum level (ng/ml) × weight (kg)]/100 infused in 0.9% saline over 15–30 min; repeat if toxicity persists
Ethylene glycol	Ethanol[d]	0.6 g/kg of ethanol in 5% D/W IV (PO) over 30–45 min, followed initially by 110 mg/kg/hr to maintain a blood alcohol level of 100–150 mg/dl
Extrapyramidal signs	Diphenhydramine hydrochloride	25–50 mg IV (IM, PO) prn
	Benztropine mesylate	1–2 mg IV (IM, PO) prn

Heavy metals (e.g., arsenic, copper, gold, lead, mercury)	Chelators[c]	
	Calcium disodium edetate (EDTA)	1 g IV (IM) in saline over 1 hr q12h
	Dimercaprol (BAL)	2.5-5.0 mg/kg IM q4-6h
	Penicillamine	250-500 mg PO q6h
	2,3-dimercaptosuccinic acid (DMSA, Succimer)	10 mg/kg PO tid × 5 days then bid × 14 days
Iron	Deferoxamine mesylate	1 g IM (IV at a rate ≤15 mg/kg/hr if hypotension) q8h prn
Isoniazid (INH)	Pyridoxine	Amount equal to estimated INH ingestion up to 5 g over 30-60 min; any remainder by IV drip over 1-2 hr
Methanol	Ethanol[d]	See Ethylene glycol
Methemoglobinemia	Methylene blue	1-2 mg/kg (0.1-0.2 ml/kg of 1% solution) IV over 5 min, repeated in 1 hr prn
Opioids	Naloxone hydrochloride	0.4-2.0 mg IV (IM, SC, endotracheally) prn
Warfarin and related drugs	Vitamin K_1 (phytonadione)	10 mg IM, SC, or IV[e]
	Fresh-frozen plasma	Variable

Note: This table is only a guide. Antidote usage and dosage will depend on the specific clinical situation. The regional poison control center should be contacted for specific therapeutic recommendations.

[a] Pralidoxime is indicated in severe organophosphate poisoning with muscle weakness, fasciculations, or respiratory depression.

[b] Nitrites probably have an antidotal effect in hydrogen sulfide poisoning.

[c] The use of a specific chelating agent or combination of agents will depend on the heavy metal involved and on the clinical situation.

[d] The requisite ethanol dose will depend on prior alcohol use, liver function, and dialysis. Consult the regional poison control center for assistance.

[e] Caution should be used when giving vitamin K_1 IV. It should be given over 20 min.

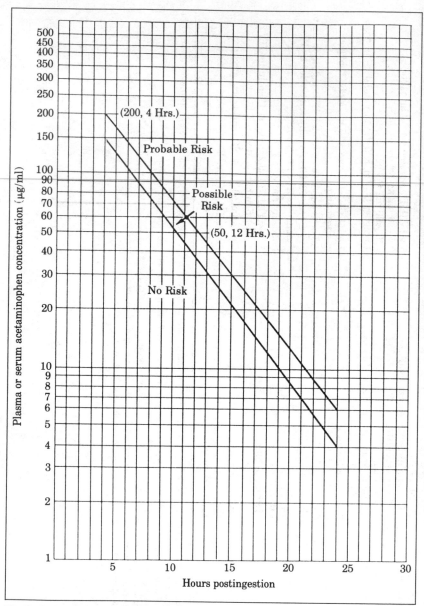

Fig. 9-1. Nomogram for acetaminophen hepatotoxicity. (Adapted from BH Rumack et al. Acetaminophen overdose: 662 cases with evaluation of oral acetylcysteine treatment. *Arch Intern Med* 141:380, 1981.)

b. **Therapy** includes immediate rinsing of the oral cavity with copious cold water. **Emesis should not be induced** because it may increase injury; charcoal administration, cathartic administration, and lavage are not indicated. Administration of milk obscures anatomic detail for subsequent endoscopy. Diluents are controversial and may induce emesis (*Vet Hum Toxicol* 31:338, 1989). *Poisindex* currently recommends administration of diluents (*Poisindex* Editorial Board Consensus Opinion, December 1988), although other experts disagree. Attempting to neutralize the alkaline agent with a weak acid will result in an exothermic reaction and increase tissue damage. The **airway** should be rapidly protected if necessary, oxygen administered, and fluids given as appropriate. Endotracheal intubation or early tracheostomy may be required. Examination and appropriate radiographs for evidence of perforation (pneumomediastinum, pleural effusion, pneumoperitoneum) should be obtained. **Endoscopy** should be performed immediately when the patient has drooling, stridor, or odynophagia; it may be deferred 12–24 hours otherwise. Nasogastric tubes should be avoided. Glucocorticoid treatment of esophageal burns for the prevention of stricture is controversial; glucocorticoids have not been shown to be helpful in one small controlled trial (*N Engl J Med* 323:637, 1990). Surgical consultation should be obtained. Prophylactic antibiotics are not appropriate. Barium swallow should be performed at 2–4 weeks (*South Med J* 81:724, 1988) to assess for esophageal stricture.

2. **Acids.** Tissue injury is less deep than that produced by alkaline agents. Gastric injury may be more common than esophageal injury due to rapid transit of liquid and resistance of squamous esophageal epithelium to acid injury. However, serious esophageal injury, including perforation, may occur.

a. **Symptoms** and signs include oral pain, drooling, odynophagia, and abdominal pain. Occasionally respiratory distress, DIC, hemolysis, and systemic acidosis may occur.

b. **Therapy** consists of airway maintenance and circulatory support. Diluent administration has no demonstrated clinical efficacy. The patient's mouth should be copiously washed with cold water. Neutralization with a weak base is contraindicated. **Induction of emesis, lavage, or charcoal administration is contraindicated,** and a nasogastric tube should be avoided. Sucralfate (1 g PO qid) may decrease symptoms but does not appear to decrease complications or perforation. Unsuspected esophageal and gastric burns and duodenal injury are commonly seen with endoscopy. The likelihood of stricture formation (gastric or esophageal) and perforation depends on the severity of ingestion (*Gastroenterology* 97:702, 1989). Surgical consultation should be obtained. The administration of glucocorticoids is controversial, but their use is probably of no added benefit. Prophylactic antibiotics are not recommended. Upper GI series should be obtained in 2–4 weeks.

C. **Ethanol and other alcohols**

1. **Ethanol.** The toxicity of ethanol (EtOH) is dose-related, but tolerance varies widely among individuals. Blood levels greater than 100 mg/dl define legal intoxication and are typically associated with ataxia, while at 200 mg/dl patients are drowsy and confused. At levels greater than 400 mg/dl there is often respiratory depression, and death is possible.

a. **Laboratory studies** should include electrolytes, glucose, serum osmolality, and blood EtOH level. The blood EtOH level may be rapidly estimated by calculating the **osmolal gap** (measured osmolality minus calculated osmolality).

$$2[Na^+] + \frac{BUN}{2.8} + \frac{[glucose]}{18} \approx \text{calculated osmolality}$$

The blood alcohol level in milligrams/deciliter divided by 4.3 equals the osmolal gap, in the absence of other low-molecular-weight toxins (*Am J Clin Pathol* 60:690, 1973):

Blood alcohol level = 4.3 (measured osmolality − calculated osmolality)

    b. Therapy. If the patient's mental status is severely depressed, an endotracheal tube should be placed followed by gastric lavage. Charcoal is not helpful due to the rapid absorption of EtOH from the stomach (*Clin Toxicol* 24:225, 1986). For life-threatening overdoses, hemodialysis may be useful. **In the comatose alcoholic,** 50 ml of 50% dextrose should be administered IV after 100 mg of thiamine IV. Patients with alcohol intoxication should be admitted when there is severe underlying illness or requirement for ventilatory support. Other patients should be observed until they are sober (blood alcohol level <100 mg/dl).

2. Isopropyl alcohol (IPA). Rubbing alcohol is 70% IPA. It has more toxicity than EtOH at any blood level (50 mg/dl = intoxication, 100–200 mg/dl = stupor and coma). Respiratory depression and hypotension occur at high blood levels. Nausea, vomiting, and abdominal pain occur frequently; hypoglycemia may occur.

    a. Laboratory evaluation commonly reveals ketosis without acidosis (IPA is metabolized to acetone). Metabolic acidosis is usually related to associated hypotension. IPA concentration in the blood may be measured directly or may be estimated in the same fashion as for EtOH, substituting a multiplier of 5.9 for 4.3 (*Top Emerg Med,* July 1984, 14–29).

    b. Therapy. Emesis is not recommended, as mental status may decline rapidly, with subsequent aspiration. Gastric lavage followed by charcoal administration may be useful if performed within 30 minutes of ingestion. For cutaneous exposures, the patient's skin should be washed and contaminated clothes should be removed (*Vet Hum Toxicol* 28:233, 1986). An adequate airway and blood pressure must be maintained. Hemodialysis is reserved for patients with hypotension.

3. Methanol (MeOH) is in gas-line antifreeze and windshield washer fluid. Sterno contains both EtOH and MeOH, and the EtOH present may delay manifestations of MeOH toxicity. The toxicity of MeOH is due to its conversion by alcohol dehydrogenase to formaldehyde and formic acid. EtOH delays this metabolism by competing for this enzyme. The patient may have initial symptoms of lethargy and confusion, followed by an apparent "hangover." Delayed toxic symptoms consisting of headache, visual symptoms, nausea, vomiting, abdominal pain, tachypnea, and respiratory failure may ensue. Coma and convulsions may occur in severe cases.

    a. Examination typically reveals an uncomfortable patient who may be remarkably tachypneic with decreased visual acuity; optic disk hyperemia may be difficult to appreciate. Laboratory studies should include CBC, electrolytes, BUN, creatinine, amylase, EtOH level, MeOH level, and ABGs, which will reveal a severe anion gap metabolic acidosis. The range of toxic ingestion is 15–400 ml. In general, pH and acid-base status are better predictors of toxicity than absolute level. The MeOH level in mg/dl may be estimated in the same way as for EtOH (see sec. **IV.C.1.a**), substituting a multiplier of 2.6 for 4.3.

    b. Therapy for MeOH intoxication includes gastric lavage and charcoal administration. A cathartic may be given once.

        (1) Folinic acid (leucovorin), 1 mg/kg (maximum 50 mg) IV, with folic acid, 1 mg/kg IV q4h for 6 doses, increases the metabolism of formate.

        (2) 4-Methylpyrazole (an alcohol dehydrogenase antagonist) is not yet available in the United States (*J Emerg Med* 8:455, 1990).

        (3) EtOH should be administered for any peak MeOH level greater than 20 mg/dl, for a suspicious ingestion while awaiting levels, for a suspicious anion gap metabolic acidosis, or to any symptomatic patient with an appropriate history. The **loading dose of EtOH** is 7.6–10.0

Table 9-11. Maintenance ethanol dosage regimens for ethylene glycol and methanol intoxication

	10% ethanol IV (ml/kg/hr)	40% ethanol PO (ml/kg/hr)	95% ethanol PO (ml/kg/hr)	Hemodialysis with 10% ethanol IV* (ml/kg/hr)
Moderate drinker	1.39	0.29	0.15	3.29
Chronic drinker	1.95	0.41	0.21	3.85
Nondrinker	0.83	0.17	0.09	2.73

* Dialysate bath concentration 100 mg/dl preferable.
Source: Modified from JP Duffy. Methanol (management/treatment protocol). In BH Rumack and DG Spoerke (eds), *Poisindex Information System*. Denver: Micromedex, Inc., 1994.

ml/kg of a 10% solution given IV or 0.8–1.0 ml/kg of 95% alcohol, administered PO in orange juice. Ethanol (10%) for IV infusion can be prepared by removing 50 ml from a stock 5% ethanol solution and replacing this with 50 ml of absolute alcohol. Maintenance dosage varies depending on previous alcohol exposure (Table 9-11). The goal is achievement of a blood alcohol level of 100–150 mg/dl to saturate the available alcohol dehydrogenase and prevent formation of MeOH's toxic metabolites. EtOH levels should be checked after the loading dose, and 2–3 times daily during maintenance infusion. EtOH is administered continuously until the MeOH level is less than 10 mg/dl, the formate level is less than 1.2 mg/dl, there is resolution of acidosis, CNS symptoms abate, and normal anion gap is restored. If MeOH levels cannot be readily measured, EtOH should be administered for at least 5 days without dialysis or 1 day with dialysis and until clinical findings resolve (*Poisindex*, 1994).

    (4) **Hemodialysis** is generally indicated for a MeOH level greater than 50 mg/dl, severe and resistant acidosis, renal failure, or visual symptoms.

  D. **Ethylene glycol (EG) and diethylene glycol** are commonly used in antifreeze and windshield de-icer. Various metabolites are responsible for toxicity. **Initial symptoms** resemble alcohol intoxication. Vomiting is common. CNS depression or coma may be seen. Congestive heart failure and pulmonary edema may occur 12–36 hours after ingestion. Death is most likely in this stage. Oliguric renal failure (from oxalate crystal deposition) may be seen 36–72 hours after ingestion. Associated flank pain may be prominent.

    1. **Laboratory findings** include a severe metabolic acidosis with an anion gap, an osmolal gap, and oxalate and hippurate crystalluria. Fluorescein is often added to antifreeze, and urine fluorescence detected with a Wood's lamp is diagnostic (*Ann Emerg Med* 19:663, 1990).

    2. **Treatment** is supportive (e.g., correction of acidosis with IV sodium bicarbonate).

      a. **Gastric lavage** may be useful if performed within 30 minutes of ingestion followed by charcoal and a single dose of magnesium-free cathartic.

      b. **Indications for IV EtOH** include an EG level greater than 20 mg/dl, suspicion of ingestion pending level, or an anion gap metabolic acidosis with a history of EG ingestion, regardless of level. An EtOH level of at least 100 mg/dl should be maintained (see sec. **VI.C.3.b**, Table 9-11).

      c. **Pyridoxine** (100 mg IV qd) and **thiamine** (100 mg IV qd) promote the conversion of glyoxylate to glycine.

      d. **Dialysis** is highly effective in severe cases; EtOH infusion should be continued during dialysis. Indications for dialysis include a glycol level greater than 50 mg/dl, congestive heart failure, renal failure, or severe persistent acid-base abnormalities. Dialysis may be discontinued when the glycol level is less than 10 mg/dl, the glycolic acid level is nondetectable, and the acidosis, clinical status, and anion gap have returned to normal. EG levels can be estimated as for alcohol (see sec. **IV.C.1.a**), using 6.3 as the multiplier of the osmolal gap. When levels cannot be measured easily, EtOH administration should continue for at least 3 days without hemodialysis or 1 day with hemodialysis and until clinical findings resolve, whichever is longer (*Poisindex*, 1994). EtOH levels are measured after the loading dose and 2–3 times daily during maintenance therapy.

E. **Hydrocarbon ingestions** (e.g., petroleum products, kerosene, turpentine, mineral spirits, and mineral seal oil) are characterized by GI upset, pulmonary aspiration, and CNS alterations. Morbidity and mortality are usually attributed to pulmonary aspiration. Low viscosity is associated with greater aspiration potential. Motor oil, transmission oil, mineral oil, baby oil, and suntan oil are usually nontoxic.

1. **Clinical manifestations** are usually apparent within the first 6 hours and include vomiting, chest or abdominal pain, cough, dyspnea, low-grade fever, arrhythmias, seizures, an altered sensorium, and radiographic evidence of aspiration pneumonitis or pulmonary edema.

2. **Treatment of nontoxic hydrocarbon ingestion** is not required in the absence of symptoms. Gastric emptying is never required, and chest x-rays are obtained only in patients with pulmonary symptoms. Such patients may be discharged if they are asymptomatic in 6 hours. Those with an abnormal chest x-ray or ABG, or both, should be hospitalized and treated supportively.

3. **Treatment of toxic hydrocarbon ingestion** is initiated by removing contaminated clothing and washing the affected skin to prevent dermatitis and percutaneous absorption. Supplemental oxygen is indicated in all significant aspiration injuries. Gastric emptying, followed by administration of activated charcoal, although controversial, is recommended for ingestion of toxic hydrocarbons, particularly halogenated hydrocarbons (trichloroethylene, carbon tetrachloride, methylene chloride), or those containing toxic additives (e.g., heavy metals, insecticides, nitrobenzene, aniline, or camphor). Other potentially toxic hydrocarbons (gasoline, benzine, kerosene, lighter fluid, turpentine, naphtha, paint thinner, xylene, and fluorene) do not require gastric emptying except for large, suicidal ingestions. In alert patients, gastric emptying should be performed by emesis induced with ipecac. In patients with CNS depression, a depressed gag reflex, or seizures, gastric lavage is indicated but should be performed only after a cuffed endotracheal tube is in place. Following gastric decontamination, observation for at least 6 hours is required. Hospitalization is recommended for patients who are symptomatic (including cough), have an abnormal pulmonary examination, are lethargic, or have an abnormal ABG or chest radiograph. Prophylactic antibiotics or glucocorticoids are not indicated; seizures may be managed with diazepam and phenytoin.

F. **Methemoglobinemia** may be caused by nitrites, nitroprusside, nitroglycerin, chlorates, sulfonamides, aniline dyes, nitrobenzene, antimalarials, sexual stimulant inhalants (containing butyl or amyl nitrite), and phenazopyridine. Reports have noted occurrence after benzocaine topical anesthesia for endoscopy (*Gastroenterology* 98:211, 1990); dapsone, now used more widely for *Pneumocystis* prophylaxis and in therapy of brown recluse spider bite, may also cause methemoglobinemia (*J Emerg Med* 3:285, 1985). Symptoms include headache, fatigue, dyspnea, tachycardia, and dizziness.

1. **The diagnosis** is suggested in patients with a normal PO_2 and generalized cyanosis (suggesting a methemoglobin level of 15%) that does not respond to oxygen. Final confirmation rests with measurement of a methemoglobin level. Blood levels greater than 50% indicate severe toxicity, often associated with CNS depression, seizures, coma, and arrhythmias; levels greater than 70% are often fatal.

2. **Treatment** includes gastric decontamination, supplemental oxygen, and administration of **methylene blue**, 1–2 mg/kg in a 1% solution given IV over 5 minutes, if there are signs of hypoxia or if the methemoglobin level exceeds 30%. The dose may be repeated in 1 hour if there are persistent signs of hypoxia and q4h thereafter to a total dose of 7 mg/kg. The patient should be hospitalized in an ICU with continuous monitoring if there are symptoms or if the methemoglobin level is greater than 20%. Hyperbaric oxygen and exchange transfusion are extreme measures for severely symptomatic patients.

G. **Organophosphates.** Parathion and malathion are the most common insecticides involved in human poisonings; they are often contained in hydrocarbon solvent. Suicidal ingestion and agricultural exposure occur.

1. **Diagnosis and routine laboratory measurements.** Nonketotic hyperglycemia and glucosuria are common. Hyperamylasemia may reflect pancreatitis. Red cell cholinesterase and plasma pseudocholinesterase levels are decreased; depression of greater than 50% from baseline is associated with poor outcome. **Toxic manifestations** are due to inhibition of acetylcholinesterase in the nervous system. **Muscarinic manifestations** include miosis, increased lacrimation, blurred vision, bronchospasm, bronchorrhea, diaphoresis, salivation, bradycardia, hypotension, urinary incontinence, and increased GI motility. **Nicotinic manifestations** include fasciculations, muscle weakness, hypotension, cramps, and respiratory paralysis. CNS toxicity includes anxiety, slurred speech, mental status changes (e.g., delirium, coma, and seizures), and respiratory depression. Complications of ingestion include pulmonary edema, aspiration pneumonia, chemical pneumonitis, and ARDS.

2. **Treatment** includes measures to support ventilation and circulation, decontamination of the skin, and gastric emptying by lavage (performed only after a cuffed endotracheal tube is placed when there is respiratory depression); **emesis is contraindicated.** These measures should be followed with activated charcoal.

   a. **Atropine** (preservative-free) is the drug of choice in organophosphate toxicity. An initial dose of 1 mg IV is given; if there are no adverse effects, a 2-mg dose is repeated every 15 minutes until atropinization (as manifested by drying of secretions, flushing, dry mouth, and dilated pupils) occurs. The average patient requires approximately 40 mg/day (*Ann Emerg Med* 16:193, 1987), but larger doses (500–1,500 mg/day) may be required. Intermittent administration may need to be continued for at least 24 hours until the organophosphate is metabolized. Severe cases may require several days or more of therapy, because of slow regeneration of acetylcholinesterase activity. Atropine will not reverse the muscle weakness.

   b. **Pralidoxime**, 1–2 g IV given over 30 minutes, reactivates the cholinesterase and counteracts weakness, muscle fasciculations, and respiratory depression. It may be repeated q6–12h to a maximum of 12 g in 24 hours. An alternative is continuous infusion at 500 mg/hour, with continuation as needed for several days.

   c. **Hemoperfusion** should be considered for severe parathion overdoses.

H. **Opioids**

1. **Symptoms.** Overdose causes respiratory depression, depressed level of consciousness, and miosis. However, the pupils may be dilated with acidosis or hypoxia, or following overdoses with meperidine and diphenoxylate plus atropine. Less common complications include hypotension, bradycardia, and pulmonary edema.

2. **Treatment** includes airway maintenance, ventilatory and circulatory support, and prevention of further drug absorption by gastric emptying and charcoal administration. **Naloxone hydrochloride** specifically reverses opioid-induced respiratory and CNS depression and hypotension. The initial dose is 2 mg IV; large doses may be required to reverse the effects of propoxyphene, diphenoxylate, or pentazocine. In the absence of an IV line, it can be administered

sublingually (*Ann Emerg Med* 16:572, 1987) or via endotracheal tube. Isolated opioid overdose is unlikely if there is no response after a total of 10 mg of naloxone. Repetitive doses may be required (duration of action is 45 minutes), and this should prompt hospitalization despite return to an alert status. Methadone overdose may require therapy for 24–48 hours. A continuous IV drip providing two-thirds of the initial dose hourly, diluted in 5% dextrose, may be necessary to maintain an alert state (*Ann Emerg Med* 15:566, 1986).

I. **Phencyclidine (PCP)** is a dissociative anesthetic and is available illicitly mislabeled as LSD, mescaline, psilocybin, and tetrahydrocannabinol.

   1. **Symptoms** include agitation, bizarre or violent behavior, hypertension, tachycardia, and horizontal or vertical nystagmus when ingested in small amounts. Patients are relatively impervious to pain and may be catatonic or self-destructive and difficult to subdue (*Ann Emerg Med* 10:290, 1981). Stupor progressing to coma, hypertension, hyperpyrexia, hypertonicity, and bronchospasm characterize moderate ingestions. Massive ingestions may lead to hypotension, respiratory failure, rhabdomyolysis, and acute tubular necrosis. Hypoglycemia is frequent and death may occur (*Ann Emerg Med* 10:237, 1981).

   2. **Treatment** is primarily supportive. Sensory input should be minimized and potentially injurious objects removed from the area. Haloperidol or diazepam may be used to control agitation; dystonic reactions may be treated with diphenhydramine. Adrenergic manifestations (e.g., hypertension) may be controlled with beta-adrenergic blockade if bronchospasm is not present (see Chap. 4); sodium nitroprusside may be required in severe cases. Gastric emptying may provoke violent behavior and is recommended only in severe poisonings and only after the airway is protected; in that case, repeated charcoal administration is also recommended. Restraints should be avoided as they may increase rhabdomyolysis. Patients with low-dose intoxication can be discharged from the emergency department after symptoms resolve and psychiatric consultation is obtained. More severe intoxication requires hospitalization.

J. **Phenothiazines.** Chlorpromazine, thioridazine, prochlorperazine, haloperidol, and thiothixene are the most common agents.

   1. **Overdoses** are characterized by agitation or delirium, which may rapidly progress to coma. Pupils are miotic, and deep tendon reflexes are depressed. Seizures and disorders of thermoregulation may occur. Hypotension (due to strong alpha-adrenergic antagonism), tachycardia, arrhythmias (including torsades de pointes), and depressed cardiac conduction occur. Measuring blood levels is not helpful. Abdominal radiographs may reveal pill concretions present in the stomach despite apparently effective gastric emptying.

   2. **Treatment** includes airway protection, respiratory and hemodynamic support, and gastric emptying followed by administration of activated charcoal. The stomach should be emptied by gastric lavage, which may be effective hours later due to delay in gastric emptying caused by the phenothiazines. Arrhythmias are treated with lidocaine and phenytoin; class Ia agents (e.g., procainamide, quinidine, disopyramide) are contraindicated. Hypotension is treated by fluid administration and alpha-adrenergic vasopressors (norepinephrine). Paradoxic vasodilation may occur in response to epinephrine administration because of unopposed beta-adrenergic response in the setting of strong alpha-adrenergic antagonism. Recurrent torsades de pointes may require magnesium, isoproterenol, or overdrive pacing (see Chap. 7). Seizures are treated with diazepam and phenytoin. Hemodialysis is not useful. Patients with significant overdosage require cardiac monitoring for at least 48 hours.

K. **Salicylate** toxicity may result from acute ingestion or chronic intoxication. Toxicity is mild for acute ingestions less than 150 mg/kg, moderate for ingestions of 150–300 mg/kg, and generally severe at levels of 300–500 mg/kg. Toxicity from chronic ingestion is typically due to ingestions of more than 100 mg/kg/day over a period of several days and usually occurs in elderly patients with chronic underlying illness. Diagnosis is often delayed in this group of patients, and mortality is about 25% (*Ann Intern Med* 85:745, 1976). Significant toxicity due to chronic ingestion may be present at blood levels lower than those associated with acute ingestions.

1. **Symptoms** include nausea, vomiting, tinnitus (implying levels >30 mg/dl), and malaise. Fever may occur and is a bad prognostic sign in adults. More severe intoxications are associated with lethargy, convulsions, and coma. Noncardiogenic pulmonary edema may occur in up to 30% of adults and is more common with chronic ingestion, cigarette smoking, neurologic symptoms, and older age (*Ann Intern Med* 95:405, 1981).

2. **Laboratory data** should include CBC, electrolytes, BUN, creatinine, blood glucose, and coagulation parameters. ABGs may reveal an early respiratory alkalosis, followed by metabolic acidosis. Approximately 20% of patients will have either respiratory alkalosis or metabolic acidosis alone (*J Crit Illness* 1·77, 1986). Most adults with pure salicylate overdose have both a primary metabolic acidosis and a primary respiratory alkalosis. Following mixed overdoses, respiratory acidosis may become prominent (*Arch Intern Med* 138:1481, 1978). Hypoglycemia, common in children, is rare in adults. Blood levels must be drawn 6 hours or more after ingestion to allow prediction of severity and disposition (Fig. 9-2). Earlier levels are appropriate in severely intoxicated patients to guide intervention. Levels greater than 70 mg/dl at any time represent moderate to severe intoxication; levels greater than 100 mg/dl are very serious and often fatal. This information is of use only for acute overdoses; estimation of severity is invalidated by the use of enteric-coated aspirin or chronic ingestion.

3. **Therapy** includes induced emesis followed by administration of charcoal and a cathartic. Multidose charcoal may be of use in severe overdose (*Pediatrics* 85:594, 1990). **Alkaline diuresis** is indicated for levels above 40 mg/dl and is achieved by administering 88 mEq (2 ampules) of sodium bicarbonate in 1,000 ml D5W at a rate of 10–15 ml/kg/hour if the patient is clinically volume depleted, until urine flow is achieved. Alkalinization is maintained using the same solution at 2–3 times maintenance fluid requirement, following urine output, urine pH (target 7–8), and serum potassium. Achievement of alkaline diuresis often requires the simultaneous administration of at least 20 mEq/liter of potassium chloride. Vigorous fluid therapy is problematic in the elderly, as it may promote pulmonary edema. Although acetazolamide will cause urine alkalinization, the associated acidemia increases salicylate toxicity, and it should not be used. **Hemodialysis is indicated for levels greater than 100–130 mg/dl** but may be useful in chronic overdoses at levels as low as 40 mg/dl, if other indications for dialysis exist, including refractory acidosis, severe CNS symptoms, progressive clinical deterioration, pulmonary edema, and renal failure. In addition to dialysis, treatment of pulmonary edema may require mechanical ventilation with high FiO_2 and PEEP. Cerebral edema is treated with hyperventilation and osmotic diuresis. Patients with minor symptoms (nausea, vomiting, tinnitus), an acute ingestion less than 150 mg/kg, a first blood level less than 65 mg/dl, and documented subsequent decline in blood level may be treated in the emergency department; these patients are often medically stable for discharge, and disposition should be determined based on psychiatric evaluation. Moderate symptomatology mandates admission for at least 24 hours; severe overdoses, manifested by tachypnea, dehydration, altered mental status, or a total dose greater than 300 mg/kg, require admission, usually to the ICU. The elderly are at high risk. Repeated blood levels that fail to decline should prompt contrast x-ray of the stomach; concretions should be subjected to lavage.

L. **Sedative-hypnotics** include a diverse spectrum of frequently abused compounds.
1. **Barbiturates**. Toxic manifestations of barbiturates vary with the amount of ingestion, type of drug, and length of time since ingestion. Short-acting barbiturates (e.g., amobarbital, butabarbital, secobarbital, and pentobar-

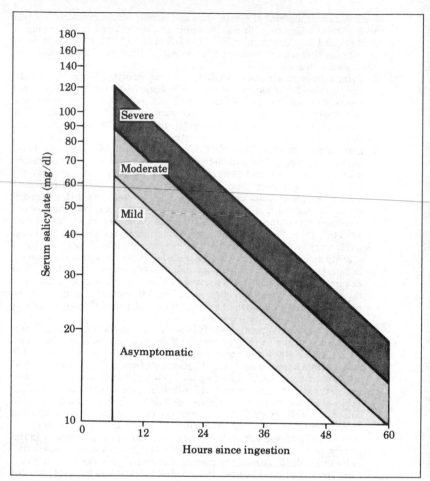

Fig. 9-2. Severity of salicylate intoxication. (Adapted from AK Done. Salicylate intoxication. *Pediatrics* 26:800, 1960.)

bital) generally cause toxicity with lower doses than the long-acting barbiturates (e.g., phenobarbital, barbital, and primidone), but fatalities are more common with the latter.

  a. Clinical manifestations. Mild intoxication resembles alcohol intoxication. Moderate intoxication is characterized by greater depression of mental status, response only to painful stimuli, decreased deep tendon reflexes, and slow respirations. Severe intoxication causes coma and a loss of all reflexes (except pupillary light reflex). Plantar reflexes are extensor. Characteristic bullae ("barb burns") may be seen over pressure points, as well as on the dorsum of the fingers (*Br Med J* 1:835, 1965). Hypothermia and hypotension may occur. In severe cases, there is no electrical activity seen on an EEG.

  b. Treatment. Maintenance of a patent airway and adequate ventilation and tissue perfusion are essential. Efficacy of GI decontamination for short-acting barbiturates is unclear; longer-acting barbiturate overdoses should be treated by **gastric emptying** and **activated charcoal administration.**

Multidose activated charcoal (50 g PO or via gastric tube q4h) markedly decreases the half-life of phenobarbital (*JAMA* 251:3104, 1984; *Q J Med* 235:997, 1986). A single dose of cathartic may be useful. Pill concretions may require repeated lavage. **Forced alkaline diuresis,** similar to that used for salicylate intoxication, is effective for phenobarbital, but not short-acting barbiturates. **Hemoperfusion** may be effective for both. Charcoal or resin hemoperfusion should be used for stage IV coma with high blood levels and is more effective than hemodialysis. Norepinephrine or dopamine may be necessary to correct hypotension, although fluid administration is usually effective. For short-acting barbiturates, charcoal or resin hemoperfusion appears to be more effective than hemodialysis. Multidose activated charcoal and alkalinization have not shown any benefit.

2. **Benzodiazepines** depress mental and respiratory function when taken in overdose. Fatalities are rare (*J Intern Med* 226:117, 1989). Mixed overdoses are common.

   a. **Symptoms** include drowsiness, dysarthria, ataxia, and confusion.

   b. **Treatment** should include gastric emptying, activated charcoal administration, a cathartic, and general supportive measures. Rarely, respiratory depression may require intubation. **Flumazenil,** a benzodiazepine antagonist, reverses toxicity without causing respiratory depression (*Eur J Anaesth* 2[Suppl.]:295, 1988); 0.2 mg (2 ml) is administered IV over 30 seconds followed by 0.3 mg at 1 minute, 0.5 mg at 2 minutes, and repeated doses of 0.5 mg each minute to a total dose of 3 mg. If, at this point, no response has been observed, benzodiazepines are unlikely to be the cause of the sedation. If a partial response has occurred, further 0.5-mg increments may be given to a total of 5 mg. Rarely, as much as a 10-mg total dose may be necessary for full reversal. Recurrence of sedation or respiratory depression, or both, may be treated by repeating the above regimen or by continuous infusion of 0.1–0.5 mg/hour. If mixed overdose with cyclic antidepressants is suspected, or the patient has a known seizure disorder, flumazenil should not be used.

M. **Stimulants** include amphetamines and cocaine.

1. **Amphetamine** toxicity is manifested by hyperactivity, irritability, delirium, hallucinations, psychosis, mydriasis, hyperpyrexia, hypertension, arrhythmias, vomiting, and diarrhea. Less common manifestations include acute renal failure secondary to rhabdomyolysis, seizures, CNS hemorrhage, coma, and circulatory collapse. **Treatment** includes early administration of activated charcoal and a cathartic. **Emesis is contraindicated,** as it may induce seizures. Gastric lavage may be useful in the comatose patient, followed by charcoal and a cathartic. Hemodialysis is not clearly effective. Agitation and psychosis are treated with haloperidol or chlorpromazine, which may also be useful in treating hypertension. Severe hypertension may require administration of nitroprusside or a beta-adrenergic antagonist (see Chap. 4). Diazepam is the drug of choice for seizures. Arrhythmias usually respond to propranolol or lidocaine. Hyperthermia may require cooling blankets or paralysis; if unsuccessful, dantrolene or bromocriptine may be useful.

2. **Cocaine**

   a. **Symptoms.** Cocaine causes short-lived CNS and sympathetic stimulation, hypertension, tachypnea, tachycardia, and mydriasis. Depression of the higher nervous centers follows rapidly and may result in death. Mortality may also result from drug-induced seizures, subarachnoid hemorrhage, stroke, or direct cardiac effects (e.g., coronary artery spasm, myocardial injury, and precipitation of lethal arrhythmias) (*N Engl J Med* 315:1495, 1986). **MI** may be precipitated in individuals without underlying heart disease. Rhabdomyolysis may occur. **Pulmonary edema** may develop abruptly after smoking the alkaloid form ("crack"). Pneumomediastinum may occur after smoking crack and may progress to pneumothorax. Other pulmonary complications include alveolar hemorrhage, obliterative bronchiolitis, hypersensitivity pneumonitis, and asthma (*Am J Med* 87:664, 1989).

b. Treatment includes maintenance of a patent airway and support of respiration and circulation. MI should be managed as outlined in Chap. 5; calcium channel antagonists and nitrates may be useful for coronary artery spasm. Beta-adrenergic antagonists should be avoided, as they allow unopposed alpha-adrenergic vasospasm (*Ann Intern Med* 112:897, 1990). Labetalol may be preferable, and phentolamine may be useful in selected cases. Urgent catheterization and thrombolysis may be necessary. Benzodiazepines are helpful in decreasing the stimulatory effect of cocaine and should be used to treat seizures. Noncoronary manifestations (e.g., hypertension, tachycardia, tachypnea) of adrenergic stimulation may be treated with labetalol; severe or sustained hypertension may require treatment with nitroprusside. Rhabdomyolysis and hypotension are treated supportively. Hyperthermia may require a cooling blanket, sedation, or paralysis. Patients with marked toxicity require hospitalization for observation. Suspected "body-packers" should have abdominal radiographs to detect continued presence of cocaine-containing condoms in the intestinal tract (*Gastrointest Radiol* 11:351, 1986). If present, gentle catharsis with charcoal and mineral oil should be performed (*Ann Intern Med* 100:73, 1984). Whole-bowel irrigation and surgery are probably not necessary, although they have been recommended, but ICU admission and monitoring are recommended. With appropriate care, mortality is less than 1% (*Am J Med* 88:325, 1990).

N. Cyclic antidepressants. Traditional tricyclics include amitriptyline, imipramine, desipramine, nortriptyline, doxepin, and protriptyline. Pharmacologic actions include central and peripheral anticholinergic activity, depression of myocardial contractility, slowing of intraventricular and atrioventricular conduction, and CNS effects similar to phenothiazines. Newer cyclic antidepressants include amoxapine and loxapine (tricyclics with diminished cardiovascular toxicity but increased propensity to severe seizures), maprotiline (a tetracyclic with seizure proclivity and cardiovascular toxicity similar to older tricyclics), mianserin (a tetracyclic with low propensity for cardiovascular or neurologic toxicity), and trazodone (a noncyclic with minimal cardiovascular and CNS toxicity). Overdose with cyclic antidepressants is the leading cause of drug-related death in the United States (>100 deaths reported to the American Association of Poison Control Centers in 1992). Overdoses less than 20 mg/kg cause few fatalities; 35 mg/kg is the approximate median lethal dose; and overdoses greater than 50 mg/kg are likely to cause death.

1. Clinical manifestations include evidence of cholinergic blockade (mydriasis, ileus, urinary retention, and hyperpyrexia). **Cardiovascular toxicity** occurs as a result of anticholinergic, catecholamine-related, quinidine-like, and alpha-antagonist effects; these include supraventricular and ventricular arrhythmias, conduction blocks, hypotension, hypoperfusion, and pulmonary edema. **CNS manifestations** range from initial agitation to confusion, stupor, and coma. Seizures may occur, and the resultant metabolic acidosis may worsen cardiac toxicity.

2. Laboratory evaluation. Plasma levels correlate poorly with severity of symptoms, although blood levels greater than 1,000 ng/ml have a higher risk of cardiac toxicity. ABGs are useful for ensuring adequate gas exchange and monitoring alkalinization. ECGs showing limb lead QRS duration greater than 100 msec are predictive of seizures and cardiac toxicity; a terminal 40-msec QRS axis greater than 120 degrees is even more sensitive (*N Engl J Med* 313:474, 1985; *Ann Emerg Med* 18:348, 1989).

3. Treatment includes supportive measures and GI decontamination. Ipecac syrup is not recommended, as obtundation may occur rapidly and promote aspiration. **Gastric lavage** should be performed regardless of time of presentation, as gastric emptying is delayed by the drug. Repetitive administration of activated charcoal, 50 g PO or per tube q2–4h, is useful. One dose of cathartic should be given. Charcoal given q1h may reduce the half-life from 36 to 14 hours. Gastric suction between charcoal instillations may promote further removal. Forced diuresis and hemodialysis are not indicated. **Resin or charcoal hemoperfusion** removes less than 1–3% of body burden, but this reduction may be associated with improvement of life-threatening cardiac or CNS complications.

   a. **Cardiac toxicity. Continuous cardiac monitoring is mandatory.** Cyclic antidepressants are protein-bound in an alkaline environment and are toxic in an acid environment. Cardiac (and CNS) toxicity is therefore enhanced by metabolic or respiratory acidosis. Treatment should be initiated prophylactically, as toxic complications are often refractory to therapy once they have developed. **Alkalinization** with IV sodium bicarbonate, 1–2 mEq/kg, to maintain an arterial pH of 7.45–7.55, is effective in preventing and treating hypotension, arrhythmias (including ventricular and supraventricular arrhythmias), and conduction disturbances. For the intubated patient, hyperventilation to a PCO_2 equal to or greater than 25 and arterial pH of 7.45–7.55 is an effective means of alkalinization and avoids the administration of large amounts of sodium. Physostigmine, because of its narrow margin of safety, should virtually never be used to treat dysrhythmias. Refractory ventricular arrhythmias may be managed with lidocaine or phenytoin. **Class Ia antiarrhythmics** (procainamide, quinidine, or disopyramide) **are contraindicated** because of additive toxicity. Phenytoin's ability to reverse heart conduction abnormalities is largely anecdotal, and objective studies do not support its use (*Ann Emerg Med* 15:876, 1986). Temporary ventricular pacing is used for complete heart block. Hypotension unresponsive to alkalinization and fluid administration should be treated with norepinephrine.

   b. **CNS complications.** Alkalinization does not reverse CNS complications. Physostigmine (2 mg IV over 1 minute) reverses CNS depression rapidly in patients with pure cyclic antidepressant overdose. However, because repeated doses are necessary and physostigmine may cause seizures, its use is generally not recommended. Supportive care of coma is usually adequate. Seizures may be treated with diazepam and phenytoin; status epilepticus (particularly common with amoxapine) should be treated aggressively, including high-dose barbiturates, paralysis, and general anesthesia, to prevent permanent neurologic damage (*JAMA* 250:1069, 1983).

   c. **Respiratory depression is common** and is treated with mechanical ventilation. Pulmonary edema and aspiration are common (*Clin Toxicol* 25:443, 1987) as is charcoal aspiration (*Chest* 96:852, 1989).

4. **Disposition.** Patients who have a depressed level of consciousness, respiratory depression, hypotension, arrhythmia, conduction blocks (including QRS >100 msec), or seizures must be admitted to an ICU. Asymptomatic individuals with a normal ECG may be observed in the emergency department with cardiac monitoring for 6 hours following intestinal decontamination and repeated charcoal. If they remain asymptomatic, the ECG remains normal, and they have normal bowel sounds, they may undergo psychiatric disposition (*JAMA* 257:521, 1987; *J Emerg Med* 6:121, 1988). If any signs or symptoms are present, they must be admitted. Caution is imperative; 25% of fatal cases are awake and alert at the time of presentation, and three-fourths of those are in normal sinus rhythm. After admission, criteria for discharge from an ICU include lack of all cyclic antidepressant symptoms, normal mental status, and no ECG abnormalities (including sinus tachycardia) for 24 hours. Patients fully meeting these criteria rarely develop subsequent significant arrhythmias.

O. **Selective serotonin re-uptake inhibitors**
   1. **Forms.** These compounds are noncyclic antidepressants. The prototype is fluoxetine, but paroxetine and sertraline share many characteristics.
   2. **Symptoms** are usually minimal. Patients may occasionally become agitated,

drowsy, or confused. Tachycardia is noted frequently. However, seizures are very rare, as is significant cardiovascular toxicity (*Am J Emerg Med* 10:115, 1992; *Vet Hum Toxicol* 32:153, 1990). Fatalities are rare (*J Anal Toxicol* 14:327, 1990). ECG changes are rare. Simultaneous ingestion with tricyclic antidepressants may raise plasma levels of the tricyclic antidepressant.

3. **Emesis** is not recommended. GI lavage, charcoal, and a cathartic may be indicated for the occasional unconscious patient or the patient who arrives soon after ingestion. Although cardiovascular and CNS toxicity is rare, an ECG as baseline should be obtained, and patients with large overdoses should be admitted to a medical floor, particularly if symptomatic or if there are coingestants. In the absence of symptoms and if the patient is medically stable, psychiatric evaluation and disposition should be made.

P. **Cardiovascular drugs**
   1. **Beta-adrenergic antagonists**
      a. **Symptoms** of beta-adrenergic antagonist overdose usually occur within 2 hours of ingestion. Cardiovascular manifestations include bradycardia, atrioventricular block, hypotension, and depression of cardiac function. Sotalol may cause torsades de pointes. Bradycardia occurs early but does not predict progression to more serious cardiac disturbances. While some beta$_1$-specific agents may have little respiratory effect in patients with asthma or COPD, severe bronchospasm may result from ingestion of any beta-adrenergic antagonist because beta$_1$ selectivity is lost at high doses. CNS manifestations include drowsiness, coma, hypoventilation, and seizures (caused most frequently by propranolol). Nausea and vomiting may occur, and mesenteric ischemia may be severe, particularly with propranolol ingestion, as a result of decreased cardiac output and unopposed alpha-agonist activity. Beta-adrenergic antagonist overdose may cause hypoglycemia by blockade of counter-regulatory mechanisms and may also make detection of hypoglycemia more difficult.

      b. **Laboratory studies.** Measurement of serum drug levels is not useful. Serum glucose and electrolyte levels should be measured; a baseline electrocardiogram should be performed, with subsequent continuous cardiac monitoring.

      c. **Therapy.** An IV line should be established before any other therapy is administered. Gastric decontamination should be performed with gastric lavage and charcoal administration. **Ipecac should not be administered** because cardiac compromise may occur rapidly and increased vagal tone associated with emesis may promote cardiovascular collapse. If bradycardia or other manifestations of a vagal reaction are present, atropine (up to 2 mg IV) should be administered and placement of an external or transvenous cardiac pacing device should be considered. Multidose charcoal administration may increase the clearance of some beta-adrenergic antagonists, particularly those with an enterohepatic circulation (atenolol, nadolol, and sotalol). A cathartic should be administered only once, after the first charcoal dose. Hypotension should be treated with IV saline; hemodynamic monitoring may be necessary to guide optimal fluid resuscitation. Isoproterenol (2–20 μg/minute) may be useful, but high doses (up to 200 μg/minute) may be necessary (*Am J Med* 80:755, 1986). If the BP does not improve or falls, norepinephrine should be added. **Epinephrine should be used with caution,** particularly in propranolol overdoses, because of the propensity for hypertension and reflex bradycardia. Glucagon (50–150 μg/kg IV over 1 minute, followed by 1–5 mg/hour in 5% dextrose) increases cardiac contractility, and heart rate (*Ann Emerg Med* 13:1123, 1984; *Adverse Drug React Acute Poisoning Rev* 9:75, 1990). For the torsades de pointes associated with sotalol overdose, isoproterenol, magnesium, and overdrive pacing may be useful (see Chap. 7). Pacemaker therapy may be useful for severe bradycardia or heart block unresponsive to medications. Ten percent calcium chloride, 10 ml IV, may also be useful for refractory propranolol overdose. Beta-adrenergic agonists and theophylline may be

used for bronchospasm. Seizures should be treated with IV benzodiazepine
followed by IV phenytoin (see Chap. 25). Hypoglycemia should be treated
with IV glucose and, if resistant, IV glucagon. Severe respiratory depression may require mechanical ventilation. Dialysis may be useful in removing nadolol, sotalol, atenolol, and acebutalol but is ineffective for propranolol, metoprolol, and timolol.

d. Disposition. Any history of beta-adrenergic antagonist ingestion should
prompt a baseline electrocardiogram and continuous electrocardiographic
monitoring for at least 6 hours, even in the absence of symptoms. If there
are any cardiovascular, respiratory, or neurologic symptoms, the patient
should be admitted to an ICU for therapy and continuous monitoring. If,
however, there are no toxic symptoms 6 hours following ingestion,
disposition guided by psychiatric consultation may be made.

2. **Calcium channel antagonists** (*Adverse Drug React Acute Poisoning Rev* 9:75,
1990)

a. Symptoms. Manifestations of calcium channel blocker overdose depend
on the drug ingested. Hypotension is common to each of the 3 most
commonly prescribed agents. Severe bradycardia, atrioventricular block,
and asystole are most common following verapamil and diltiazem overdose
and are uncommon with the dihydropyridines (e.g., nifedipine). Pulmonary edema is most likely following verapamil, as is hypocalcemia.
Seizures are most often due to verapamil, are less common with diltiazem,
and occur rarely with nifedipine. Cardiovascular manifestations are
usually apparent within 1–5 hours after ingestion but may persist for
more than 24 hours. Sustained-release preparations, particularly verapamil, may cause rhythm disturbances up to 7 days postingestion.

b. Laboratory studies should include serum calcium, magnesium, electrolytes, and glucose. Serum drug levels are not routinely available or useful.
An electrocardiogram should be obtained and continuous cardiac monitoring should be performed.

c. Therapy. Emesis should be avoided because of the potential for rapid
cardiovascular collapse. **Gastric lavage** should be followed by administration of activated charcoal and a cathartic. Gastroscopy and whole bowel
irrigation with polyethylene glycol solution may be considered for
sustained-release product ingestion. Hypotension should be treated with
IV 0.9% saline, and volume-resistant hypotension may be treated with IV
dopamine or dobutamine (see Appendix C). Ten percent **calcium chloride**
(10–20 ml IV) may be administered for hypotension, bradycardia, or heart
block. Calcium gluconate is preferred when the patient is severely
acidotic. **Glucagon** (50–150 μg/kg IV over 1 minute followed by 1–5
mg/hour) may also be useful for heart block and hypotension. Atropine (up
to 2 mg IV) may also be given for bradycardia or atrioventricular block,
although it is rarely successful. Isoproterenol is a less desirable alternative; a transvenous pacemaker should be placed for medication-resistant
heart block. Seizures should be treated with a benzodiazepine and phenytoin (see Chap. 25). Hemodialysis and hemoperfusion are not useful for
accelerated drug removal.

d. Disposition. All patients who have cardiovascular symptoms or seizures
or who have ingested a sustained-release preparation should be admitted
for continuous cardiovascular monitoring. For the asymptomatic patient
who has taken an immediate-release preparation, a baseline electrocardiogram should be obtained and continuous electrocardiographic monitoring performed for at least 8 hours. If, at that point, the patient is
asymptomatic with a normal electrocardiogram, discharge after psychiatric consultation may be considered.

3. **Digoxin** (see Chap. 6)

a. Symptoms of digoxin overdose include nausea, vomiting, and a wide
variety of dysrhythmias including bradycardia and atrioventricular block,
paroxysmal atrial tachycardia (PAT) with block, and ventricular dys-

rhythmias. In severe overdoses, the patient may be drowsy. Onset of symptoms typically occurs within 30 minutes and reaches a peak in 3–12 hours. Marked hyperkalemia may occur due to a severe overdose.

b. **Laboratory studies** should include digoxin levels, electrolytes (specifically potassium), and a baseline electrocardiogram. Continuous electrocardiographic monitoring should be performed. If antidigitalis FAB fragments have been administered, serum digoxin levels will be markedly elevated due to measurement of digoxin-FAB complexes (inactive) and are not useful. Free serum digoxin levels should be measured in this situation if necessary (*DICP Ann Pharmacother* 25:1047, 1991; *Clin Toxicol* 30:259, 1992). A single digoxin dose of 2–3 mg is likely to result in toxicity; a smaller ingestion may cause symptoms if the patient is already taking a digitalis preparation. Severe toxicity occurs at a level greater than 10 ng/ml, but as little as 3.5 ng/ml has been associated with severe toxicity. Peak levels may be delayed up to 6 hours after ingestion.

c. **Therapy** should begin with establishment of **IV access and gastric decontamination.** Emesis or gastric lavage are equally acceptable, although atropine should be available for vagally induced cardiovascular complications. Charcoal and a cathartic should be administered at least once, and multiple doses of charcoal may be necessary. Cholestyramine, 4 g q6h, may decrease the half-life of digoxin, especially in patients with renal failure. Serum digoxin levels should be measured frequently if anti-digitalis FAB fragments are not administered. **Digoxin-immune FAB fragments** should be administered for ventricular tachycardia, ventricular fibrillation, severe bradyarrhythmia, second- or third-degree atrioventricular block (which is atropine unresponsive), hyperkalemia, an ingestion greater than 10 mg, or a level greater than 10 ng/ml (see Table 9-10 for dosage). The FAB fragments should be administered over 30 minutes through a 0.22-μm filter. Insulin, glucose, and bicarbonate may also be used acutely for hyperkalemia, but calcium salts should not be administered, as **calcium increases the toxicity of digitalis.** Sodium polystyrene sulfonate (Kayexalate) should be avoided, as it lowers total body potassium; in this situation, the major problem is shift of potassium between the intracellular and the extracellular compartments. Atropine may be useful for bradycardia and atrioventricular block. Ventricular arrhythmias may be treated with phenytoin, lidocaine, and magnesium (see Chap. 7); hypokalemia should be corrected if present. Because heart block is more likely to develop after beta-adrenergic antagonist administration, their use should be limited to IV esmolol because of its very short half-life (*Postgrad Med* 69:337, 1993; see Chap. 6). A transcutaneous or transvenous pacemaker may be necessary for second- or third-degree atrioventricular block or severe bradycardia. Hemodialysis and hemoperfusion are of no benefit.

d. **Disposition.** All symptomatic patients should be admitted to an ICU for continuous cardiovascular monitoring. Asymptomatic patients with nontoxic levels should have all studies repeated at 12 hours. If the electrocardiogram remains normal and the patient is asymptomatic, disposition may be guided by psychiatric consultation.

Toxic Inhalants

Toxic inhalants comprise a variety of noxious gases and particulate matter capable of producing local irritation, asphyxiation, and systemic toxicity. In managing exposure victims, it is important to identify the offending agent and contact the regional poison control center for specific therapeutic guidelines.

I. **Irritant gases** produce cutaneous burns, mucosal irritation, laryngotracheitis, bronchitis, pneumonitis, bronchospasm, and pulmonary edema (which may be delayed up to 24 hours after exposure). The more water-soluble gases (e.g., chlorine, ammonia, formaldehyde, sulfur dioxide, ozone) primarily produce inflammation of the eyes, throat, and upper respiratory tract, whereas the less soluble gases (e.g., phosgene, nitrogen dioxide) tend to cause more damage to the terminal airways and alveoli. Household exposure may result from inadvertent mixture of bleach (sodium hypochlorite) with toilet bowl cleaner (sulfuric acid), producing chlorine gas, or bleach with ammonia, producing chloramine gas.

A. **Treatment.** A patent airway and adequate oxygenation are essential. Bronchospasm should be treated with bronchodilators. Noncardiogenic pulmonary edema should be treated with oxygen, mechanical ventilation, and PEEP as needed (see Respiratory Failure). Skin burns are treated by copious irrigation, removal of contaminated clothing, and tetanus prophylaxis (see Appendix E), if needed. Chemical contact with the eyes requires immediate, copious irrigation with water or saline. Ophthalmologic consultation is recommended for caustic eye burns.

B. **Disposition.** Because pulmonary edema may develop, asymptomatic patients with normal ABGs and chest radiographs should be observed for at least 6 hours. Patients with symptoms or signs of upper airway edema or pulmonary involvement warrant hospitalization.

II. **Simple asphyxiants** (e.g., acetylene, argon, ethane, helium, hydrogen, nitrogen, methane, butane, neon, carbon dioxide, natural gas, and propane) cause hypoxia by displacing oxygen from the inspired air. Morbidity and mortality are related to the extent and duration of the hypoxia. **Treatment** consists of supplemental oxygen for symptomatic patients and supportive care.

III. **Systemic toxic inhalants** are those gases capable of producing prominent systemic toxicity, including hydrogen sulfide, methyl bromide, organophosphates (see Overdosage, sec. VI.G), carbon monoxide, and hydrogen cyanide. Treatment consists of supportive care and specific therapy directed toward the offending agent.

A. **Carbon monoxide** displaces oxygen from hemoglobin, shifts the oxyhemoglobin dissociation curve to the left, and depresses cellular respiration by inhibiting the cytochrome oxidase system. Direct binding to cardiac myoglobin depresses cardiac function. Toxic manifestations are a consequence of tissue hypoxia. Poisoning usually occurs in poorly ventilated areas in which carbon monoxide is released by fires, combustion engines, or faulty stoves or heating systems. **Arterial PO$_2$ is usually normal; thus the diagnosis of carbon monoxide poisoning requires a high level of suspicion and direct measurement of arterial oxygen saturation or carbon monoxide (carboxyhemoglobin) levels.**

1. **Symptoms** correlate, albeit imperfectly, with the carboxyhemoglobin level. Levels of 20–40% are associated with dizziness, headache, weakness, disturbed judgment, nausea and vomiting, and diminished visual acuity. Examination may reveal retinal hemorrhages. Levels of 40–60% are associated with tachypnea, tachycardia, ataxia, syncope, and seizures. The ECG may reveal ST segment changes, conduction blocks, and atrial or ventricular arrhythmias. Levels greater than 60% are associated with coma and death. Cherry-red coloration of the lips or skin is a relatively rare, late manifestation. Late complications include basal ganglia infarction and parkinsonism. Less severe, delayed neuropsychiatric symptoms may also occur.

2. **Treatment** consists of supportive care and administration of **100% oxygen** delivered by tight-fitting mask or endotracheal tube. The latter ensures tissue oxygen delivery and decreases the half-life of carboxyhemoglobin to 90 minutes from 4–5 hours. Carboxyhemoglobin levels should be measured q2–4h, and oxygen should be continued until blood levels are less than 10%. **Hyperbaric oxygen** (3 atm) is strongly recommended for patients who present with neurologic signs or symptoms, ECG changes consistent with ischemia, severe metabolic acidosis, pulmonary edema, or shock. It is also recommended for carboxyhemoglobin levels greater than 25–30%, but this recommendation is controversial. Transfer to a hyperbaric oxygen facility should occur only after the patient is stabilized. Seizures are treated with diazepam and phenytoin (see Chap. 25).

B. Hydrogen cyanide may be present in industrial fumigants, insecticides, and products of combustion of synthetics and plastics from house fires. The gas has a characteristic "bitter almond" odor, which many people are unable to smell. Toxic amounts are rapidly absorbed through the bronchial mucosa and alveoli, and symptoms usually appear seconds after inhalation. Concentrations of 0.2–0.3 mg/liter of air are almost immediately fatal. Oral exposures to **potassium cyanide** may occur with rodenticides, insecticides, silver polish, artificial fingernail remover (acetonitrile), film developer, laboratory reagents, and amygdalin (*N Engl J Med* 300:238, 1979).

1. **Toxic manifestations** are due to inhibition of cytochrome oxidase and include palpitations, dyspnea, and mental status depression, which may quickly progress to coma and death. ECG changes include atrial fibrillation, ventricular ectopy, and abnormal ventricular repolarization. Severe lactic acidosis is present, and venous oxygen content is approximately equal to arterial oxygen content. Measurement of whole-blood cyanide levels will delay therapy for at least 2 hours.

2. **Therapy.** Specific antidote kits are available to treat cyanide poisoning. **Amyl nitrite** (one pearl held under the nostril for 15–30 seconds/minute, repeated every minute, with a new pearl every 3 minutes) produces a methemoglobin level of approximately 5% and should be followed by 10 ml of 3% sodium nitrite (0.3 g IV over 3–5 minutes). This antidote also converts hemoglobin to methemoglobin, which binds to the cyanide ion, sparing vital oxidative enzymes. One-half of this dose of **sodium nitrite** may be repeated in 30 minutes if there is an inadequate response. The goal is a measured methemoglobin level of 30%. Methylene blue should not be given. **Sodium thiosulfate** (50 ml of a 25% solution IV) converts the cyanide into thiocyanate. One-half the dose may be repeated in 30 minutes if there is an inadequate response. **Oxygen (100%)** must be administered at all times during treatment to ensure adequate tissue oxygen delivery despite methemoglobinemia. Continuous ECG monitoring is mandatory. Endotracheal intubation will protect the airway; mechanical ventilation may be needed. **Sodium bicarbonate,** 1 mEq/kg, is administered after the above measures are undertaken for severe, persistent acidosis (pH <7.2). Seizures are treated with diazepam and phenytoin. In the event of an oral ingestion, the stomach should be emptied by gastric lavage after the above measures have been undertaken, and activated charcoal and cathartic should be administered. The efficacy of **hyperbaric oxygen** is controversial but may be considered for those who respond poorly to the above. **Hydroxycobalamin** binds cyanide but a clinically useful preparation is not currently available in the United States. Dicobalt ethylenediametetraacetic acid (EDTA) is similarly effective but unavailable.

C. Hydrogen sulfide is a colorless gas with a characteristic "rotten egg" odor. It is found in mines and sewers as well as petrochemical, agricultural, and tanning industries. As with hydrogen cyanide, toxicity is secondary to inhibition of cytochrome oxidase.

1. **Symptoms.** Exposure to low concentrations causes eye irritation and visual changes, including blurred vision and scotomata. Higher concentrations cause cyanosis, confusion, pulmonary edema, coma, and convulsions. Rapid death occurs in approximately 6% of cases.

2. **Treatment** is similar to that used for hydrogen cyanide. Oxygen (100%) and nitrites are used; thiosulfate is not. The efficacy of nitrites is controversial.

IV. Smoke inhalation. Smoke is a suspension of small particles in a heated gas. More than 50% of fire-related deaths are due to smoke inhalation. Thermal injury is usually confined to the upper airway because of the rapid cooling of inhaled gases that occurs proximal to the larynx. Toxic gases released by pyrolysis include carbon dioxide, carbon monoxide, hydrogen chloride, phosgene, chlorine, benzene, isocyanate, hydrogen cyanide, aldehydes, oxides of sulfur and nitrogen, ammonia, and numerous organic acids. Carbon monoxide accounts for 80% of mortality in the first 12 hours. The other toxins produce epithelial injury resulting in airway edema, increased capillary permeability, and mechanical obstruction from desquamated tissue and secretions. Patients who have been exposed to a large quantity of smoke in a closed space, had prolonged inhalation, had steam exposure, were involved in an explosion, were with other persons who died or were severely injured, or have sustained facial burns or singed nasal vibrissae are at risk for developing respiratory complications, which may be delayed in onset for up to 3 days. High-risk patients should undergo upper airway endoscopy to rule out immediately life-threatening airway injury; bronchoscopy or xenon lung scanning is useful in confirming the diagnosis. A positive xenon scan predicts increased mortality. Carboxyhemoglobin levels greater than 15% are indicative of severe exposure.

A. **Clinical manifestations.** Asphyxiation, expectoration of carbonaceous sputum, hoarseness, dyspnea from upper airway edema, stridor, bronchospasm, and noncardiogenic pulmonary edema are characteristic features of smoke inhalation. Upper airway burns may also be noted. Late complications include bacterial pneumonia and pulmonary embolism.

B. **Treatment. Scrupulous airway care is essential,** with frequent suctioning as needed. Endotracheal intubation is required in patients with evidence of significant upper airway edema or respiratory insufficiency. Bronchoscopy may be necessary to remove endotracheal debris. **Humidified oxygen** should be administered to all patients. Bronchodilators are indicated for bronchospasm. For those who develop ADRS, mechanical ventilation with PEEP is indicated. Prophylactic antibiotics and glucocorticoids are not indicated. Specific toxins, such as cyanide and carbon monoxide, should be treated.

C. **Disposition.** Patients who have minor smoke inhalation and are asymptomatic at 4–6 hours with none of the above-noted risk factors may be safely discharged home. Patients who are asymptomatic but have any of the above-noted risk factors should be admitted for a minimum of 24 hours. Patients who have symptoms, significant laboratory abnormalities, or abnormal $P(A-a)O_2$ gradient should be admitted to an ICU.

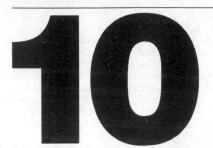

Pulmonary Diseases

Dan Schuller

Asthma

Asthma is a chronic illness characterized by airway inflammation and increased responsiveness of the tracheobronchial tree to diverse stimuli that result in varying degrees of airway obstruction. The clinical course of asthma is one of exacerbation and remission but typically is without the inexorable progression of other chronic obstructive disease (e.g., emphysema).

I. **Diagnosis**
   A. **Clinical presentation.** Patients typically have a history of dyspnea, wheezing, cough, and chest tightness. Severity ranges from intermittent, mild symptoms requiring no therapy to continuous, disabling respiratory symptoms despite intensive therapy.
   B. **Pulmonary function tests** are often normal during remissions. During an acute attack, and occasionally when symptoms are absent, there is a reduction in the forced expiratory volume in 1 second (FEV_1) and often a proportionally smaller reduction in the forced vital capacity (FVC), producing a decreased FEV_1/FVC ratio (<0.75). Hyperinflation, with increased residual volume (RV) and functional residual capacity (FRC), may be observed. The diagnosis of asthma can be confirmed by demonstrating an improvement in the FEV_1 following the inhalation of a bronchodilator. Bronchial provocation testing (e.g., methacholine challenge) is occasionally useful in the evaluation of patients with normal spirometry.

II. **Assessment of severity of an asthma attack** is critical for proper management of the patient. Identification of factors associated with fatal asthma allows for appropriate triage, close monitoring, and more aggressive treatment of the patient at risk.
   A. **History.** Patients with a prolonged history of asthma can often compare the present attack to prior attacks. Previous or current use of corticosteroids, frequent hospitalizations, previous need for mechanical ventilation, or recent emergency room visits may be indicative of a more severe or unresponsive attack that requires hospitalization.
   B. **Physical examination.** A severe attack is suggested by respiratory distress at rest, difficulty speaking in sentences, diaphoresis, or use of accessory respiratory muscles. A respiratory rate greater than 28 breaths/minute, pulse greater than 110 beats/minute, and pulsus paradoxus greater than 12 mm Hg indicate a severe episode (*Arch Intern Med* 145:321, 1985). The intensity of wheezing is an unreliable indicator. Subcutaneous emphysema suggests an associated pneumothorax or pneumomediastinum. Impending respiratory muscle fatigue may become apparent as decreased respiratory effort, exhaustion, paradoxic diaphragmatic movement, and alternation between abdominal and rib-cage breathing (respiratory alternans) occur.
   C. **Laboratory studies**
      1. **Spirometry.** Objective measurements of airflow are essential in evaluating and treating an attack. Hospitalization is recommended if the initial FEV_1 is less than 30% of the predicted value or does not increase to at least 40% of the predicted value after 1 hour of vigorous therapy (*Am J Med* 72:416, 1982). When spirometry is not readily available, peak expiratory flow rates can be

easily obtained with a peak flowmeter. Generally, hospitalization is recommended if peak flow is less than 60 liters/minute initially, or does not improve to greater than 50% of the predicted value after 1 hour of treatment.

2. **Arterial blood gases.** Mismatching of ventilation and perfusion ($\dot{V}/\dot{Q}$ mismatch) due to airway obstruction results in an increased alveolar-arterial oxygen tension difference ($P[A-a]O_2$), which correlates roughly with the severity of the attack. An arterial oxygen tension (PaO_2) less than 60 mm Hg may be a sign of a severe attack or a complicating condition. With a severe or prolonged attack, the $PaCO_2$ may rise as a result of a combination of severe airway obstruction, areas of high $\dot{V}/\dot{Q}$ ratio causing increased dead-space ventilation, and respiratory muscle fatigue. A "normal" or increased $PaCO_2$ may be a sign of impending respiratory failure and should be managed in a hospital with careful and frequent evaluation for the need for intubation and mechanical ventilation.

3. **Chest radiography** contributes little information. Although a chest radiograph may suggest or confirm a diagnosis of pneumonia, atelectasis, pneumothorax, pneumomediastinum, or other conditions that mimic asthma, its performance should not delay initial therapy.

III. **Management of asthma** consists of reducing chronic airway inflammation, alleviating symptoms of the disease, preventing exacerbations, and identifying asthma triggers and associated conditions. **Specific asthma therapies must be individualized.** Asthma treatment should be based not only on disease severity, as defined primarily by the frequency of acute episodes, but also on the intensity and duration of obstruction, the circadian variations, the state of functional limitation between exacerbations, the presence of concomitant diseases, and the presence of adverse drug reaction. The optimal therapeutic approach to asthma integrates pharmacologic therapy, patient and family education, and environmental control to minimize trigger factors. Guidelines for asthma therapy have been developed that provide a framework for evaluation and therapy (NIH Publication No. 91-3042). **During an acute exacerbation** of asthma, the goals of therapy are to ensure adequate gas exchange and to reduce airway obstruction and the work of breathing. Early recognition of worsening lung function, followed by prompt and appropriate triage, intensification of anti-asthma therapy, and removal of the allergen or irritant if one is identified are the best measures to prevent deterioration. In contrast, during **maintenance therapy**, the goals are to maintain pulmonary function close to normal, prevent chronic or recurrent symptoms, prevent asthma exacerbations, and avoid side effects of medications. The use of oxygen and airway and ventilator management for the most severe cases of asthma are described in Chap. 9.

A. **Pharmacologic therapy** includes both antiinflammatory agents and bronchodilators.

1. **Antiinflammatory agents**

a. **Glucocorticoids** have an important role as first-line maintenance therapy. The major use of steroids for asthma appears to be for reduction of airway inflammation. In addition, steroids may augment a patient's responsiveness to beta-adrenergic agonists and may prevent the down regulation of beta-receptors. Steroids may be administered parenterally, orally, or as aerosols. **Systemic glucocorticoids** speed the resolution of severe asthma exacerbations refractory to bronchodilator therapy and should be used as first-line therapy for patients admitted to the hospital with acute, severe asthma. Methylprednisolone is the drug of choice for IV therapy. The amount of glucocorticoid needed to ensure a remission in acute or chronic asthma exacerbation is still undefined. However, methylprednisolone, 40–60 mg IV q6h, is recommended. **Oral glucocorticoid** administration may be as effective as IV administration when given at equivalent dosages (e.g., prednisone 60 mg q6–8h PO). For maximum therapeutic benefit, treatment with the above doses should continue for 36–48 hours followed by tapering of prednisone to 40–60 mg PO qd when airflow improves and the patient is comfortable. A 2-week prednisone dosage reduction to 0 is usually successful, particularly when inhaled glucocorticoids are instituted at the beginning of the oral glucocorticoid taper (*Am Rev Respir Dis* 147:1306, 1993). Prolonged daily use of oral prednisone is reserved for patients with severe asthma despite use of maximal bronchodilators and inhaled glucocorticoids. **Inhaled glucocorticoids** (e.g., beclomethasone, triamcinolone, and flunisolide) delivered by metered-dose inhalers (MDIs) are safe and effective for the treatment of asthma. They have been shown to reduce the frequency of asthma exacerbations, the need for chronic oral glucocorticoids, the frequency of airway hyperresponsiveness, and the need for additional concurrent medication. The usual dose is 2 puffs qid (bid for flunisolide) 5–10 minutes after administration of inhaled bronchodilators. Larger doses of inhaled glucocorticoids (up to 4 times the starting dose) may be required to control some patients. At usual dosages, inhaled glucocorticoids have minimal side effects (e.g., oropharyngeal candidiasis and dysphonia) that can be prevented by rinsing and gargling the mouth with water after each use. However, larger dosages of inhaled glucocorticoids have been reported to produce systemic side effects, but the incidence of untoward effects can be controlled by lowering the dose.

b. **Cromolyn sodium,** 2 puffs qid by MDI, is a nonsteroidal antiinflammatory drug effective in the maintenance therapy of asthma, particularly when exercise is a precipitating factor (*Am Rev Respir Dis* 139:694, 1989). A clinical trial of 4–6 weeks is necessary to determine efficacy in individual patients. Cromolyn is virtually free of side effects and thus combining cromolyn with inhaled glucocorticoids in selected patients whose asthma is difficult to control may be beneficial.

c. **Nedocromil sodium,** 2 puffs qid by MDI, is a pyranoquinoline derivative available for the prevention and maintenance therapy of asthma. Like cromolyn, it is not indicated for the reversal of acute bronchospasm. Nedocromil inhibits allergen-induced acute and late-phase asthmatic reactions and decreases bronchial hyperresponsiveness. Its use is associated with an improvement of maximal expiratory airflow. Side effects attributable to nedocromil therapy include taste disturbance, cough, headache, and pharyngitis. Its optimal role in the treatment of asthma remains to be defined (*Chest* 97:1299, 1990).

d. **Methotrexate, gold salts, cyclosporine, and other immunomodulators** have been used in the management of severe, glucocorticoid-dependent asthma in an effort to stabilize the disease and allow a reduction in glucocorticoid dosage (*Ann Intern Med* 112:577, 1990; *Lancet* 339:324, 1992). These therapies should only be considered for patients who are not well controlled on moderate doses of glucocorticoids or patients who experience unacceptable side effects from chronic glucocorticoid use. A thorough assessment of the factors potentially contributing to the persistent bronchospasm should be undertaken before administration of these agents (Table 10-1). **Troleandomycin,** 250 mg qd PO, has also been reported to have glucocorticoid-sparing activity in asthma. Troleandomycin can induce severe hepatic injury, so its use in asthma may be limited.

2. **Bronchodilators**

a. **Beta-adrenergic agonists** continue to be first-line therapy for rapid symptomatic improvement in patients with acute bronchoconstriction. Although oral and parenteral forms are available, reversal of airflow obstruction is most effectively achieved by the repetitive administration of inhaled beta$_2$-agonist bronchodilators. In situations in which parenteral therapy is necessary, aqueous epinephrine, 0.3–0.5 ml of a 1 : 1,000 solution SC q20–30min for up to 3 doses, may be considered. Epinephrine can cause tachycardia and should be used with caution in older patients and those with cardiovascular disease. **Inhaled beta$_2$-selective agonists** administered by aerosol are rapid, effective bronchodilators that minimize cardiac side effects. Use of an MDI with a spacer device or reservoir is as effective as delivery of the drug by a nebulizer (*Chest* 98:822, 1987). A

Table 10-1. Conditions that can present as "refractory asthma"

Upper airway obstruction
  Tumor
  Epiglottitis
  Vocal cord dysfunction
  Obstructive sleep apnea
Tracheomalacia
Endobronchial lesion
Foreign body
Congestive heart failure
Gastroesophageal reflux
Sinusitis
Herpetic tracheobronchitis
Adverse drug reaction
  Aspirin
  Beta-blocker
  Angiotensin-converting enzyme inhibitors
  Inhaled pentamidine
Allergic bronchopulmonary aspergillosis
Hyperventilation with panic attacks
Factitious asthma

spacer device minimizes the need for coordination between canister activation and inspiration, decreases oropharyngeal particle deposition, and allows effective drug delivery even during tidal breathing. There is equivalent effectiveness of the various beta$_2$-agonists available for inhalation. Usual dosages of the aerosolized bronchodilators are given in Table 10-2. However, in severe cases, 2–4 initial puffs can be followed by 1–2 puffs q10–20min until improvement is obtained or significant toxicity such as unacceptable tremor, tachycardia, or cardiac arrhythmia is noted. Patient instruction and supervised administration are essential to ensure that effective delivery is achieved (*Br Med J* 303:1426, 1991). It may be prudent to minimize the use of beta-agonists when patients are faring well and to reevaluate patients that are requiring maximal therapy to exclude alternative diagnoses (see Table 10-1), or the possibility of adverse reaction to beta$_2$-agonists. **Oral beta-adrenergic agonists** available include terbutaline, 2.5–5.0 mg q6–8h; albuterol, 2–4 mg q6–8h; albuterol extended-release, 4–8 mg q12h; and metaproterenol, 10–20 mg q6–8h. Although their use has been associated with higher toxicity and side effects than inhaled beta-agonists, they may play a role in the management of nocturnal asthma (*Am Rev Respir Dis* 174:525, 1993), or in patients who cannot use inhaled medications.

b. **Theophylline and aminophylline** are the principal xanthines used in asthma therapy. Although their mechanism of action is still uncertain, it is clear that the therapeutic effects are not only due to bronchodilation but may also include an antiinflammatory effect, improved mucociliary clearance, ventilatory drive, and contractility of the diaphragm. In addition, they may enhance diuresis, improve cardiac output, reduce systemic and pulmonary vascular resistance, and decrease microvascular permeability (*Am Rev Respir Dis* 147:S33, 1993). Despite these beneficial effects, the use of theophylline has waned due to its controversial clinical efficacy and narrow therapeutic window, with adverse effects that range from tremor, nausea, anxiety, and palpitation to life-threatening arrhythmias and seizures. When used alone, IV aminophylline is less effective in relieving airflow obstruction than repetitive beta-agonist administration (*Am Rev Respir Dis* 122:365, 1980). When used in combination with aerosolized

Table 10-2. Aerosolized bronchodilators

Drug	Formulation	Adult dosage	Duration (hours)
Beta$_2$-adrenergic agonists			
Isoetharine (Bronkosol)	Nebulized 1% solution	0.3–0.5 ml	2–3
Metaproterenol (Alupent, others)	Nebulized 5% solution	0.2–0.3 ml	3–6
	MDI (650 µg/puff)	2–3 puffs q3–4h prn	
Albuterol (Proventil, Ventolin, others)	Nebulized 5% solution	2.5–5.0 mg	4–6
	MDI (90 µg/puff)	2–3 puffs q4–6h prn	
	Powder inhaler (200 µg Ventolin Rotacaps)	1–2 caps q4–6h prn	
Terbutaline (Brethaire)	MDI (200 µg/puff)	2–3 puffs q4–6h prn	4–6
Pirbuterol (Maxair)	MDI (200 µg/puff)	2–3 puffs q4–6h	4–6
Bitolterol mesylate (Tornalate)	MDI (370 µg/puff)	2–3 puffs q4–6h	4–6
Salmeterol* (Serevent)	MDI (21 µg/puff)	2 puffs q12h	12
Formoterol*	MDI	2 puffs q12h	12
Anticholinergics			
Atropine sulfate	Nebulized 1% solution	0.5–2.5 mg	4–6
Ipratropium bromide (Atrovent)	MDI (18 µg/puff)	2 puffs q4–6h	4–6
	Nebulized 0.02% solution	500 µg/vial	6–8
Glycopyrrolate (Robinul)	Solution (0.2 mg/ml)	0.8–2.0 mg q6–8h	6–8

MDI = metered-dose inhaler.
* Not available in the United States.

Table 10-3. Dosage of methylxanthines

Intravenous administration
  Loading dose of aminophylline (80% anhydrous theophylline)
    If no previous theophylline use: aminophylline 6 mg/kg (ideal body weight) over 20 min
    If previously taking theophylline (level not available): 3 mg/kg over 20 min
    If theophylline level known: aminophylline 1.25 mg/kg bolus for every 2 µg/ml desired increase in theophylline level
  Maintenance IV infusion (mg/kg/hr)

Smoking adult	0.8
Nonsmoking adult	0.5
Elderly	0.3
Cor pulmonale	0.3
Pregnant	0.3
Congestive heart failure	0.1–0.2
Liver disease	0.1–0.2

Oral administration
  Daily theophylline dose (mg) = total dose (mg) of aminophylline/24h ($\times$ 0.8).
  Start therapy at relatively low dose (400–600 mg/day). Increase by 100–200 mg/day following serum levels and therapeutic response.

Drugs that decrease theophylline clearance
  Cimetidine
  Macrolide antibiotics
  Ciprofloxacin and other quinolones
  Isoniazid
  Propranolol
  Calcium channel antagonists
  Mexiletine
  Allopurinol
  Oral contraceptives
  Caffeine
  Influenza vaccine

Drugs that increase theophylline clearance
  Phenytoin
  Phenobarbital
  Rifampin
  Carbamazepine
  Furosemide

beta-agonists, it has increased toxicity without additive benefit. Therefore, aminophylline therapy should not be used as a first-line agent but may be considered for hospitalized patients who do not respond to maximal inhaled bronchodilators (*Ann Intern Med* 119:1161, 1993). To minimize adverse effects, **theophylline dosages should be individualized** and serum levels should be monitored frequently (Table 10-3). In the outpatient (maintenance) management of asthma, sustained-release theophylline preparations can be particularly useful in the control of nocturnal asthma. However, the potential for significant adverse effects mandates appropriate dosing and monitoring.

  c. **Anticholinergic agents** (see Chronic Obstructive Pulmonary Disease, sec. **III.B.1**). Ipratropium bromide by MDI (2–4 puffs qid) may be useful in cases of refractory asthma or when there are intolerable side effects from other agents. Because of its adverse systemic side effects, atropine is no longer recommended in the treatment of asthma.

  d. **Magnesium sulfate,** 1.2 g IV over 20 minutes, has been reported to cause significant bronchodilation and subjective improvement in patients with severe and acute asthma exacerbation. Although the data are limited, it appears to be safe and effective when used in conjunction with beta$_2$-agonists and glucocorticoids (*Chest* 97:323, 1990; *JAMA* 262:1210, 1989).

B. Environmental control to reduce exposure to indoor and outdoor allergens is a critical component of asthma management. There is increasing evidence that the most important allergens associated with asthma are encountered indoors (i.e., house dust mite, cat, dog, cockroach, and indoor molds) and that measures to decrease the exposure to specific allergens can reduce asthma symptoms and decrease bronchial hyperreactivity (*Am Rev Respir Dis* 148:553, 1993).

Chronic Obstructive Pulmonary Disease

Chronic obstructive pulmonary disease (COPD) is a syndrome of chronic dyspnea with expiratory airflow obstruction that, unlike asthma, does not fluctuate markedly over periods of several months of observation. The term COPD includes chronic bronchitis and emphysema. However, other diseases such as cystic fibrosis (CF), bronchiectasis, or bronchiolitis obliterans are associated with chronic airflow limitation. Airflow obstruction may be worsened by airway inflammation, bronchospasm, mucus plugging, and fibrosis of small airways.

I. **Diagnosis and evaluation**

A. **History and physical examination.** Patients typically have a chronic productive cough for many years, followed by slowly progressive breathlessness with decreasing amounts of exertion. COPD is unusual in the absence of a history of cigarette smoking. Alpha$_1$-antitrypsin deficiency should be considered in non-smokers or young patients (age <50 years) with emphysema. On examination, tachypnea, pursed-lip breathing, and use of accessory muscles of respiration are commonly observed. The chest may be hyperresonant to percussion, breath sounds may be decreased, and adventitious sounds (wheezes, midinspiratory crackles, and large airway sounds) may be present. Signs of cor pulmonale may be present in severe or long-standing disease (see sec. **III.E**).

B. **Chest radiographs** often show low, flattened diaphragms. In severe emphysema, the lung fields may be hyperlucent, with diminished vascular markings and bullae. Disease is often most prominent in the upper lung zones except in alpha$_1$-antitrypsin deficiency, which may show a basilar predominance. Chest radiographs are of value during an acute exacerbation to exclude complications such as pneumonia and pneumothorax.

C. **Pulmonary function testing.** The FEV$_1$ and all other measurements of expiratory airflow are reduced. The FEV$_1$ is not only the standard way of assessing objectively the clinical course and response to therapy but also an important predictor of prognosis and mortality in patients with COPD (*Am Rev Respir Dis* 133:14, 1986). When the FEV$_1$ falls to less than 1 liter, the 5-year survival is approximately 50%. Total lung capacity (TLC), FRC, and RV may be increased. The diffusion capacity of carbon monoxide (DL$_{CO}$), although reduced in the presence of emphysema, is not specific.

D. **Arterial blood gases.** Gas exchange abnormalities vary with the type and severity of $\dot{V}/\dot{Q}$ abnormalities. Perfusion of poorly ventilated areas of the lungs (i.e., areas with low $\dot{V}/\dot{Q}$) results in an increased $P(A\text{-}a)O_2$ gradient and hypoxemia. A subpopulation of patients with severe airway obstruction will have chronically increased arterial PaCO$_2$, but metabolic compensation (increased serum bicarbonate) will maintain the arterial pH near normal. During an acute exacerbation of COPD, worsening airway obstruction, increased dead-space ventilation, and respiratory muscle fatigue may lead to rapid rises in PaCO$_2$, with subsequent acute respiratory acidosis (*Am Rev Respir Dis* 138:1006, 1988).

II. **Management of acute exacerbations.** A variety of insults may provoke bronchospasm or an increase in mucus secretion with plugging. The resulting increase in airway obstruction may cause worsening dyspnea, fatigue, and, sometimes, respiratory failure. Infections are the most common identifiable cause of acute exacerbations; the most common organisms implicated are *Streptococcus pneumoniae*, *Haemophilus influenzae*, *Mycoplasma pneumoniae*, *Moraxella (Branhamella) catarrhalis*, and viruses such as influenza and adenovirus. In addition, pulmonary emboli, pulmonary edema, and pneumothorax may all worsen gas exchange and increase breathlessness in patients with COPD. The therapeutic goals in the acute management of COPD exacerbations are to improve oxygenation, facilitate the clearance of secretions, decrease the resistive mechanical load, improve respiratory muscle force and endurance, treat precipitating factors such as infection or thromboembolism, correct electrolyte abnormalities, and avoid complications.

A. **Maintenance of adequate gas exchange**
   1. Oxygen should be administered to achieve and maintain a PaO_2 of 55–60 mm Hg (88–90% oxyhemoglobin saturation). The effectiveness of supplemental oxygen should be evaluated by serial arterial blood gas (ABG) determinations. Low-flow oxygen (1–3 liters/minute by nasal cannula or 24–35% oxygen by Venturi mask) is usually adequate. **Adequate oxygenation must be maintained, even in the face of increasing hypercapnia** (see Chap. 9). The requirement for high concentrations of supplemental oxygen suggests a complicating condition.
   2. **Mechanical ventilation** should be considered in patients with acute ventilatory failure (see Chap. 9).

B. **Inhaled beta$_2$-adrenergic agonists.** As in asthma, inhaled medications are best given by MDI (with a spacer device or reservoir if appropriate) with careful patient instruction. Inhaled beta$_2$-adrenergic agonists such as metaproterenol, terbutaline, or albuterol, 2–4 puffs initially, followed by 2 puffs q4h, are the mainstay of treatment for acute exacerbations of COPD (see Table 10-2).

C. **Anticholinergic agents** (see sec. III.B.1). Ipratropium bromide and beta-adrenergic agonists are equally efficacious in the treatment of acute exacerbations of COPD, but no further benefit is achieved with combination therapy (*Chest* 98:835, 1990). During acute exacerbations, the usual dose of ipratropium, 2 puffs qid, may be increased to 4–6 puffs q4–6h to produce maximal bronchodilation. These dosing regimens are well tolerated without added toxicity. Ipratropium is now available in solution for nebulization (see Table 10-2).

D. **Glucocorticoids.** Methylprednisolone, 0.5 mg/kg IV q6h for 3 days, may be used in patients with COPD. Improvement in airflow has been demonstrated in some patients (*Ann Intern Med* 92:753, 1980). Oral prednisone, 40–60 mg PO qd, is usually substituted after a few days and tapered as tolerated. The role of glucocorticoids for acute exacerbations in outpatients with COPD is controversial.

E. **Theophylline** administration in patients with COPD is controversial. There is considerable evidence to suggest that theophylline provides therapeutic benefit to some patients, improving airway function and dyspnea. Theophylline may also improve mucociliary clearance and central respiratory drive. The decision to use theophylline or IV aminophylline in the acute setting **should be individualized.** Dosage and administration are similar to those for asthma (see Table 10-3).

F. **Antimicrobial therapy.** For routine exacerbations of COPD in the absence of pneumonia, no reliable method of differentiating exacerbations caused by bacteria from exacerbations caused by other agents currently exists. A benefit from antibiotic therapy is most often seen in patients who have more severe underlying lung disease and in those who experience more severe exacerbations (*Ann Intern Med* 106:196, 1987). First-line antibiotic regimens for acute bacterial exacerbations of chronic bronchitis (see Chap. 13) consist of a 7- to 10-day course of oral therapy (e.g., (1) trimethoprim-sulfamethoxazole, 160 mg/800 mg [one double-strength tablet] PO bid; (2) amoxicillin, 250 mg PO tid; or (3) doxycycline, 100 mg PO bid).

G. **Chest physiotherapy** may improve clearance of secretions in patients with copious respiratory secretions (>50 ml/day). However, increased hypoxemia during chest percussion or postural drainage may occur (*Chest* 78:559, 1980).

III. **Long-term management** is aimed not only at relieving the main symptoms and managing acute exacerbations when they occur but, more important, slowing the progression of airflow obstruction and loss of vital capacity, preventing morbidity, and prolonging survival. Although the therapeutic armamentarium is extensive, only smoking cessation and the correction of hypoxemia improve survival.

   A. **Smoking cessation.** Interventions that may be beneficial include (1) repetitive counseling on the preventable health risks of smoking and advice to stop smoking, (2) encouraging patients to make further attempts to stop smoking even if they have failed previously, and (3) providing smoking cessation materials to patients. Nicotine-containing chewing gum, 2 mg chewed slowly over 20–30 minutes, repeated up to 60 mg/day, may reduce nicotine withdrawal symptoms and promote abstinence in some patients. It is most effective when used short-term in conjunction with formal smoking cessation programs or close medical follow-up. Transdermal nicotine patches are more convenient and better tolerated than nicotine polacrilex gum. The usual regimen is 6 weeks of the high-dose patch, 15–22 mg/day, followed by 2–4 weeks of the intermediate-dose patch, 10–14 mg/day, and 2–4 weeks of the low-dose patch, 5–7 mg/day. As with the nicotine gum, transdermal nicotine is only effective when used in combination with an organized smoking cessation program (*Clin Chest Med* 12:631, 1991; *JAMA* 272:1497, 1994).

   B. **Bronchodilators.** The optimal bronchodilator regimen for long-term management of COPD has not been established. **Inhaled anticholinergic agents and inhaled beta-adrenergic agonists** may be beneficial in stable COPD.

   1. **Anticholinergic agents** are now considered the **first-line drug for most patients with stable COPD**, based on studies showing that ipratropium is as effective as beta-adrenergic agonists and has a longer duration of action and less toxicity. The usual dosage of 2 puffs q4–6h can be doubled or tripled to achieve maximal bronchodilation (*N Engl J Med* 328:1017, 1993); minor side effects include cough and dry mouth.

   2. **Beta-adrenergic agonists** are still commonly used; however, safety of long-term administration of beta-adrenergic agonists is controversial. In addition to the well-known adrenergic side effects, concerns regarding tolerance (tachyphylaxis), acute or long-term rebound bronchoconstriction, and deterioration of pulmonary function have been suggested (*Arch Intern Med* 153:814, 1993) (see Asthma, sec. **III.A.2** and Table 10-2).

   3. **Oral theophylline preparations** provide therapeutic benefit to some COPD patients (see sec. **II.E**). Administration of long-acting preparations in the evening may improve the overnight decline in lung function and morning respiratory symptoms (*Am Rev Respir Dis* 145:540, 1992) (see Table 10-3).

   C. **Glucocorticoids.** A minority of outpatients with stable COPD have a response to glucocorticoids. Many of those who respond have significant improvements (e.g., greater than 50% improvement in FEV_1). However, there is no way to predict glucocorticoid-responsiveness with certainty. A trial of glucocorticoids (prednisone 30–60 mg/day for 2 weeks) with spirometric evaluation before and after the trial may help identify these patients (*Med Clin North Am* 74:661, 1990) and therapy should be continued only if pulmonary function test (PFT) values improve significantly (e.g., 15% improvement in FEV_1 or 20% improvement in FVC) on repeat testing in 2–3 weeks. The lowest effective dose should be used, and alternate-day therapy is preferred. Inhaled glucocorticoids should be substituted for systemic glucocorticoids when possible (*Am Rev Respir Dis* 146:389, 1992).

   D. **Oxygen therapy** has been shown to improve survival and quality of life in patients with COPD and chronic hypoxemia. Results are best with continuous oxygen administration (*Ann Intern Med* 93:391, 1980; *Lancet* 1:681, 1981). PaO_2 should be maintained at approximately 60 mm Hg. Increased oxygen supply may be required with exercise and sleep. Criteria for continuous or intermittent long-term oxygen therapy include (1) a PaO_2 consistently less than 55 mm Hg or oxyhemoglobin saturation less than 88% by pulse oximetry at rest, with exercise, or during sleep despite optimal medical therapy or (2) PaO_2 of 55–59 mm Hg with evidence of cor pulmonale or secondary polycythemia (hematocrit >55%). A 1- to 3-month period of observation with reassessment of oxygenation to ensure clinical stability is recommended prior to committing a patient to long-term oxygen therapy. The type of oxygen delivery system prescribed should be individualized.

E. **Pulmonary hypertension and cor pulmonale in patients with COPD** may present clinically as a progressive decrease in exercise tolerance in the absence of worsening airflow limitation. Physical examination may reveal a parasternal heave, an accentuated P_2 heart sound, a right parasternal S_4, or later in the course an S_3 or a murmur of tricuspid insufficiency in association with a pulsatile liver and lower extremity edema. An ECG, echocardiography with Doppler measurement of the tricuspid jet, and radionuclide ventriculography can provide useful information regarding right ventricular function. The primary approach to treatment is to optimize the use of inhaled bronchodilators and provide oxygen therapy. Digoxin should only be considered for patients in whom left ventricular failure is also present (*Ann Intern Med* 95:283, 1981). Diuretics should be used cautiously, since they may be poorly tolerated in patients dependent on preload. In addition, diuretics may precipitate a metabolic alkalosis that can be deleterious in the hypercapnic patient. Phlebotomy should be considered when the hematocrit, despite supplemental oxygen, is greater than 50% in the presence of pulmonary vascular or central nervous system compromise. Vasodilator therapy trials have not shown a survival benefit and are not recommended (*Am Rev Respir Dis* 148:1414, 1993).

F. **A general rehabilitation program**, including exercise training and proper nutrition, may help improve the patient's exercise tolerance and sense of well-being.

G. **Influenza vaccine and pneumococcal vaccine** are recommended for patients with COPD (see Appendix E, Table E-1).

H. **Psychoactive drugs** should be used with caution in patients with COPD. Buspirone (5–10 mg PO tid) is an anxiolytic agent not related to benzodiazepines that is usually well tolerated; however, it takes several weeks to become effective. Doxepin (25–100 mg/day) is the agent of choice in agitated depression, and it can contribute a minor bronchodilating effect. Protriptyline (20 mg/day, taken at bedtime) is a nonsedating tricyclic antidepressant that improves diurnal and nocturnal hypoxemia in patients with COPD (*Ann Intern Med* 113:507, 1990).

I. **Alpha₁-proteinase inhibitor** administration may be appropriate in patients older than 18 years, with documented alpha₁-antitrypsin deficiency (<11 μm of alpha ₁-antitrypsin/liter) and airflow obstruction (FEV_1 between 30 and 65% of normal) who have stopped smoking. Weekly IV administration of Prolastin, 60 mg/kg, is safe and effective in achieving normal plasma levels of antitrypsin; however, its long-term benefit has not been established (*Am Rev Respir Dis* 140:1494, 1989; *Ann Intern Med* 111:957, 1989).

Cystic Fibrosis

Cystic fibrosis (CF) is the most common lethal genetic disease in white populations. It is inherited in an autosomal-recessive fashion, with heterozygotes being asymptomatic carriers. The median survival of those with the disease has improved to approximately 29 years, and nearly one-third of the CF population consists of adolescents and adults (*Science* 256:774, 1992). The genetic defect responsible for CF has been identified (*Science* 245:1073, 1989) as a mutation that leads to abnormal chloride permeability at epithelial surfaces.

I. **Diagnosis**

A. **Clinical manifestations** of CF reflect the profound alteration of exocrine secretions such that mucus becomes excessively thick and tenacious and sweat becomes salty. **Pulmonary disease** accounts for most of the morbidity and mortality and is characterized by a chronic progressive course with acute exacerbations. The presenting symptoms of cough, purulent sputum, hemoptysis, wheezing, and dyspnea are variable and depend on the extent of supraimposed infection. The **extrapulmonary manifestations** of CF are intestinal (constipation, volvulus, intussusception, fecal impaction, rectal prolapse); pancreatic (malabsorption, malnutrition, pancreatitis, diabetes mellitus); hepatobiliary (fatty liver, cholelithiasis, cholecystitis, biliary cirrhosis, portal hypertension); genitourinary (sterility, infertility, epididymitis); and skeletal (hypertrophic osteoarthropathy, retardation of growth and bone age, demineralization).

B. **Laboratory studies**
1. **Sweat testing** using the pilocarpine iontophoresis method remains the gold standard for the diagnosis of CF. A sweat test diagnostic for CF has chloride greater than 60 mEq/liter.
2. **Chest radiography** usually reveals increased interstitial, reticular marking, bronchiectasis, and hilar adenopathy. The upper lobes are generally more involved than the lower lobes.
3. **Pulmonary function tests** are consistent with an obstructive abnormality, with evidence of air trapping and bronchial hyperreactivity in some patients. Later in the course, hypoxemia and progressive hypercapnia occur.
4. **Sputum culture and sensitivities of the cultured organisms** are mandatory during exacerbations. Although the most characteristic organism associated with CF is *Pseudomonas aeruginosa*, organisms such as *Staphylococcus aureus*, *H. influenzae,* and *P. cepacia* are also common.

II. **Therapy.** The goals of therapy for CF pulmonary disease are to decrease the burden of infection, to provide bronchopulmonary hygiene, to aid in the clearance of secretions, to maintain adequate nutrition, and to improve airflow. As the disease progresses, supplemental oxygen is required and referral for lung transplantation should be considered.

A. **Antibiotics. IV antibiotics** are the treatment of choice for acute exacerbations of CF. Since *P. aeruginosa* is the most frequent pathogen, a combination of a semisynthetic penicillin or a third-generation cephalosporin with antipseudomonal activity and an aminoglycoside are usually selected, pending results from sputum cultures. Mild exacerbations may be treated with oral antipseudomonal antimicrobials. The use of chronic prophylactic and suppressive oral and inhaled antibiotics remains controversial. **Direct aerosolized tobramycin** in patients with clinically stable disease has been shown to improve pulmonary function and decrease the density of *P. aeruginosa* (*N Engl J Med* 328:1740, 1993). However, the long-term impact on emergence of resistant strains and overall outcome is still uncertain.

B. **Bronchial hygiene**
1. **Chest physiotherapy** consisting of postural drainage with percussion, breathing exercises, vigorous coughing, and participation in an exercise program have been shown to have short-term clinical utility in removing mucus secretions and improving pulmonary function and physical performance; however, oxygen desaturation and exercise-induced bronchospasm may occur with its use.
2. **Bronchodilators** are used for patients with bronchial hyperreactivity (see Asthma, sec. **III.A.2** and Table 10-2).
3. **Glucocorticoid** use in patients with CF is controversial. Limited data available suggest a beneficial effect without worsening of bacterial infection or growth retardation (*Lancet* 2:686, 1985; *Pediatrics* 87:245, 1991). Due to the adverse effects of glucocorticoids, chronic use is not recommended.
4. **Recombinant human deoxyribonuclease I (rhDNase),** has been approved for the treatment of CF. By digesting extracellular DNA, rhDNase decreases the viscoelasticity of the sputum and has been shown in clinical studies to improve pulmonary function and decrease the risk of respiratory tract infections that require parenteral antibiotics (*N Engl J Med* 326:812, 1992; *Am Rev Respir Dis* 148:145, 1993). The recommended dosage is Pulmozyme, 2.5 mg/day inhaled using a jet nebulizer. Adverse effects reported with

rhDNase include pharyngitis, laryngitis, voice alteration, rash, chest pain, and conjunctivitis.

C. **Oxygen therapy** is indicated in patients with hypoxemia at rest, at night, during exercise, or if there is evidence of pulmonary hypertension.

D. **Lung transplantation.** The majority of patients with CF die of pulmonary disease. Thus, when the clinical course of patients with CF has progressed to cause resting hypoxemia, hypercapnia, and increasing frequency or severity of exacerbations, transplantation should be considered. The actuarial 1-year survival for CF patients after lung transplantation is 58–65% (*J Thorac Cardiovasc Surg* 103:287, 1992).

Pulmonary Embolism

Pulmonary thromboembolism is an important cause of morbidity and mortality, especially among hospitalized patients. The majority of clinically significant pulmonary emboli arise from deep venous thromboses (DVTs) in the iliofemoral system; many of the remainder arise in the pelvic venous plexus as postsurgical or gynecologic complications. Predisposing factors for thromboembolic disease include venous disease of the lower extremities, carcinoma, heart failure, recent pelvic or lower abdominal surgery, prolonged immobilization, pregnancy, and administration of estrogens. The clinical manifestations of acute pulmonary embolism may be nonspecific and vary widely, ranging from tachycardia to hypotension and sudden death. The most common symptoms are dyspnea, pleuritic chest pain, apprehension, and cough; frequent physical findings include tachypnea, tachycardia, accentuation of the pulmonic component of the second heart sound, and inspiratory crackles (*Am Heart J* 103:239, 1982). Pleuritic chest pain and hemoptysis suggest pulmonary infarction.

I. **Diagnosis** of pulmonary embolism is based on clinical suspicion, ancillary laboratory data, and the results of specific diagnostic studies. It is important to consider pulmonary embolism and the antecedent DVT as one clinical entity, wherein the diagnosis of either component establishes the indication for treatment.

A. **A general diagnostic evaluation** should include ABG analysis, which may demonstrate an increased $P(A-a)O_2$ gradient. Arterial hypoxemia with a PaO_2 below 80 mm Hg occurs in the majority of patients without underlying cardiopulmonary disease (*Chest* 81:495, 1982) and is usually accompanied by hypocapnia. The ECG most often demonstrates sinus tachycardia and may show signs of right heart strain; rhythm disturbances such as atrial fibrillation or flutter occur less frequently. Chest radiographs are generally unremarkable or demonstrate subsegmental atelectasis. Pleural effusion occurs in 30–50% of cases but is often small. Although uncommon, pleural-based infiltrates may be present, especially in the lower lobes. Areas of hyperlucency in the lung fields may result from oligemia.

B. **Specific diagnostic studies** are necessary in patients suspected of having pulmonary emboli. The patient's clinical status and previously obtained data determine which tests to order and the sequence in which they should be performed.

1. **Ventilation-perfusion ($\dot{V}/\dot{Q}$) lung scans** should be performed in all clinically stable patients with suspected pulmonary emboli. The information obtained, however, depends not only on the quality and interpretation of the scan but also on the clinician's estimation of the probability of pulmonary emboli in the patient being studied (pretest probability) (Table 10-4). Thus, a $\dot{V}/\dot{Q}$ scan is most useful when the $\dot{V}/\dot{Q}$ result category is either normal, low, or high probability and is concordant with the clinician's pretest suspicion of pulmonary embolism. Further evaluation is usually indicated in patients with intermediate probability $\dot{V}/\dot{Q}$ scans and in patients with low-probability studies when the clinical suspicion of pulmonary embolism is high (*Ann Intern Med* 114:300, 1991; *JAMA* 263:2753, 1990).

Table 10-4. Presence of pulmonary embolism (%) by angiogram combining pretest probability and ventilation-perfusion ($\dot{V}/\dot{Q}$) lung scan results

$\dot{V}/\dot{Q}$ scan category	Clinical science pretest probability			
	80–100	20–79	0–19	All
High probability	96	88	56	87
Intermediate probability	66	28	16	30
Low probability	40	16	4	14
Near normal/normal	0	6	2	4
Total	68	30	9	28

Source: Data from PIOPED Investigators. Value of the ventilation/perfusion scan in acute pulmonary embolism: Results of the Prospective Investigation of Pulmonary Embolism Diagnosis (PIOPED). *JAMA* 263:2753, 1990.

2. **Evaluation for deep venous thrombosis** may support a diagnosis of thromboembolic disease in patients in whom a $\dot{V}/\dot{Q}$ scan is nondiagnostic. Impedance plethysmography and Doppler ultrasonography are noninvasive techniques for the diagnosis of DVT in the thigh. However, both of these methods have a low sensitivity (24–38%) in asymptomatic patients (*Arch Intern Med* 151:2167, 1991; *Ann Intern Med* 117:735, 1992), and even in the setting of symptomatic DVT their sensitivity is only 66% in detecting DVT (*Ann Intern Med* 118:25, 1993). Venous duplex scanning, which provides ultrasonic venous imaging with Doppler blood-flow imaging, may have greater accuracy than either technique. These noninvasive tests can be used individually or in combination, depending on availability and expertise in interpretation. Venography may be needed to make a definitive diagnosis.

3. **Pulmonary angiography** should be performed whenever clinical data and noninvasive tests are equivocal or contradictory (*Circulation* 85:462, 1992). When reasonable clinical suspicion of pulmonary emboli exists, the risks of untreated pulmonary embolism or of complications from unnecessary anticoagulation outweigh the morbidity and mortality of pulmonary angiography (*Am J Med* 70:17, 1981). In addition, pulmonary angiography is appropriate in patients with a high probability of pulmonary embolism by $\dot{V}/\dot{Q}$ scan, if the risks of anticoagulation are high, or if vena caval interruption or thrombolytic therapy is being considered. Pulmonary angiography may be the appropriate initial diagnostic test in patients who are hemodynamically unstable.

II. **Treatment**
   A. **Supportive care.** Supplemental oxygen should be given to correct hypoxemia. Patients with hypotension and reduced cardiac output that do not rapidly respond to IV saline infusion should be treated with norepinephrine or dopamine and should be considered for thrombolytic therapy or surgical intervention (see sec. **II.C**).
   B. **Prevention of recurrent emboli** is the major therapeutic goal.
      1. **Anticoagulation** (see Chap. 17) with IV heparin should be started immediately based on the clinical suspicion of pulmonary embolism without waiting for definitive studies to be obtained, unless there is an absolute contraindication for anticoagulation. A bolus of heparin, 5,000 IU, followed by a continuous infusion (e.g., 1,200 units/hour) titrated individually to an activated partial thromboplastin time (aPTT) between 1.5 and 2.5 times the control value is continued for 5–10 days. Adjusted-dose SC heparin is also acceptable. Oral warfarin therapy can be initiated once the aPTT is therapeutic, or concurrently with the initiation of heparin. An overlap of 3–5 days with an international normalized ratio (INR) system of 2.0–3.0 and a therapeutic aPTT is recommended. Adopting this approach is not associated

with any greater risk of recurrent thromboembolism or bleeding complications and may lead to a shorter hospitalization (*Arch Intern Med* 152:1589, 1992). Warfarin is then continued for approximately 3 months, or indefinitely if risk factors are still present or thromboembolism is recurrent (*Chest* 102:408S, 1992). Although not yet approved by the U.S. Food and Drug Administration for the treatment of proximal DVT, low-molecular-weight fractions of commercial heparin have equal (or greater) antithrombotic efficacy, with less hemorrhagic complications (see Chap. 17).

   2. **Inferior vena caval interruption** should be considered in the following settings: (1) pulmonary embolism in patients in whom anticoagulants are absolutely contraindicated (e.g., active bleeding, immediate postoperative state, neurosurgical patients, severe diastolic hypertension), (2) documented recurrent embolic events in patients who are adequately anticoagulated, (3) massive pulmonary emboli with hemodynamic compromise, especially if there is evidence of residual thrombus in a lower extremity, (4) patients with compromised cardiac or pulmonary function who may not survive a recurrent event, (5) patients undergoing pulmonary embolectomy, (6) patients with paradoxic emboli via a patent foramen ovale, or (7) septic pulmonary emboli from lower extremities or pelvic veins. If a transvenous filter device is placed in the vena cava, heparin therapy should be continued (unless otherwise contraindicated), since heparin will prevent extension of an already existing clot and development of postphlebitic venous insufficiency.

C. **Specific therapy**
   1. **Systemic thrombolytic therapy** with streptokinase, urokinase, or recombinant tissue plasminogen activator hastens the resolution of thrombi but has not yet been shown to reduce mortality in patients with pulmonary emboli. Thrombolytic therapy should be considered in the treatment of patients with acute massive embolism who are hemodynamically unstable and do not appear prone to bleeding.
   2. **Pulmonary embolectomy** should be considered only in the rare patients with angiographically proven pulmonary emboli (1) who remain in shock despite thrombolytic therapy and supportive care, or (2) in whom thrombolytic therapy would be appropriate but is contraindicated.

III. **Chronic thromboembolic pulmonary hypertension** is a complication that occurs in a minority of patients who fail to resolve a thromboembolic pulmonary event, with resultant pulmonary vascular obstruction and consequent pulmonary hypertension. The syndrome should be considered in patients with unexplained dyspnea on exercise in association with physical findings of pulmonary hypertension (see Chronic Obstructive Pulmonary Disease, sec. **III.E**). The lung perfusion scan may help differentiate this condition from primary pulmonary hypertension. Subsequent invasive evaluation including cardiac catheterization, angiography, or angioscopy are best referred to experienced medical teams who can perform surgical thromboendarterectomy (*Circulation* 81:1735, 1990).

Adult Respiratory
Distress Syndrome

The adult respiratory distress syndrome (ARDS) is a form of acute lung injury attributable to a wide variety of insults. The predominant medical risk factor for ARDS is sepsis, particularly from an abdominal source (*Am Rev Respir Dis* 132:485, 1985). Other predisposing conditions include major trauma, aspiration of gastric contents, and drug overdose (including heroin, methadone, and barbiturates). The common end result is disruption of the alveolar capillary membrane, leading to increased vascular permeability and accumulation of neutrophils and protein-rich edema in the alveolar space.

I. **Diagnosis** requires exclusion of other causes of pulmonary edema. Patients with ARDS have respiratory distress with severe hypoxemia despite a high fractional concentration of inspired oxygen (F_IO_2). Chest radiographs demonstrate diffuse infiltrates without cardiomegaly or pulmonary vascular redistribution. Significant pleural effusions are unusual in ARDS unless there is a complicating illness.

II. **Therapy** centers on maintaining adequate tissue oxygen delivery while minimizing the risk of oxygen toxicity from prolonged exposure to high concentrations of supplemental oxygen (i.e., F_IO_2 >0.5). Additional goals of therapy include identification and treatment of the underlying disorder and prevention of complications. Empiric antimicrobial therapy is often appropriate until infection can be excluded.

A. **Oxygenation.** Mechanical ventilation with positive end-expiratory pressure (PEEP) usually allows maintenance of an adequate PaO_2 with an acceptably low F_IO_2 (see Chap. 9). Because of the possibility of adverse hemodynamic consequences with high levels of PEEP (i.e., >10 cm H_2O), invasive hemodynamic monitoring may be indicated. Patients must also be monitored carefully for other complications of mechanical ventilation, especially barotrauma (see Chap. 9).

B. **Invasive monitoring** (see Chap. 9) with a pulmonary artery catheter may be useful for (1) ensuring adequate cardiac output and mixed venous oxygen content when using high levels of PEEP, and (2) obtaining the lowest pulmonary artery occlusive pressure (PAOP) or lung water compatible with an adequate cardiac output (*Am Rev Respir Dis* 145:990, 1992).

C. **Intravascular volume.** Pulmonary edema may be minimized by maintaining the lowest intravascular volume compatible with adequate tissue perfusion (*Chest* 100:1068, 1991). Blood hemoglobin should be kept greater than 10 mg/dl to optimize oxygen delivery.

D. **Complications.** Despite supportive measures, mortality remains high (50% overall and higher when associated with sepsis). If the patient survives the acute phase, multiple organ dysfunction and secondary pulmonary infections are the most frequent causes of death (*Chest* 101:320, 1992). Superimposed pneumonia is difficult to diagnose in patients with diffuse pulmonary infiltrates. Therefore, if clinical and radiographic changes consistent with pneumonia develop, aggressive antimicrobial therapy is indicated.

E. **Antiinflammatory therapy.** Since interstitial and alveolar inflammation are prominent features of ARDS, the use of agents that can decrease the magnitude of the inflammatory response or block specific substances thought to mediate tissue damage seems attractive (*Chest* 103:932, 1993). However, their use has not been demonstrated to improve the outcome in ARDS. In addition, several clinical trials have not shown benefit with the use of glucocorticoids in the acute phase of ARDS (first 72 hours) (*N Engl J Med* 317:653, 1987; *N Engl J Med* 317:1565, 1987; *Am Rev Respir Dis* 138:62, 1988).

F. **Nitric oxide (NO)**, a potent gaseous vasodilator given by inhalation in patients with severe ARDS, has been shown to reduce pulmonary arterial pressure and improve oxygenation (*N Engl J Med* 328:399, 1993). However, large-scale clinical trials will be required to define its impact on outcome.

Pneumonia, Pulmonary Aspiration Syndromes, and Lung Abscess

I. **Pneumonia**

A. **Pneumonia in the immunocompetent host.** Diagnosis and treatment of community-acquired and nosocomial pneumonia in the normal host are discussed in Chap. 13.

B. **Pulmonary infiltrates in the immunocompromised host.** Immunocompromised patients include those with severe defects in lymphocyte or granulocyte number or function. Host defenses are significantly impaired in patients with AIDS (see sec. I.C and Chap. 14), in those with hematologic malignancy, and in those undergoing immunosuppressive therapy for malignancy or organ transplantation (*Am Rev Respir Dis* 144:213, 1991).

1. **Causes of pulmonary infiltrates** in this population are diverse, but the differential diagnosis may be narrowed by noting the specific host immune defect and the rate of onset and radiographic appearance of the pulmonary process (*Ann Intern Med* 117:415, 1992). **Noninfectious etiologies** include spread of malignancy, cytotoxic drug reactions, radiation pneumonitis, pulmonary hemorrhage, pulmonary edema, and pulmonary embolus. **Infectious etiologies,** however, account for the majority of infiltrates and have a mortality approaching 50%. During the first month following **organ transplantation,** bacterial infections and herpes simplex virus predominate; over the next several months, when immunosuppression is greatest, opportunistic infections are common and are due to organisms such as *Nocardia* species, fungi (e.g., *Aspergillus* species, *Cryptococcus*), viruses (e.g., cytomegalovirus [CMV] and varicella-zoster), and *Pneumocystis carinii*. Patients with **severe neutropenia** (absolute granulocyte count <500/μl) are also at markedly increased risk for infection with these organisms and are particularly susceptible to infection with *P. aeruginosa* and *Aspergillus* species (see Chap. 14). Specific pulmonary problems related to **AIDS** are discussed in sec. **I.C** (see Chap. 14).
2. **Diagnostic evaluation.** Empiric antimicrobial therapy should be initiated after a rapid clinical evaluation is performed and cultures are obtained. In patients without rapid clinical improvement (e.g., within 1–3 days), invasive procedures (e.g., bronchoscopy, lung biopsy) are generally pursued because of the large differential diagnosis, the necessity for effective antimicrobial therapy, and the potential toxicity of unnecessary therapy.
   a. **Fiberoptic bronchoscopy (FOB)** with bronchoalveolar lavage and transbronchial lung biopsies are complementary and have a combined diagnostic yield of 60–90% in the presence of diffuse pulmonary involvement (*Ann Intern Med* 117:415, 1992). Bacteria, atypical mycobacteria, and fungi recovered from washings may reflect upper airway colonization, and confirmation with quantitative cultures and special stains of biopsy specimens is helpful in identifying true pathogens. FOB is less sensitive in diagnosing noninfectious causes of pulmonary infiltrates. Transbronchial biopsy is relatively contraindicated in the presence of uncorrected coagulopathy, severe hypoxemia, uremia, and mechanical ventilation.
   b. **Open lung biopsy** requires a thoracoscopy or thoracotomy but allows for better control of bleeding and air leaks. Diagnostic yield, particularly for noninfectious etiologies, is higher than with FOB. This procedure is generally reserved for patients who are rapidly deteriorating, have contraindications to transbronchial biopsy, or have had nondiagnostic FOB and are not improving clinically.
3. **Treatment of pneumonia in immunocompromised patients.** Therapy includes supportive measures, supplemental oxygen, antibiotics, and mechanical ventilation if respiratory failure develops. Empiric broad-spectrum antimicrobial therapy should include coverage for *P. aeruginosa* and *Staph. aureus* (see Chap. 12). Amphotericin is often added if the patient fails to respond to initial antimicrobial therapy, especially if there is evidence of superficial fungal colonization or infection; however, a tissue diagnosis of invasive fungal infection should be pursued (*Am J Med* 72:101, 1982). Therapy should be adjusted if a specific etiologic diagnosis is obtained. The greatest impact on ultimate outcome is the response to therapy or resolution of the underlying disorder that initially produced the patient's immunodeficiency.
C. **Pulmonary infiltrates in patients with AIDS.** Almost 50% of AIDS patients initially present with pulmonary disease, most commonly on the basis of an opportunistic pulmonary infection (*Am Rev Respir Dis* 135:504, 1987) (see Chap. 14). The most common pulmonary infection is *P. carinii* pneumonia, although prophylactic therapy has been effective in reducing the incidence of this diagnosis.
   1. **Clinical manifestations of PCP** often include the acute or insidious onset of nonproductive cough and dyspnea. The lung examination may be normal, or

scattered crackles may be present. The chest radiograph often demonstrates diffuse interstitial or alveolar infiltrates. Occasionally, focal infiltrates are seen or the radiograph appears normal. In patients who have been receiving prophylactic aerosolized pentamidine, PCP may occur as upper lobe infiltrates. Gas exchange abnormalities are usually present.

2. **Differential diagnosis**
   a. **Opportunistic infections** account for the majority of pulmonary complications in patients with AIDS. Other common opportunistic infections besides PCP that occur alone, or more often in addition to PCP, include those due to *Mycobacterium avium-intracellulare* (MAI) and CMV. *Cryptococcus neoformans, Histoplasma capsulatum, Toxoplasma gondii, Coccidioides immitis, Blastomyces dermatitidis,* and herpes simplex virus pneumonia also occur but are less common (see Chap. 14).
   b. **Nonopportunistic pathogenic organisms** associated with HIV infection include pyogenic bacteria (e.g., *Strep. pneumoniae* and *H. influenzae*) and *Mycobacterium tuberculosis.* Tuberculosis often presents with atypical, noncavitary infiltrates and mediastinal and hilar adenopathy in this patient population.
   c. **Neoplasms.** Kaposi's sarcoma (KS) is common and may cause pulmonary symptoms and radiographic infiltrates in HIV patients with cutaneous KS (*Thorax* 47:726, 1992). Pulmonary involvement of patients with non-Hodgkin's lymphoma may also complicate AIDS and implies a poor prognosis.
   d. **Lymphocytic and nonspecific interstitial pneumonitis** may be seen on biopsy, but the implications of these diagnoses are unclear.

3. **Diagnostic evaluation** of patients with pulmonary symptoms who have or are at high risk for AIDS should be performed if an infiltrate is seen on chest radiograph, or gas exchange abnormalities are present. IV drug abuse may produce similar abnormalities as a result of either infectious etiologies or from a reaction to IV contaminants and particles from injected materials. Evaluation should be directed toward identifying treatable infections.
   a. **Induced sputum samples** can be used to detect *P. carinii;* the reliability of this method depends on expertise in collection and interpretation of these specimens. **Stains and cultures** of sputum for mycobacteria, fungi, and bacteria should also be performed. **Cytology** is occasionally diagnostic.
   b. **Fiberoptic bronchoscopy** with bronchoalveolar lavage (BAL) and transbronchial biopsy have a 90% sensitivity for diagnosing infectious processes in patients with AIDS and have a higher yield for *P. carinii* pneumonia. Kaposi's sarcoma may also be diagnosed by FOB.
   c. **Open lung biopsy** is generally reserved for patients who are unable to safely undergo transbronchial biopsy and in whom BAL is nondiagnostic.

4. **Therapy.** Empiric therapy for PCP is recommended while awaiting completion of FOB and interpretation of the results. Glucocorticoid therapy appears to have benefit in patients with moderately severe *P. carinii* pneumonia (defined by PaO_2 <75 mm Hg on room air) (*N Engl J Med* 323:1500, 1990) (see Table 14-2). Specific treatment should be instituted for documented *P. carinii,* fungal, bacterial, and *M. tuberculosis* infections (see Chap. 13). MAI may be resistant to therapy, although the clinical significance of this infection is unclear. Neoplasms causing symptomatic airway obstruction or hemoptysis may be controlled with radiotherapy.

II. **Pulmonary aspiration syndromes** occur most often in patients with decreased level of consciousness, impaired pharyngeal or laryngeal function (e.g., myopathy, neuropathy, immediately postextubation), increased intragastric pressure or volume (e.g., nausea, vomiting, ileus, tube feeding), or esophageal disorders that predispose patients to reflux (*Clin Chest Med* 12:269, 1991).
   A. **Aspiration of gastric contents** may have a variety of consequences.
      1. **Aspiration of inert liquids or foreign bodies** may cause a syndrome of airway obstruction and manifest clinically as acute respiratory distress or hypoxemia. Radiographic evidence of pulmonary infiltrates, atelectasis, or lobar

collapse may be present. The possible presence of aspirated food particles must always be considered in patients with known aspiration of gastric contents and focal infiltrates. Early bronchoscopy is frequently indicated, especially if the patient has signs of parenchymal volume loss, or localized wheezing.

2. **Chemical pneumonitis** occurs if the pH of the aspirate is low (<2.5) or the volume of acidic aspirate is large. Symptoms of cough, dyspnea, and wheezing will vary depending on the patient's level of consciousness. Tachypnea, tachycardia, hypotension, and fever may be seen in association with rales, increased $P(A-a)O_2$, and pulmonary infiltrates. If aspiration is massive, ARDS may develop. With the exception of aspiration associated with intestinal obstruction, severe gingivitis and periodontitis, or immunocompromised status, antibiotics should be withheld until there is evidence of bacterial superinfection (see sec. **II.A.3**) (*Clin Chest Med* 12:269, 1991).

3. **Aspiration pneumonia** occurs in approximately 40% of patients who aspirate, most commonly 2–5 days after the initial event, and is often caused by **mixed aerobic-anaerobic organisms.** It may be difficult to discriminate between bacterial pneumonia and chemical pneumonitis. Penicillin G or clindamycin is usually effective, but broader coverage should be considered in hospitalized patients because they are more likely to be colonized with gram-negative bacilli and *Staph. aureus* (see Chap. 13).

III. **Lung abscess** most often follows aspiration of oropharyngeal contents containing large numbers of anaerobes. Extensive gingival and dental disease facilitate the growth of anaerobic organisms and thus predispose to such infections. The onset of illness may be insidious with constitutional symptoms, fever, and weight loss. Foul-smelling sputum suggests infection with anaerobic bacteria.

A. **Evaluation.** Other causes of cavitary lung disease should be considered, including tuberculosis, fungal disease, acute necrotizing pneumonia (e.g., gram-negative bacilli and *Staph. aureus*), carcinoma, vasculitis, septic embolism, and pulmonary embolism with infarction. Sputum should be cultured for mycobacteria and fungi, and skin testing with an intermediate-strength purified protein derivative (PPD) should be performed. Bronchoscopy is indicated if an obstructing tumor or foreign body is suspected.

B. **Therapy.** Postural drainage of the involved segment is performed to facilitate removal of secretions. Antibiotic treatment with aqueous penicillin G, 1.5–2.0 million units IV q4h, is satisfactory, although treatment with clindamycin may hasten the resolution of anaerobic lung abscesses (*Ann Intern Med* 98:486, 1983). Therapy can be switched to oral penicillin VK, 500 mg PO q6h, once there is a definite clinical response, and should be continued until the cavity closes. Healing may take 6–12 months. Surgical resection or percutaneous drainage of a lung abscess is only rarely required for a nonresolving abscess with persistent fevers and leukocytosis despite appropriate medical therapy, the development of a bronchopleural fistula, empyema, persistent hemoptysis, evidence of an enlarging cavity, or mechanical ventilation dependence (*Ann Thorac Surg* 44:356, 1987; *Radiology* 178:347, 1991).

Interstitial Lung Disease

The interstitial lung diseases are a heterogeneous group of disorders. Pathologically, these diseases are characterized by acute, subacute, or chronic infiltration of the alveolar walls by cells, fluid, and connective tissue. The initial intraalveolar and interstitial inflammation, if left untreated, may progress to irreversible fibrosis, altered alveolar architecture, and impaired gas exchange. The differential diagnosis of interstitial lung disease is extensive (Table 10-5).

I. **Clinical manifestations**

A. **General.** Patients typically present with breathlessness and a nonproductive cough. The physical examination, chest radiograph, PFTs, and ABG abnormalities vary depending on the underlying etiology.

Table 10-5. Common causes of interstitial lung disease

Known etiologies
  Occupational or environmental inhalants
    Dusts (organic, inorganic); gases (oxygen toxicity); fumes
  Drugs (e.g., cytotoxic agents, amiodarone, nitrofurantoin, gold)
  Radiation
  Infections (viral, bacterial, fungal, parasites)
  Hypersensitivity pneumonitis
  Pulmonary edema (cardiogenic or noncardiogenic)
  Neoplasms (e.g., lymphangitic spread of carcinoma, lymphoma, alveolar-cell
    carcinoma)
  Metabolic causes
Unknown etiologies
  Sarcoidosis
  Idiopathic pulmonary fibrosis (cryptogenic fibrosing alveolitis)
  Interstitial disease associated with collagen-vascular disorders
  Pulmonary vasculitis
  Pulmonary hemorrhage syndromes (e.g., Goodpasture's, idiopathic
    hemosiderosis)
  Eosinophilic granuloma
  Alveolar proteinosis
  Amyloidosis
  Veno-occlusive disease
  Microlithiasis
  Neurofibromatosis, tuberous sclerosis, lymphangioleiomyomatosis
  Bronchiolitis obliterans organizing pneumonia

    B. Clinical manifestations of idiopathic pulmonary fibrosis (IPF). Physical examination reveals bibasilar end-inspiratory crackles; clubbing of the digits is present in 40–80%. Evidence of pulmonary hypertension develops in about 30–40% of cases. Chest radiographs usually demonstrate diffuse bilateral reticular infiltrates; however, 14% of patients may have normal chest radiographs (*N Engl J Med* 289:934, 1978). Early gas exchange abnormalities include a decrease in the DL_{CO} and oxygen desaturation during exercise. ABGs may show variable degrees of hypoxemia at rest and a chronic respiratory alkalosis; with more severe disease, $PaCO_2$ may rise and acidosis may occur. PFTs demonstrate a restrictive abnormality with decreased lung volumes (especially total lung capacity), but usually no evidence of airflow obstruction (FEV_1/FVC >0.75).

  II. Initial evaluation should include a careful history focusing on possible reversible causes of lung injury. Particular attention should be given to exposure to dusts, fumes, and drugs with known pulmonary toxicity. In addition, the duration of illness should be estimated by noting the rate of progression of symptoms, and especially by reviewing previous chest radiographs. High-resolution, thin-section computed tomography may be useful for the radiographic detection of interstitial lung disease, to guide the optimal biopsy site, and to assess suspected etiologies (e.g., infection, malignancy) (*Clin Chest Med* 12:97, 1991). Although the etiology may be suspected from the initial evaluation, diagnosis often requires microscopic examination of lung tissue. A pathologic diagnosis should be obtained before initiation of glucocorticoid or immunosuppressive therapy. The method of lung biopsy used depends on the suspected diagnosis.

    A. FOB with transbronchial lung biopsy provides small samples but should be the initial procedure if the leading diagnostic possibilities are infection, cancer, sarcoidosis, or other conditions with specific, well-defined, widespread histologic abnormalities.

    B. Open lung biopsy requires thoracoscopy or thoracotomy but provides an opportunity to study a relatively large amount of tissue for diagnosis. This is the procedure of choice when transbronchial lung biopsy is nondiagnostic or contraindicated or when IPF or another syndrome with a variable and patchy histologic appearance is likely.

C. **Monitoring of disease activity.** Serial evaluation of the severity of breathlessness, radiographic changes (including high-resolution thin-section CT), and physiologic derangements as judged by PFTs, ABGs, and physiologic response to exercise are used to assess the rate of progression of disease, and to facilitate decisions concerning the initiation, continuation, and termination of therapy.

III. **Therapy**

A. **General therapy.** Potentially injurious occupational, environmental, and drug exposures should be discontinued if possible. Appropriate therapy should be directed toward management of heart failure, infection, or other treatable etiologies of interstitial lung disease.

B. **Supplemental oxygen.** PaO_2 or oxygen saturation should be evaluated both while the patient is at rest and during exercise. Supplemental oxygen, with appropriate increases during exercise, should be prescribed when appropriate.

C. **Treatment of specific interstitial lung diseases**

1. **Sarcoidosis** is a granulomatous disease of unknown etiology with protean clinical manifestations and an unpredictable natural course. Up to two-thirds of patients who present with sarcoidosis will have resolution or improvement in symptoms or radiographic abnormalities over the following several years, with chronic disease developing in only a minority of patients. Because of the waxing and waning nature of the illness and the lack of controlled studies, it has been difficult to prove that glucocorticoids actually improve outcome. Glucocorticoids are, however, indicated for ophthalmologic disease (i.e., uveitis), or for significant dysfunction of a vital organ (e.g., heart, brain, kidney, or progressive liver involvement). In an asymptomatic patient with parenchymal infiltrates and a mild to moderate restrictive defect, **decisions regarding initiation of therapy should be individualized**. Bilateral hilar lymphadenopathy (stage I) seldom requires glucocorticoid therapy. When pulmonary infiltrates with or without lymphadenopathy (stages II and III) occur in patients with sarcoidosis, the appropriate therapy is controversial. In the asymptomatic patient with no evidence of clinical or radiologic progression, it is prudent to follow the patient closely without treatment. Symptomatic patients and those with progressive objective deterioration warrant a trial of glucocorticoids (prednisone 30–40 mg/day for 4–8 weeks). When therapy is effective, a clinical and radiologic response is obtained in 2–4 weeks. If no response is obtained in 4–8 weeks, it is reasonable to discontinue treatment gradually (*Am Rev Respir Dis* 147:1598, 1993). If a clinical response is obtained, prednisone should be tapered to the lowest dose that maintains the clinical response (usually >15 mg every other day) and maintained for approximately 1 year before discontinuing therapy completely. Serial evaluation should be performed every 2 months initially, gradually lengthening the intervals to about 4–5 months; patients should be carefully followed for at least 2 years after glucocorticoids have been discontinued. Relapse occurs in up to 20–50% of cases after discontinuation of the treatment. Immunosuppressive agents and inhaled glucocorticoids have not been shown to be beneficial in sarcoid lung disease. However, chloroquine, hydroxychloroquine, and methotrexate have all been used successfully in the management of severe mucocutaneous sarcoidosis and in patients who either do not respond to prednisone or who have severe side effects (*Am J Med Sci* 299:153, 1990).

2. **IPF** has a highly variable but progressive course, with a median survival of less than 5 years from presentation. Relatively good prognostic factors include young age; recent onset of symptoms; less severe breathlessness and infiltrates at presentation and predominantly cellular histology (as opposed to fibrosis); and initial responsiveness to glucocorticoids (*Thorax* 35:171, 1980).

    a. Glucocorticoids (prednisone, 1.0–1.5 mg/kg PO qd) should be initiated early in the course of the illness and the dosage decreased to 0.5–1.0 mg/kg/day after 3–6 months if there has been a response, and then to 0.25 mg/kg/day for 6 additional months. After 1 year, prednisone is slowly tapered to the minimal dosage that maintains clinical stability (*J Respir Dis* 14:1244, 1993). Fifty percent of treated patients have a subjective improvement, whereas 25% demonstrate objective improvement (*Thorax* 38:349, 1983).

    b. Cyclophosphamide, 1–2 mg/kg/day, not to exceed 200 mg/day PO (adjusted to maintain a white blood cell count >3,000/μl), or azathioprine, 3 mg/kg/day, not to exceed 200 mg/day, in combination with low-dose glucocorticoids, may result in improvement in some cases that are unresponsive to glucocorticoids alone (*Am Rev Respir Dis* 144:291, 1991; *Chest* 102:1090, 1992).

    c. Unilateral lung transplantation for IPF appears promising in patients with end-stage disease who are young and free of infection (see Lung Transplantation).

  3. Radiation pneumonitis is a subacute inflammatory pneumonitis that occurs in response to radiation exposure to the lung, most commonly in the form of radiotherapy for malignant diseases. **Symptoms** are nonspecific—usually cough, dyspnea, and low-grade fevers. Radiographically, the presence of an infiltrate corresponding to the region of radiation exposure is characteristic. The incidence, severity, and time of onset of symptoms depend on several factors, the most important of which are the total radiation dose, fractionation schedule, volume of lung irradiated, and concomitant administration of bleomycin or other cytotoxic therapy. In general the onset of symptoms occurs 6–12 weeks after completion of radiotherapy; however, the onset can range from 1–6 months. **Management** of radiation pneumonitis involves first excluding other causes of pulmonary infiltrates, especially infections, recurrent tumors, and lymphangitic carcinomatosis. Mild symptoms can be managed with cough suppressants, antipyretics, and rest. Patients with more severe symptoms and a deterioration in gas exchange should be treated with glucocorticoids. Prednisone is started at 60–100 mg/day, is continued until symptoms and gas exchange improve (usually 3–5 days), and then is tapered to 20–40 mg/day. After 4 weeks of treatment, attempts should be made to gradually taper the patient completely off prednisone. Only half of patients with radiation pneumonitis will respond to glucocorticoid therapy.

Pulmonary Hypertension

Pulmonary hypertension may result from a variety of underlying diseases, including pulmonary venous hypertension (e.g., mitral stenosis), chronic hypoxemia (e.g., COPD, see sec. **III.E**), left-to-right shunts (e.g., atrial septal defects), or vascular diseases of the lungs (e.g., thromboembolic disease). Primary pulmonary hypertension (PPH) is an uncommon disease of unknown etiology characterized by dyspnea, fatigue, and occasionally syncope. It is a diagnosis of exclusion. It occurs most often in young women and usually results in death within several years of diagnosis (*Ann Intern Med* 107:216, 1987). Evaluation of the patient should include chest radiography, PFTs, echocardiography, V̇/Q̇ scanning, and pulmonary artery catheterization. Pulmonary angiography and open lung biopsy may be appropriate in some patients. Treatment should include therapy for the underlying disease in cases of secondary pulmonary hypertension.

  I. Supplemental oxygen is beneficial in patients who are hypoxemic.

 II. Vasodilator therapy is effective in some patients with PPH but is usually not helpful in secondary pulmonary hypertension. The potential direct benefits of vasodilator therapy for PPH include improved pulmonary hemodynamics, right ventricular function, and oxygen delivery, which may lead to clinical improvement and prolonged survival (*Chest* 105:17S, 1994). However, potential deleterious effects of vasodilators, including worsening gas exchange, mandate invasive hemodynamic monitoring when this therapy is initiated. Calcium channel antagonists (e.g., nifedipine or diltiazem) titrated individually to the maximum tolerated dose have been the preferred agents (*Circulation* 76:135, 1987).

III. **Anticoagulation** is of questionable benefit unless thromboembolic disease is present. Some evidence suggests that, at least in a subset of patients with PPH, chronic microvascular thrombosis in the abnormal pulmonary vascular bed is involved in the pathophysiology of this disease (*Circulation* 82:841, 1990; *Circulation* 70:580, 1984). In addition, heparin has an inhibitory effect on smooth muscle cell proliferation. Because of this evidence, many centers advocate anticoagulation in patients with PPH (*Chest* 105:17S, 1994).

IV. **Lung transplantation or heart-lung transplantation** is the ultimate therapeutic alternative for selected patients (see Lung Transplantation).

Sleep Apnea Syndrome

Sleep apnea syndrome, clinically defined by frequent episodes of apnea, hypopnea, and symptoms of functional impairment, is associated with significant adverse health effects and increased mortality (*Chest* 97:27, 1990). Approximately 2% of women and 4% of men between 30 and 60 years of age meet diagnostic criteria for sleep apnea syndrome (*N Engl J Med* 328:1230, 1993). Obstructive sleep apnea (OSA) is caused by repetitive inspiratory occlusion of the upper airway during sleep. This occlusion results in respiratory efforts without airflow, hypoxemia, disrupted sleep pattern, and an array of potentially serious physiologic consequences (*Am Rev Respir Dis* 134:791, 1986).

I. **Diagnosis.** Disorders commonly associated with OSA include obesity, nasal obstruction, adenoidal or tonsillar hypertrophy, micrognathia, retrognathia, macroglossia, acromegaly, hypothyroidism, vocal cord paralysis, and bulbar involvement from neuromuscular disease (*Otolaryngol Clin North Am* 23:727, 1990).

A. **Clinical presentation.** Snoring and excessive daytime sleepiness are the cardinal features of OSA. Patients may also complain of personality changes, intellectual deterioration, morning headaches, automatic behavior, and loss of libido. Systemic hypertension, pulmonary hypertension, and cardiac arrhythmias are the consequences of repetitive oxygen desaturation. Hypoxemia, hypercapnia, polycythemia, and cor pulmonale may complicate the late stage of the disease, especially when obesity and chronic lung disease are present (*Mayo Clin Proc* 65:1087, 1990).

B. **Polysomnography** performed at night in a qualified sleep laboratory by a trained technician is the diagnostic gold standard (*Am Rev Respir Dis* 139:559, 1989). The indications for a sleep study include (1) excessive daytime sleepiness, (2) unexplained pulmonary hypertension or polycythemia, (3) disturbances of respiratory control in patients with daytime hypercapnia, (4) titration of optimal nasal CPAP therapy, and (5) assessment of objective response to therapeutic interventions.

II. **Management.** The therapeutic approach to OSA depends on the severity of the disease, underlying medical condition, cardiopulmonary sequelae, and expected degree of patient compliance. The treatment needs to be highly individualized, with special attention to correcting potentially reversible exacerbating factors. These include weight reduction when appropriate, avoidance of alcohol and sedatives, nasal decongestants if needed, assessment of nighttime oxygenation, and specific therapy for other conditions (e.g., COPD, HTN, hypothyroidism). All patients should have a thorough nose and throat examination to detect sources of upper airway obstruction that are surgically correctable (e.g., septal deviation, enlarged tonsils, uvulopalatopharyngopasty). **Nasal CPAP**, with its level optimized individually in the sleep laboratory, is the treatment of choice for most patients with OSA. Side effects, including nasal and eye complaints, discomfort, and intolerance to machine noise, affect compliance. Newer mask designs, variable inspiratory and expiratory airway pressure devices, and quite smaller CPAP units have improved long-term tolerance to nasal CPAP (*Chest* 98:317, 1990). **Tracheostomy** is the most effective treatment for OSA. However, it is invasive and interferes with speech, exercise, social interactions, and mucociliary clearance. Suitable patients for tracheostomy are these who have life-threatening hypoxemia or cardiac arrhythmias, disabling hypersomnolence, and intolerance or noncompliance with other therapies.

Hemoptysis

Hemoptysis is a nonspecific sign associated with many pulmonary diseases, including infection (e.g., bronchitis, lung abscess, tuberculosis, pneumonia), neoplasm (e.g., carcinoma, bronchial adenoma), cardiovascular disease (e.g., mitral stenosis, pulmonary embolus, pulmonary vascular malformations), and autoimmune disorders (e.g., Wegener's granulomatosis, Goodpasture's syndrome). Often, the specific etiology of hemoptysis is never determined.

I. **Diagnosis**
   A. **History and physical examination.** The source of bleeding should be confirmed to be the lower respiratory tract and not the GI tract or nasopharynx (see Chap. 15). An attempt should be made to estimate the amount of bleeding, although quantification is often difficult. The remainder of the clinical evaluation should focus on obtaining clues to the cause of hemoptysis.
   B. **Laboratory studies** include a chest radiograph, sputum cytology, appropriate sputum stains and cultures, ABGs, tests of hemostasis, and urinalysis to detect red cells or red-cell casts that may be associated with Wegener's granulomatosis or Goodpasture's syndrome.
   C. **Bronchoscopy** is indicated in patients with hemoptysis who have a risk factor for carcinoma, even if hemoptysis is minor and the radiograph is normal. Risk factors include (1) age greater than 40 years, (2) significant smoking history, (3) hemoptysis of greater than 1-week duration, and (4) unexplained abnormality on chest radiograph (*Chest* 87:142, 1985). If bleeding is brisk, rigid bronchoscopy is required.

II. **Therapy** is tailored to the severity of the episode and the underlying cause.
   A. **Minor hemoptysis.** Therapy for minor bleeding or blood-streaked sputum should be directed at the underlying etiology.
   B. **Massive hemoptysis** is defined as greater than 600 ml over 48 hours, or quantities sufficient to impair gas exchange. The primary goals of therapy are to provide cardiopulmonary support and control bleeding while preventing asphyxiation (*Clin Chest Med* 13:69, 1992).
      1. **Supportive care.** While awaiting surgical consultation, clinically stable patients should be positioned with the bleeding side in a dependent position to reduce aspiration of blood into the contralateral lung. Supplemental oxygen should be supplied. Sedatives aid patient cooperation, but excessive sedation may suppress airway protection and mask signs of respiratory decompensation. Bed rest, mild cough suppression, and avoidance of excessive thoracic manipulation (e.g., chest percussion, incentive spirometry) are helpful.
      2. **Definitive therapy.** Prompt surgical resection of the bleeding site is the therapy of choice. Rigid bronchoscopy should be performed first to localize the site of bleeding if possible, and to isolate and ventilate the uninvolved lung. Contraindications to surgical resection include inoperable lung cancer and previous pulmonary function studies precluding pulmonary resection (e.g., a predicted postoperative FEV_1 of <800 ml). Potential therapeutic maneuvers in inoperable patients include tamponade of the bleeding bronchial segment with a balloon catheter, endobronchial cold saline or fibrinogen-thrombin solution lavage, IV vasopressin, and embolization of the bronchial artery supply to the bleeding segment.

Pleural Effusion

Transudative pleural effusions are formed when the normal hydrostatic or oncotic pressures are perturbed (e.g., increased mean capillary pressure [heart failure]; or decreased oncotic pressure [cirrhosis or nephrotic syndrome]). **Exudative pleural effusions** occur when there is damage or disruption of the normal pleural membranes or vasculature leading to increased capillary permeability or decreased lymphatic drainage (e.g., tumor involvement of the pleural space, infection, inflammatory conditions, or trauma).

I. **Diagnosis.** Most pleural effusions require further evaluation unless their origin is clear (e.g., heart failure) and the patient is responding well to therapy (*Am Rev Respir Dis* 140:257, 1989).

A. **Thoracentesis** can be safely performed, in the absence of disorders of hemostasis (see Chap. 17), on effusions demonstrating a thickness of greater than 10 mm on lateral decubitus films. Loculated effusions can be localized with ultrasonography or CT. Proper technique and sonographic guidance minimize the risk of pneumothorax and other complications (*Arch Intern Med* 150:873, 1990).

1. **The etiology of an effusion** can be reasonably deduced from the clinical circumstances (e.g., congestive heart failure or hepatic failure with ascites). **Exudates** have at least one (and transudates none) of the following: (1) pleural fluid protein to serum protein ratio more than 0.5, (2) pleural fluid lactic dehydrogenase (LDH) to serum ratio more than 0.6, and (3) pleural fluid LDH more than two-thirds of the upper limit of normal for serum LDH. **Parapneumonic effusions** are exudates with a leukocyte count usually more than $10,000/mm^3$ and a predominance of polymorphonuclear leukocytes. The pleural fluid glucose, pH, and LDH are helpful in differentiating **complicated** (i.e., pH <7.10, glucose <40 mg/dl, and LDH >1,000 IU/liter), from **uncomplicated** (pH >7.30, glucose >60 mg/dl, and LDH of <500 IU/liter) parapneumonic effusions and are useful to identify the patients who will usually require chest tube drainage (*Am J Med* 69:507, 1980).

2. **Other studies** involving pleural fluid that may be useful in specific clinical settings include cell count and differential, amylase, triglycerides, microbiologic stains, cultures, and cytology. Some useful observations regarding the results of studies on pleural fluid include the following: (1) **gross blood** is seen with pulmonary infarction, tumor, or trauma; a pleural fluid/blood hematocrit ratio more than 0.5 establishes the diagnosis of a hemothorax; (2) a **pH** less than 7.3 is seen with empyema, tuberculosis, malignancy, collagen vascular disease, or esophageal rupture; (3) a **glucose** concentration less than 40 mg/dl is associated with an empyema, rheumatoid arthritis, tuberculosis; or malignancy; (4) an elevation of **amylase** occurs with pancreatitis, pancreatic pseudocyst, renal failure, malignancy, esophageal rupture, or ruptured ectopic pregnancy; (5) elevation of **triglycerides** (>110 mg/dl) indicates chylous effusions, which are caused by thoracic duct rupture from trauma, surgery, or malignancy (usually lymphoma); and (6) **cytology** is positive in approximately 60% of malignant effusions (*Mayo Clin Proc* 60:158, 1985). Priming the fluid collection bag with 300–1,000 IU of heparin and submitting a large pleural fluid volume will maximize the diagnostic yield.

B. **Closed pleural biopsy** should be performed when the cause of an exudative pleural effusion cannot be determined by thoracentesis. For tuberculous effusions, pleural fluid cultures alone are positive in only 20–25% of cases; however, the combination of pleural fluid studies and pleural biopsy (demonstrating granulomas or organisms) is 90% sensitive in establishing tuberculosis as the etiology of the effusion (*Arch Intern Med* 144:325, 1984). For malignant effusions, pleural biopsies add a small but significant diagnostic yield to fluid cytology alone.

C. **Other diagnostic procedures** useful in establishing a diagnosis of pleural effusion when the above are normal include biopsy of other abnormal sites (e.g., a mediastinal or lung mass), diagnostic thoracoscopy under local anesthesia with mild sedation, and evaluation for pulmonary emboli.

II. Treatment

A. Symptomatic pleural effusions may require removal of large amounts of pleural fluid. The rapid removal of more than 1 liter of pleural fluid may rarely result in ipsilateral pulmonary edema, especially when re-expansion of the lung is accomplished with suction. When frequent or repeated thoracentesis is required for effusions that reaccumulate, early consideration should be given to tube drainage and pleurosclerosis.

B. Parapneumonic effusions are pleural effusions associated with bacterial pneumonia. Thoracentesis is required both as a reliable means of identifying a pathogen and as a guide to further management of the pleural space.

1. **Uncomplicated parapneumonic effusions** should resolve with antimicrobial therapy for the underlying pneumonia. If the volume of fluid does not progressively decrease, the pleural fluid should be reevaluated.

2. **Complicated parapneumonic effusions** should be considered for immediate drainage (*Am Rev Respir Dis* 148:813, 1993). However, occasional patients (e.g., *Streptococcus pneumoniae* infections) appear to do well without drainage, even with positive pleural fluid bacteriology (*Chest* 97:731, 1990; *Chest* 100:963, 1991). Chronic empyemas may not drain completely with closed chest tubes; in these cases, thoracotomy with decortication is the most effective intervention. However, this procedure is generally reserved for young, otherwise healthy patients or those in whom more conservative measures such as open drainage fail. Instillation of streptokinase into the pleural cavity may occasionally promote chest tube drainage (*Am Rev Respir Dis* 145:680, 1992). There is **no established role for repeated therapeutic thoracenteses** in the treatment of complicated parapneumonic effusions.

C. Malignant pleural effusions arise from tumor involvement of the pleura or mediastinum. Patients with malignancy are also at increased risk for pleural effusions from postobstructive pneumonia, pulmonary emboli, chylothorax, and drug or radiation reactions. If pleural tissue or cytology is positive for malignancy, or if other causes of effusion are reasonably excluded in a patient with malignancy, several therapeutic options exist (*Clin Chest Med* 14:189, 1993).

1. **Therapeutic thoracentesis** may improve patient comfort and relieve dyspnea. The subjective response to drainage and the rate of fluid reaccumulation should be monitored. Repeated thoracenteses are reasonable if they achieve symptomatic relief and if fluid reaccumulation is slow.

2. **Complete drainage via chest tube** followed by sclerosis is an effective therapy for recurrent effusions. This treatment is recommended in patients whose symptoms are relieved with initial drainage but who have rapid reaccumulation of fluid. Talc pleurodesis appears to be the most effective and least expensive agent; however, it requires thoracoscopy and general anesthesia. Doxycycline, 500 mg in 50 ml normal saline (NS), or minocycline, 300 mg in 50 ml NS, can be instilled in the pleural space. If, after 48 hours, the chest tube drainage remains high (>100 ml/day), a second dose of the sclerosing agent can be administered. The efficacy of these two agents is 72% and 86%, respectively. Bleomycin appears to be less effective and more expensive. The use of lidocaine in the sclerosing agent solution (3 mg/kg to a maximum of 150 mg) helps decrease the discomfort associated with the procedure (*Ann Intern Med* 120:56, 1994).

3. **Pleurectomy or pleural abrasion** requires thoracotomy and should be reserved for patients with a good prognosis when sclerosis has been ineffective.

4. **Chemotherapy and mediastinal radiation therapy** may control effusions in responsive tumors such as lymphoma or small-cell bronchogenic carcinoma but are seldom useful in metastatic carcinoma.

5. **Observation** may also be appropriate.

Lung Transplantation

The results of lung transplantation have steadily improved over the last several years to the point that it is a viable option for patients with end-stage lung disease (*Clin Chest Med* 11:347, 1990).

I. **Selection criteria.** Patients with IPF, COPD, antitrypsin deficiency emphysema, CF, PPH, and selected forms of Eisenmenger's syndrome have had successful transplants. Single lung transplantation (SLT) is the procedure of choice for fibrotic, restrictive disease, but suitable for COPD, emphysema, and PPH. Double lung transplantation (DLT) is mandatory for CF and generalized bronchiectasis because of the risk of spillover infection from a remaining native lung. Heart-lung transplantation (HLT) should be reserved for patients with combined cardiopulmonary disease. In general, selection criteria include the following: (1) a limited life expectancy based on the severity of the lung disease, (2) the absence of underlying systemic disease or dysfunction of other organs, (3) no mitigating psychosocial problems, and (4) a good emotional support structure. The age of the patient is also a consideration, with approximately 50 and 60 years being the upper limits for HLT and SLT, respectively. Early referral of a prospective transplant candidate is suggested. The time to consider referral for transplant evaluation is variable depending on the underlying disease, pulmonary function, gas exchange abnormality, and severity of pulmonary hypertension. Lung transplantation is not a therapy for acutely ill patients in respiratory failure.

II. **Transplant complications** include the typical postthoracotomy problems not unique to transplantation. In addition, dehiscence of airway anastomosis (early), airway stenosis (late), acute and chronic rejection, and infectious complications (see Pneumonia, Pulmonary Aspiration Syndromes, and Lung Abscess and Chap. 14) require close surveillance by physicians experienced in the care of these patients (*Clin Chest Med* 11:195, 1990; *Chest* 103:1566, 1993).

11

Renal Diseases

Steven B. Miller

Evaluation of the Patient with Renal Disease

The patient with renal disease may present with a variety of signs and symptoms. A careful history and physical examination will often lead to the correct diagnosis. Initial evaluation should emphasize identifying reversible causes of renal dysfunction.

I. **Initial studies** should include a **urinalysis** of a freshly voided specimen to look for proteinuria, hematuria, and pyuria, and to assess urine pH. Dirty brown sediment with epithelial cells and granular casts is seen with ischemic damage of the tubules. WBC casts are seen in pyelonephritis and RBC casts are seen in glomerulonephritis (GN). **Serum chemistries** should include electrolytes, creatinine (Cr), BUN, calcium, magnesium, phosphate, uric acid, and protein. If the serum Cr is stable (i.e., steady state), the **glomerular filtration rate** (GFR) can be estimated by using the following empiric formula for creatinine clearance (Cl_{Cr}):

$$Cl_{Cr} \text{ (ml/min)} = [(140 - \text{age}) \times \text{weight (kg)}/72 \times \text{serum Cr (mg/dl)}] \times$$
$$(0.85 \text{ for women})$$

This equation provides only a rough estimate of GFR and should not be used in place of a 24-hour-urine collection for Cl_{Cr}. Weight should reflect ideal body weight.

II. **Supplementary studies** can be useful to further assess renal function and may aid in identifying specific disorders.

A. Twenty-four-hour urine studies include measurement of **urine volume, Cr, and protein.** The GFR can be estimated by measurement of the Cl_{Cr}, which is calculated as follows:

$$Cl_{Cr} \text{ (ml/min)} = [\text{urine Cr (mg/dl)} \times \text{volume (ml)}/\text{plasma Cr (mg/dl)} \times$$
$$\text{time (min)}]$$

This value is useful in predicting remaining renal function, timing placement of dialysis access, and adjusting drug dosage in renal insufficiency. When the GFR is markedly reduced, measurement of Cl_{Cr} may actually overestimate the true GFR. If the 24-hour Cr is less than 15–20 mg/kg lean body weight, the collection may be incomplete, leading to an underestimate of the GFR. Twenty-four-hour protein studies are necessary for diagnosis of the nephrotic syndrome and are useful for following the response of certain glomerular diseases to treatment. Measurements of **24-hour urinary calcium, phosphate, oxalate, and uric acid** are indicated in the evaluation of some patients with nephrolithiasis.

B. **Supplementary blood tests.** Erythrocyte sedimentation rate, antinuclear and antiglomerular basement membrane antibody studies, antineutrophil cytoplasmic antibodies, angiotensin-converting enzyme (ACE) level, complement levels, cryoglobulin studies, hepatitis B and C serology, and antistreptococcal antibody titers are often useful for laboratory evaluation of glomerular disease. Serum protein electrophoresis should also be performed in selected patients with proteinuria to exclude multiple myeloma.

C. **Renal ultrasonography** noninvasively assesses kidney size and evaluates the collecting system. Small kidneys generally reflect chronic renal disease, although kidney size may not be diminished in some common chronic processes such as diabetes, amyloidosis, and multiple myeloma. Ultrasound is also useful in the evaluation of acute renal failure, as the presence of hydronephrosis suggests obstructive nephropathy.

D. **Radionuclide scanning** uses predominantly technetium isotopes to define renal filtration and tubular secretion. The renal scan allows an assessment of the relative contribution of each kidney to overall renal function and provides important information if unilateral nephrectomy is being considered. Renal scanning is useful when disruption of renal blood flow is suspected; the absence of perfusion of either kidney on scan should prompt further investigation of the renal vasculature. In addition, radionuclide studies can be used to follow renal function and rejection in transplanted kidneys.

E. **MRI** can be useful in the evaluation of renal disorders. It provides images similar in format to CT scans but without the use of ionizing radiation or the requirement of potentially nephrotoxic contrast material. MRI uses include the evaluation of renal masses and atherosclerotic disease involving the proximal renal arteries (*J Vasc Surg* 13:311, 1991).

F. **Renal biopsy** is an invasive procedure that may be indicated in patients with proteinuria (or nephrotic syndrome), hematuria, or casts suggestive of glomerular disease. Biopsy may also be useful in guiding the therapy of some glomerular diseases (e.g., systemic lupus erythematosus [SLE]) and often provides prognostic information. Finally, biopsy may be useful in patients with renal failure and kidneys of normal size when other studies fail to reveal a diagnosis. Prior to biopsy, the presence of two kidneys should be established, sterility of the urine ensured, and hypertension and abnormalities of hemostasis corrected. Packed RBCs should be available for transfusion. The patient should not take drugs that interfere with platelet function (e.g., aspirin) before or immediately following the biopsy. Patients on dialysis who require a biopsy should have their dialysis sessions planned to avoid heparin anticoagulation immediately following the biopsy.

Acute Renal Failure

Although there are many causes of acute renal failure (ARF) (Table 11-1), the syndrome uniformly presents with a sudden decline in the ability of the kidney to maintain homeostasis, resulting in failure to clear metabolic wastes, as well as electrolyte, acid-base, and volume disturbances. Renal failure may be oliguric (urine output <500 ml/day) or nonoliguric. The approach to patients with ARF is simplified by classifying it as prerenal, intrinsic, or postobstructive. Table 11-2 includes laboratory tests that are helpful in differentiating oliguric prerenal azotemia from oliguric, intrinsic acute tubular necrosis (ATN). Serum and urine should be obtained simultaneously before a fluid challenge or diuretic use is initiated. A fresh urine sample is essential, as urine retained in the bladder may not reflect current renal function. Temporary bladder catheterization is recommended to exclude lower urinary tract obstruction, but the catheter should be removed promptly unless obstruction is present.

I. **Prerenal azotemia** is a functional disorder that results from a decrease in effective arterial blood volume. Early correction of decreased renal perfusion, with volume expansion, BP support, or treatment of heart failure, may result in reversal of renal insufficiency; prolonged hypoperfusion may cause permanent renal damage. In prerenal states, the kidney attempts to reabsorb filtered sodium and the fractional excretion of sodium (FE_{Na}) is usually less than 1%. Intrinsic renal failure with damaged tubules results in sodium loss and a FE_{Na} greater than 1%. This calculation may not be diagnostic in patients who are elderly, who have received diuretics, or who have preexisting renal disease, acute GN, vasculitis, radiocontrast-induced renal failure, or cirrhosis.

A. **Hemodynamic monitoring** is sometimes necessary to assess intravascular

Table 11-1. Causes of acute renal failure

I. Prerenal (ischemic)
  A. Volume contraction
  B. Hypotension
  C. Heart failure (severe)
  D. Liver failure (?)
II. Intrinsic renal failure
  A. Acute tubular necrosis (prolonged ischemia; nephrotoxic agents such as heavy metals, aminoglycosides, radiographic contrast media)
  B. Arteriolar injury
    1. Accelerated hypertension
    2. Vasculitis
    3. Microangiopathic (thrombotic thrombocytopenic purpura, hemolytic-uremic syndrome)
  C. Glomerulonephritis
  D. Acute interstitial nephritis (drug induced)
  E. Intrarenal deposition or sludging (uric acid, myeloma)
  F. Cholesterol embolization (especially postarterial procedure)
III. Postrenal
  A. Ureteral obstruction (clot, calculus, tumor, sloughed papillae, external compression)
  B. Bladder outlet obstruction (neurogenic bladder, prostatic hypertrophy, carcinoma, calculus, clot, urethral stricture)

volume, especially in patients with poor cardiac function. There is danger of excessive volume expansion in oliguric patients and a risk of inadequate volume replacement in prerenal patients. Invasive monitoring with a central venous pressure (CVP) or Swan-Ganz catheter is indicated if an accurate assessment of intravascular volume cannot be obtained by physical examination and an initial volume challenge.

  B. Fluid challenge may be appropriate in oliguric patients who are not volume overloaded. **The quantity of fluid to be given must be determined on an individual basis,** but typically 500–1,000 ml of normal saline is infused over 30–60 minutes. Frequent cardiopulmonary examination is necessary. Such a volume challenge may result in increased urine flow in prerenal azotemia, but some cases of intrinsic renal failure may also respond with increased urine output; therefore, the response to volume challenge must be interpreted with caution. If there is no response, volume infusion can be followed by 100–400 mg IV furosemide to promote urine flow. Occasionally, the addition of metolazone, 5–10 mg PO, will facilitate initiation of diuresis induced by volume repletion and furosemide. If successful, the lowest effective dose of furosemide can be continued in the volume-repleted patient, with careful monitoring to avoid volume depletion. Diuretic administration may convert oliguric ARF to non-oliguric ARF, which simplifies management and may improve prognosis. However, large doses of furosemide given intravenously for prolonged periods may cause hearing loss, particularly when renal function is impaired. To avoid the use of high doses of furosemide, 20% mannitol can be given as a continuous infusion through a separate IV line at a rate of 10–20 ml/hour. An effect is usually observed within the first 6 hours. If no effect is seen by 12 hours, then the infusion should be discontinued.

  C. Dopamine (less than 3 μg/kg/minute), a dosage that preferentially dilates the renal vasculature, may occasionally initiate natriuresis and diuresis. A response is usually seen within the first 6–12 hours of therapy. If the patient remains oliguric, therapy with low-dose dopamine should be discontinued.

II. Obstructive nephropathy. ARF may be secondary to upper or lower urinary tract obstruction. Early diagnosis and relief of obstruction are essential to prevent

Table 11-2. Laboratory examination in oliguric acute renal failure

Diagnosis	U/P Cr	U_{Na}	$FE_{Na}(\%)$	U osmolality
Prerenal azotemia	>40	<20	<1	>500
Oliguric ATN	<20	>40	>1	<350

U = urine; P = plasma; FE_{Na} = fractional excretion of sodium = $100 \times$ (U/P sodium)/(U/P creatinine).

permanent renal damage. Lower tract obstruction can be assessed (and relieved) by temporary bladder catheterization, while renal ultrasonography will aid in the diagnosis of upper tract obstruction. Urine flow often increases dramatically after relief of obstruction. This postobstructive diuresis is often physiologic and reflects excretion of fluid, urea, and sodium accumulated during the period of obstruction; however, inappropriate loss of volume and electrolytes may occur after relief of severe acute bilateral obstruction. If the **postobstructive diuresis** appears excessive, replacement of fluid and electrolytes should be guided by daily weights, urine output, orthostatic BP changes, and serum and urine electrolyte concentrations. The appropriate initial replacement fluid in such cases is usually 0.45% saline.

III. **Intrinsic renal failure** results from a variety of injuries to the renal blood vessels, glomeruli, tubules, or interstitium (see Table 11-1). These insults may be toxic, immunologic, or idiopathic; they may be iatrogenic and may develop as part of a systemic disorder or as a primary renal disease. Specific syndromes that are preventable or treatable are discussed in the following paragraphs.

A. **Radiocontrast nephropathy** occurs with increased frequency in patients with long-standing diabetes mellitus or preexisting renal insufficiency. Volume depletion, multiple myeloma, heart failure (HF), and age greater than 65 years may also be risk factors. The ARF of contrast nephropathy tends to be oliguric and the serum Cr peaks in the first 72 hours. Patients often recover renal function over 7–14 days. Preventive measures may decrease the incidence of ARF. Patients at risk who require contrast studies should be adequately volume expanded, preferably for 24 hours prior to the study. Patients with normal cardiac function can receive mannitol, 25 g in 1 liter of 0.45% saline IV. Infusion rates need to be individualized but should be approximately 100–150 ml/hour for 4 hours prior to the study followed by the same infusion for an additional 2–4 hours after the study. Subsequently, urinary volume loss should be replaced by infusion of 0.45% saline for 24 hours. Serum electrolytes should be monitored.

B. **Aminoglycoside nephrotoxicity** may cause ARF that is often nonoliguric and results from direct toxicity to the proximal tubules. Predisposing factors include large dosages, prolonged exposure to these drugs, advanced age, volume depletion, liver disease, and preexisting renal disease. Patients in whom ARF develops from aminoglycoside therapy have usually received the medication for at least 5 days. The risk of aminoglycoside nephrotoxicity may be minimized by frequent monitoring of drug levels with appropriate dosage adjustments to keep levels in the therapeutic range.

C. **Pigment-induced renal injury** occurs during **hemolysis** or **rhabdomyolysis.** With rhabdomyolysis, early aggressive volume expansion to replace the fluid that is lost into necrotic muscle may be beneficial. Diuresis to decrease tubular pigment reabsorption may be promoted by mannitol, 25 g IV. If sufficient urine flow can be established, IV infusion of bicarbonate, 2–3 ampules in 1 liter of 5% dextrose in water (D/W), to maintain urine pH greater than 6.5 may also be useful by preventing dissociation of myoglobin and hemoglobin into potentially toxic compounds.

D. **Acute uric acid nephropathy** may result from cell lysis with consequent hyperuricemia during the course of cytotoxic therapy of hematologic malignancies. Renal failure results from intratubular precipitation of uric acid. Prevention involves decreasing uric acid production prior to cytotoxic therapy with allopurinol, 600 mg PO initially, followed by 100–300 mg/day if renal function is normal. In addition, forced alkaline diuresis to maintain a urine pH of 6.5–7.0 will help prevent uric acid precipitation; this may be accomplished with acetazolamide, 250 mg PO qid, or infusion of sodium bicarbonate, 2–3 ampules in 1 liter of 5% D/W. If tumor lysis results in hyperphosphatemia, alkalinization should be avoided because of the increased risk of calcium phosphate precipitation.

E. **Allergic interstitial nephritis** secondary to drugs is often unrecognized and may result in classic signs that include fever, rash, and renal dysfunction. When present, eosinophilia, elevated serum immunoglobulin E (IgE), and eosinophiluria suggest the diagnosis. A high index of suspicion for interstitial nephritis must be maintained in patients taking drugs such as the **penicillins, sulfonamides**, and **nonsteroidal antiinflammatory drugs** (NSAIDs). In most cases, renal insufficiency will resolve with discontinuation of the offending agent. In severe or prolonged cases, however, a 1-week course of prednisone, 60 mg PO qd, may hasten recovery (*Ann Intern Med* 93:735, 1980).

F. **Glomerular disease** of a rapidly progressive nature can result in ARF. Histologically, glomeruli demonstrate extensive crescent formation on biopsy, but this morphologic end point is shared by a variety of antecedent events (see The Glomerulonephropathies).

IV. **Management of ARF** can often be accomplished with conservative measures alone. Dialysis may be required depending on the severity of renal impairment, the resulting complications, and the presence of other diseases.

A. **Conservative medical management** of ARF is facilitated by weighing the patient daily, accurately recording fluid intake and output, and frequently (at least 3 times/week) measuring serum electrolyte, BUN, Cr, calcium, and phosphate levels.

1. **Fluid management** requires accurate clinical assessment of intravascular volume. Volume depletion may contribute to ARF by decreasing renal perfusion and must be corrected, occasionally with the aid of invasive hemodynamic monitoring (see sec. **I.A**). Once any volume deficit has been corrected, fluid and sodium balance must be carefully regulated to avoid volume overload. Fluid replacement should be equal to insensible loss (about 500 ml/day in afebrile patients) plus urinary and other drainage losses. Increased urine output and diuretic responsiveness in nonoliguric ARF allow more liberal administration of fluids (and nutrients), facilitating the general care of the patient. Because patients with nonoliguric ARF may lose significant amounts of fluid and electrolytes in the urine, careful attention to volume status and serum electrolyte levels is necessary to avoid electrolyte and water depletion. Hyponatremia in patients with ARF is usually secondary to volume expansion with hypotonic fluid, whereas hypernatremia is most often caused by overly aggressive diuresis with inadequate intake of free water.

2. **Dietary modification. Protein intake** should be limited to approximately 0.5 g/kg/day to decrease nitrogenous waste production. Total caloric intake should be 35–50 kcal/kg/day to avoid catabolism. Patients who are highly catabolic (e.g., postsurgical and burn patients) or malnourished require higher protein intake and should be considered for early institution of dialysis (see sec. **IV.B**). Restricting intake of salt to 2–4 g/day NaCl will facilitate volume management. **Potassium** intake should be restricted to 40 mEq/day and **phosphorus** should be restricted to 800 mg/day. Ingestion of **magnesium-containing compounds** should be avoided.

3. **Blood pressure. Hypotension** should be promptly evaluated and corrected with volume expansion or vasopressors, depending on the patient's intravascular volume status. Volume overload is frequently a contributing factor to **hypertension**, which should be managed aggressively. Antihypertensive medications that do not decrease renal blood flow (e.g., clonidine, prazosin) or calcium channel antagonists are preferred. Hypertensive crisis can be managed with IV sodium nitroprusside (see Chap. 4), but thiocyanate, a toxic metabolite of nitroprusside, is excreted by the kidneys and may accumulate

in renal failure. Thiocyanate levels should be closely monitored during therapy with this agent. IV labetalol is an effective alternative and avoids potential thiocyanate toxicity (*N Engl J Med* 323:1177, 1990).

4. **Phosphate and calcium.** Serum phosphate levels may remain elevated despite dietary restriction. Aluminum hydroxide–containing antacids such as Basaljel or Amphojel, 15–30 ml PO tid with meals, are used to decrease intestinal absorption of phosphate. Concomitant with elevated phosphate, serum calcium is often low but usually does not require specific treatment. The calcium phosphate product should be kept less than 60 to avoid metastatic calcification. Once the phosphate level is controlled, calcium carbonate (500–1,000 mg PO tid–qid) given with meals can be substituted as a phosphate binder.

5. **Uric acid.** Mild elevations of serum uric acid levels are frequent in ARF but do not have any clearly deleterious effect on the kidneys. In some types of ARF (e.g., associated with rhabdomyolysis), however, uric acid may be quite elevated (>20 mg/dl) and should be treated with allopurinol, 100 mg PO qd.

6. **Hyperkalemia** is common and, if mild (<6 mEq/liter), can be treated with dietary restriction and potassium-binding resins (e.g., sodium polystyrene sulfonate [Kayexalate]). More marked hyperkalemia or hyperkalemia accompanied by ECG or neuromuscular abnormalities, requires immediate medical therapy (e.g., insulin and glucose, calcium chloride) (see Chap. 3). Hyperkalemia refractory to medical therapy is an indication for dialysis.

7. **Metabolic acidosis.** Mild acidosis (serum bicarbonate level ≥16 mEq/liter) does not require therapy. More marked acidosis should be corrected with sodium bicarbonate, 325–650 mg PO tid. Severe uncompensated acidosis (serum pH <7.2) requires prompt medical therapy with parenteral sodium bicarbonate (see Chap. 3). Caution must be exercised with sodium bicarbonate therapy, because the additional sodium may exacerbate volume overload. In addition, excessive alkali use may decrease the ionized calcium concentration and cause tetany. Correctable causes of metabolic acidosis should be sought and treated. Acidosis unresponsive to medical therapy is an indication for dialysis.

8. **Drug dosages** of agents excreted by the kidney must be adjusted for the level of renal function (see Appendix D).

9. **Infection** is common and accounts for a significant proportion of deaths associated with ARF. Antimicrobial therapy is dictated by the infectious process; potentially nephrotoxic agents should not be withheld if clinically necessary. Most antimicrobial dosages need to be adjusted for the degree of renal failure (see Appendix D).

10. **GI bleeding** may occur in ARF, reflecting both mucosal changes and altered platelet function secondary to uremia. Major bleeding sources should be excluded (see Chap. 15).

11. **Anemia** is common and usually is caused by decreased RBC production and increased blood loss. The hematocrit often falls below 30%. Transfusion is appropriate for patients with active bleeding or symptoms referable to anemia (see Chap. 18). Erythropoietin is not effective as short-term therapy for anemia.

B. **Dialysis** for ARF is indicated when **severe hyperkalemia, acidosis,** or **volume overload** cannot be controlled by conservative measures. Additional indications include **uremic pericarditis, encephalopathy,** or **nutritional requirements** that would precipitate volume overload or uremia. A patient may not need dialysis early in the course of ARF but should be evaluated daily to assess the need for such intervention. Technical aspects of dialysis are considered under Renal Replacement Therapies.

1. **Uremic signs and symptoms** become prominent as BUN and Cr rise. Morbidity and mortality may be reduced if the BUN is maintained below 100 mg/dl, and dialysis is often started empirically as the BUN approaches this level. **Neurologic manifestations** (e.g., lethargy, seizures, myoclonus, asterixis, and peripheral polyneuropathies) may develop with uremia and are an indication for dialysis. **Uremic pericarditis** is often manifested only as a pericardial

friction rub and should be treated with dialysis; heparin use during dialysis should be minimized in these patients (see Renal Replacement Therapies, sec. I.C). Patients with pericarditis who do not respond to dialysis or in whom signs of pericardial tamponade develop require pericardial drainage.

2. **Nutritional considerations.** Patients with ARF are often highly catabolic or need dietary supplementation to promote wound healing. Dialysis is indicated in patients who need aggressive nutritional therapy (e.g., hyperalimentation) that cannot be provided within the limitations imposed by the volume and dietary restrictions of conservative management.

V. **Management of the recovery phase of ARF** is best accomplished by careful monitoring of serum electrolytes, volume status, and urinary fluid and electrolyte loss. As with obstructive nephropathy, a diuretic phase may occur during recovery. Management is similar to that for postobstructive diuresis (see sec. II). Renal function may continue to improve over several weeks to months after the patient enters the recovery phase.

The Glomerulonephropathies

Glomerular disease may be **primary** or **secondary** to a systemic process and can present in a variety of ways. **Acute GN** is often characterized by hematuria, RBC casts, proteinuria, hypertension, edema, and deteriorating renal function. Other glomerulonephropathies may present with significant proteinuria, an unremarkable urine sediment, and a relatively preserved GFR. Renal biopsy often provides useful diagnostic, therapeutic, and prognostic information in glomerular disease. Treatment usually involves the use of glucocorticoids. In the following sections, cytotoxic therapy (e.g., cyclophosphamide) is recommended for certain types of GN in consultation with a nephrologist or other physician experienced with their use. Initial dosages of these agents are suggested, but these may require adjustment to keep the WBC count above 3,000–3,500 µl. WBC counts should be checked at least weekly in outpatients while cytotoxic agents are administered to decrease the potential for excessive immunosuppression and infectious complications.

I. **Minimal change disease** (MCD) presents with nephrotic syndrome (see The Nephrotic Syndrome). The pathologic diagnosis is confirmed by normal light microscopy, negative immunofluorescence, and foot process fusion on electron microscopy. About 80% of adults with MCD respond to prednisone, 1 mg/kg/day PO, with a decrease in proteinuria to less than 3 g/day, or a remission of the nephrotic syndrome. Patients who respond should have steroids tapered over 3 months and discontinued. Failure to respond may reflect an error in diagnosis; MCD is most commonly confused with early focal segmental glomerulosclerosis. Urinary protein should be carefully monitored during steroid taper. If relapse is documented, reinstitution of prednisone is often effective. Treatment with cytotoxic agents may be indicated in patients who relapse frequently or who do not respond to or cannot be tapered off high dosages of glucocorticoids. Cyclophosphamide, 2 mg/kg/day PO for 8 weeks, or chlorambucil, 0.2 mg/kg/day PO for 8–12 weeks, are typical regimens. Progression to chronic renal failure (CRF) is unusual. Certain neoplastic disorders such as Hodgkin's disease and non-Hodgkin's lymphoma have been associated with the development of MCD and should be considered in the appropriate setting.

II. **Focal segmental glomerulosclerosis** is an idiopathic glomerular disorder usually characterized by hypertension, hematuria, renal insufficiency, and nephrotic syndrome. Histologic findings include foot process fusion and segmental sclerosis of glomeruli. The disease slowly progresses to chronic renal failure within 5–10 years of diagnosis. No therapy has proven benefit in the treatment of this disorder, but a trial of prednisone, 60 mg PO qd, for at least 1 month may be appropriate in an effort to reduce proteinuria and slow progression to CRF (*Medicine* 65:304, 1986). Likewise, as in the treatment of MCD, some authors recommend a combination of glucocorticoids and cytotoxic agents to induce a remission (*Adv Nephrol* 17:127, 1988).

III. **Membranous glomerulonephropathy** characteristically presents with the nephrotic syndrome, although some patients have nonnephrotic proteinuria. The GFR is usually normal or near normal, and the urinary sediment is often unremarkable. Biopsy demonstrates thickening of the glomerular capillary wall secondary to subepithelial deposits of IgG and C3. Membranous nephropathy may be a primary renal disease or may be associated with systemic diseases (e.g., malignancy, SLE) or drug ingestions (e.g., penicillamine, gold). The natural history of the disease includes spontaneous remissions and exacerbations, making evaluation of potential therapy difficult. About 20% of patients will progress to end-stage renal disease, whereas the remainder will have variable degrees of remission. The optimal therapy for membranous glomerulonephropathy has not been established. Treatment options include high-dose alternate-day glucocorticoids (*N Engl J Med* 320:210, 1989) and the combination of a cytotoxic agent (e.g., chlorambucil) and glucocorticoids (*N Engl J Med* 320:8, 1989). Not all patients require treatment and patient selection is important (*Ann Intern Med* 116:672,1992). **Renal vein thrombosis** with potential systemic thromboembolism may complicate this disease. A sudden decrease in GFR should prompt evaluation for renal vein thrombosis with Doppler ultrasonography or MRI; venography may be required in some cases.

IV. **Membranoproliferative glomerulonephritis** (MPGN) has a variety of clinical presentations, including acute GN, nephrotic syndrome (see The Nephrotic Syndrome), and asymptomatic hematuria and proteinuria. The diagnosis should be suspected if these clinical findings are associated with low complement levels. Histologic findings include mesangial proliferation and alterations of the glomerular basement membrane (GBM) with subendothelial (type I) or intramembranous (type II) deposits. MPGN progresses slowly to renal failure. No therapy has been shown to improve disease-free survival, despite a trend toward better outcome in some studies (*Am J Kidney Dis* 14:445, 1989).

V. **Idiopathic rapidly progressive glomerulonephritis** (RPGN) presents with an acute deterioration in renal function, proteinuria (sometimes nephrotic range), and an active urinary sediment with hematuria and RBC casts. Oliguria may be present. Many patients note a preceding viral-like illness. As many as 75% of patients with idiopathic RPGN may respond to high-dose pulse glucocorticoid therapy, methylprednisolone, 30 mg/kg (up to 3 g) IV every 48 hours for 3 doses, followed by prednisone, 2 mg/kg PO qod for 2 months, with a subsequent taper over 4 months (*Am J Kidney Dis* 11:449, 1988). In patients with extrarenal disease suggestive of vasculitis or a renal biopsy demonstrating necrotizing GN, the addition of cyclophosphamide, 2 mg/kg PO qd, may be beneficial.

VI. **Anti-GBM antibody disease** may present with lung and renal involvement (Goodpasture's syndrome) or with renal disease alone. Diagnosis is based on either the presence of anti-GBM antibodies in the serum or the linear deposition of antibody along the basement membrane on renal biopsy. Anti-GBM disease is often rapidly progressive, requiring urgent diagnosis and treatment. Therapy may not be effective if the patient is already oliguric or receiving dialysis, or has a Cr greater than 6.5 mg/dl. The accepted therapeutic strategy in this disease is clearance of anti-GBM antibodies from the serum with concomitant suppression of formation of new antibodies. Daily total volume plasmapheresis for approximately 2 weeks, in combination with cyclophosphamide, 2 mg/kg PO qd for 8 weeks, and prednisone, 60 mg PO qd tapered over 8 weeks, may be effective. Progress is monitored by frequent clinical evaluation and measurement of anti-GBM antibody titers. Immune suppression should be continued until the anti-GBM antibody is undetectable. Relapse is common and tends to occur within the first several months.

VII. **Systemic lupus erythematosus** (SLE) may involve the kidney and can present as slowly progressive azotemia with urinary abnormalities, as nephrotic syndrome, or as rapidly progressive renal insufficiency. A wide variety of histologic changes may be seen on renal biopsy, including mesangial, membranous, focal or diffuse proliferative, and crescentic GN. Renal biopsy is useful in SLE for evaluating disease activity and assessing irreversible changes such as glomerular sclerosis, tubular atrophy, and interstitial fibrosis. A predominance of irreversible changes with little acute inflammation portends a poor response to therapy and should modify the aggressiveness of immunosuppressive treatment. Glucocorticoids are the mainstay of treatment. Patients with severe renal disease are initially treated with methylprednisolone, 500 mg IV q12h for 3 days, followed by oral prednisone, 0.5–1.0 mg/kg PO qd. Prednisone should then be tapered over 6–8 weeks to the lowest dosage that controls disease activity, preferably using an alternate-day regimen. The addition of cytotoxic agents to maintenance glucocorticoid therapy may result in better preservation of renal function and may decrease the progression of renal scarring (*Am J Kidney Dis* 21:239, 1993).

VIII. **Systemic vasculitides** (see Chap. 24) often present with clinical features of acute GN that may be rapidly progressive. Wegener's granulomatosis usually responds to a combination of cyclophosphamide, 2 mg/kg/day PO continued for at least 1 year beyond induction of remission with subsequent taper, plus prednisone, 1 mg/kg PO qd for 4 weeks followed by slow taper and conversion to alternate-day therapy over the next 6–9 months (*Ann Intern Med* 98:16, 1983). The combination of prednisone and cyclophosphamide may also be effective in other forms of necrotizing GN, such as microscopic polyarteritis nodosa.

IX. **Infection-related GN** may occur in association with a variety of infectious processes, including bacterial endocarditis, visceral abscesses, and infected shunts. Treatment of the underlying infection (e.g., antimicrobials, drainage) may result in improvement or resolution of renal disease. **Poststreptococcal GN** may follow group A beta-hemolytic streptococcal infection of the upper respiratory tract or skin. There is no specific therapy, and treatment consists of supportive measures. **Human immunodeficiency virus (HIV)–associated GN** is characterized by proteinuria, edema, and hematuria with or without azotemia. The histologic appearance on biopsy is similar to focal segmental glomerulosclerosis and is usually seen in patients who abuse IV drugs. Patients may respond to zidovudine therapy with stabilization of renal function and reduction of proteinuria (*N Engl J Med* 323:1775, 1990).

The Nephrotic Syndrome

The nephrotic syndrome is a glomerulonephropathy that is characterized by proteinuria (>3.5 g/day), hypoalbuminemia, hyperlipidemia, and edema. It may appear as a manifestation of primary glomerular disease or may be associated with systemic diseases such as diabetes mellitus, amyloidosis, multiple myeloma, SLE, or many other disorders. Therapy includes treatment of the underlying disease and symptomatic management. The nephrotic syndrome increases the risk of cardiac (e.g., atherosclerosis, coronary heart disease, myocardial infarction [MI]) and noncardiac (e.g., infection) complications and thus therapy that lowers urinary protein excretion may be indicated (*Kidney Int* 44:638, 1993). ACE inhibitors reduce proteinuria in diabetic and nondiabetic patients and seem to have long-term beneficial effects (*Am J Kidney Dis* 20:240, 1992).

I. **Edema** should be controlled with bed rest, salt restriction (2–3 g/day), and judicious use of diuretics. Despite massive edema, these patients are subject to intravascular volume depletion, and diuretic therapy may lead to severe volume contraction with decreased renal perfusion. Nevertheless, diuretic therapy is appropriate for controlling edema that is causing respiratory compromise, skin breakdown, or difficulty in ambulation. Furosemide alone or in combination with metolazone is often effective; the dosage must be individualized. Occasionally, parenteral furosemide is necessary, with or without prior infusion of albumin to mobilize fluid into the vascular space.

II. **Hyperlipidemia.** Dietary restriction of cholesterol and saturated fat seems prudent. Hepatic hydroxymethyl glutaryl coenzyme A reductase inhibitors (see Chap. 22) are effective in improving the lipoprotein profile in patients with the nephrotic syndrome. The efficacy and long-term benefit of treatment with lipid-lowering drugs has not been established (*Am J Kidney Dis* 22:143, 1993).

III. **Thromboembolic complications.** The nephrotic syndrome produces a hypercoagulable state, and the clinician should maintain a high index of suspicion for

Table 11-3. Causes of rapid deterioration of renal function in chronic renal failure

I. Decrease in effective arterial blood volume
   A. Volume depletion
   B. Worsening congestive heart failure
II. Alterations in BP
   A. Hypertension
   B. Hypotension, including that induced by antihypertensive medications
III. Infection
IV. Urinary tract obstruction
V. Nephrotoxic agents
VI. Renal vascular events
   A. Renal vein thrombosis
   B. Progression of renal artery stenosis
   C. Cholesterol embolization (especially postarterial procedure)

thromboemboli. Renal vein thrombosis is common. If embolization occurs, anticoagulation with heparin followed by long-term warfarin therapy is indicated (see Chap. 17).

IV. **Dietary protein restriction,** 0.6–0.7 g/kg, may be appropriate for nephrotic patients with renal insufficiency (see Chronic Renal Failure, sec. **II.A.1**), but an amount of protein equal to that lost in the urine should be added to the calculated protein restriction to give the total daily protein intake.

Chronic Renal Failure

CRF may result from many different etiologies. Because of the compensatory ability of remaining nephrons, declining renal function is often asymptomatic until the very late stages of the process. When CRF progresses to end-stage renal disease (ESRD), renal replacement therapy may be required. The decline in GFR may be followed by recording the reciprocal of serum Cr versus time. The resulting plot is usually linear, unless there is a superimposed renal insult, and is useful in end-stage planning and predicting the time when dialysis is needed (usually when GFR is <10 ml/minute). Conservative medical treatment of CRF and attention to factors that are known to cause an acute decline in renal function may postpone the need for dialysis in these patients.

I. **Acute deterioration in CRF** (Table 11-3). A sudden decline in GFR that is more rapid than expected should prompt a search for a superimposed, reversible process.
   A. **Volume depletion** resulting in decreased renal perfusion is a common cause of deterioration of renal function in CRF. Ideally, patients with CRF should be volume expanded as suggested by the presence of a small amount of pedal edema.
   B. **Depression of cardiac output** may impair renal perfusion, thereby worsening CRF. Treatment that increases cardiac output may improve renal function through enhanced renal blood flow. Afterload reduction may be particularly useful in these patients, but caution should be taken to avoid decreased renal perfusion (see Chap. 6).
   C. **Drugs** may exacerbate CRF through direct toxicity to renal structures (e.g., aminoglycosides) or decreased renal perfusion (e.g., NSAIDs). Careful attention to drug dosing in patients with decreased GFR and avoidance of unnecessary use of nephrotoxic agents is appropriate.
II. **Conservative management of CRF** includes measures intended to prevent and correct the metabolic derangements of renal failure and to preserve remaining renal function.
   A. **Dietary modification** is important in controlling metabolic abnormalities and possibly for slowing progression of renal failure.

1. **Protein restriction** will reduce accumulation of nitrogenous waste products. In addition, a low-protein diet may slow the progression of renal failure. Intake should be reduced to 0.6–0.7 g/kg/day of high biologic value protein when GFR falls below 30 ml/minute. Adequate caloric intake (35–50 kcal/kg/day) must be provided to avoid endogenous protein catabolism; thus, patients should be followed carefully for evidence of malnutrition.

2. **Potassium** should be restricted to 40 mEq/day when GFR falls below 20 ml/minute.

3. **Phosphate and calcium.** Renal failure results in phosphate retention with elevation of serum phosphate and a reciprocal fall in serum calcium. Decreased generation of 1,25-dihydroxyvitamin D_3 and skeletal resistance to the action of parathyroid hormone (PTH) further exacerbate hyperphosphatemia and hypocalcemia. These alterations result in increased PTH concentration and secondary hyperparathyroidism, which contributes to renal osteodystrophy seen in CRF (see sec. III). Hyperphosphatemia may also play a role in the progression of renal failure. Dietary phosphorus should be restricted to 800–1,000 mg/day when GFR is less than 50 ml/minute. As GFR falls further, phosphate restriction becomes less effective and the addition of phosphate binders that prevent GI phosphate absorption is indicated. These include aluminum (Al) hydroxide antacids, such as Amphojel or Basaljel, 15–30 ml or 1–3 capsules PO with meals, and calcium carbonate, 1–2 g PO with meals. The disadvantage of Al-containing phosphate binders is accumulation of Al in patients with CRF. Elevated tissue Al levels can cause osteomalacia and have been implicated as a cause of encephalopathy in patients with CRF. Although use of calcium carbonate avoids these problems, large doses may be required to control phosphate levels and may result in hypercalcemia with potential extraskeletal calcification. Calcium carbonate should not be used until serum phosphate is less than 7 mg/dl, and a calcium-phosphate product less than 60 should be maintained to avoid the possibility of metastatic calcification. Vitamin D metabolites may be required in the treatment of hypocalcemia (see Chap. 23).

4. **Sodium and fluid restriction** must be determined on an individual basis, taking the patient's cardiovascular status into consideration. For most patients, a no-added salt diet (8 g NaCl/day) is palatable and adequate. If necessary, 24-hour urinary sodium loss can be determined to aid in sodium intake planning. Once a patient has reached an acceptable volume status, fluid intake should equal daily urine output plus an additional 500 ml for insensible losses. Fluid restriction is appropriate in patients with dilutional hyponatremia or excessive weight gain, and the presence of heart failure or refractory hypertension requires greater restriction of salt and water.

5. **Magnesium** is excreted by the kidney and accumulates in CRF. Extradietary intake of magnesium (e.g., some antacids and cathartics) should be avoided.

B. **Hypertension** may accelerate the rate of decline of renal function in patients with CRF and should be treated aggressively (see Acute Renal Failure, sec. IV.A.3, and Chap. 4). Diuretic use must be carefully monitored to avoid volume depletion. Loop diuretics (e.g., furosemide) remain efficacious when GFR is less than 25 ml/minute.

C. **Acidosis** is treated with oral sodium bicarbonate, 300–600 mg PO tid, when serum bicarbonate falls below 16 mEq/liter. The additional sodium load from such therapy may require further dietary sodium restriction or administration of a diuretic.

D. **Anemia** is responsible for many symptoms of CRF and can be corrected with use of recombinant human erythropoietin, both in dialysis and predialysis patients. Treatment should be initiated in patients with symptoms secondary to anemia and should be considered prior to the onset of symptoms in patients with underlying cardiovascular disease. The starting dose is 50 U/kg SC 3 times/week (*Am J Nephrol* 10:128, 1990) (see Chap. 18). Hypertension may complicate therapy and should be aggressively treated.

III. **Renal osteodystrophy** (*Kidney Int* 38:193, 1990) refers to the skeletal disorders seen in CRF. The major histologic categories are (1) **secondary hyperparathyroidism** (high-turnover bone disease, osteitis fibrosa), due to hyperphosphatemia, hypocalcemia, deficient production of calcitriol [1,25(OH)$_2$D$_3$], and skeletal resistance to PTH; (2) **low-turnover bone disease** (osteomalacia and aplastic bone disease), most often due to Al retention from Al-containing phosphate binders and dialysate; and (3) **mixed renal osteodystrophy**, with features of both.

A. **Clinical manifestations** include bone pain, fractures, skeletal deformity, proximal muscle weakness, pruritus, and extraskeletal calcification. Serum phosphorus is elevated and serum calcium is usually low. Hypercalcemia may develop in Al-related bone disease, marked parathyroid hyperplasia, or during treatment with calcium and calcitriol. Serum PTH, measured by immunoassay for intact hormone, is markedly elevated in osteitis fibrosa and much less elevated in low-turnover bone disease. X-ray findings of osteitis fibrosa include subperiosteal resorption and patchy osteosclerosis; pseudofractures may be seen in osteomalacia.

B. **Diagnosis.** Certain clinical features suggest a particular histologic category. Pruritus or periarticular calcification suggests hyperparathyroidism as the dominant lesion, whereas spontaneous fractures, relatively low serum PTH levels, or hypercalcemia suggest Al-related bone disease. Serum Al levels do not reflect tissue Al content; definitive diagnosis of Al-related bone disease requires bone biopsy.

C. **Management.** Therapy should be started early in the course of progressive renal failure. Goals include (1) maintenance of normal serum calcium and phosphorus levels, (2) suppression of secondary hyperparathyroidism, (3) prevention of extraskeletal calcification, (4) reversal of histologic abnormalities of bone, and (5) prevention and therapy of Al toxicity.

1. **Correction of hyperphosphatemia** (see Chap. 23). Dietary phosphate should be restricted to 0.6–0.9 g/day. Calcium carbonate is the phosphate binder of choice. Calcium citrate and other citrate preparations (e.g., Shohl's solution) should not be used because they promote intestinal Al absorption. The goal is to maintain predialysis serum phosphorus levels between 4.5 and 6.0 mg/dl. Use of Al-containing phosphate binders should be kept to a minimum.

2. **Calcitriol, or 1,25(OH)$_2$D$_3$** (see Chap. 23), is often required to suppress hyperparathyroidism despite control of hyperphosphatemia. The usual dose is 0.25–1.0 μg PO qd, which is adjusted to maintain serum calcium between 10.5 and 11.0 mg/dl. Serum calcium should be measured twice a week and the dose can be adjusted at 2–4-week intervals. The major side effect is hypercalcemia, which is especially likely if Al-related bone disease is present. If low doses of oral calcitriol cause hypercalcemia, substitution of IV calcitriol, 1.0–2.5 μg 3 times a week, may suppress hyperparathyroidism more effectively, with less hypercalcemia (*N Engl J Med* 321:274, 1989).

3. **Parathyroidectomy** may be required to control severe hyperparathyroidism (*Am J Med* 84:23, 1988). A bone biopsy must be done to confirm the presence of osteitis fibrosa and exclude Al-related bone disease. Indications include (1) persistent severe hypercalcemia (after other causes of hypercalcemia are excluded), (2) pruritus unresponsive to dialysis or medical therapy, (3) progressive extraskeletal calcification, (4) severe skeletal pain or fractures, and (5) calciphylaxis (ischemic necrosis of skin or soft tissue associated with vascular calcification). The risk of Al toxicity is increased after parathyroidectomy and, thus, only calcium carbonate should be used as a phosphate binder.

4. **Management of Al toxicity.** Asymptomatic patients with evidence of Al-related bone disease should avoid Al-containing phosphate binders. In symptomatic patients with biopsy-proven Al-related bone disease, deferoxamine (Desferal), 1–3 g infused IV over 2 hours weekly, increases removal of Al by dialysis and improves symptoms over a period of 6–12 months. Side effects of deferoxamine include nausea, vomiting, hypotension, cataracts and other visual abnormalities, and predisposition to bacteremia and mucormycosis.

Renal Replacement Therapies

As CRF progresses and metabolic abnormalities can no longer be controlled with conservative management, signs and symptoms of uremia develop, and the patient requires renal replacement therapy. The indications for dialysis in CRF are similar to those for ARF (see Acute Renal Failure, sec. **IV.B**). The patient with ESRD now has a variety of therapeutic options.

I. **Hemodialysis** (HD) works by diffusion of small-molecular-weight solutes across a semipermeable membrane. Fluid removal occurs via ultrafiltration (see sec. **III.A**). To perform HD, access to the vasculature for blood outflow and return is necessary. Temporary access can be achieved via internal jugular, subclavian, or femoral venous catheters. Permanent vascular access requires creation of a primary arteriovenous (AV) anastomosis or a synthetic (e.g., polytetrafluorethylene) AV graft. Since these grafts must heal before use, they should be placed when Cl_{Cr} is 10–15 ml/minute. The frequency and duration of dialysis and type of artificial kidney used are based on the patient's metabolic, nutritional, and volume status. When HD is instituted, dietary protein should be increased to 1.0–1.2 g/kg/day, and fluid intake should be adjusted to permit a weight gain of about 2 kg between dialysis sessions. Antihypertensive medication may no longer be needed and often should be withheld on dialysis days. **Complications** of HD are described below.

A. **Active bleeding and coagulopathies** may be exacerbated by the systemic anticoagulation needed in HD. The heparin dosage used for hemodialysis should be minimized in these patients or a switch to peritoneal dialysis should be considered. When uremic patients require therapy for active bleeding, the use of IV diamino-8-D-arginine-vasopressin (DDAVP; 0.3 µg/kg in 50 ml saline every 4–8 hours), IV conjugated estrogen (0.6 mg/kg/day for 5 days), or intranasal DDAVP (3.0 µg/kg every 4–6 hours) may shorten the bleeding time (see Chap. 17).

B. **Dialysis disequilibrium** is a syndrome that may occur during the first few treatments of profoundly uremic patients and is attributed to CNS edema from rapid osmolar shifts. Symptoms include nausea, emesis, and headache, with occasional progression to confusion and seizures. This complication may be prevented or ameliorated by using low blood flows and shortened treatment duration during initial dialysis sessions.

C. **Pericarditis** may occur in patients undergoing dialysis and appears to be different than uremic pericarditis. Treatment involves intensification of dialysis to 6–7 times a week. If this therapy fails or if there is evidence of tamponade, pericardiectomy is indicated. Anticoagulation during HD must be minimized or discontinued until pericarditis resolves.

D. **Hypotension** during dialysis may be the result of many factors, including volume depletion, low dialysate sodium content, use of antihypertensive medications before dialysis, allergic reactions to the dialyzer, intolerance to acetate-containing dialysate, left ventricular dysfunction, and autonomic insufficiency. Acute treatment includes infusion of normal saline, reduction of dialyzer blood flow, and reduction of the ultrafiltration rate. Other causes of hypotension such as MI, cardiac tamponade, sepsis, and bleeding should be excluded. In patients exhibiting acetate intolerance, a switch to bicarbonate-based dialysate is often beneficial.

E. **Vascular access complications**

1. **Vascular access infections** may produce local or systemic signs but are often clinically "silent." Prompt therapy with IV antibiotics should be started after blood cultures are obtained. Careful examination and ultrasound of the access site may reveal a local abscess, which should be cultured and drained. Initial therapy must include coverage for staphylococci and should be continued for at least 4 weeks. Removal of an infected access is often necessary.

2. **Vascular access thrombosis.** A clotted access can be recanalized by balloon catheter embolectomy. The access can usually be used immediately after declotting.

F. **Dialysis dementia** is a progressive syndrome occurring secondary to CNS accumulation of Al. Hesitant, nonfluent speech is frequently the presenting sign. Awareness of the potential toxicity of Al has led to monitoring of blood and dialysate levels, and to careful use of Al-containing phosphate binders. Chelation therapy with deferoxamine may improve or stop progression of dialysis dementia in some patients.

II. **Peritoneal dialysis (PD)** uses the peritoneum as a dialysis membrane. It can be performed acutely for ARF by bedside placement of a temporary peritoneal catheter, or on a chronic basis after surgical placement of a catheter. Solutes are removed by diffusion into the dialysate. Fluid removal is controlled by the addition of dextrose to the dialysate to create an osmotic gradient. Dextrose concentrations are usually 1.50–4.25 g/dl. Higher dextrose concentrations and more frequent exchanges increase the rate of fluid removal. A typical dialysis exchange is performed by infusion of 2 liters of fluid into the peritoneal cavity, followed by an equilibration period and dialysate drainage. In acute PD, exchanges can be performed as often as every hour. **Continuous ambulatory peritoneal dialysis** (CAPD) usually involves 4–5 exchanges/day performed by the patient. A modification of CAPD uses an automatic cycler to perform exchanges during sleep (continuous cyclic peritoneal dialysis, or CCPD). Peritoneal dialysis should be avoided in patients with recent abdominal surgery or a history of multiple surgeries with adhesions. Strict sterile technique is mandatory when performing exchanges. Compared with HD, PD is less efficient and less useful in highly catabolic patients. Because PD does not require systemic anticoagulation and produces less stress on the cardiovascular system, it may offer advantages over HD in certain situations. In addition, PD causes fewer abrupt changes in BP and electrolytes and allows patients greater independence than HD. Complications of PD are as follows.

A. **Infections** are the most significant problem in PD and include peritonitis, infection of the catheter tunnel, and infection of the catheter exit site. Peritonitis is usually secondary to a break in sterile technique during fluid exchanges. Most episodes of peritonitis are mild and can be treated on an outpatient basis, with the patient initiating therapy; however, patients should save infected dialysate for culture. Initial treatment is accomplished with two rapid exchanges, followed by exchanges q1–2h until abdominal pain stops. Antimicrobials and heparin (500 units/liter) should be added to the dialysate after the first two exchanges. Fluid balance must be closely monitored and dialysate concentration adjusted to avoid dehydration or volume overload. Treatment is continued for 14 days. Antimicrobial therapy should include coverage for skin organisms, especially staphylococci. Intraperitoneal ceftazidime or an aminoglycoside in combination with vancomycin, are appropriate choices (Table 11-4). Hospitalization is indicated in patients with frank sepsis, resistant or recurrent infections, or suspicion of organ perforation or abscess formation. Tunnel or exit site infections also involve skin organisms, are frequently difficult to treat, and may require catheter removal and temporary HD until the infection resolves (*Peritoneal Dialysis Int* 13:14, 1993).

B. **Hyperglycemia** may occur from absorption of glucose in PD fluid. If necessary, regular insulin can be added directly to the dialysate (e.g., 2 units to 2 liters of 1.5% dextrose, 6 units to 2 liters of 4.25% dextrose). In diabetic patients, intraperitoneal insulin is effective in controlling blood sugar. Conversion from SC insulin to intraperitoneal insulin is best accomplished in the hospital, where proper glucose monitoring can be ensured. Initially, the patient's usual total daily SC insulin dose is divided by the number of exchanges he or she will receive and is given as regular insulin in each CAPD exchange. Additional insulin to cover glucose in the PD fluid (see above) should be included. Insulin must be added using sterile technique to avoid contamination and peritonitis.

C. **Protein loss** in PD can be excessive, and dietary protein intake should be increased to 1.2–1.4 g/kg/day.

Table 11-4. Intraperitoneal antibiotics in peritoneal dialysis

Antibiotic	Dose
Ceftazidime	Loading dose of 500 mg/liter IP; maintenance dose of 125 mg/liter with each exchange
Vancomycin	2 g IP every 7 days × 2
Gentamycin	20 mg/liter IP for 1 exchange daily; 4–8 mg/liter in all other exchanges
Tobramycin	20 mg/liter IP for 1 exchange daily; 4–8 mg/liter in all other exchanges
Imipenem	Loading dose of 500 mg/liter IP; maintenance dose of 100 mg/liter with each exchange
Flucytosine	Loading dose of 2 g PO; maintenance dose of 1 g PO qd and 150 mg/liter IP every 2 days

III. Ultrafiltration and hemofiltration remove large volumes of fluid with minimal removal of metabolic wastes. These filtration techniques are useful for removing fluid in patients with renal insufficiency and volume overload who do not need concomitant dialysis.

 A. **Ultrafiltration** is performed with standard hemodialysis cartridges and equipment. A blood pump perfuses the cartridges with the patient's blood, but no dialysate is used. By manipulation of the transmembrane pressure gradient, an ultrafiltrate of plasma is formed and removed. Because large volumes of fluid are removed in a short period of time, the patient may experience hypotension. Ultrafiltration can be performed alone or in combination with hemodialysis.

 B. **Continuous arteriovenous hemofiltration** (CAVH) or hemodialysis (CAVHD) uses a highly permeable membrane to filter blood from a femoral or extremity artery. Blood is returned to the patient through a femoral or extremity vein. The driving force for filtration is the patient's BP; no blood pump is needed. CAVH is better tolerated than ultrafiltration in hemodynamically unstable patients because fluid removal is slow and continuous. Another advantage of this technique is the simplicity of the equipment. However, the patient must be continuously heparinized and is virtually bed-bound. In addition, fluid balance must be closely monitored to avoid massive volume depletion. Fluid removal rates can be adjusted frequently to compensate for fluid input. This procedure should be carried out only in an intensive care setting. Continuous venovenous hemofiltration (CVVH) or hemodialysis (CVVHD) is now possible with special equipment. The advantage is that the only access required is a double-lumen dialysis catheter, thus avoiding the need for an arterial line.

IV. Renal transplantation has enjoyed considerable success as a result of improved donor-recipient selection, immunosuppressive drug regimens, and methods of treating allograft rejection. One-year graft survival rates are 80% for cadaver allografts and 90% for living-related donor grafts (*Am J Kidney Dis* 22:58, 1993). Transplantation represents the only therapeutic option that may allow patients with ESRD to return to their premorbid life-styles. Selected medical aspects of transplant therapy are described below.

 A. **Pretransplant evaluation** of the recipient includes assessment of cardiovascular status, structural abnormalities of the urinary tract, correction of potential sources of infection (e.g., dental hygiene problems), human lymphocyte antigen typing, and evaluation for preformed antibodies against potential donor antigens. The latter, along with blood group compatibility testing, should prevent hyperacute rejection in most cases.

 B. **Immunosuppression** after transplantation is essential for prevention of allograft rejection. A variety of immunosuppressive regimens have been used, and the choice of immune suppression varies with the type of transplant (i.e., cadaver versus living-related donor). The most frequently used regimens employ a combination of prednisone and either cyclosporine (CsA) or azathioprine, but some regimens use all three agents. The advent of CsA has improved cadaver allograft survival rates by 10–20% and has reduced rejection episodes. Its major toxicities are ARF and CRF. A rising Cr in a patient receiving CsA may thus indicate rejection or CsA nephrotoxicity. Acute nephrotoxicity often responds to a decrease in dosage or discontinuation of CsA. CsA may rarely produce a hemolytic-uremic–like syndrome, which results in significant allograft loss. Chronic CsA nephrotoxicity produces irreversible interstitial fibrosis. Other adverse effects of CsA include hypertension, hyperkalemia, predisposition to lymphoproliferative malignancy, tremor, seizure, and hepatotoxicity. CsA levels can be measured and the incidence of toxic side effects is increased when trough levels are elevated. CsA is metabolized by the liver. Concomitant drug use may affect CsA metabolism. Use of erythromycin or ketoconazole increases CsA blood levels, whereas use of phenytoin decreases CsA levels. Such drug interactions should be considered and appropriate dosage adjustments made in patients taking CsA (see Appendix B).

C. **Allograft rejection** may be acute or chronic and is suggested by rising Cr, allograft tenderness, and decreasing urine output. Other causes of renal impairment such as volume depletion, obstruction, problems of vascular supply, drug nephrotoxicity, and recurrent or de novo renal disease should be excluded. Evaluation of suspected rejection generally requires allograft biopsy. Therapy of rejection is best carried out by an experienced transplant team.

1. **Acute cellular rejection.** Currently used modalities for treatment of acute rejection include high-dose IV methylprednisolone, antilymphocyte globulin, and anti–T-lymphocyte monoclonal antibody (OKT3) administration.

2. **Chronic rejection** generally progresses to allograft failure over months to years. There is no specific treatment for chronic rejection; general measures for conservative management of chronic renal insufficiency should be instituted.

D. **Infections** are a major cause of morbidity and mortality in the transplant patient and must be excluded when fever is present (see Chap. 14).

Nephrolithiasis

I. **Clinical manifestations** of nephrolithiasis include hematuria, predisposition to urinary tract infection, and pain (usually flank) with passage of the stone. Renal stones may also be an incidental finding on radiographic studies. Oliguria and ARF may occur when both collecting systems are blocked by stones.

II. **Diagnostic evaluation** of an acute episode of flank pain and hematuria should include a plain abdominal roentgenogram, as the majority of renal stones are radiopaque. Exceptions include cystine stones, which may be of intermediate opacity, and uric acid stones, which are radiolucent. IVP should be performed acutely if renal colic is severe and obstruction is suspected. IVP is also useful in evaluating the anatomy of the kidneys and collecting systems. Urine should be examined for pH and crystals and cultured. Other initial studies include serum electrolytes, Cr, calcium, uric acid, and phosphorus. All passed stones should be saved for analysis. After resolution of the acute episode, further diagnostic evaluation can be guided by stone composition. The extent of the metabolic evaluation that should be undertaken for the patient with a single calcium stone has not been established, but recurrent calcium nephrolithiasis warrants complete investigation. Patients with noncalcium stones should undergo complete evaluation after the first episode. Further studies may include PTH levels (if hypercalcemia is present) and 24-hour urine studies for measurement of calcium, phosphate, urate, oxalate, citrate, Cr, sodium, urea nitrogen, and cystine. Yearly follow-up examination of the patient with nephrolithiasis includes abdominal roentgenograms to check for new stone formation or growth of existing stones and repeat metabolic studies to assess the effects of specific therapies.

III. Treatment. Acute management of patients with stones includes analgesia and hydration. If the stone is obstructing outflow or is accompanied by infection, removal is indicated. After passage of a stone, treatment is directed at prevention of recurrent stone formation. In most patients, the foundation of general therapy is maintenance of high urine output (>2.5 liters/day) through oral hydration and avoidance of dietary excesses. Specific treatments (*N Engl J Med* 327:1141, 1992) are described below.

A. Calcium stones account for about 80% of all stones and are composed of calcium oxalate and phosphate. Hypercalciuria is usually present and may be idiopathic or secondary to an identifiable disease. Calcium stones may also precipitate around a uric acid nidus in patients with hyperuricosuria, even in the absence of hypercalciuria (see sec. III.B). Other conditions associated with calcium stone formation include hyperoxaluria (commonly seen in patients with inflammatory bowel disorders), distal renal tubular acidosis, medullary sponge kidney, and sarcoidosis.

   1. Hypercalciuria (calcium excretion >4 mg/kg/day with a normal calcium intake [800–1,000 mg/day]) may be due to increased GI absorption of calcium, impaired renal tubular calcium reabsorption, or excessive skeletal resorption as in primary hyperparathyroidism. Hypercalciuria can be treated conservatively by modest limitations of calcium intake to 800 mg/day and protein to 1 g/kg/day and by maintaining a high fluid intake. Severe restrictions of calcium may be counterproductive because of increased urinary oxalate excretion and the risk of bone mineral depletion. Excess sodium intake (i.e., >10 g salt/day) should be avoided, and restriction of salt intake to less than 6 g/day may be beneficial. If dietary measures are not effective, addition of a thiazide diuretic (hydrochlorothiazide, 25–50 mg PO bid) to increase calcium reabsorption by the kidney is often useful. Careful follow-up is important in these patients to ensure that therapy has decreased calcium excretion and has not caused adverse alterations in serum electrolyte concentrations.

   2. Hyperparathyroidism resulting in renal stone formation should be treated with parathyroidectomy.

   3. Hyperoxaluria (urinary oxalate excretion >0.7 mg/kg/day) requires dietary oxalate restriction. Patients with malabsorption by the small bowel due to intrinsic disease, postresection, or jejunoileal bypass absorb excessive oxalate, resulting in hyperoxaluria. Dietary restriction of oxalate along with supplemental oral calcium and cholestyramine may be useful.

   4. Hypocitraturia. Urine citrate (an inhibitor of calcium oxalate precipitation) is frequently low in patients with calcium stones. Therapy with potassium citrate, 20 mEq PO tid, is often effective.

B. Uric acid stone formation is favored by conditions of uric acid overproduction (urine uric acid excretion >11 mg/kg/day), low urinary volume, and persistently acid urine pH. Conservative therapy involves maintenance of urine volume greater than 2 liters/day through oral hydration and alkalinization of urine to pH 6.5–7.0 with an oral alkali preparation (e.g., Shohl's solution, 20 ml PO bid–tid). Patients should be instructed in the home measurement of urine pH so that the oral alkali dose can be appropriately titrated. If these measures fail, administration of allopurinol, 300 mg PO qd, is indicated. Probenecid and other uricosuric drugs should be avoided as they may increase the risk of uric acid or calcium oxalate stone formation.

C. Cystine stones arise from an inborn error in amino acid transport with consequent cystinuria. Cystine crystals are hexagonal on microscopic examination of the urine. Treatment includes maintenance of urine volume of greater than 3 liters/day and alkalinization of urine to a pH greater than 7.0 with Shohl's solution, 30 ml PO qid. D-penicillamine, 1–2 g/day PO, or tiopronin can be used in refractory cases, but this therapy is often complicated by side effects such as nephrotoxicity, allergic reactions, and hematologic abnormalities (see Chap. 24).

D. Struvite stones (staghorn calculi) occur under conditions of high urinary pH, reflecting infection with urea-splitting organisms (e.g., *Proteus mirabilis*). For antimicrobial therapy to be effective, the infected stone material must be removed.

Antimicrobials

Jay R. Erickson and
Wm. Claiborne Dunagan

Principles of Antimicrobial Therapy

Use of antimicrobial agents. The decision to institute antimicrobial chemotherapy should be made carefully. Antimicrobials may have serious adverse effects and are often expensive. In addition, antimicrobial resistance continues to increase. Antimicrobials should be selected to provide the desired clinical improvement while minimizing the prevalence of resistant organisms in the patient and in the community. When antimicrobial therapy is indicated, a number of factors must be considered.

I. **Choice of initial antimicrobial therapy.** The infecting organism is often unknown when therapy is initiated. In these cases, empiric therapy should be directed against the most likely pathogens. Therapy should then be altered in accordance with the patient's course and laboratory results. It is generally prudent to use the regimen that possesses the narrowest antimicrobial spectrum that adequately covers the predicted infecting organisms.

   A. **Gram's stain.** During the initial evaluation, all accessible potentially infected material should be examined with a Gram's stain. A careful examination often permits a rapid presumptive etiologic diagnosis and may be essential for interpretation of subsequent culture results.

   B. **Local susceptibility** patterns must be considered in selecting empiric therapy because patterns vary widely among communities and individual hospitals.

   C. **Cultures** are necessary for precise diagnosis and for susceptibility testing. Specimens obtained for culture should be delivered promptly to the laboratory, as delays may allow fastidious pathogens to die and contaminating flora to overgrow. Whenever organisms with special growth requirements are suspected, the microbiology laboratory should be consulted to ensure appropriate transport and processing. If anaerobes are suspected, specimens must be handled in a manner that minimizes exposure to air and should be cultured as soon as possible.

   D. **Antimicrobial susceptibility testing.** Susceptibility testing facilitates a rational selection of antimicrobial agents. Disk-diffusion susceptibility testing is usually sufficient. In serious infections, such as infective endocarditis, quantification of the drug concentrations that inhibit and kill the pathogen may be useful. The antimicrobial activity of a treated patient's serum can be estimated by measuring **serum bactericidal titers.** Peak serum bactericidal titers of $\geq 1 : 8$ have been associated with improved outcomes in the treatment of intravascular infections (*N Engl J Med* 312:968, 1985).

   E. **An acute-phase serum specimen** is often valuable when the diagnosis is uncertain. Serum should be collected and stored for comparison with a convalescent sample. Demonstration of a high-antibody titer or of changing titers against an infectious agent may be diagnostic.

II. **Status of the host.** The clinical status of the patient determines the speed with which therapy must be instituted, as well as the route of administration and type of therapy. Patients should be promptly evaluated for hemodynamic stability, rapidly progressive or life-threatening infections, and immune defects.

   A. **Timing of the initiation of antimicrobial therapy.** When the clinical situation is acute, empiric therapy is usually begun immediately after appropriate cultures have been obtained. However, if the patient's condition is stable, delaying empiric antimicrobials may permit specific therapy based on the results of culture and susceptibility testing and may prevent adverse effects from the use of unnecessary drugs. **Urgent therapy** is indicated in febrile patients who are neutropenic, asplenic, or otherwise immunosuppressed (see Chap. 14). Sepsis, meningitis, and rapidly progressive anaerobic or necrotizing infections should always be treated with antimicrobial therapy as quickly as possible.

B. **Route of administration.** Patients with serious infections should be given antimicrobial agents intravenously. In less urgent circumstances, intramuscular or oral therapy is often sufficient. Oral therapy is acceptable when it can be tolerated by the patient and when it produces adequate drug concentrations at the site of infection.

C. **Type of therapy.** Bactericidal therapy is indicated for patients with immunologic compromise or life-threatening infection. It is also preferred for infections characterized by impaired regional host defenses, such as endocarditis, meningitis, and osteomyelitis (*Infect Dis Clin North Am* 3:389, 1989).

D. **Underlying renal or hepatic disease.** Renal and hepatic metabolism and excretion are the major pathways of antimicrobial elimination. Many antimicrobials are excreted by the kidney and require dosage adjustment in patients with renal insufficiency (see Appendix D). Likewise, hepatically metabolized drugs may require dosage adjustment in patients with significant liver disease, though precise guidelines for individual drugs are lacking. Measurement of serum drug levels is especially helpful in the treatment of patients with hepatic or renal failure.

E. **Pregnancy and the puerperium.** Although no antimicrobial is known to be completely safe in pregnancy, the penicillins and cephalosporins are used most often. Tetracyclines and quinolones are among the agents specifically contraindicated, and the sulfonamides and aminoglycosides should not be used if alternative agents are available. Dosages of most antimicrobials should be increased to compensate for an increased maternal volume of distribution in pregnancy. In addition, most antibiotics administered in therapeutic dosages will appear in breast milk and should be used with caution in patients who are breast-feeding.

III. **Drug interactions.** The possibility of chemical incompatibilities or in vivo drug interactions should be considered each time a new drug is prescribed (see Appendix B).

IV. **Antimicrobial combinations.** The empiric use of multiple antimicrobials to provide broader coverage is justified in seriously ill patients when (1) the identity of an infecting organism is not apparent, (2) the suspected pathogen has a variable antimicrobial susceptibility, or (3) failure to initiate effective antimicrobial therapy will significantly increase morbidity or mortality. In addition, antimicrobial combinations are specifically indicated (1) to produce synergism (e.g., in enterococcal endocarditis or gram-negative sepsis in neutropenic patients), (2) to treat polymicrobial infections (e.g., peritonitis following rupture of a viscus), and (3) to prevent the emergence of antimicrobial resistance (e.g., tuberculosis). The indiscriminate use of antimicrobial combinations should be avoided because of the potential for increased toxicity, pharmacologic antagonism, and the selection of resistant organisms.

V. **Duration of therapy.** Treatment of acute, uncomplicated infections should be continued until the patient has been afebrile and clinically well for a minimum of 72 hours. Infections at certain sites (e.g., endocarditis, septic arthritis, osteomyelitis) require long-term therapy; periodic cultures may be useful in these cases to assess the response to treatment.

Antibacterial Agents

I. **Beta-lactam antimicrobials** include the penicillins, cephalosporins, cephamycins, carbacephems, carbapenems, and monobactams. These highly effective antimicrobials bind to penicillin-binding proteins on the bacterial cytoplasmic membrane and interfere with cell wall physiology. Beta-lactam resistance may result from alterations in penicillin-binding proteins, antimicrobial degradation by beta-lactamases, or decreased antimicrobial permeation of the outer membrane.

A. Penicillins (PCNs) remain among the most effective and least toxic antimicrobials available and are often the drugs of choice for treatment of susceptible pathogens. Most PCNs are rapidly excreted by the kidney; therefore, dosages must be adjusted in patients with renal insufficiency. **Probenecid** (500 mg PO q6h) interferes with renal tubular secretion of PCNs and can be used to increase their serum half-lives. **Hypersensitivity** reactions are among the most common side effects of the PCNs, and they may produce fever, eosinophilia, serum sickness, or anaphylaxis (*Ann Intern Med* 107:204, 1987). Penicillins have a common immunogenicity, and persons known to be allergic to one PCN preparation should not be given another if an acceptable alternative is available. When there is no alternative to the use of a PCN, **skin testing** can be performed. A negative reaction makes anaphylaxis unlikely if the PCN is given immediately but does not preclude other allergic reactions or the possibility of anaphylaxis if the patient is rechallenged with PCN at a later date. **Desensitization** is rarely required and should be performed only in a closely monitored setting (*J Allergy Clin Immunol* 69:275, 1982). Coombs'-positive hemolytic anemia, leukopenia, and thrombocytopenia are rare complications of PCN therapy. Seizures may occur with very high dosages of PCN, particularly in patients with renal failure. Interstitial nephritis is an unusual side effect, most commonly seen with ampicillin and the penicillinase-resistant PCNs (see Chap. 11).

  1. Penicillin G (benzyl penicillin) is hydrolyzed by gastric acid and in general is ineffective when taken orally. Penicillin G is active against most gram-positive and gram-negative aerobic cocci (beta-lactamase–negative) and many anaerobes, including anaerobic cocci and *Clostridium* spp. Penicillin resistance is increasing, and resistance among once uniformly susceptible species (e.g., *Streptococcus pneumoniae*) is not uncommon (*Clin Infect Dis* 15:77, 1992). The decision to use penicillin should therefore be based on local resistance patterns and susceptibility testing. Dosages vary depending on the disease being treated.

   a. Aqueous penicillin G (IM or IV) is usually supplied as the potassium salt (1.7 mEq K$^+$/million units), although sodium salts are available and may be useful for patients with hyperkalemia or renal failure.

   b. Procaine penicillin G is a repository form of penicillin G that yields sustained serum levels when given intramuscularly. It is useful for treatment of streptococcal infections, particularly when compliance with oral therapy may be a problem. Procaine hypersensitivity is a contraindication to its use.

   c. Benzathine penicillin G (IM) is another repository penicillin mixture that produces low sustained serum levels of penicillin G for 1–3 weeks. Its use is largely limited to treatment of streptococcal pharyngitis, prophylaxis of rheumatic fever, and treatment of syphilis. CSF penetration is unreliable.

  2. Penicillin V (250–500 mg PO q6h) is relatively resistant to hydrolysis by gastric acid and can be taken orally. In general, food diminishes its absorption. Penicillin V is the oral drug of choice for infections caused by gram-positive cocci that do not produce beta-lactamase (e.g., group A streptococci).

  3. Penicillinase-resistant semisynthetic penicillins (PRSP) are indicated for the treatment of infections caused by penicillinase-producing staphylococci. They are less active than penicillin G and penicillin V against non–beta-lactamase–producing gram-positive cocci. Staphylococci that are resistant to one of the PRSPs are also generally resistant to other PRSPs, the cephalosporins, and imipenem. Notable toxicities of these agents include interstitial nephritis, elevations of serum transaminases, cholestatic jaundice, and neutropenia.

    a. Oxacillin (1–2 g IV q4–6h) and **nafcillin** (1–2 g IV q4–6h) are the preferred agents for parenteral therapy.

    b. Dicloxacillin (125–500 mg PO q6h) and **cloxacillin** (250–500 mg PO q6h) are similar to oxacillin but possess superior oral bioavailability and are preferred for oral use. These agents should be given on an empty stomach.

    c. Methicillin may be associated with a higher incidence of interstitial nephritis than the other semisynthetic PCNs. Therefore, many physicians avoid its use.

4. Amino PCNs are also semisynthetic PCN derivatives that provide enhanced activity against many gram-negative bacilli.

    a. Ampicillin (500 mg PO q6h, 1.0–2.0 g IV q4–6h) is active against many community-acquired Enterobacteriaceae, *Haemophilus influenzae,* and *Neisseria* spp. Ampicillin retains much of the gram-positive activity of penicillin G, and it is slightly less active against group A streptococci and pneumococci. It possesses good activity against *Listeria monocytogenes* and gram-positive anaerobes including *Clostridium* spp and *Actinomyces israelii.* However, ampicillin is hydrolyzed by many beta-lactamases and is inactive against most strains of *Staphylococcus, Klebsiella,* 25–50% of *H. influenzae,* and most nosocomial gram-negative bacilli. For optimal bioavailability, ampicillin should be taken on an empty stomach.

    b. Amoxicillin (250–500 mg PO q8h) is an analog of ampicillin with a similar antibacterial spectrum. Amoxicillin has superior oral bioavailability and it is generally preferred for oral therapy.

5. Carboxy and acylamino PCNs are extended-spectrum agents indicated primarily for treatment of infections due to *Pseudomonas aeruginosa* and other gram-negative bacilli. They are also effective against many strains of *Bacteroides fragilis.* All these drugs are susceptible to staphylococcal beta-lactamase and should not be used to treat infections caused by staphylococci. In treating serious infections due to susceptible gram-negative organisms such as *P. aeruginosa, Enterobacter* spp, and *Serratia,* these agents should be **combined with an aminoglycoside** for potential synergy. CNS penetration of these agents is modest (10% of serum levels), and they are not recommended for the treatment of gram-negative bacillary meningitis. **Adverse effects** of these agents are similar to those of other PCNs. In addition, phlebitis, hypokalemia, and prolongation of the bleeding time may occur (*Ann Intern Med* 105:924, 1986). Carboxy and acylamino PCNs may chemically inactivate aminoglycosides and therefore should not be administered simultaneously through the same IV line (*J Pharmacol Exp Ther* 217:345, 1981).

    a. Ticarcillin (3 g IV q4h or 4 g IV q6h) is a carboxy PCN with activity against many gram-negative rods. It is not generally active against enterococci and most *Klebsiella* spp. Ticarcillin contains 5.2 mEq sodium/g, which must be considered when used in patients susceptible to volume overload.

    b. Acylamino PCNs include **mezlocillin** and **piperacillin** (both 3 g IV q4h or 4 g IV q6h). These acylamino PCNs have activity against *Enterococcus* spp approaching that of ampicillin. In addition, mezlocillin and piperacillin are active in vitro against most strains of *Klebsiella.* The acylamino PCNs may inhibit *P. aeruginosa* strains that are resistant to the carboxy PCNs.

    c. Indanyl carbenicillin (1–2 tablets PO q6h), an oral carboxy PCN, is effective for urinary tract infections (UTIs) caused by susceptible *Pseudomonas* spp and some other ampicillin-resistant organisms. Since it produces low serum levels, it should not be used for the treatment of systemic infections.

6. Amdinocillin (mecillinam) is an amidino PCN with a high degree of activity in vitro against many gram-negative bacilli but is inactive against gram-positive cocci, *Pseudomonas* spp, and anaerobes. Amdinocillin offers no advantage over other antimicrobial regimens.

B. Cephalosporins, cephamycins, and **carbacephems.** These agents can be classified by generations, the members of which share similar antibacterial activity and pharmacokinetics. Newer generations of cephalosporins tend to have increased activity against gram-negative bacilli, usually at the expense of gram-positive activity. The use of these broad-spectrum second- and third-generation agents has been accompanied by the development of bacteria with clinically significant drug resistance (*Rev Infect Dis* 10:830, 1988). Cross-resistance with other beta-lactam agents also occurs. Resistance is particularly common with *Enterobacter, Pseudomonas,* and *Citrobacter* spp. **None of these agents are indicated for treatment of enterococcal infections.** These drugs may produce **hypersensitivity** reactions, and some PCN-allergic patients are also allergic to the cephalosporins. Other **adverse reactions** include phlebitis (with IV administration), sterile abscesses (when given IM), and diarrhea. In addition, cephalosporins that contain an *N*-methylthiotetrazole (MTT) side chain (cefamandole, cefoperazone, and cefotetan) may produce a coagulopathy by interfering with the synthesis of vitamin K–dependent clotting factors. This effect is reversed by administration of vitamin K. Ingestion of ethanol may also induce a disulfiram-like reaction in patients receiving agents with the MTT side chain. Most cephalosporins are renally excreted, and dosages should be adjusted in renal failure (see Appendix D).

1. **First-generation cephalosporins** have activity against most gram-positive cocci, including beta-lactamase–producing strains, and against the gram-negative bacilli that cause most community-acquired infections, including *Escherichia coli* and *Klebsiella* spp. However, *B. fragilis, P. aeruginosa,* and *Enterobacter* spp are typically resistant, as are methicillin-resistant staphylococci. None of these agents cross the meninges in concentrations sufficient for the treatment of meningitis.

   a. **Cephalothin, cephapirin,** and **cephradine** (all 0.5–2.0 g IV, IM q4–6h) have similar pharmacokinetics and toxicity. Oral cephradine is equivalent to cephalexin (see sec. **I.B.1.c**).

   b. **Cefazolin** (1–2 g IV or IM q8h) produces higher and more sustained serum levels and is less painful when given IM than the other first-generation cephalosporins.

   c. **Cephalexin** (250–500 mg PO q6h) and **cefadroxil** (1–2 g/day PO in 1 or 2 doses) are used primarily in the treatment of UTI and may not be optimal for systemic infections at standard doses because achievable serum levels are low.

2. **Second-generation cephalosporins** offer expanded coverage against gram-negative bacilli compared to first-generation agents. There are sufficient differences among their antibacterial spectra to require individual susceptibility testing of clinical isolates. Their major role is in the treatment of infections due to cephalothin-resistant gram-negative bacilli. **Aside from cefuroxime, none of the second-generation agents has reliable CSF penetration and they should not be used to treat meningitis.**

   a. **Cefamandole** (1–2 g IM or IV q4–6h) and **cefonicid** (1–2 g IM or IV qd) are active in vitro against most Enterobacteriaceae and *H. influenzae*. They are not active against *P. aeruginosa, B. fragilis,* or *Serratia marcescens*. Cefamandole may produce MTT side chain–associated toxicities (see sec. **I.B**). **Ceforanide** (0.5–1 g IV or IM q12h) is similar to cefamandole but is less active in vitro against *Staph. aureus* and *H. influenzae*; it has no advantage over other agents in this class.

   b. **Cefuroxime** (0.75–1.5 g IV or IM q8h) has a spectrum of activity similar to that of cefamandole but is more resistant to beta-lactamases, including those produced by *H. influenzae*. Cefuroxime enters the CSF in sufficient concentration to be useful in the treatment of meningitis due to susceptible organisms, although data suggest that third-generation cephalosporins may be more effective (*J Pediatr* 114:1049, 1989).

   c. **Cefoxitin** (1–2 g IM or IV q4–8h), **cefotetan** (1–3 g IM or IV q12h), and **cefmetazole** (2 g IV q6–12h) are cephamycins that are particularly resistant to certain beta-lactamases and are active against many gram-positive and gram-negative aerobes, anaerobes including *B. fragilis*, and beta-lactamase–producing *Neisseria gonorrhoeae*. They are not active against most strains of *P. aeruginosa* or *Enterobacter* spp. Cefotetan and cefmetazole also possess the MTT side chain (see sec. **I.B**). Despite minor differences in in vitro activity, there is no clear therapeutic advantage among any of these agents for treatment of infections due to susceptible bacteria, and choices can usually be made based on local cost considerations.

  d. Cefuroxime axetil (250 mg PO q12h) and **cefprozil** (250–500 mg PO q12h–24h) are oral cephalosporins with activity against beta-lactamase–producing *H. influenzae, Moraxella catarrhalis*, and gram-positive cocci. They can be used to treat otitis media, UTI, and some soft-tissue and respiratory infections, but equally effective and less expensive drugs are often available.

  e. Cefaclor (250–500 mg PO q8h) has a spectrum of activity similar to that of cephalexin but with enhanced activity against *H. influenzae*, including beta-lactamase–producing strains. Serum sickness has been associated with cefaclor, usually in children during the second course of therapy.

  f. Loracarbef (200–400 mg PO q12–24h) is a carbacephem with a spectrum of activity similar to the second-generation cephalosporins. It can be used to treat infections of the upper and lower respiratory tract, skin, and urinary tract due to susceptible pathogens, although it offers no clear advantage over many other agents. Food interferes with absorption of loracarbef, so it should be taken at least 1 hour before or 2 hours after meals.

3. Third-generation cephalosporins are generally more active in vitro against gram-negative bacilli and less active against gram-positive cocci (especially *Staph. aureus*) than the first- and second-generation agents. Most third-generation agents are not effective for infections due to *Pseudomonas* spp, and none are effective for enterococcal infections, even if used in combination with an aminoglycoside. **The third-generation cephalosporins are the drugs of choice for gram-negative bacillary meningitis.** They are also useful for treatment of other gram-negative bacillary infections, but widespread use may lead to the emergence of resistant flora and superinfection with enterococci and other resistant bacteria and fungi. These agents are not indicated for routine surgical prophylaxis.

  a. Cefotaxime (1–2 g IV q4–12h), **ceftizoxime** (1–4 g IV q8–12h), and **ceftriaxone** (1–2 g IV q12–24h) have similar spectra of activity. The dosages of cefotaxime and ceftizoxime should be adjusted in renal insufficiency (see Appendix D). The dosage of ceftriaxone needs to be adjusted only in patients with combined renal and hepatic dysfunction. Ceftriaxone is useful for the treatment of gonorrhea due to penicillinase-producing *N. gonorrhoeae*. Its long half-life may also facilitate long-term parenteral therapy. These agents may also be administered IM.

  b. Ceftazidime (1–2 g IV or IM q8–12h) is the most active of the cephalosporins against *P. aeruginosa*. Its activity against most other gram-negative rods is equivalent to that of cefotaxime, but it is less active than other third-generation agents against gram-positive cocci.

  c. Cefoperazone (1–4 g IV q6–12h) is less active than other third-generation agents against most gram-negative pathogens. It does not penetrate the CSF well and is **not recommended for the treatment of meningitis.** Because of its hepatic excretion, dosage reduction may be necessary in severe liver disease. Cefoperazone also possesses the MTT side chain (see sec. **I.B**).

  d. Cefixime (400 mg PO q24h in 1 or 2 doses) and **cefpodoxime proxetil** (100–400 mg PO q12h) are oral third-generation cephalosporins active against many streptococci, Enterobacteriaceae, *N. gonorrhoeae, H. influenzae*, and *M. catarrhalis*. They have generally poor activity against anaerobes and *Pseudomonas* and *Enterobacter* spp. Neither drug offers a clear advantage over the older, often less expensive, agents in treating most cases of otitis media, upper or lower respiratory infections, or UTI. The bioavailability of cefpodoxime proxetil is increased when taken with food.

C. **Aztreonam** (0.5–2.0 g IV q6–12h) is a monobactam, with activity exclusively against aerobic gram-negative bacilli, including most strains of *P. aeruginosa* and *Serratia* spp. It is inactive against gram-positive cocci and anaerobes. **Aztreonam may be useful in patients allergic to PCN, as there is no apparent cross-reactivity in these patients** (*Ann Intern Med* 107:204, 1987). Otherwise, it has no clear advantage over other broad-spectrum beta-lactam agents. **Aztreonam should not be used in place of aminoglycosides when synergistic therapy is desired** (e.g., treatment of pseudomonal or enterococcal infections). Resistance may occur, often with cross-resistance to third-generation cephalosporins.

D. **Imipenem** (0.5–1.0 g IV q6–8h), a carbapenem antimicrobial, given in a fixed combination with cilastatin (an inhibitor of imipenem metabolism) has potent broad-spectrum activity against many bacteria, including anaerobes, most gram-positive cocci (except *Enterococcus faecium* and methicillin-resistant staphylococci), and gram-negative bacilli (excluding *Xanthomonas maltophilia* and some *Pseudomonas cepacia*). As with other beta-lactam antimicrobials, resistance may emerge during imipenem therapy, particularly among strains of *P. aeruginosa*. Whether concurrent use of an aminoglycoside will prevent the emergence of resistance has not yet been determined. The dosage should be adjusted in patients with renal dysfunction (see Appendix D). IM administration (0.50–0.75 g q12h) can be used for certain less severe infections.

1. **Indications.** Imipenem is useful for the treatment of infections due to multiply resistant organisms, including *P. aeruginosa* and *Enterobacter* and *Acinetobacter* spp, and is also useful as empiric single-drug therapy for mixed aerobic/anaerobic infections when the potential toxicity of alternative antimicrobial combinations is unacceptable.

2. **Adverse reactions.** Toxicity is similar to that of the PCNs, and there may be immunologic cross-reactivity in some PCN-allergic patients. Seizures occur more frequently than with the PCNs, especially in patients with predisposing factors or renal insufficiency.

E. **Inhibitors of beta-lactamase. Clavulanic acid, sulbactam,** and **tazobactam** are beta-lactam molecules that have minimal intrinsic antibacterial activity but are potent inhibitors of many beta-lactamases, including some of those produced by *Staph. aureus, H. influenzae, E. coli,* and *Klebsiella pneumoniae*. None of these beta-lactam/beta-lactamase inhibitor combinations are indicated for the treatment of infections due to broadly beta-lactam–resistant *P. aeruginosa* or *Enterobacter* spp. In addition, methicillin-resistant staphylococci are not susceptible to the beta-lactam/beta-lactamase inhibitor combinations. CSF penetration of these agents is unreliable, and they should not be used to treat meningitis.

1. **Amoxicillin with clavulanic acid** (250–500 mg PO q8h) is useful in the treatment of UTI, otitis media, sinusitis, and bite wounds. There is an increased incidence of GI side effects compared with amoxicillin alone.

2. **Ampicillin with sulbactam** (1.5–3.0 g IV or IM q6h) may be useful for therapy of community-acquired soft-tissue, intraabdominal, or pelvic infections, as well as polymicrobial upper and lower respiratory infections.

3. **Ticarcillin with clavulanate** (3.1 g IV q4–6h) and **piperacillin with tazobactam** (3.375 g IV q6h) may be useful in the treatment of polymicrobial soft-tissue, intraabdominal, pelvic, and lower respiratory infections.

II. **Macrolide and azalide antimicrobials** are agents with a large volume of distribution producing high tissue concentrations but **unreliable CSF penetration.** Azithromycin, erythromycin, and troleandomycin undergo significant hepatic elimination, whereas clarithromycin excretion is primarily renal. Macrolide and azalide antimicrobials may **increase plasma levels of theophylline, carbamazepine, cyclosporine, digoxin, and warfarin** as well as other drugs, so special attention to drug interactions is necessary (see Appendix B). Erythromycin can interfere with the hepatic metabolism of terfenadine, which may result in prolongation of the QT interval and life-threatening ventricular arrhythmias in susceptible individuals. Although there are limited data for the other macrolides or azalides, concurrent administration of these agents with the H_1-antagonists, terfenadine, or astemizole should probably be avoided. Gastric irritation and diarrhea are common side effects with erythromycin; azithromycin and clarithromycin produce fewer GI symptoms.

A. Erythromycin (250–500 mg PO q6h or 0.5–1.0 g IV q6h) is used most frequently as an alternative to PCNs for PCN-allergic patients with infections caused by streptococci or staphylococci. Erythromycin is the drug of choice for infections due to *Legionella* or *Mycoplasma* spp and can be used in the treatment of chlamydial infections, chancroid, and *Campylobacter jejuni* enteritis. Phlebitis is common with IV administration. Reversible ototoxicity is a rare complication of erythromycin use. The erythromycin estolate formulation is associated with cholestatic hepatitis in adults.

B. Clarithromycin (250–500 mg PO q12h) is a semisynthetic macrolide antimicrobial with a spectrum of activity similar to erythromycin but with improved coverage of *H. influenzae* and *M. catarrhalis*. It can be used for treatment of mild to moderately severe upper and lower respiratory tract infections and skin and soft-tissue infections. Clarithromycin also has in vitro activity against mycobacteria and may be useful in the treatment of infections caused by *Mycobacterium avium* complex and other nontuberculous mycobacteria. **Clarithromycin is contraindicated in pregnancy.** The dosage should be adjusted for severe renal insufficiency, with or without coexisting hepatic dysfunction (see Appendix D).

C. Azithromycin (250–500 mg PO qd) is an azalide antimicrobial chemically related to erythromycin but with a longer half-life and greater tissue penetration. Azithromycin has an extended spectrum similar to clarithromycin and additional activity against genitourinary pathogens, including *Chlamydia trachomatis*. Azithromycin can be used for respiratory tract infections, skin and soft-tissue infections, and cervicitis or urethritis due to chlamydia. Azithromycin should not be given concurrently with ergot alkaloids due to the risk of precipitating ergotism. Food decreases the bioavailability of azithromycin; thus, it should be taken on an empty stomach.

D. Clindamycin (150–450 mg PO q6h or 600–900 mg IV q8h) and **lincomycin** (500 mg PO q8h or 600–1,000 mg IV q8h) are lincosamides with gram-positive spectra similar to that of erythromycin and activity against most anaerobes, including *B. fragilis*. Clindamycin is generally the preferred agent as it has superior oral absorption. The most common side effects of these agents are rashes and diarrhea. **Pseudomembranous colitis** occurs in a significant number of patients treated with these agents (see Chap. 13).

III. Vancomycin (1 g IV q12h) is a tricyclic glycopeptide antimicrobial that is bactericidal against most gram-positive organisms. It is bacteriostatic against enterococci.

A. Indications include treatment of infections due to methicillin-resistant staphylococci and infections due to susceptible organisms in patients allergic to both PCNs and cephalosporins. Vancomycin in combination with an aminoglycoside is also effective for the treatment of enterococcal endocarditis. Vancomycin is particularly well suited for use in dialysis patients, since 1 g IV provides adequate blood levels for up to 7–10 days. Oral vancomycin (125–500 mg PO q6h for 10 days) is not well absorbed but is useful in the treatment of *Clostridium difficile* diarrhea (see Chap. 13).

B. Administration. Vancomycin should be given intravenously at a rate that does not exceed 1 g/hour to avoid the "red man" syndrome (see sec. **III.C**). Vancomycin is excreted by the kidney, and its dosage must be adjusted in the presence of renal insufficiency (see Appendix D). Serum levels should be monitored routinely to ensure adequate therapy and to minimize toxicity.

C. Adverse effects. Rapid administration of vancomycin often results in a histamine-mediated reaction characterized by tingling and flushing of the face, neck, and upper torso **(the "red man" syndrome),** sometimes associated with hypotension. Skin rash, phlebitis, chills, and, rarely, reversible neutropenia have also been described. Although reported, **ototoxicity** is a rare complication of vancomycin therapy. Significant nephrotoxicity is not clearly associated with current preparations, but limited data suggest concurrent vancomycin administration may increase the risk for aminoglycoside nephrotoxicity (*J Antimicrob Chemother* 25:679, 1990).

IV. Tetracyclines are bacteriostatic agents with a broad spectrum of activity, including *Rickettsia, Chlamydia, Mycoplasma, Nocardia,* and *Actinomyces* spp. However, resistance is widespread, especially among *Staph. aureus,* group A streptococci, pneumococci, and gram-negative bacilli.

  A. Indications include treatment of nongonococcal urethritis, rickettsial disease, exacerbations of chronic bronchitis, early Lyme disease, and acne. The tetracyclines are alternatives for the PCN-allergic patient with syphilis or *Pasteurella multocida* infection.

  B. Pharmacokinetics. The tetracyclines are well absorbed when taken on an empty stomach. Their absorption may be decreased if they are taken with milk, antacids, calcium, or iron. The absorption of doxycycline and minocycline is not significantly affected by food. Tetracyclines are distributed throughout the extracellular fluid compartment.

  C. Preparations and dosages. Tetracycline hydrochloride (250–500 mg PO q6h) and **minocycline** (200 mg, then 100 mg q12h IV, PO) are excreted primarily by the kidney. **Doxycycline** (100 mg PO or IV q12h) is well absorbed orally and has a prolonged serum half-life (17–20 hours). Because it is excreted by the liver, doxycycline is preferred in patients with renal insufficiency.

  D. Adverse effects include GI upset, photosensitivity (especially with doxycycline), elevation of BUN, and, with prolonged use, oral or vaginal candidiasis. Tetracyclines should not be administered to pregnant women or to children younger than 10 years of age because of adverse effects on developing teeth and bones.

V. Chloramphenicol (500–750 mg PO q6h or 50–100 mg/kg/day IV divided q6h) is a bacteriostatic agent active against a wide variety of gram-negative and gram-positive organisms, including anaerobes.

  A. Indications include the treatment of infections due to ampicillin-resistant *H. influenzae, Salmonella* (especially typhoid fever), *Rickettsia,* and anaerobes including *B. fragilis.* Because of potentially serious toxicity, use of chloramphenicol should be restricted to seriously ill patients in whom this risk can be justified.

  B. Pharmacokinetics. Chloramphenicol can be given orally or intravenously; IM administration results in unreliable absorption. This agent penetrates into all body tissues, including the CSF (where concentrations 30–50% of serum levels are attained), the eye, and the fetal circulation. Chloramphenicol is metabolized in the liver; dosage adjustment is necessary in the presence of significant liver disease.

  C. Adverse effects. Hematopoietic toxicity, including reversible bone-marrow suppression and irreversible aplasia, may occur. Aplastic anemia is a rare (approximately 1 : 25,000 cases) but usually fatal late idiosyncratic reaction to the drug. Reversible leukopenia, thrombocytopenia, and suppression of erythropoiesis are dose related and can usually be avoided by maintaining peak serum levels below 25 µg/ml. Other adverse effects include hemolysis (in glucose-6-phosphate dehydrogenase [G-6-PD]-deficient patients), allergic reactions, and peripheral neuritis.

VI. Aminoglycoside antimicrobials are bactericidal for numerous gram-positive and gram-negative organisms and mycobacteria. They are not active in an oxygen-poor environment or at a low pH and are therefore ineffective against anaerobes and unsuitable for the treatment of abscesses. Aminoglycosides demonstrate concentration-dependent bacterial killing. Their antibacterial efficacy is proportional to their peak serum concentration over a broad range. Aminoglycoside resistance primarily results from plasmid-mediated aminoglycoside-modifying enzymes that vary in their ability to inactivate different aminoglycosides. Consequently, susceptibility testing should be used when selecting an aminoglycoside for therapeutic use. Resistance to streptomycin is widespread among the Enterobacteriaceae, and neither streptomycin nor kanamycin has reliable activity against *Pseudomonas* spp.

A. **Pharmacokinetics.** Aminoglycosides are distributed throughout the extracellular space, excluding the CSF, and are rapidly excreted by normally functioning kidneys. Parenteral administration is necessary to produce therapeutic levels because of poor GI absorption. Factors that increase the volume of distribution (e.g., pregnancy, burns, ascites, septic shock) increase the amount of aminoglycoside necessary to achieve an effective peak serum level. In contrast, renal failure prolongs the serum half-life of aminoglycosides and necessitates a decrease in dose or a lengthening of the dosing interval. Measurements of serum drug levels are invaluable for ensuring appropriate dosing (see sec. **VI.C**).

B. **Indications.** Aminoglycosides are useful (usually in combination with a beta-lactam antibiotic) for the treatment of serious infections caused by susceptible gram-negative bacilli, especially *Pseudomonas* spp. Aminoglycosides are also useful for therapy of streptococcal (especially enterococcal) endocarditis when used with penicillin or ampicillin. The limited indications for streptomycin include plague, tularemia, brucellosis, serious enterococcal infections, and tuberculosis. Parenteral aminoglycosides are not effective for meningitis because they do not cross the blood-brain barrier. These agents are not used for most gram-positive infections because the PCNs and cephalosporins possess more favorable therapeutic indices. Systemic aminoglycosides are not recommended for monotherapy of staphylococcal infections even when such organisms display in vitro susceptibility.

C. **Dosage.** Aminoglycosides may be given intravenously or intramuscularly. The **loading dose** for gentamicin, tobramycin, and netilmicin is 1.5–2.0 mg/kg, and for amikacin and kanamycin is 5.0–7.5 mg/kg. Critically ill patients may require larger loading doses (3 mg/kg for gentamicin and 9 mg/kg for amikacin) to achieve therapeutic serum levels (*Ann Pharmacother* 27:351, 1993). The **maintenance dosage** is 3–5 mg/kg/day in 3 divided doses for gentamicin and tobramycin, 4–6 mg/kg/day in 3 doses for netilmicin, and 15 mg/kg/day in 2–3 doses for amikacin and kanamycin. Peak and trough serum levels should generally be measured within 48 hours of the start of therapy and repeated every 3–4 days in patients with stable renal function. Peak levels indicate adequacy of dosing and should be obtained 30 minutes following the end of IV infusion or 1 hour following IM injection. Peak serum levels of 4–6 μg/ml for gentamicin and tobramycin, 6–10 μg/ml for netilmicin, and 20–35 μg/ml for amikacin are usually adequate. Peaks at the upper end of the therapeutic range are often desirable in pulmonary infections as aminoglycosides penetrate lung tissue poorly. Trough levels gauge drug accumulation and are obtained just prior to the next dose. To minimize toxicity, appropriate trough levels should be less than 2 μg/ml for gentamicin and tobramycin and less than 10 μg/ml for amikacin. **Maintenance dosages often must be adjusted in patients with renal insufficiency and in the elderly** (see Appendix D). Single daily administrations of larger doses of aminoglycosides have been associated with efficacy and toxicity profiles comparable to traditional dosing regimens and may reduce costs associated with administration and serum level determination (*Ann Intern Med* 119:584,1993).

D. **Adverse effects.** Nephrotoxicity and ototoxicity are the major adverse effects of the aminoglycosides. Nephrotoxicity is usually reversible, but **acute renal failure** with azotemia may occur. Consequently, renal function should be closely monitored during therapy. **Ototoxicity** may be cochlear or vestibular and is more likely to occur with prolonged use (>14 days), in patients with baseline renal insufficiency, and with concurrent use of other ototoxic drugs, especially loop diuretics. Serial audiometry should be conducted on patients treated for extended periods. **Neuromuscular blockade** is a rare complication of aminoglycoside use.

VII. **Inhibitors of folic acid metabolism (sulfonamides** and **trimethoprim)**

A. **Sulfonamides** are useful in the treatment of uncomplicated UTI, nocardiosis, and chancroid, and in the topical therapy of burns and ocular infections.

1. **Pharmacokinetics.** GI absorption is rapid and **therapeutic CSF levels are achieved.** Only oral preparations are currently available in the United

States. Sulfonamides are excreted by the kidney, and their dosages should be adjusted in renal failure (see Appendix D).

2. **Selected preparations and dosages. Sulfisoxazole** (1 g PO q6h) is used in the treatment of UTI. **Sulfamethoxazole** (2-g load, then 1 g PO q12h) has a longer half-life that allows twice daily dosing. **Sulfadiazine** (1.0–1.5 g PO q6h) is often used for nocardiosis and toxoplasmosis.

3. **Adverse effects** occur in 5–10% of treated patients. **Hypersensitivity** reactions are common and include skin rashes, vasculitis, and drug fever. Crystalluria may occur, especially in patients taking larger doses of the less soluble sulfonamides (e.g., sulfadiazine, sulfathiazole). This complication can be minimized by ensuring adequate urine flow and, in some cases, by urine alkalinization. Erythema multiforme and the Stevens-Johnson syndrome may occur. These agents can induce hemolytic anemia in patients with G-6-PD deficiency. The sulfonamides are contraindicated in the last month of pregnancy because of the risk of neonatal kernicterus.

B. **Trimethoprim** (100 mg PO bid) has a slow bactericidal effect against many gram-negative bacteria, though not *P. aeruginosa*. It can be used alone for prophylaxis and therapy of UTI. **Side effects** include megaloblastic anemia, bone marrow suppression, and skin rashes.

C. **Trimethoprim/sulfamethoxazole (cotrimoxazole, TMP/SMX)** is a fixed-dose combination of trimethoprim and sulfamethoxazole in a ratio of 1:5 (by weight). The antibacterial spectrum of TMP/SMX includes most gram-positive and gram-negative pathogens, except *P. aeruginosa* and enterococci. Both agents are excreted by the kidney, and the dosage should be adjusted in patients with renal dysfunction (see Appendix D).

1. **Indications.** TMP/SMX is useful in the treatment of UTI, prostatitis, acute and chronic bronchitis, acute otitis media, sinusitis, nocardiosis, shigellosis, and salmonellosis. It is the agent of choice in the treatment of *Pneumocystis carinii* infection. TMP/SMX can also be used to treat serious infections (e.g., meningitis, osteomyelitis) caused by susceptible gram-negative bacilli that are resistant to other antimicrobials.

2. **Administration.** Typical dosing includes 1 double-strength tablet (160 mg TMP/800 mg SMX) PO q12h for mild to moderate infections; 8–20 mg/kg/day (based on TMP component) PO or IV in 2–4 doses for serious infections. Monitoring SMX or TMP levels is useful when using high dosages, particularly in patients with renal insufficiency.

3. **Adverse effects.** This combination shares all the potential toxicities of its component drugs (see sec. **VII.A.3** and sec. **VII.B**). Megaloblastic anemia, leukopenia, or thrombocytopenia may occur as a result of the inhibition of folate metabolism. Generalized bone marrow suppression can occur, especially at high dosages. Patients with AIDS seem particularly susceptible to drug toxicity from TMP/SMX. The large fluid volumes required for parenteral TMP/SMX may complicate the care of patients with renal or cardiac disease.

VIII. **Quinolones** (quinolone carboxylic acids) effect bactericidal activity through inhibition of DNA gyrase. Most agents in this class have good oral absorption and are widely distributed. They are generally well tolerated. Their most frequent adverse effects are GI symptoms such as nausea, vomiting, diarrhea, and abdominal pain. Rashes, phototoxicity, and CNS side effects (e.g., drowsiness, headache, insomnia, restlessness, dizziness, subjective visual disturbances, and, rarely, seizures) are less common. These drugs should be avoided in pregnant women and children. The fluoroquinolones (primarily enoxacin and ciprofloxacin) may interfere with hepatic metabolism of theophylline and caffeine and may increase levels of these drugs in some patients. Aluminum- and magnesium-containing antacids and oral iron preparations interfere with absorption of the quinolones.

A. **Nalidixic acid** (1 g PO q6h) is the prototype of this family. Its spectrum of activity includes most gram-negative bacilli except *P. aeruginosa*. Poor oral absorption and a high frequency of acquired resistance have limited its utility to the treatment of UTI.

B. Fluoroquinolones. Norfloxacin, ciprofloxacin, ofloxacin, lomefloxacin, and enoxacin are effective against most gram-negative bacilli, including *P. aeruginosa*, and many gram-positive cocci, including some *Staph. aureus*. They have variable activity against streptococci, especially *Enterococcus* spp, and generally have poor activity against anaerobic bacteria and most nonaeruginosa strains of *Pseudomonas*. Reports of treatment failures and pneumococcal superinfections during fluoroquinolone therapy raise concern about their use as monotherapy for community-acquired pneumonia. These agents are highly active against *N. gonorrhoeae* and *Haemophilus ducreyi*, but none are effective for syphilis. Ciprofloxacin and ofloxacin are also active against *Mycoplasma pneumoniae*, *Legionella pneumophila*, *Chlamydia trachomatis*, *Mycobacterium tuberculosis*, and atypical mycobacteria. Resistance to fluoroquinolones has arisen, however, especially among methicillin-resistant *Staph. aureus* and *P. aeruginosa*. **The dosage of all of these drugs should be reduced in renal failure.**

1. **Norfloxacin** (400 mg PO q12h) and **enoxacin** (200–400 mg PO q12h) are useful for the treatment of UTI due to susceptible (primarily gram-negative) organisms. Achievable serum levels of these compounds are relatively low; therefore, they are not recommended for systemic or serious local infections. **Enoxacin has particularly pronounced effects on methylxanthine elimination,** so close monitoring of theophylline levels is warranted in patients receiving both agents.

2. **Ofloxacin** (200–400 mg PO or IV q12h) has excellent oral bioavailability, so PO and IV dosing are equivalent. It can be used in the treatment of acute uncomplicated gonococcal and chlamydial urethritis or cervicitis. Ofloxacin may also be useful in the treatment of uncomplicated skin and soft-tissue infections, UTI, prostatitis, or respiratory infections due to susceptible pathogens.

3. **Ciprofloxacin** (250–750 mg PO q12h or 200–400 mg IV q12h) also achieves significant serum concentrations after oral administration. Of the available quinolones, ciprofloxacin has the greatest in vitro activity against gram-negative aerobic bacilli, including *P. aeruginosa*. Ciprofloxacin may be useful in the treatment of UTI, osteomyelitis, pneumonia, and skin infections due to susceptible organisms. It is also approved for the treatment of infectious diarrhea (*Campylobacter*, toxigenic *E. coli*, and *Shigella*).

4. **Lomefloxacin** (400 mg PO qd) may be useful for the treatment of bacterial exacerbations of chronic bronchitis or UTI due to susceptible organisms. Phototoxic reactions have occurred with lomefloxacin therapy, and exposure to sunlight should be avoided during and for several days after completion of therapy. It is not indicated in infections due to *Strep. pneumoniae*.

IX. Metronidazole (250–500 mg PO or IV q8h; a 1-g loading dose can be used for serious infections) is a nitro-imidazole active against most gram-negative anaerobic bacteria, including *Bacteroides* spp and many *Clostridium* spp. Many anaerobic streptococci are resistant to this agent. Metronidazole is also active against several protozoa and parasites, including *Trichomonas vaginalis*, *Giardia lamblia*, *Entamoeba histolytica*, and *Dracunculus medinensis*.

A. Indications. Metronidazole is useful in the treatment of anaerobic bacterial infections, including abdominal and pelvic infections, brain abscesses, osteomyelitis, and endocarditis. Oral metronidazole is effective for the treatment of pseudomembranous colitis. Metronidazole must be combined with other antimicrobials when treating mixed aerobic and anaerobic infections.

B. Pharmacokinetics. The GI absorption of metronidazole is excellent. Its tissue distribution is widespread, including CSF, where therapeutic levels are obtained. Metronidazole is metabolized in the liver before excretion by the kidney, and the dosage should be reduced in patients with severe hepatic or renal dysfunction.

C. Adverse effects include nausea, dry mouth, alterations in taste, disulfiram-like effects with alcohol, and uncommon neurologic reactions. Because of potential teratogenicity, metronidazole should not be used in pregnant women.

Antituberculous Agents

Combination chemotherapy designed to prevent the emergence of resistant organisms is essential for the effective therapy of *M. tuberculosis* infections. This therapy requires a **minimum of two active drugs** for treatment of a given isolate. Increases in the frequencies of resistance to the conventional antituberculous agents have led to the use of more complex empiric regimens and have made susceptibility testing an integral part of tuberculosis management (see Chap. 13).

I. **Primary drugs**
  A. **Isoniazid (INH)** (300 mg PO qd) is bactericidal for *M. tuberculosis, M. kansasii,* and *M. bovis.*
    1. **Administration.** Isoniazid is well absorbed orally and is widely distributed throughout the body, including the CSF. To ensure compliance, INH can be given twice weekly (15 mg/kg PO; maximum dose, 900 mg) in supervised regimens. Larger dosages (10 mg/kg/day) have been used in more severe disease but are associated with increased toxicity.
    2. **Adverse effects**
      a. **Hepatotoxicity.** Asymptomatic elevations of serum transaminases occur during the first few months of therapy in up to 20% of patients receiving INH but usually resolve as drug therapy continues. **Hepatitis** is an idiosyncratic toxicity. The incidence of INH-induced hepatitis increases with age from 0.3% for patients 20–34 years old to approximately 2.3% for patients 50 years of age or older (*Am Rev Respir Dis* 117:991, 1978). Daily alcohol consumption and alcoholic liver disease increase the risk of INH-induced hepatitis; however, a prior history of nonalcoholic liver disease may not. Isoniazid-induced hepatitis usually resolves after discontinuation of the drug.
      b. **Peripheral neuropathy** is a dose-related complication of INH therapy probably due to enhanced excretion of pyridoxine. Poorly nourished patients and those predisposed to neuropathy by diabetes, uremia, or alcoholism are at particular risk and should receive **pyridoxine, 50 mg PO qd.** Patients receiving large dosages of INH, pregnant women, and those with seizure disorders should also receive pyridoxine. Other nervous system toxicities are not clearly related to pyridoxine deficiency but have been reported to respond to supplementation.
  B. **Rifampin** (600 mg PO qd) is bactericidal for gram-positive cocci, many gram-negative bacilli, and most species of *Mycobacterium.* Alternatively, rifampin may be given as 600 mg PO twice weekly in supervised regimens. Absorption and distribution, including CNS penetration, are excellent. Rifampin undergoes enterohepatic circulation and is progressively metabolized by the liver. Rifampin induces hepatic microsomal enzymes and may alter the metabolism of many drugs. Patients should be warned about the orange-red discoloration of secretions (e.g., tears, urine, and sweat) that occurs with rifampin; it is harmless but will permanently discolor soft contact lenses. **Toxicities** include rash, CNS side effects, mild GI disturbances, and hepatitis that may be potentiated by other types of liver disease. A rare influenza-like syndrome associated with a variety of hematologic and renal abnormalities has been reported.
  C. **Pyrazinamide (PZA)** (15–30 mg/kg/day PO; maximum 2 g/day) is bactericidal for intracellular mycobacteria. A dosage of 50–70 mg/kg PO twice a week can be used to facilitate supervised therapy. PZA is well absorbed from the GI tract and is widely distributed to body fluids and tissues including CSF. The drug is excreted by the kidneys. The major side effect is hepatotoxicity.
  D. **Ethambutol** is typically dosed at 15 mg/kg PO daily, although an initial dosage of 25 mg/kg/day can be used for more serious disease. Ethambutol may be administered as 50 mg/kg twice weekly in supervised regimens. In vitro testing suggests the activity of ethambutol is concentration dependent, with bactericidal activity seen at higher levels (*Am Rev Respir Dis* 141:1478, 1990). The drug is

excreted primarily by the kidneys, and the dosage should be reduced in patients with renal failure. The only significant dose-related toxicity is **optic neuritis,** which occurs in fewer than 1% of patients treated with 15 mg/kg/day but is seen more frequently at higher dosages. The earliest manifestations may include decreased green color perception, reduced visual acuity, or visual field deficits. Routine eye examinations should be included in the care of these patients because the ophthalmologic complications are often reversible with early drug withdrawal.

   E. Streptomycin (15 mg/kg/day IM) is an aminoglycoside that is tuberculocidal in vitro but may only be suppressive in animal models. A dosage of 25–30 mg/kg IM twice/week can also be used in supervised settings. Toxicities include rash, vestibular and cochlear dysfunction, paresthesias, and, rarely, nephrotoxicity (see Antibacterial Agents, sec. **VI.D**).

II. Second-line agents have narrower therapeutic windows than primary drugs for the treatment of mycobacterial disease and should be administered by clinicians familiar with their use.

   A. Ethionamide (0.5–1.0 g/day PO in 2 doses) is widely distributed, including the CSF. Adverse effects include gastric irritation, hepatotoxicity, and peripheral neuropathy.

   B. Cycloserine (0.5–1.0 g/day PO in 2–3 divided doses) is widely distributed with good CSF penetration. Side effects include behavioral disturbances, as well as seizures, somnolence, and muscle twitching.

   C. Other aminoglycosides. Although experience is limited, **amikacin** may be preferable as a second-line aminoglycoside for the treatment of tuberculous disease, including *Mycobacterium avium* complex, as drug assays for monitoring amikacin levels are readily available. Kanamycin can also be used.

Antiviral Agents

Current antiviral agents suppress viral replication; viral containment or elimination requires an intact host immune response.

I. Amantadine and **rimantadine**, its alpha-methyl derivative, block an early step in replication of the influenza A virus. They have no effect against infections caused by influenza B or C.

   A. Indications. Uncomplicated influenza A infection usually resolves within 3–7 days, and most patients do not need prophylaxis or treatment with antiviral agents. However, these drugs should be used for patients at high risk of complications (e.g., immunocompromised patients, the elderly, and patients with pulmonary or cardiac disease) when they have influenza. During an epidemic, prophylactic amantadine or rimantadine should be strongly considered for nonimmune patients and staff members of nursing homes or hospitals, where epidemic spread of influenza can be devastating.

   B. Dosage. Amantadine (100 mg PO bid) is excreted by the kidneys, and its use should be restricted to patients with adequate renal function. Dosage should be adjusted for patients 65 years or older (100 mg PO qd). Rimantadine (200 mg PO qd in 1–2 doses) undergoes extensive hepatic metabolism, and dosage adjustment may be warranted in patients with liver dysfunction or the elderly. **Prophylaxis** should begin when influenza A is documented in the community. These agents can be started concurrently with vaccination for influenza A and discontinued 14 days later when protective antibodies have developed. Administration to nonimmune individuals should begin as soon as possible after exposure or within 48 hours of the onset of symptoms and can be discontinued after 10 days or 48 hours after symptoms disappear. Amantadine or rimantadine prophylaxis may be indicated for longer periods in individuals who are unable to receive the vaccine or those who are unlikely to mount appropriate antibody responses.

   C. Adverse effects are uncommon, although both agents have been associated with GI complaints such as nausea and vomiting. Amantadine has a higher incidence of neurologic side effects including confusion, slurring of speech, blurred vision, and sleep disturbance; rimantadine may be preferred for use in patients at increased risk for CNS side effects. Resistant isolates may arise during treatment with either agent and may be transmitted to nonimmune contacts despite concurrent amantadine or rimantadine prophylaxis. Both drugs have been associated with adverse pregnancy outcomes in animals and therefore should probably not be given to pregnant women.

II. Nucleoside analogs

A. Acyclovir (acycloguanosine) is most active against herpes simplex virus (HSV) types 1 and 2 and varicella-zoster virus (VZV). It has no effect on latency of the herpes viruses. Although high doses of acyclovir will inhibit Epstein-Barr virus (EBV) and cytomegalovirus (CMV) in vitro, the clinical utility of this activity is questionable.

1. Indications. Acyclovir is indicated for treatment of primary and recurrent genital herpes, severe herpes stomatitis, and herpes simplex encephalitis in normal hosts. Acyclovir can modestly reduce the duration and severity of primary varicella and localized zoster in immunocompetent adults. There is no consensus on antiviral therapy of uncomplicated VZV infections in normal adults, and the potential benefits must be weighed against the risks and costs of therapy. However, varicella pneumonitis, disseminated zoster, and herpes zoster ophthalmicus are indications for acyclovir therapy. In immunocompromised hosts, acyclovir is also effective for therapy and prophylaxis of HSV infections and in the therapy of VZV.

2. Pharmacokinetics. Acyclovir is distributed throughout the extracellular fluid compartment; CSF levels are about 50% of plasma. Acyclovir is excreted by the kidney, and its dosage must be reduced in renal failure. Each infusion of acyclovir should be given over 1 hour to minimize the risk of crystalline nephropathy.

3. Dosage. For severe systemic infections, the dosage is 5 mg/kg IV q8h for most HSV infections and 10 mg/kg IV q8h for HSV encephalitis or VZV infections. The oral dosage is 200 mg PO 5 times/day for HSV infection and 800 mg PO 5 times/day for localized herpes zoster infections. Acyclovir, 800 mg PO qid for 5 days, may be used for the treatment of uncomplicated varicella in immunocompetent adults.

4. Adverse effects are uncommon. Reversible crystalline nephropathy may occur; preexisting renal failure, dehydration, and bolus infusion enhance the risk of nephrotoxicity. Elevation of serum transaminases and phlebitis also occur. CNS toxicity (delirium, tremors) has been reported, particularly with high dosages, in patients with renal failure, and in the elderly.

B. Ganciclovir is considerably more active than acyclovir against CMV and EBV. It is equivalent to acyclovir in its ability to inhibit HSV and VZV.

1. Indications. Ganciclovir is indicated for therapy of sight-threatening CMV retinitis in immunocompromised patients and may be useful for prophylaxis or preemptive therapy of CMV disease in certain transplant patients (see Chap. 14). Bone marrow and solid organ transplant patients with CMV disease may also benefit from ganciclovir therapy, but data are limited. CMV disease may progress despite ganciclovir therapy, and ganciclovir resistance has been reported. Patients whose conditions worsen on therapy sometimes respond to increased dosages of ganciclovir. Indefinite maintenance therapy is generally required to suppress CMV disease in patients with AIDS.

2. Administration. The dosage for initial **induction therapy** is 5 mg/kg q12h for 14–21 days. Usual **maintenance regimens** are 6 mg/kg/day for 5 days every week or 5 mg/kg/day every day. Ganciclovir is currently available only as an IV preparation and should be given as a 1-hour infusion. It is widely distributed in body tissues and CSF. The dosage must be adjusted for patients with renal dysfunction (see Appendix D).

3. Adverse effects include reversible neutropenia and thrombocytopenia, which may require dosage reduction or discontinuation. Bone marrow suppression is particularly severe when ganciclovir is used in conjunction with zidovudine (AZT), and few patients tolerate concurrent use of both drugs. Rash, confusion, headache, and GI side effects have also been reported.

C. Foscarnet (trisodium phosphonoformate) has antiviral activity against herpes viruses and HIV.

1. **Indications.** Foscarnet is indicated for CMV retinitis in patients with AIDS (see Chap. 14). Its safety and efficacy have not been established for CMV infection at other sites, nor for infections caused by other viruses. Foscarnet is an alternative for immunocompromised patients with CMV infections in whom ganciclovir therapy is ineffective or who cannot tolerate ganciclovir. Foscarnet may also be useful in patients with serious infections due to acyclovir-resistant HSV or VZV and ganciclovir-resistant CMV. Like ganciclovir, foscarnet is virustatic, so maintenance therapy is necessary for AIDS patients with CMV retinitis.

2. **Administration.** Initial induction therapy for CMV retinitis infection in patients with AIDS is 60 mg/kg IV over 1 hour q8h for 2–3 weeks, depending on the clinical response. The recommended maintenance dose is 90–120 mg/kg/day IV over 2 hours. For acyclovir-resistant HSV and VZV infections, 40 mg/kg IV q8h can be used. **The dosage should be carefully adjusted for the patient's renal function according to the manufacturer's instructions.** To minimize nephrotoxicity, patients should also be given normal saline prior to and during the infusion. An infusion pump should be used to control the rate of infusion. The concomitant use of other nephrotoxic agents (e.g., aminoglycosides, amphotericin, pentamidine) should be avoided.

3. **Adverse effects.** Nephrotoxicity occurs in up to 30% of patients treated with foscarnet. Nausea is also common. Other complications include disturbances of calcium, magnesium, and phosphorus levels, as well as seizures.

D. Famciclovir is an oral prodrug of penciclovir that has demonstrated activity versus VZV, HSV-1, HSV-2, and EBV.

1. **Indications.** Famciclovir is currently approved for the treatment of acute herpes zoster (shingles). Its efficacy in reducing the time to cutaneous healing and relieving acute pain appears comparable to that of acyclovir. Like acyclovir, it may shorten the duration of postherpetic neuralgia. It has not been evaluated in the treatment of herpes zoster ophthalmicus and disseminated zoster, or in immunocompromised patients.

2. **Administration.** The dosage of famciclovir is 500 mg PO q8h for 7 days in the treatment of acute zoster. Dosage adjustment is necessary in patients with renal insufficiency (see Appendix D).

3. **Adverse effects** are uncommon. Headache, nausea, and diarrhea have been reported.

E. Zidovudine (AZT), dideoxyinosine (ddl), and zalcitabine (dideoxycytidine, ddC) are antiretroviral agents used for therapy of HIV disease (see Chap. 14).

Antifungal Agents

I. Amphotericin B is a polyene antimicrobial that disrupts the fungal cell by binding to ergosterol in the plasma membrane. It is indicated for most systemic mycoses except *Pseudallescheria boydii* infections.

A. Pharmacokinetics. Amphotericin B is poorly absorbed and must be administered intravenously. Low concentrations are achieved in the CSF. Although the metabolism and excretion of amphotericin B are poorly defined, its dosage need not be adjusted in patients with preexisting renal failure, because only a small percentage of the administered dose is excreted by the kidneys.

B. Administration

1. **Intravenous infusion.** The initial amphotericin B dose and the rate at which the dosage is increased should be dictated by the severity of the infection and the occurrence and nature of adverse effects. **Test doses** have been advocated

to identify patients prone to severe infusion-related adverse events and should be performed in a manner that does not significantly delay therapy. A 1-mg test dose may be given over 30 minutes and, if tolerated, can be followed by a separate infusion of 0.2–0.5 mg/kg. Alternatively, 1–2 mg of the initial therapeutic dose may be infused over 30 minutes. With the infusion interrupted, the patient is then observed (30 minutes is generally adequate), and if there are no serious adverse reactions (e.g., hypotension), the remainder of the dose can be given. The dosage can be increased each day until a therapeutic or maximum tolerated dosage is reached, usually 0.5–1.0 mg/kg/day over 2–4 hours in adults and 1.0–1.5 mg/kg/day in children. Initial dosage increases of 0.1–0.2 mg/kg/day are typical, although more rapid escalations may be required for severe infections. The maintenance dosage can be doubled and given on alternate days, but a single dose should not exceed 1.5 mg/kg.

2. **Intraventricular infusion** of amphotericin B is occasionally used in the treatment of fungal meningitis, but it often produces significant toxicity. This route of administration should only be used with expert consultation.

3. **Bladder irrigation** may be useful in the treatment of fungal cystitis. Regimens include continuous irrigation with amphotericin B, 50 mg in 1 liter sterile water daily for 3–5 days.

C. **Adverse effects.** Acute side effects, including fever, chills, headache, myalgias, nausea, and vomiting, often occur but can be reduced by **premedicating** the patient with aspirin or acetaminophen and diphenhydramine, 25–50 mg PO or IV, or with hydrocortisone, 25–100 mg IV. Meperidine, 25–50 mg IV, is often effective in the treatment of infusion-related chills. Patients often become tolerant to these adverse effects and may not require premedication for the entire course of therapy. **Thrombophlebitis** may be minimized by administering amphotericin B via a central catheter or by adding heparin, 1,000 units, to a peripheral infusion. **Nephrotoxicity** develops in most patients treated with amphotericin B and may consist of distal renal tubular acidosis, hypokalemia, hypomagnesemia, and impairment of glomerular filtration. Significant irreversible renal damage usually does not occur unless underlying renal disease is present or the cumulative dose exceeds 3–4 g. As there is evidence that sodium or volume depletion may potentiate amphotericin B–associated nephrotoxicity, these conditions should be avoided in patients receiving amphotericin B when possible. In addition, sodium loading with 250–500 ml of 0.9% saline infused over 30 minutes before and after each amphotericin B dose may decrease nephrotoxicity in patients who are able to tolerate volume expansion. Patients with serious renal dysfunction due to amphotericin B generally require a reduction in dosage or temporary cessation of therapy. If possible, other nephrotoxic drugs should be avoided during therapy with amphotericin B. **Other toxicities** include anemia, neuritis, and arachnoiditis, which may occur with intrathecal administration.

II. **Flucytosine (5-FC)** (37.5 mg/kg PO q6h) is effective orally against some isolates of *Candida* and *Cryptococcus neoformans*. If used alone, resistance to 5-FC develops during prolonged treatment. 5-FC is used in combination with amphotericin B in the treatment of cryptococcal meningitis or alone in short courses for persistent candidal UTI.

A. **Pharmacokinetics.** 5-FC is well absorbed from the GI tract and reaches therapeutic levels in the CSF. The drug is excreted by the kidney, and the dosage must be reduced in renal insufficiency. Serum levels of 5-FC should be monitored during therapy.

B. **Adverse effects.** Bone marrow suppression is dose related and associated with peak serum levels greater than 100 μg/ml. Other adverse effects include GI toxicity ranging from nausea and diarrhea to colitis with intestinal perforation. Hepatic dysfunction may occur and liver function tests should be monitored during 5-FC therapy.

III. **Azoles.** These agents are generally fungistatic against most organisms.

A. **Ketoconazole** (200–600 mg PO qd) is an orally active imidazole effective in treating mucocutaneous candidiasis, localized pulmonary histoplasmosis, blastomycosis, chromomycosis, and paracoccidioidomycosis. It is inactive against *Aspergillus* spp. **CSF penetration is unreliable.** Ketoconazole should not be used for rapidly progressive or severe fungal infections in immunosuppressed patients.

1. **Administration.** Absorption depends on gastric acidity and may be impaired in patients with achlorhydria or those taking antacids, omeprazole, or H_2-receptor antagonists. A serum level should be obtained 2 hours after a dose to ensure adequate absorption. Ketoconazole is principally eliminated by the liver and generally does not require dosage reduction in renal failure.

2. **Adverse effects** include nausea and fever and effects due to decreased testosterone levels, including oligospermia, gynecomastia, decreased libido, and impotence. Inhibition of adrenal steroid synthesis may occur with prolonged use. Hepatotoxicity has been reported. Ketoconazole may impair the hepatic metabolism of a variety of compounds (see Appendix B). Coadministration of ketoconazole with the antihistamines terfenadine and astemizole may result in prolongation of the QT interval and ventricular tachycardia and should be avoided. Ketoconazole may increase cyclosporine levels and should be used with caution in patients receiving this agent.

B. **Fluconazole** is more reliably absorbed than ketoconazole, even with achlorhydria. It is available both as oral and IV preparations. Fluconazole is widely distributed in the body and **penetrates readily into the CSF.** The dosage should be reduced in patients with renal dysfunction. Fluconazole may interfere with metabolism of phenytoin, cyclosporine, and warfarin. Concurrent therapy with rifampin lowers fluconazole levels (see Appendix B).

1. **Administration.** Fluconazole (200-mg load, 100 mg/day PO or IV) is useful for oropharyngeal and esophageal candidiasis and as maintenance therapy for cryptococcal meningitis in patients with AIDS. Higher doses (400-mg load, 200 mg/day PO or IV) are recommended for therapy of cryptococcal meningitis. Fluconazole has been effective in the treatment of candidal UTI, peritonitis, and hepatosplenic candidiasis. Its role in the treatment of other fungal infections, especially acute disseminated candidiasis and candidemia, is unclear.

2. **Adverse effects.** Headache, GI side effects, elevated serum transaminases, and rashes have been reported most frequently. Stevens-Johnson syndrome and hepatic necrosis have been reported infrequently.

C. **Itraconazole** is a triazole with a broad antifungal spectrum. It is available in an oral formulation and is approved for therapy of histoplasmosis and blastomycosis in immunocompetent and immunocompromised hosts.

1. **Administration.** Itraconazole (200 mg PO q12–24h) is best absorbed when given with food. For life-threatening infections, a loading dose of 200 mg PO tid can be used for the first 3 days. Itraconazole undergoes extensive hepatic metabolism, and plasma concentrations should be monitored in patients with hepatic impairment.

2. **Adverse effects** include nausea, vomiting, rash, and, rarely, hepatitis. Itraconazole may interfere with hepatic metabolism of phenytoin, cyclosporine, and warfarin (see Appendix B). Itraconazole should not be concurrently prescribed with terfenadine or astemizole, as increased levels of these antihistamines may lead to cardiac arrhythmias. Concurrent rifampin administration may significantly lower itraconazole levels.

D. **Miconazole** is generally a second-line antifungal agent. It is the drug of choice for *Pseudallescheria* infection. Miconazole has some efficacy in the treatment of coccidioidomycosis and systemic candidiasis but is ineffective against *Aspergillus* and *Histoplasma* spp. Cerebrospinal penetration is poor. A **test dose** of 200 mg is recommended, followed by gradual escalation of the dosage up to 200–1,200 mg IV q8h as tolerated. **Adverse effects** include phlebitis, pruritus, nausea and vomiting, fever, rash, and CNS abnormalities. Transient decreases in hematocrit and serum sodium have been reported with IV infusion. Rare but serious toxicities include anaphylaxis and cardiac arrhythmias.

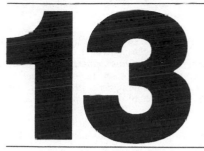

Treatment of Infectious Diseases

Timothy J. Henkel and
Victoria J. Fraser

Principles of Therapy

I. **General principles of therapy.** In addition to the selection of antimicrobials, several aspects of care are important in the treatment of patients with infectious diseases.

   A. **Treatment of protected sites** of infection involves the removal of foreign bodies, drainage of purulent material, and relief of obstruction.

   B. **Predisposing conditions** to infection, such as diabetes mellitus, uremia, hepatic failure, chronic lung disease, asplenia, renal failure, and malignancy should influence the initial selection of antimicrobials, and medical therapy should be optimized when possible. Iatrogenic immunosuppression should be minimized.

   C. **Renal and hepatic function** should be evaluated before initiating therapy since dosages may need to be adjusted.

   D. **Supportive care** should include the maintenance of circulation, oxygenation, and electrolyte balance and provision of adequate nutrition.

   E. **Passive immunization** is indicated for hepatitis A and B, rabies, tetanus, and diphtheria (see Appendix E) and decreases the risk of infection in patients with immunoglobulin deficiency and chronic lymphocytic leukemia.

   F. **Treatment of fever** is **not** required unless (1) complications of fever are present, (2) there is a significant probability of cardiac or respiratory insufficiency, or (3) there is a possibility of CNS damage. Care must be taken not to obscure fever due to inadequate therapy or emerging complications of infection. Antipyretics should not be administered indiscriminately.

   G. **Empiric therapy** should take into consideration the prevalence of particular pathogens in a given host and region, and local susceptibility patterns of those organisms.

   H. **Isolation techniques.** Communicable diseases may be asymptomatic or undiagnosed (e.g., human immunodeficiency virus [HIV], herpes simplex virus, or hepatitis); therefore, body fluids from all patients should be considered potentially infectious. **Body substance Isolation (BSI)** involves the use of barrier protection (e.g., gloves, mask, gown, or protective eyewear as appropriate) whenever direct contact with any body fluid is anticipated and should be employed for **all** patients (see Appendix F). Patients with diseases that are transmitted by the airborne route such as tuberculosis, measles, chicken pox (varicella), disseminated herpes zoster, invasive meningococcal infection, and pertussis need respiratory precautions in addition to BSI. These include a private room with negative-pressure ventilation and the use of properly fitted masks.

II. **Assessment of therapy.** Some infections respond slowly, even when optimal therapy is used. A premature change in therapy in such cases may confound the care of the patient. However, **when the expected response to treatment does not occur, the following questions should be asked:** (1) Is the isolated organism really the etiologic agent? (2) Is adequate antimicrobial therapy being given (i.e., the appropriate drug, dosage, and route)? (3) Is the antimicrobial penetrating to the site of infection (e.g., is drainage necessary)? (4) Have resistant or superinfecting pathogens emerged? (5) Is a persistent fever due to an underlying disease, an iatrogenic complication (e.g., phlebitis), a drug reaction, or another process?

III. Upper respiratory infections

A. Pharyngitis. Most cases of pharyngitis are viral. Treatable nonviral etiologies include group A *Streptococcus, Neisseria gonorrhoeae, Corynebacterium diphtheriae,* group C and G streptococci, *Haemophilus influenzae, Arcanobacterium haemolyticum, Mycoplasma pneumoniae,* and *Chlamydia pneumoniae.* Noninfectious causes include pemphigus and systemic lupus erythematosus. Viral and bacterial pharyngitis may be indistinguishable on clinical grounds.

1. Diagnosis

a. Throat cultures in adults can be reserved for patients with a previous history of rheumatic fever, symptomatic patients exposed to a patient with streptococcal pharyngitis, and patients with significant infection (i.e., fever, pharyngeal exudate, and cervical adenopathy). Patients who fail to clear a pharyngeal infection despite symptomatic therapy should also be cultured. Cultures for *N. gonorrhoeae* should be performed if indicated by sexual history. If diphtheria or *A. haemolyticum* is suspected, specific culture techniques are required. Group A beta-hemolytic *Streptoooccus,* which requires therapy to prevent acute pyogenic complications or rheumatic fever, can be identified by either culture or antigen detection tests. Antigen detection tests, although specific, vary in sensitivity. A positive test permits early diagnosis and treatment, but a negative test does not safely exclude group A streptococcal disease, making a culture necessary. Thus, the cost-effectiveness of rapid antigen detection tests is yet to be proved.

b. Serology for infectious mononucleosis (e.g., a test for heterophil agglutinin) and differential WBC count to detect atypical lymphocytes should be performed when infectious mononucleosis is suspected. Pharyngitis, atypical lymphocytosis, and a negative heterophil test should suggest the possibility of primary cytomegalovirus (CMV) infection or acute HIV infection.

2. Treatment. Most cases of pharyngitis are self-limited and do not require antimicrobial therapy. (For treatment of gonococcal pharyngitis, see Sexually Transmitted Diseases, sec. II.C.3.)

a. Treatment for group A beta-hemolytic *streptococcus* should be given (1) for a positive culture or antigen detection test, (2) if the patient is at high risk for development of rheumatic fever, or (3) if the diagnosis is strongly suspected, pending the results of culture. **Treatment schedules** include penicillin (PCN) VK, 250 mg PO qid for 10 days; erythromycin, 250 mg PO qid for 10 days; or benzathine PCN G, 1.2 million units IM.

b. Hospitalization and parenteral therapy are indicated when the patient is unable to take oral fluids or airway obstruction is present. Surgical treatment may be necessary in the latter case.

3. Prophylaxis against streptococcal infection is indicated for the prevention of **recurrent rheumatic fever** in patients at high risk of streptococcal infection (e.g., children, parents of young children, school teachers, medical and military personnel, patients in crowded living conditions) and those who have had rheumatic fever within the previous 5 years. Prophylaxis can be provided by several regimens (*Circulation* 70:118A, 1984). **Benzathine PCN G,** 1.2 million units IM q4wk, is the regimen of choice. **PCN V,** 125–250 mg PO bid, can also be used, but compliance should be monitored. **Sulfadiazine,** 1 g PO qd, for adults with normal renal function is effective in patients with PCN allergy. **Erythromycin,** 250 mg PO bid, may also be effective.

B. Epiglottitis should be considered in the febrile, toxic patient who complains of severe sore throat and dysphagia but has minimal findings on inspection of the pharynx.

1. Diagnosis. If epiglottitis is suspected, a lateral soft-tissue radiograph of the neck should be performed under close supervision. Throat and blood cultures should also be obtained.

2. Treatment. Hospitalization and prompt otolaryngology consultation for airway management are suggested in all suspected cases. Close observation for the possibility of airway obstruction is indicated. Antibacterial therapy should include an agent that is active against *H. influenzae*. In areas where ampicillin resistance is common, ceftriaxone, 1–2 g IV q12–24h; cefotaxime, 1–2 g q4–6h; or cefuroxime, 0.75–1.5 g IV q8h are appropriate agents.

C. **Acute sinusitis** in adults is most often caused by *Strep. pneumoniae, H. influenzae* (unencapsulated), rhinoviruses, and anaerobes. Cough and purulent postnasal discharge occur in the majority of patients, but fever occurs in less than 50%. Pain over the affected sinus that worsens with percussion or movement may be present. First-line empiric therapy includes amoxicillin, 500 mg PO tid, or trimethoprim and sulfamethoxazole (TMP/SMX), 160 mg/800 mg PO bid. The use of agents resistant to beta-lactamases such as amoxicillin-clavulanic acid, cefaclor, and cefuroxime axetil should be reserved for patients who have persistent symptoms after 10–14 days of first-line therapy, who have severe symptoms, or who are immunocompromised. Useful adjunctive measures include systemic decongestants, topical decongestants (phenylephrine or oxymetazoline) for no more than 3–5 days, and nasal irrigation with saline spray.

D. **Influenza** infection presents during the winter months with abrupt onset of high fever, severe myalgias, and a nonproductive cough. The elderly may have a more subtle presentation. Hospitalized patients with suspected influenza should be placed in respiratory isolation to prevent nosocomial transmission.

1. **Prevention.** High-risk patients and health care workers should be immunized yearly to prevent infection (see Appendix E). Either amantadine or rimantadine may be given prophylactically to unimmunized patients following exposure to influenza A, preferably in conjunction with immunization. Both drugs should be given at a dosage of 100 mg PO bid for 2–3 weeks to allow the development of an adequate immune response to vaccination. The dosage of both drugs should be reduced in the elderly and in patients with renal insufficiency. Rimantadine dosage must also be decreased in the setting of hepatic insufficiency.

2. **Diagnosis** is often clinical. However, a rapid diagnosis by immunofluorescence assay of a nasopharyngeal swab or a viral culture may be useful in limiting unnecessary diagnostic tests and antimicrobial therapy.

3. **Treatment.** Amantadine or rimantadine, when begun within 24–48 hours of initial symptoms and given for 7 days, can shorten the course of influenza A. Both drugs are given in the same dosages as for postexposure prophylaxis. Treatment is otherwise supportive. Vigilance for complications such as primary influenza pneumonia, secondary bacterial pneumonia, and rhabdomyolysis should be maintained.

IV. **Pneumonia** accounts for about 10% of admissions to medical wards and remains a common cause of death. Although *Strep. pneumoniae* is the most common etiologic agent identified, many bacteria, viruses, and fungi can cause pneumonia. Clinical criteria have historically been used to subdivide pneumonias into "typical" (i.e., *Strep. pneumoniae*) and "atypical" (i.e., *M. pneumoniae, C. pneumoniae, Legionella* spp, and influenza). However, the usefulness of such clinical features to determine the etiology of pneumonia is often misleading (*Medicine* 69:307, 1990).

A. **Diagnosis**

1. **Sputum examination. Specimens containing more than 5 epithelial cells/low-power field on a Gram's stain represent oral rather than pulmonary secretions and are not satisfactory.** Inducing sputum with inhalation of a warmed saline aerosol or nasotracheal suction can be helpful.

2. **Cultures.** In patients with a productive cough, **sputum** should always be cultured and results compared with those of a simultaneous Gram's stain. Sputum should not be cultured anaerobically, because contaminating pharyngeal organisms may produce misleading results. Hospitalized patients should have **blood cultures** collected, because they are often positive in patients with pneumococcal pneumonia. A diagnostic **thoracentesis** should be performed when a significant pleural effusion is present.

3. **A chest radiograph** is helpful in confirming the diagnosis of pneumonia,

although it is not specific. It is particularly valuable in detecting parapneumonic effusions, abscesses, and cavities.

4. **The leukocyte count** may be low or normal in the elderly, in immunocompromised patients, and in patients with overwhelming infections. A leukocyte count less than $10,000/mm^3$ is common in mycoplasma pneumonia.

5. **Invasive procedures,** such as transtracheal aspiration, transthoracic needle aspiration, bronchial brushings, bronchoalveolar lavage, transbronchial biopsy, and open lung biopsy are usually not indicated in community-acquired pneumonias. However, they may be required to diagnose severe pneumonias, especially in patients who (1) are immunocompromised, (2) fail to respond to therapy, or (3) are likely to have a nonbacterial etiology for their infiltrate (see Chap. 10).

B. **Supportive measures.** Adequate **hydration** is essential. **Oxygen** should be administered when indicated; occasionally, intubation and mechanical ventilation are required (see Chap. 9). **Antitussives** are unnecessary unless continued coughing exhausts the patient. **Control of pleuritic pain** may be achieved with antiinflammatory agents, analgesics, or intercostal nerve blocks.

C. **Empiric antimicrobial therapy.** Initial therapy of pneumonia is often empiric, but a properly performed Gram's stain may allow more specific therapy. If a specific etiologic agent is subsequently identified, antimicrobial therapy can be adjusted accordingly. The otherwise healthy patient with community-acquired pneumonia will usually have subjective improvement and resolution of fever 2–4 days after initiation of therapy. **Delayed clearing of the chest radiograph** should not be cause for concern in a patient who is improving clinically (*N Engl J Med* 293:798, 1975).

1. **Community-acquired pneumonia in adults.** Empiric antimicrobial therapy should be directed against the most likely pathogens in a given host. Rational choices can be made on the basis of several factors, including the severity of illness and the need for hospitalization, the age of the patient, and the presence of coexisting illnesses (*Am Rev Respir Dis* 148:1418, 1993). Examples of such coexisting illnesses include chronic obstructive lung disease, diabetes mellitus, renal failure, congestive heart failure, chronic liver disease, and malnutrition. Fluoroquinolones are not recommended for the empiric treatment of community-acquired pneumonias given their unreliable activity against *Strep. pneumoniae.*

a. **Outpatient community-acquired pneumonia in patients under the age of 60 without comorbidity** is most often caused by *Strep. pneumoniae, M. pneumoniae,* respiratory viruses, *C. pneumoniae,* and *H. influenzae.* Initial empiric therapy with a macrolide such as erythromycin is appropriate. In smokers, clarithromycin or azithromycin may be used because of their activity against *H. influenzae.* A tetracycline should be used only if the patient cannot tolerate a macrolide.

b. **Outpatient community-acquired pneumonia in patients with comorbidity or who are older than 60 years, or both,** is most commonly caused by *Strep. pneumoniae,* respiratory viruses, *H. influenzae,* and aerobic gram-negative bacilli, and *Staphylococcus aureus.* Initial empiric therapy should consist of an oral second-generation cephalosporin, TMP/SMX, or amoxicillin/clavulanic acid. Erythromycin may be added when infection with *Legionella, Mycoplasma,* or *Chlamydia* is a concern. Alternatively, clarithromycin or azithromycin can be used as a single agent in this setting.

c. **Patients with community-acquired pneumonia who require hospitalization** have an increased chance of having polymicrobial infection (including anaerobes), gram-negative aerobes, *Legionella,* and *Chlamydia* spp relative to their less severely ill counterparts. Risk factors that have been associated with increased morbidity and mortality include age greater than 65 years, coexisting illnesses (see sec. **IV.C.1**), immunosuppression, altered mental status, aspiration, malnutrition, alcohol abuse, tachypnea (respiratory rate >30 respirations/minute), systolic BP less than 90 mm Hg, evidence of extrapulmonary disease, hypoxemia, and multilobar involvement. Therefore, hospitalization to begin treatment should be considered for patients with any of these risk factors. Ceftriaxone and cefotaxime are appropriate agents for initial therapy. When infection with *Legionella, Mycoplasma,* or *Chlamydia* is suspected, or for severe disease, a macrolide should be added.

2. **Nosocomial pneumonia.** Gram-negative and, less frequently, staphylococcal organisms are important pathogens in patients who develop pneumonia in the hospital. *Legionella* is also a nosocomial pathogen in some locations. In most patients, a combination of a broad-spectrum beta-lactam antimicrobial with gram-positive activity (e.g., ceftriaxone or cefotaxime) and an aminoglycoside is effective. If *Pseudomonas aeruginosa* or other resistant gram-negative organisms are of particular concern, such as in an ICU setting or in an immunocompromised host, an antipseudomonal beta-lactam antimicrobial (e.g., mezlocillin or ceftazidime) plus an aminoglycoside should be used.

3. **Aspiration pneumonia.** See Chap. 10.

4. **Pneumonia in adults with cystic fibrosis.** See Chap. 10.

D. **Antimicrobial therapy for pneumonias caused by specific organisms**

1. *Streptococcus pneumoniae* (pneumococcus). In uncomplicated infection, procaine PCN G, 600,000 units IM, followed by PCN V, 250–500 mg PO q6h for a total of 7–10 days, is an appropriate outpatient regimen. Seriously ill patients should be treated with PCN G, 1–2 million units IV q4h in areas where high-level PCN resistance is not problematic. Erythromycin, 500 mg PO or IV q6h, can be used in patients who are allergic to PCN. Vancomycin, 1,000 mg IV q12h, may be preferable to erythromycin in seriously ill or immunocompromised patients who are allergic to PCN. Vancomycin may also be used in seriously ill patients pending susceptibility data when PCN-resistant or multiply resistant *Strep. pneumoniae* is present.

2. *Staphylococcus aureus.* Diabetics, patients with a recent history of influenza, and institutionalized or hospitalized patients are at increased risk of *Staph. aureus* pneumonia. A beta-lactamase–resistant PCN (e.g., oxacillin, 6–12 g/day IV) or vancomycin when the risk of methicillin-resistant organisms is high should be used initially. Serious complications include bacteremia and abscess formation. Treatment of staphylococcal pneumonia should usually be continued for a minimum of 3–4 weeks.

3. *Klebsiella pneumoniae* causes a virulent, necrotizing pneumonia often seen in alcoholic or otherwise debilitated patients. Abscess formation is common. Third-generation cephalosporins (e.g., ceftriaxone or cefotaxime) are the drugs of choice.

4. *Haemophilus influenzae* pneumonia may be treated in outpatients with TMP/SMX, amoxicillin/clavulanic acid, oral second- and third-generation cephalosporins, clarithromycin, azithromycin, or a fluoroquinolone. A third-generation cephalosporin (ceftriaxone or cefotaxime) is the treatment of choice for serious illness, though ampicillin, 1–2 g IV q6h, may be used if the isolate is susceptible.

5. *Pseudomonas aeruginosa* pneumonia is a severe necrotizing infection requiring intensive parenteral therapy with a combination of an aminoglycoside and an antipseudomonal beta-lactam agent (see Chap. 12). **Combination therapy** should be used for synergy and because resistance may develop with single-agent therapy. The choice of individual agents should be made according to the local antimicrobial susceptibility patterns of *P. aeruginosa*. Empyema is a common complication in *Pseudomonas* pneumonia.

6. *Moraxella (Branhamella) catarrhalis* is a gram-negative diplococcus that typically causes pneumonia in patients with underlying lung disease. It can be treated with TMP/SMX, amoxicillin-clavulanic acid, a second- or third-generation cephalosporin, clarithromycin, or azithromycin.

7. *Mycoplasma pneumoniae.* The treatment of choice is a macrolide antimicrobial (erythromycin, clarithromycin, or azithromycin). Tetracycline or doxycycline are effective alternatives.

8. *Chlamydia pneumoniae* (TWAR agent) is a recently described pathogen that

causes a spectrum of illnesses from mild upper respiratory symptoms to pneumonia. Comparative studies of therapy are lacking, but tetracycline, 500 mg PO qid, or doxycycline, 100 mg IV or PO bid, are most likely to be effective. A macrolide antimicrobial is an alternative.

9. **Legionnaires' disease** (*Legionella pneumophila* and other *Legionella* spp) occurs in debilitated and immunocompromised hosts. It is treated with erythromycin, 500 mg PO q6h for mild cases and 1,000 mg IV q6h for severe cases. Therapy should be continued for 21 days. Critically ill patients should be given high-dose IV therapy initially. The addition of rifampin (RIF), 600 mg PO qd, may be synergistic.

10. *Pneumocystis carinii.* See Chap. 14, sec. II.E.

E. **Complications** of pneumonia include effusion, empyema, abscess formation, purulent pericarditis, and the adult respiratory distress syndrome (ARDS). Significant pleural effusions should be tapped to exclude an empyema. Empyema requires chest tube drainage. Drainage by repeated thoracenteses has been associated with a significant failure rate and is not recommended. See Chap. 10 for the management of lung abscess and ARDS.

V. **Urinary tract infections (UTIs)** can be classified as lower UTI (urethritis or cystitis) or upper UTI (pyelonephritis). **Lower UTI** is characterized by pyuria, often with dysuria, urgency, or frequency. A rapid, presumptive diagnosis can be made by microscopic examination of a **fresh, unspun, clean-voided urine specimen.** A urine Gram's stain can be helpful in guiding initial antimicrobial choices. Bacteriuria (>1 organism/oil-immersion field) or pyuria (>8 leukocytes/high-power field) correlates well with the presence of infection. Quantitative culture often yields more than 10^4 bacteria/ml, but colony counts of 10^2-10^4 coliforms/ml may also indicate infection in women with acute dysuria. **Pyelonephritis** represents infection of the renal parenchyma. Presenting symptoms include fever and flank pain, as well as lower tract symptoms. Urine specimens characteristically demonstrate significant bacteriuria, pyuria, and occasional leukocyte casts. Other sites of infection within the genitourinary tract (e.g., epididymis, prostate, perinephric areas) are often associated with less than 10^3 bacteria/ml and have different clinical manifestations. Special techniques, such as quantitative cultures before and after prostatic massage, may be necessary to diagnose these infections.

A. **The diagnostic and therapeutic approach to adults with UTIs** can be simplified by dividing patients into the groups described below (*N Engl J Med* 329:1328, 1993).

1. **Acute uncomplicated cystitis in women** is caused by *Escherichia coli* in 80% of cases and *Staphylococcus saprophyticus* in another 5–15%. Because the spectrum of organisms responsible for these infections is small, and their antimicrobial susceptibilities are relatively predictable, a limited laboratory evaluation followed by empiric therapy is advocated. If pyuria is present microscopically or by leukocyte esterase testing, treatment with a 3-day regimen of TMP/SMX, 160 mg/800 mg PO bid, is recommended without the need for a urine culture. In patients intolerant of sulfa, trimethoprim, 100 mg PO bid, may be used. Fluoroquinolones are more costly than TMP/SMX but are very effective alternatives when given for 3 days. Because single-dose regimens are associated with higher relapse rates, 3-day regimens are more cost-effective. In diabetics, patients who are symptomatic for more than 7 days, those with a recent UTI, women who use a diaphragm, and those older than 65 years, a pretreatment culture is recommended and therapy should be extended to 7 days.

2. **Recurrent cystitis in young women** is rarely the result of a persistent focus of infection or due to anatomic or functional abnormalities of the urinary tract. Exogenous reinfection accounts for over 90% of recurrences. Relapses with the original infecting organism that occur within 2 weeks of cessation of therapy should be treated for 2 weeks or more and may indicate a urologic abnormality. An alternative method of contraception may decrease the frequency of reinfection in women who use a diaphragm and spermicide. **Prophylaxis** may also be helpful for patients with frequent reinfection.

Sterilization of the urine with a standard treatment regimen is necessary before prophylaxis is initiated. For women with relapses that correlate with sexual intercourse, TMP/SMX, 80 mg/400 mg, or cephalexin, 250 mg, after coitus may provide adequate prophylaxis. TMP/SMX, 40 mg/200 mg qd or qod, is usually sufficient to decrease recurrences unrelated to coitus.

3. **Acute uncomplicated pyelonephritis in young women** is usually due to uropathogenic strains of *E. coli*. Urine cultures should be obtained in all patients suspected of having pyelonephritis, and blood cultures should be obtained in those who are hospitalized, since bacteremia will be detected in 15–20%. Patients with mild to moderate illness who are able to take oral medication may be safely treated as outpatients with TMP/SMX or fluoroquinolones for 10–14 days. Patients with more severe illness, those with nausea and vomiting, and pregnant patients should be treated initially with parenteral therapy. Appropriate empiric parenteral regimens include TMP/SMX, third-generation cephalosporins, fluoroquinolones, or aminoglycosides (with or without a beta-lactam antimicrobial). If enterococcal infection is suspected on the basis of urine Gram's stain, ampicillin, 1 g IV q6h, plus gentamicin, 1 mg/kg IV q8h, is appropriate.

4. **UTIs in men younger than 50 years** are rare; however, they do not necessarily indicate urologic abnormalities. Uropathogenic strains of *E. coli* capable of causing pyelonephritis in women can cause cystitis in men as well. In men, risk factors for UTI include anal intercourse, lack of circumcision, and having a sexual partner whose vagina is colonized by uropathogens (*N Engl J Med* 329:1328, 1993). A pretreatment urine culture should be obtained, and if no complicating factors are present, a 7-day course of TMP/SMX, trimethoprim, or a fluoroquinolone may be prescribed. If there is a prompt response to therapy, a urologic evaluation is unlikely to be useful. Urologic studies are appropriate with treatment failures, recurrent infections, or when pyelonephritis occurs.

5. **Asymptomatic bacteriuria** in adults is defined as two successive cultures with (greater than or equal to 10^5 colony-forming units/ml). Screening for asymptomatic bacteriuria can be justified only before urologic surgery and in pregnant women. No evidence supports the practice of routine screening or treatment in other settings.

6. **Catheter-associated bacteriuria** is the most common source of gram-negative bacteremia in hospitalized patients (*Am J Med* 68:332, 1980). Therefore, bladder catheters should be used only when absolutely necessary. Effective preventive measures include aseptic technique for catheter insertion, use of a closed drainage system, and removal of the catheter as soon as possible. With **chronic indwelling catheters**, the development of bacteriuria is inevitable, and long-term antimicrobial suppression simply selects for multiply resistant bacteria. Such patients should be treated with systemic antimicrobials only when symptomatic infection is evident. Condom catheters may be associated with less frequent UTIs in cooperative or paralyzed patients when patency of the outflow can be ensured.

B. **Adjunctive measures** such as hydration and analgesia with phenazopyridine, 200 mg PO tid, may provide symptomatic relief during the first 24–48 hours. Analgesia should not be given for longer periods because it may obscure persistent infection.

C. **Acute urethral syndrome (AUS)** is a condition of women who have lower UTI symptoms and pyuria with fewer than 10^5 bacteria/ml of urine. These patients may have bacterial cystitis or urethritis caused by *Chlamydia trachomatis, Ureaplasma urealyticum,* or, less frequently, *N. gonorrhoeae*. Specific cultures of the endocervix for *N. gonorrhoeae* should be performed. Vaginitis and genital herpes should be excluded. If no specific etiology is found, doxycycline, 100 mg PO bid, should be given for at least 7 days. Azithromycin, 1 g in a single dose, is an alternative. Erythromycin, 500 mg PO qid for 7 days, should be used for pregnant women with nongonococcal urethritis.

D. **Prostatitis** is usually caused by enteric gram-negative bacilli. TMP/SMX, 160 mg/800 mg PO bid for 14 days, is an effective, economical treatment for acute infections. Quinolones are useful alternatives. Patients with chronic bacterial prostatitis should receive prolonged therapy (for at least 1 month with the quinolones or 3 months with TMP/SMX).

E. Epididymitis is usually caused by *N. gonorrhoeae* or *C. trachomatis* in sexually active young men and by gram-negative enteric organisms in older men. Diagnosis and therapy should be directed accordingly (see Sexually Transmitted Diseases).

VI. Central nervous system infections

A. Acute bacterial meningitis is a medical emergency. The prognosis in bacterial meningitis depends on the interval between the onset of disease and the initiation of antimicrobial therapy. Therefore, when bacterial meningitis is suspected, diagnostic procedures (e.g., lumbar puncture) should be completed and therapy instituted within 1 hour of presentation. Adjunctive radiographic studies, such as sinus x-rays and CT of the brain, can be performed electively **after the initiation of antimicrobial therapy** when they are indicated. Meningitis should be considered in any patient with fever and neurologic symptoms, especially if there is a history of other infection (e.g., pneumonia) or head trauma. CSF pleocytosis with negative cultures may be associated with viral meningoencephalitis, parameningeal infection, neoplastic disease, subarachnoid hemorrhage, trauma, and partially treated bacterial meningitis. Chronic meningitis due to fungi or mycobacteria should be considered if initial cultures for bacteria are negative. *Strep. pneumoniae* **and** *Neisseria meningitidis* **are responsible for most cases of bacterial meningitis in adults.** *Listeria monocytogenes, H. influenzae,* other gram-negative bacilli, streptococci, and staphylococci are less frequent causes.

1. Diagnostic measures. In the absence of focal neurologic signs, a lumbar puncture should be performed immediately. CSF pressure should be measured and a CSF specimen should be obtained. Head CT, preferably with contrast, is indicated in the patient with focal neurologic signs or diminished level of consciousness. **However, in the seriously ill patient, antimicrobial therapy should be instituted without delay, and appropriate diagnostic procedures (lumbar puncture or head CT) should follow.**

a. Cultures. CSF specimens should be taken to the laboratory immediately. Blood, nasal swabs, and aspirates of skin lesions should be handled similarly. If viral meningitis is a possibility, CSF specimens should be cultured promptly. If this is not possible, CSF and serum should be frozen at −70°C for subsequent viral culture and serologic investigation; viral cultures of the throat and stool may provide additional evidence for the cause of the meningitis.

b. CSF examination should include cell counts with differential and Gram's stain of the centrifuged sediment. Neutrophilic pleocytosis is usually seen in bacterial meningitis but may also be present early in viral meningitis (*N Engl J Med* 289:571, 1973). In very early bacterial meningitis, pleocytosis may be absent. **A cryptococcal antigen test** or **India ink preparation** and an **acid-fast stain** should be examined if Gram's stain does not yield a diagnosis. A wet-mount examination of the sediment may reveal motile amebas in amebic meningoencephalitis.

c. CSF protein and glucose. The CSF protein is commonly elevated (>100 mg/dl) and glucose decreased (<45 mg/dl or <50–66% of blood glucose) in bacterial meningitis, as well as tuberculous and fungal meningitis.

d. Detection of capsular polysaccharide antigens is possible for *Strep. pneumoniae, H. influenzae* type B, *N. meningitidis* (groups A and C), and group B *Streptococcus*. Because false-positives and false-negatives may occur, these tests should not be the sole basis for selecting initial antimicrobial therapy. In contrast, the detection of capsular polysaccharide of *Cryptococcus neoformans* in CSF by latex agglutination is sensitive and specific when positive at a dilution of greater than or equal to 1:4.

The microbiology or serology laboratory should be consulted to determine which tests and specimens are appropriate for particular pathogens.

2. **Supportive measures** include maintenance of electrolyte balance and airway patency. Fluid intake should be restricted to 1,000 ml/m^2/day. Comatose patients may require intubation. Treatment of associated seizures is discussed in Chap. 25. Use of glucocorticoids as an adjunctive measure in the treatment of meningitis in adults is controversial. However, early administration of glucocorticoids has been essential in pediatric studies to demonstrate benefit.

3. **Initial antimicrobial therapy.** When bacterial meningitis is suspected, high-dose parenteral antimicrobial therapy should be administered. Antimicrobial combinations are reasonable if the pathogen is unknown or if polymicrobial infection (e.g., brain abscess) is suspected. Aqueous PCN G, 2 million units IV q2h, will usually provide effective initial therapy in areas where PCN-resistant *Strep. pneumoniae* is not present. However, treatment failures with both PCN and ceftriaxone have been reported with even intermediate-level PCN resistance. In areas where such PCN resistance is present, vancomycin can be combined with a third-generation cephalosporin (cefotaxime or ceftriaxone) until culture and susceptibility data are available.

   If the cause of the meningitis is unclear, additional antimicrobials should be chosen based on the clinical setting and the CSF Gram's stain. If no organisms are seen on Gram's stain, a third-generation cephalosporin (e.g., ceftriaxone, 2 g IV q12h, or cefotaxime, 2 g IV q4h) is prudent while awaiting culture results. *Listeria* should be strongly considered in the immunocompromised adult, and therapy should include appropriate doses of ampicillin (see sec. **VI.A.4.g**). Antistaphylococcal coverage is important in the postneurosurgical setting or following head or spinal trauma.

4. **Therapy for specific infections**
   a. *Streptococcus pneumoniae.* PCN G, 2 million units IV q2h for 10–14 days, is appropriate when the isolate is fully susceptible to PCN. Patients with a history of a PCN allergy may be given a skin test and may be desensitized if necessary, or treated with ceftriaxone or cefotaxime if the allergic reaction was mild. Patients with a history of a severe allergy to PCN can be treated with chloramphenicol, 1.0–1.5 g IV q6h, unless the isolate is PCN-resistant. Because a significant portion of these isolates may be resistant to chloramphenicol as well, vancomycin should be used.
   b. *Neisseria meningitidis.* PCN G, 2 million units IV q2h, should be continued for at least 5 days after the patient has become afebrile. Patients who are allergic to PCN can be given a skin test and desensitized, treated with ceftriaxone or cefotaxime, or treated with chloramphenicol, 1.0–1.5 g IV q6h. **Patients with meningococcal meningitis** should be placed in a private room on respiratory isolation for at least the first 24 hours of treatment. **Close contacts (i.e., persons living in the same household, medical personnel after CPR, and children and day care personnel) should receive prophylaxis** with rifampin, 600 mg PO bid for 2 days, or, if the pathogen is known to be susceptible to sulfa, with sulfadiazine, 1 g PO bid for 2 days. Terminal component complement deficiency (C6–C9) should be ruled out in patients with recurrent meningococcal infections.
   c. *Haemophilus influenzae* is a rare cause of meningitis in adults. Cefotaxime, 2 g IV q4h, or ceftriaxone, 2 g IV q12h, is effective as initial therapy. Chloramphenicol, 1.0–1.5 g IV q6h, is the preferred alternative for patients who are allergic to PCNs and cephalosporins. Ampicillin, 2 g IV q4h, is the drug of choice for beta-lactamase–negative strains. Treatment should be continued for a minimum of 10 days.
   d. *Staphylococcus aureus* is a rare cause of meningitis and produces high mortality despite treatment. It may result from high-grade staphylococcal bacteremia, direct extension from a parameningeal focus, a neurosurgical

procedure, or skull trauma. **Initially, nafcillin or oxacillin, 2 g IV q4h, should be given.** First-generation cephalosporins should not be used because they do not enter the CSF. Vancomycin, 1,000 mg IV q12h, is the drug of choice for PCN-allergic patients and when methicillin resistance is likely or is confirmed by culture. Documentation of adequate CSF levels may be prudent, particularly in patients who respond poorly to therapy. RIF may be beneficial in cases of methicillin-resistant *Staph. aureus* (MRSA) meningitis that does not respond to vancomycin alone.

  e. *Staphylococcus epidermidis* **meningitis** is usually secondary to an infected ventricular shunt. Vancomycin, 1,000 mg IV q12h, is the drug of choice. Intraventricular vancomycin, 10 mg qd–qod, may be a useful adjunct. A combination of RIF and vancomycin has not shown superiority over vancomycin alone. Removal of an infected shunt is often necessary for cure.

  f. **Gram-negative bacillary meningitis** occurs with head trauma and neurosurgical procedures and is also seen in neonates, the elderly, and debilitated patients (e.g., alcoholics). Third-generation cephalosporins such as cefotaxime, 2 g IV q4h, or ceftriaxone, 2 g IV q12h, are indicated for susceptible pathogens. TMP/SMX, chloramphenicol, and ampicillin are alternatives. Ceftazidime, 2 g IV q8h, has been used effectively for *P. aeruginosa* meningitis but should probably be combined with IV aminoglycoside therapy.

  g. *Listeria monocytogenes* is an important cause of meningitis in immunosuppressed adults. The treatment of choice is ampicillin, 2 g IV q4h (or PCN G, 2 million units IV q2h), in combination with a systemically administered aminoglycoside. TMP/SMX is an alternative for the PCN-allergic patient. Treatment should be continued for at least 3–4 weeks.

B. **Brain abscess** may result from the spread from a contiguous focus (e.g., mastoiditis, sinusitis), by hematogenous spread from a distant site (e.g., lung abscess, endocarditis), or by reactivation of a latent infection (e.g., toxoplasmosis).

  1. **Clinical features.** The presentation is often subacute to chronic and is usually that of an expanding mass lesion with neurologic signs or symptoms. Fever may be absent. Hematogenous abscesses or abscesses that rupture into the ventricles may present more acutely, suggesting bacterial meningitis.

  2. **Diagnosis.** Patients with a compatible clinical picture should undergo a head CT with contrast, which typically reveals ring-enhancing lesions, often with associated edema. MRI may be more sensitive in detecting small lesions or lesions in the posterior fossa. Lumbar puncture is unlikely to be helpful and is contraindicated in some patients. In patients with AIDS, multiple brain abscesses usually represent *Toxoplasma* encephalitis (see Chap. 14). The presence of pulmonary or skin lesions should suggest the possibility of nocardiosis, tuberculosis, cryptococcosis or, in endemic areas, histoplasmosis, coccidioidomycosis, or blastomycosis.

  3. **Therapy.** Most patients will require either needle aspiration or surgical drainage for microbiologic diagnosis and therapy. In the immunologically normal host, a reasonable empiric combination while awaiting bacteriologic confirmation is IV PCN G, 12–24 million units IV daily, a third-generation cephalosporin (e.g., ceftriaxone, 2 g IV q12h, or cefotaxime, 2 g IV q4h), and metronidazole, 500 mg IV q8h. If *Staph. aureus* is suspected, a penicillinase-resistant PCN (e.g., oxacillin or nafcillin) should be used. Chloramphenicol, 1 g IV q6h, is suitable for the PCN-allergic patient. Antimicrobials should be continued for 3–4 weeks after drainage.

C. **Herpes encephalitis** is the most common cause of acute sporadic encephalitis. Successful treatment depends on a high degree of suspicion and early institution of therapy.

  1. **Clinical features.** The diagnosis should be suspected in any patient who presents with the abrupt onset of fever and behavioral changes, alteration of consciousness, focal neurologic findings, or seizures, particularly if such manifestations are out of proportion to CSF abnormalities.

  2. **Diagnosis. CSF findings are nonspecific** and may be minimal or absent. CT

with contrast may demonstrate localized temporal lobe edema, mass effect, hemorrhage, and patchy contrast enhancement. MRI is more sensitive than CT scan for detecting subtle abnormalities. Brain biopsy is occasionally required but is no longer considered imperative. Examination of the CSF by the polymerase chain reaction (PCR) for HSV DNA may prove to be the most sensitive and specific noninvasive test (*Lancet* 337:189, 1991).

3. **Therapy.** In suspected cases, treatment should be instituted without delay with acyclovir, 10 mg/kg IV q8h for 10 days.

VII. **Infective endocarditis (IE)** is usually caused by gram-positive cocci. Parenteral drug abusers and patients with catheter-associated sepsis have an increased risk of staphylococcal disease. Gram-negative and fungal endocarditis are infrequent and usually occur in drug addicts or in patients with prosthetic valves. **The clinical features of IE are influenced by the causative organism.** However, although *Strep. viridans* classically produces the clinical picture of subacute bacterial endocarditis (SBE), and *Staph. aureus* produces acute bacterial endocarditis (ABE), either organism may cause either syndrome. Patients with ABE are typically symptomatic for a short time (3–10 days) and present critically ill. In contrast, patients with SBE are often chronically ill, with symptoms of fatigue, weight loss, low-grade fever, immune complex disease (nephritis, arthralgias, petechiae, Osler's nodes, Janeway lesions), and emboli (renal, splenic, and cerebral infarcts). A deformed or previously damaged valve is the usual focus of infection in SBE. Left-sided endocarditis, involving the aortic or mitral valves, occurs most commonly in middle-aged and older patients with preexisting valvular disease. Dental procedures, instrumentation of the genitourinary or GI tract, and bacteremia from distant foci of infection are frequent seeding events. Right-sided endocarditis, involving the tricuspid or pulmonic valves, is seen most frequently in parenteral drug abusers and in hospitalized patients with vascular catheters.

A. **Diagnosis.** The most reliable criterion is continuous bacteremia in a compatible clinical setting.

1. **Blood cultures** are positive in more than 90% of patients. Three sets of blood cultures taken over a 24-hour period are usually adequate in patients with SBE; however, the yield may be reduced significantly if the patient has received antimicrobial therapy within 1–2 weeks. Cultures should be incubated for 4 weeks if fastidious organisms are suspected. **Because ABE is a medical emergency,** three cultures should be taken from separate sites over a 1-hour period before empiric therapy is begun.

2. **Echocardiography.** Patients with IE and vegetations seen by conventional echocardiography are at higher risk of embolism, heart failure, and valvular disruption. A normal echocardiogram does not exclude the diagnosis of IE, and false-positive findings occur with myxomatous valvular degeneration, ruptured chordae tendineae, and atrial myxomas. Transesophageal echocardiography is more sensitive than M-mode or two-dimensional techniques. Visualization of vegetations alone does not mandate surgical intervention. Vegetations visualized by echocardiography may persist unchanged for at least 3 years after clinical cure.

B. **Treatment of bacterial endocarditis on native valves** requires high doses of antimicrobials for extended periods. Quantitative susceptibility testing (minimal inhibitory concentrations and minimal lethal concentrations), the measurement of serum drug levels and serum bactericidal activity, and serial erythrocyte sedimentation rates help assess the adequacy of therapy (see Chap. 12).

1. **ABE** requires empiric antimicrobial treatment before culture results become available. *Staph. aureus* and gram-negative bacilli are the most likely pathogens. Treatment should include oxacillin or nafcillin, 2 g IV q4h, plus gentamicin or tobramycin, 1.5–2.0 mg/kg IV q8h. Therapy can then be modified based on culture and susceptibility data.

2. **SBE is most often caused by streptococci.** PCN therapy typically results in cure rates of more than 90%. *Streptococcus bovis* bacteremia and endocarditis are associated with lower GI disease, including neoplasms. Group B streptococcal endocarditis may also be associated with lower intestinal pathology.

    a. Penicillin G, 2 million units IV q4h for 4 weeks, is effective for PCN-susceptible strains (minimal inhibitory concentration <0.1 μg/ml). Therapy with parenteral PCN and an aminoglycoside for 2 weeks is an alternative, but extended aminoglycoside treatment should be avoided in the elderly and in patients who will not tolerate the potential nephrotoxicity or ototoxicity. If the minimal inhibitory concentration (MIC) of PCN is greater than 0.1 μg/ml but less than 1.0 μg/ml, the addition of streptomycin or gentamicin may be appropriate for the first 2 weeks of therapy, followed by PCN G alone for 2 weeks. Patients with endocarditis caused by streptococci with PCN MICs greater than 1.0 μg/ml may require combination therapy similar to that given for enterococcal IE (see sec. **VII.B.3**).

    b. Patients who are allergic to PCN. PCN skin testing and desensitization should be considered. Vancomycin is an acceptable alternative.

    c. *Streptococcus pyogenes* **(group A) and** *Strep. pneumoniae* typically cause ABE and should be treated with PCN G, 2–4 million units IV q4h, for 4–6 weeks.

  3. *Enterococcus* **spp** cause 10–20% of cases of SBE. **The combination of a PCN plus an aminoglycoside** produces synergism against these bacteria and is the treatment of choice. PCN alone is usually ineffective. Recommended dosages are ampicillin, 2 g IV q4h, or PCN G, 2–3 million units IV q4h, in combination with gentamicin, 1.0–1.5 mg/kg IV q8h for 6 weeks. In susceptible strains, **vancomycin** in combination with an aminoglycoside is effective against enterococci and should be used for **PCN-allergic patients or patients with beta-lactamase–producing strains.** Aminoglycoside and vancomycin levels should be monitored. Weekly audiometry is also recommended. Serum bactericidal activity should be determined to optimize therapy.

    Antimicrobial resistance among enterococci is increasingly problematic. High-level resistance to either or both gentamicin and streptomycin (MIC >2,000 μg/ml) occurs. Streptomycin can be used instead of gentamicin for susceptible strains, but isolates resistant to both gentamicin and streptomycin are resistant to all aminoglycosides. The optimal management of IE due to enterococci with high-level resistance to all aminoglycosides is unclear. Isolates from patients with enterococcal endocarditis should also be screened for beta-lactamase production and vancomycin resistance.

  4. *Staphylococcus aureus* **endocarditis** should be treated with oxacillin or nafcillin, 2 g IV q4h, although PCN is effective against sensitive strains. An aminoglycoside can be added during the initial 3–5 days of therapy or in patients who fail to respond to beta-lactam therapy alone. Antimicrobials should be continued for 6 weeks in most cases. The prognosis is better in young parenteral drug abusers with right-sided endocarditis in whom treatment with oxacillin or nafcillin alone for 4 weeks may be sufficient and surgery is rarely required. A 2-week course of nafcillin plus an aminoglycoside has been studied as treatment for purely right-sided disease in parenteral drug abusers at one center (*Ann Intern Med* 109:619, 1988). Older patients with aortic valve infection have a high mortality and often require surgical intervention. For IE caused by MRSA, vancomycin is the drug of choice. Cephalosporins should not be used in such cases, even if the isolate is sensitive in vitro.

  5. *Staphylococcus epidermidis* is an increasingly frequent cause of IE, particularly after cardiac surgery. These organisms are often resistant to PCN, semisynthetic PCNs, and the cephalosporins. Pending susceptibility studies, the treatment of choice is vancomycin, 1 g IV q12h, in combination with rifampin, 300 mg PO q12h, and gentamicin. Cephalosporins should not be used to treat methicillin-resistant strains, even if the isolate is sensitive in vitro. Treatment should be continued for at least 6 weeks.

  6. HACEK is an acronym for a group of fastidious, slow-growing gram-negative bacteria (*Haemophilus parainfluenzae, H. aphrophilus, Actinobacillus, Cardiobacterium, Eikenella,* and *Kingella*) that have a predilection for infecting heart valves when they cause human disease. The treatment of choice is PCN or ampicillin plus an aminoglycoside until susceptibility information is available. Ceftriaxone may be substituted in patients who are unable to tolerate PCNs.

7. **Culture-negative endocarditis.** When IE is suspected and routine bacterial cultures remain negative, efforts should be made to isolate more fastidious organisms such as fungi and nutritionally deficient streptococci. If the diagnosis of IE is well established on clinical grounds, therapy may be initiated despite negative cultures. Treatment usually includes PCN G, 2–3 million units IV q4h, or ampicillin, 2 g IV q4h, plus an aminoglycoside. This regimen should be continued for 4–6 weeks.

C. **Prosthetic valve endocarditis (PVE)** occurs in 1–4% of patients after valve replacement. **Early infections** (within 2 months of surgery) are commonly caused by *Staph. aureus, Staph. epidermidis,* gram-negative bacilli, *Candida* spp, and other opportunistic organisms. The diagnosis is difficult, because fever and transient bacteremia often occur in the postoperative period; however, endocarditis must be considered in any patient with sustained bacteremia after valve surgery. Treatment should continue for at least 6 weeks and should be guided by the results of MIC and serum bactericidal studies. **Late PVE** (i.e., >2 months after surgery) is usually caused by organisms similar to those seen in SBE on native valves. Treatment should be continued for at least 6 weeks.

D. **Role of surgery.** Indications for urgent cardiac surgery include (1) uncontrolled infection as manifested by sustained bacteremia, (2) refractory heart failure, or (3) in PVE, an unstable prosthesis or valve obstruction. Surgical intervention may also be necessary when native valve endocarditis is complicated by recurrent systemic emboli, mycotic aneurysm, persistent conduction defects, chordae tendineae or papillary muscle rupture, or early closure of the mitral valve on echocardiography, or when PVE is complicated by a periprosthetic leak. In addition, **fungal endocarditis** is usually refractory to medical therapy and requires surgery. Endocarditis due to gram-negative bacilli may also be refractory to antimicrobials alone. Although a 10-day course of preoperative antimicrobials is desirable, surgery must not be delayed in patients whose condition is deteriorating.

E. **Response to antimicrobial therapy.** Appropriate antimicrobial therapy in IE frequently leads to clinical improvement within 3–10 days. Daily blood cultures should be obtained until sterility is documented. Persistent or recurrent fever usually represents extensive cardiac infection but may also be due to septic emboli or drug hypersensitivity. Such fever seldom represents the development of antimicrobial resistance, and drug therapy should be altered only if there is clear evidence of another infection or drug hypersensitivity (*Lancet* 1:1341, 1986).

F. **Prophylaxis** (Table 13-1) should be provided for those at increased risk for IE, including patients with a previous history of IE, rheumatic valvular disease, most forms of congenital heart disease, calcific aortic stenosis, hypertrophic obstructive cardiomyopathy, prosthetic valves and other intravascular prostheses, and mitral valve prolapse with mitral insufficiency. Antimicrobial prophylaxis is **not** recommended for patients with previous coronary artery bypass graft surgery, mitral valve prolapse without valvular regurgitation, or cardiac pacemakers and implanted defibrillators. Parenteral prophylaxis for oral procedures is not required for high-risk patients (e.g., those with prosthetic valves) but may still be preferred by some physicians. For high-risk patients who are undergoing genitourinary or GI procedures, parenteral prophylaxis is recommended (*JAMA* 264:2919, 1990).

VIII. **Enteric infections** are among the most common infections worldwide. They usually present with GI symptoms but may also present as enteric fever or septicemia. Most cases of enteritis, including those caused by viruses and many bacterial pathogens, are self-limited and do not require specific therapy in the normal host. **Fluid replacement** is often the only treatment needed. Usually, oral replacement is satisfactory, but IV fluids may be required if the illness is protracted or if dehydration is severe. **Antidiarrheal agents** may provide symptomatic relief but should generally be avoided if fever or symptoms of dysentery are present (see

Table 13-1. Endocarditis prophylaxis

Drug	Dosage
Dental procedures	
Standard regimens	
1. Amoxicillin	3.0 g PO 1 hour before procedure and 1.5 g PO 6 hours after initial dose
or (if PCN allergy is present)	
2. Erythromycin	Erythromycin ethyl succinate, 800 mg, or erythromycin stearate, 1.0 g PO 2 hours before procedure; then half the dose 6 hours after the initial dose
or	
3. Clindamycin	300 mg PO 1 hour before procedure and 150 mg PO 6 hours after initial dose
Alternate regimens	
4. Ampicillin	2.0 g IM or IV 30 minutes before procedure; then ampicillin, 1.0 g IM or IV, or amoxicillin, 1.5 g PO 6 hours after initial dose
or	
5. Clindamycin	300 mg IV 30 minutes before procedure; then 150 mg IV or PO, 6 hours after initial dose
For high-risk patients who are not candidates for standard regimens	
1. Ampicillin, plus	2 g IM or IV 30 minutes before procedure
Gentamicin, plus	1.5 mg/kg (maximum 80 mg) IM or IV 30 minutes before procedure
Amoxicillin	1.5 g PO 6 hours after ampicillin plus gentamicin; alternatively, the parenteral regimen can be repeated 8 hours after the initial dose
or (if PCN allergy is present)	
2. Vancomycin	1 g IV over 1 hour beginning 1 hour before procedure
Lower GI and genitourinary procedures	
Standard regimens	
1. Ampicillin, plus	2 g IM or IV 30 minutes before procedure
Gentamicin, plus	1.5 mg/kg (maximum 80 mg) IM or IV 30 minutes before procedure
Amoxicillin	1.5 g PO 6 hours after ampicillin plus gentamicin
or (if PCN allergy is present)	
2. Vancomycin, plus	1 g IV over 1 hour beginning 1 hour before the procedure
Gentamicin	1.5 mg/kg (maximum 80 mg) IM or IV 1 hour before the procedure; can be repeated once 8 hours after the initial dose
Alternate regimen for low-risk patients	
3. Amoxicillin	3 g PO 1 hour before the procedure and 1.5 g PO 6 hours after the initial dose

Chap. 15). **Diagnostic studies** are not cost-effective in acute illness of mild to moderate severity. Fever, symptoms of dysentery, a prolonged course, or an unusual exposure history should prompt further evaluation. **A detailed history, methylene blue stain** of the stool to look for **fecal leukocytes** suggesting an invasive process, stool examination for **ova and parasites,** and **sigmoidoscopy** to exclude the characteristic pseudomembranes associated with *Clostridium difficile* toxin–induced enterocolitis may be useful. **Stool cultures** may reveal many common

pathogens, but the microbiology laboratory should be notified if specific pathogens are anticipated to ensure optimal processing.

A. **Salmonella infections** may present as enteric fever, septicemia, or enterocolitis. The usual sources of nontyphoidal salmonella are contaminated meat and poultry products.

1. **Salmonella typhi is the classic cause of enteric fever,** but other serotypes may present similarly and are more common in the United States than *S. typhi*. Chloramphenicol, 500 mg IV or PO q4h, remains the drug of choice throughout much of the world. However, resistance to multiple drugs has been a problem with *S. typhi*, particularly among strains acquired in Mexico. A fluoroquinolone or a third-generation cephalosporin for 5 days is the treatment of choice. Ampicillin, 1–2 g IV q6h, and TMP/SMX, 160 mg/800 mg PO q12h, are alternatives. **Carriers** (patients who continue to excrete the organism in the stool for more than 3 months after recovery) are the reservoir of disease. Ampicillin, 2 g PO qid, amoxicillin, 2 g PO tid, TMP/SMX, 160 mg/800 mg PO bid, and ciprofloxacin, 750 mg PO bid, for 4–6 weeks can eliminate the carrier state in patients with normal gallbladder function. Carriers with cholelithiasis often need cholecystectomy to eradicate *S. typhi*.

2. **Septicemia** caused by nontyphoidal salmonella frequently presents as fever without gastroenteritis. Uncomplicated septicemia should be treated (see sec. **VIII.A.1**) for a minimum of 14 days. Treatment of complications (e.g., intravascular infection, osteomyelitis) warrants prolonged antimicrobial therapy. Patients with AIDS may have recurrent, disseminated salmonella infections despite therapy (see Chap. 14, HIV Infection and AIDS, sec. **II.B.1**).

3. **Enterocolitis** is the most common form of salmonellosis. Blood cultures are usually negative. Supportive therapy is adequate in the normal host, although antimicrobials (see sec. **VIII.A.1**) may be useful in compromised hosts, the very young, and the elderly.

B. **Shigella infections.** Bacillary dysentery primarily affects children and is transmitted by the fecal-oral route. The infection is also prevalent in male homosexuals. Diagnosis is generally made by stool culture. The majority of patients with shigellosis recover spontaneously within 1 week and require only supportive therapy. Antimicrobials may hasten recovery in more seriously ill patients. Ciprofloxacin, 500 mg PO bid, or norfloxacin, 400 mg PO bid, is the treatment of choice. TMP/SMX, 160 mg/800 mg PO or IV q12h for 5 days, or ampicillin, 500 mg IV or PO q6h for 5–7 days, is effective for susceptible strains. Amoxicillin is less effective and should not be used. **Antidiarrheal agents should be avoided, if possible,** since they may increase the duration of symptoms and the risk of bacteremia.

C. **Campylobacter enteritis** usually presents as an acute dysenteric illness with spontaneous recovery within 4–5 days. Prolonged infections may be confused with inflammatory bowel disease. The diagnosis is confirmed by a positive stool culture. When treatment is necessary, the drug of choice is erythromycin, 0.5–1.0 g PO qid. Serious infections require 3–4 weeks of therapy to prevent relapse. Tetracycline and the quinolones are also active against *Campylobacter* spp.

D. **Yersinia spp** may cause enterocolitis, mesenteric adenitis, or septicemia. Childhood infection with *Y. enterocolitica* may present as an inflammatory enterocolitis. Infection in older children and adults may mimic acute appendicitis. Isolation of the pathogen requires special techniques and should be discussed with the microbiology laboratory. Enterocolitis and mesenteric adenitis are usually self-limited and require only supportive care. Septicemia is rare.

E. **Enterohemorrhagic E. coli** (serogroup O157 : H7) produces a toxin that causes a unique syndrome characterized by hemorrhagic colitis without fever. The hemolytic-uremic syndrome, or thrombotic thrombocytopenic purpura, may develop following infection. It is transmitted almost exclusively through processed food, particularly inadequately cooked meat. Antimicrobial therapy has not been shown to be of any benefit.

F. **Aeromonas hydrophila, Vibrio parahaemolyticus,** and **Plesiomonas** *shigelloides* have all been associated with self-limited, sporadic, or epidemic diarrhea. Treatment is rarely required.

G. **Traveler's diarrhea** results from ingestion of contaminated water or food in areas of poor hygiene. It is frequently caused by enterotoxigenic *E. coli* and less often by other bacteria and viruses. Treatment begun promptly with the onset of symptoms with TMP/SMX, 160 mg/800 mg PO bid for 3–5 days; ciprofloxacin, 500 mg PO bid for 5 days; or norfloxacin, 400 mg PO bid for 5 days, is effective in decreasing the severity and length of the illness. **Prophylactic antimicrobial therapy** is effective in reducing the incidence of traveler's diarrhea, but the risk of toxicity may outweigh the benefit for most people (*N Engl J Med* 328:1821, 1993).

H. **Pseudomembranous enterocolitis** is caused by a toxin produced by *Clostridium difficile*, an anaerobe that may proliferate when antimicrobials or other factors alter the normal bowel flora. The extended-spectrum PCNs (e.g., ampicillin), cephalosporins, and clindamycin are the most common offenders, but it has been reported with most antimicrobials. Metronidazole, 250 mg PO qid, and vancomycin, 125 mg PO qid for 7–10 days, are equally effective therapies, and both agents are associated with similar relapse rates. Metronidazole is far more economical and is therefore the preferred drug. Bacitracin, 25,000 units PO qid, is also effective. In patients who are unable to take oral medication, parenteral metronidazole may be used. Relapses result from the failure to eliminate the organism from the colon or from exogenous reinfection, and patients typically respond promptly to another course of metronidazole (*N Engl J Med* 330:257, 1994).

I. **Protozoal infections**
   1. *Giardia lamblia* may cause acute or chronic GI symptoms in sporadic cases or epidemics due to the ingestion of contaminated water. Patients with hypogammaglobulinemia and achlorhydria are predisposed to giardiasis. Diagnosis can often be made by stool examination, but duodenal aspiration or small-bowel biopsy may be required. **Treatment** with quinacrine hydrochloride, 100 mg PO tid after meals for 5 days, is effective. Metronidazole, 250 mg tid PO for 5 days, and furazolidone, 100 mg qid PO for 7–10 days, are also effective.
   2. *Entamoeba histolytica* **infection (amebiasis)** is acquired by ingestion of contaminated food or water. Typical symptoms include crampy abdominal pain with dysentery; systemic symptoms are less common and imply more extensive disease. Complications include peritonitis, toxic megacolon, and hepatic abscess formation. Conversion to an asymptomatic carrier state occurs. Asymptomatic carriage can be treated with drugs such as paromomycin, 25 mg/kg/day, or iodoquinol, 650 mg PO tid for 20 days, that act on intraluminal parasites. The **treatment of choice** for intestinal disease and hepatic abscess is metronidazole, 750 mg PO tid for 10 days, followed by an intraluminal agent.
   3. *Cryptosporidium* **spp** and *Isospora belli* are related protozoa that cause acute self-limited diarrhea in normal hosts but may produce severe, chronic, watery, noninflammatory diarrhea in immunocompromised hosts such as those with AIDS. Therapy is usually unnecessary in immunologically competent patients (see Chap. 14, HIV Infection and AIDS, sec. II.F.2).

IX. **Intraabdominal infections**
   A. **Peritonitis**
      1. **Primary or spontaneous bacterial peritonitis** usually occurs in patients with cirrhosis and ascites. *E. coli, Strep. pneumoniae,* and other streptococci and Enterobacteriaceae account for the majority of infections, although anaerobic bacteria and *M. tuberculosis* may occasionally be responsible. Initial therapy with a third-generation cephalosporin with good activity against streptococci is appropriate (e.g., cefotaxime or ceftriaxone).
      2. **Secondary peritonitis.** The causes of secondary peritonitis are numerous, including traumatic or disease-induced perforation of the GI tract and contiguous spread from a visceral infection or abscess. Enterobacteriaceae,

obligate anaerobes, and enterococci are common pathogens, but staphylococci, *M. tuberculosis,* and *N. gonorrhoeae* are also seen. Empiric antimicrobial therapy should include broad-spectrum coverage while awaiting culture results. **For peritonitis from a presumed GI source,** a variety of regimens appear effective. These include (1) ampicillin or mezlocillin, an aminoglycoside, and either clindamycin or metronidazole; and (2) an aminoglycoside plus cefoxitin, clindamycin, or chloramphenicol. Cefoxitin alone may be adequate for community-acquired disease. Imipenem provides effective coverage and is used when more resistant organisms are likely to be present. **Abscess formation is common and requires surgical or percutaneous drainage in most cases.** Peritonitis complicating peritoneal dialysis is discussed in Chap. 11.

 B. **Visceral infections.** There is no evidence that antimicrobial therapy is of benefit in **uncomplicated cholecystitis or pancreatitis,** but broad-spectrum therapy is appropriate if there is evidence of sepsis, secondary peritonitis, or abscess formation (see sec. **IX.A.2**).

X. **Infectious diseases with cutaneous manifestations**

 A. **Erysipelas and cellulitis. Erysipelas** is a superficial, erythematous, edematous, sharply demarcated lesion almost always caused by group A *Streptococcus* (*Strep. pyogenes*). **Cellulitis** is typically more deep-seated with less distinct margins and, in normal hosts, is usually caused by group A *Streptococcus* or *Staph. aureus,* which are indistinguishable on clinical grounds. If staphylococcal disease cannot be excluded, initial therapy with oxacillin or nafcillin, 4.0–8.0 g/day, or cefazolin, 1.0–2.0 g IV q8h, can be used. The treatments of choice for documented streptococcal disease are PCN VK, 0.5–1.0 g PO qid; procaine PCN G, 600,000 units IM bid; or PCN G, 2–6 million units/day IV, depending on the severity of illness. In patients who are allergic to PCN, erythromycin, 500 mg PO qid, or vancomycin, 1 g IV q12h, is an alternative. **Lower extremity cellulitis associated with cutaneous ulcers in diabetic patients** may be polymicrobial in origin. Agents with activity against anaerobes (e.g., metronidazole or clindamycin) may be added when treating cellulitis in this setting. Alternatively, cefoxitin, 1–2 g IV q8h, can be used as single-agent therapy for these patients.

 B. **Petechial, purpuric, and macular skin eruptions** are associated with several important systemic infections.

 1. ***Neisseria meningitidis* septicemia (meningococcemia)** should be considered in any febrile patient with a petechial, purpuric, or macular rash because of its high mortality and potentially rapid course. The diagnosis can frequently be made from Gram's stain of petechial scrapings or a peripheral blood buffy coat specimen. As in meningococcal meningitis, the treatment of choice is PCN G, 2 million units IV q2h.

 2. **Encapsulated bacteria such as *Strep. pneumoniae* and *H. influenzae*** may produce a picture similar to that of meningococcemia in asplenic patients (see sec. **XII.A.2**).

 3. **Rocky Mountain spotted fever** due to *Rickettsia rickettsii* typically begins with fever, chills, headache, and myalgias, with the development of the characteristic macular rash 1–5 days later. With time, the rash may become petechial. The diagnosis should be suspected in patients with a compatible clinical picture and potential tick exposure. The treatment of choice is doxycycline, 100 mg IV or PO q12h. Chloramphenicol, 1.0 g IV or PO q6h, is also effective.

 4. **Other infections** associated with macular, maculopapular, or petechial rashes include typhoid fever (rose spots) (see sec. **VIII.A.1**), endocarditis (see sec. **VII**), disseminated gonorrhea (see Sexually Transmitted Diseases, sec. **II.C.5**), and disseminated candidiasis in the neutropenic host (see Systemic Mycoses, sec. **VI.C**).

 C. **Toxic shock syndrome (TSS)** is due to an exotoxin produced by *Staph. aureus,* though a similar syndrome may be seen with invasive group A streptococcal infections. TSS was first recognized in menstruating women who used tampons, but nonmenstrual TSS may complicate staphylococcal colonization of surgical wounds. The diagnosis is based on the clinical presentation of fever, a diffuse macular erythroderma involving the palms and soles that often desquamates 1–2 weeks after the illness, hypotension, conjunctivitis, vomiting, and diarrhea. **Supportive care is the mainstay of acute therapy.** Antistaphylococcal therapy does not appear to affect the acute illness but may prevent progression of local infection and decrease the rate of relapse. Discontinuation of tampon use may also reduce recurrences.

D. **Lyme disease** is due to infection with the tick-borne spirochete *Borrelia burgdorferi*. The characteristic erythematous annular lesion known as **erythema chronicum migrans** begins as a macular lesion at the site of the tick bite and may be accompanied by fever, fatigue, arthralgias, headache, and neck stiffness. Sequelae are common in untreated patients and include recurrent oligoarticular arthritis, CNS abnormalities (meningitis and cranial and peripheral neuropathies), and cardiac involvement (myopericarditis and heart block). **Treatment** of early Lyme disease with **doxycycline**, 100 mg PO bid for 10–21 days, shortens the duration of symptoms and usually prevents major sequelae. Amoxicillin, 500 mg PO tid, is appropriate for patients in whom doxycycline is contraindicated (pregnant or lactating women and children under 8 years of age). Optimal therapy of established Lyme arthritis and neurologic complications has not been established. Late manifestations of Lyme disease have been successfully treated with high-dose PCN G, 20 million units/day IV. However, ceftriaxone is preferred because of its in vitro activity and ease of administration relative to IV PCN G (*Ann Intern Med* 114:472, 1991).

XI. **Osteomyelitis** should be considered in patients with localized bone pain who are febrile or septic. The **diagnosis** is made by **culturing the pathogen from bone.** An early bone biopsy is essential for management. The radiographic changes of soft-tissue swelling, periosteal elevation, bone lysis, and sclerosis may lag several weeks behind the clinical presentation. Abnormalities on technetium bone scan are often apparent before radiographic changes, and biopsy of suspicious lesions may yield an early diagnosis. Conditions that predispose to osteomyelitis include (1) vascular insufficiency (e.g., diabetes mellitus), (2) soft-tissue infection contiguous with bone (e.g., a decubitus ulcer), (3) bacteremia, (4) hemoglobinopathy, and (5) recurrent UTI. In the absence of vascular insufficiency or a foreign body, acute osteomyelitis can usually be treated successfully with antimicrobial therapy alone. The appropriate antimicrobial agent depends on the results of culture and susceptibility testing. If a causative organism is not identified, antimicrobial therapy should be based on the most likely pathogens. Cure typically requires **at least 6 weeks of therapy** with high dosages of appropriate antimicrobials. Parenteral therapy should be given initially, but oral antimicrobials can be considered after 2–3 weeks provided the causative organism is susceptible and adequate bactericidal levels can be demonstrated.

A. **Acute hematogenous osteomyelitis** is most frequently caused by *Staph. aureus,* and blood cultures are often positive. Vertebral osteomyelitis may be due to *Staph. aureus* or gram-negative bacilli and may be associated with UTI, presumably arising by dissemination via communicating veins.

B. **Osteomyelitis associated with contiguous foci of infection** (e.g., postsurgical infections) may be due to *Staph. aureus* as well as gram-negative bacilli.

C. **Osteomyelitis in the presence of internal fixation devices** cannot usually be eradicated by antimicrobials alone. Cure typically requires the removal of the foreign material.

D. **Osteomyelitis associated with vascular insufficiency** (e.g., in diabetic patients) is seldom cured by drug therapy alone; revascularization, debridement, or amputation is often required.

E. **Osteomyelitis in patients with hemoglobinopathies** is usually caused by *Staph. aureus* but may also be caused by *Salmonella* spp.

F. **Chronic osteomyelitis** is usually associated with the presence of dead and sclerotic bone (i.e., a sequestrum) that serves as a nidus for persistent infection. Eradication requires a combined medical and surgical approach, with excision of the sequestrum. Suppressive antimicrobial therapy can be used if surgery is not feasible.

XII. **Sepsis of unknown origin**

A. **Early bactericidal treatment** is essential in the therapy of septicemia. If a probable source of infection is evident, antimicrobials can be selected to treat the most likely pathogens originating from that site. If no obvious source is uncovered, antimicrobial selection is more empiric and should be based on the clinical situation. Before therapy is initiated, specimens of potentially infected body fluids (e.g., CSF, pleural fluid) should be examined and cultured, and several sets of blood cultures should be obtained from separate venipuncture sites. The broadest coverage is usually provided by a beta-lactam antimicrobial plus an aminoglycoside, such as gentamicin or tobramycin, although amikacin can be used when resistance is suspected.

1. **Community-acquired sepsis with no obvious underlying disease.** A first-generation cephalosporin plus an aminoglycoside will cover most potential pathogens in this setting.

2. **Postsplenectomy patients or those with congenital or functional asplenia** (e.g., sickle cell anemia patients) are at particular risk for fulminant sepsis with encapsulated organisms such as *Strep. pneumoniae, H. influenzae,* and *N. meningitidis.* PCN G, 2 million units IV q2h, plus a third-generation cephalosporin (e.g., ceftriaxone, 2 g IV q12h) should be promptly administered. Gram's stain of a buffy coat specimen can subsequently be performed and will sometimes reveal a probable diagnosis.

3. **Nosocomial septicemia in patients with intravascular catheters** is usually due to *Staph. aureus,* coagulase-negative staphylococci, aerobic gram-negative bacilli, or enterococci. Vancomycin plus an aminoglycoside is appropriate therapy.

4. **Neutropenic or otherwise immunocompromised patients,** in whom *P. aeruginosa* sepsis may be likely, are usually treated with an antipseudomonal beta-lactam antimicrobial plus an aminoglycoside. The addition of an anti-staphylococcal agent such as vancomycin may be warranted in patients with **indwelling central venous catheters.**

B. **Septic shock** is usually caused by bacteremia, although it may complicate fungemia or viremia. Early recognition of bacteremic shock is critical, since delays in instituting therapy increase mortality. Cardiovascular collapse occurs in approximately 40% of gram-negative bacillary bacteremias and has an overall mortality rate of 40% (*Am J Med* 68:344, 1980). Clinically, there may be two stages of bacteremic shock. In the early, hyperdynamic phase (warm shock), the cardiac output is elevated, peripheral vascular resistance is decreased, and the patient is warm, diaphoretic, and peripherally vasodilated. A second hypodynamic phase (cold shock) is manifested by normal or increased peripheral vascular resistance and cool, vasoconstricted skin. Ultimately, decreased cardiac output may occur. Evaluation and treatment should address the underlying infection as well as the manifestations of circulatory compromise.

1. **Stabilization of the cardiovascular system** (see Chap. 9). Crystalloid fluids should be administered initially to achieve normal BP; if this is unsuccessful, vasopressor drugs should be used. The placement of a Swan-Ganz catheter may be useful for hemodynamic monitoring and fluid management. Because of the risk of catheter sepsis, these catheters should be replaced within 72 hours of insertion if they were placed under emergency conditions. Catheters placed under sterile conditions may remain in place for longer periods, if necessary.

2. **Electrolyte and acid-base disturbances** must be corrected, and adequate ventilation must be ensured.

3. **Disseminated intravascular coagulation (DIC).** Laboratory evidence of DIC may occur, but restoration of BP and appropriate antimicrobials are usually adequate to reverse this problem. Other modes of treatment (e.g., heparin, fresh-frozen plasma) are rarely necessary (see Chap. 17).

4. **The underlying infection** should be treated with antimicrobials appropriate to the clinical situation.

5. **There is little evidence that steroids,** even in high dosages and early in the course of infection, significantly **alter the ultimate outcome** (*N Engl J Med* 311:1137, 1984).
6. **Antilipopolysaccharide antibody preparations** have not been shown to reduce mortality (*Ann Intern Med* 121:1, 1994).

Sexually Transmitted Diseases

Sexually transmitted diseases (STDs) may be caused by bacterial, viral, or protozoal pathogens. Common principles should be applied when caring for any patient with a presumed STD. The patient's sexual practices may help identify risk factors for particular infections. The physical examination and microbiologic studies should be directed toward the oropharyngeal, rectal, and urogenital areas.

Because infection with multiple organisms is common, studies for gonorrhea and syphilis should be included when evaluating these patients. In addition, HIV testing and counseling are recommended by the United States Public Health Service (USPHS). When possible, cultures should also be obtained from **sexual contacts,** as treatment of asymptomatic carriers may prevent the spread of infection. Empiric treatment of sexual contacts is indicated in cases of primary and secondary syphilis. **Follow-up cultures or serologic studies** should be obtained after completion of therapy to document cure. An STD apparently refractory to treatment may represent reinfection, a concomitant previously undiagnosed STD, or antimicrobial resistance. Patients with STDs should be reported to the local health department. Most of the following guidelines are based on those from the USPHS (*MMWR* 42[No. RR-14], 1993). The Centers for Disease Control and Prevention (CDC) maintain a hot line to answer specific questions regarding STDs: 1-(800)-227-8922.

I. **Syphilis** may present in primary (chancre), secondary (disseminated), or tertiary forms. Commonly, however, infection is discovered through serologic screening tests in the latent stages (early, within 1 year of infection, or late, 1 or more years following infection). The incubation period for the primary lesion is usually 2–6 weeks. Manifestations of secondary syphilis usually appear 2–12 weeks later and may occur several times during subsequent years. Both primary and moist secondary lesions are infectious. Diagnosis can be made by dark-field microscopy of the primary or moist secondary lesions, or by serologic testing. **All patients with syphilis should be tested for HIV infection.**

A. **Serologic tests** are of major importance in diagnosis but present difficulties in interpretation, because false-positive nontreponemal tests occur in many non-syphilitic conditions.

1. **Nontreponemal tests** (e.g., Venereal Disease Research Laboratory [VDRL] test, rapid plasma reagin [RPR]) are useful for screening. They require a minimum of 1–3 weeks from the onset of infection to turn positive, are usually positive in primary syphilis, and are invariably positive in secondary syphilis. However, they are nonspecific; biologic false-positive tests (usually <1 : 8) occur in IV drug users, in many acute infections (e.g., infectious mononucleosis, mycoplasma infection), in a variety of chronic disorders (e.g., systemic lupus erythematosus) (see Chap. 24), and possibly pregnancy.

2. **Treponemal tests** (e.g., fluorescent treponemal antibody [FTA], microhemag-glutination–*Treponema pallidum* [MHA-TP]) are specific. Their greatest value is in distinguishing false-positive from true-positive reagin tests and in diagnosing late syphilis when blood and CSF reagin tests may be negative.

3. **Serologic response to therapy.** The nontreponemal test titers should decrease by at least two dilutions within 3 months of adequate treatment of primary or secondary disease, and within 6 months following therapy of early latent disease. The CSF titer should also diminish with adequate therapy of neurosyphilis. However, the serum nontreponemal test titer may not change

in patients with late latent syphilis. The FTA test is not useful in monitoring response to therapy because it typically remains positive for life.

B. Treatment

1. **Early syphilis. Benzathine PCN G,** 2.4 million units IM, is the recommended treatment for primary and secondary syphilis, latent syphilis of less than 1 year's duration, and case contacts. PCN-allergic patients can be treated with doxycycline, 100 mg PO bid, for 14 days.

2. **Syphilis exceeding 1 year's duration.** For latent syphilis of more than 1 year's duration, and for cardiovascular syphilis, recommended therapy is benzathine PCN G, 2.4 million units IM weekly for 3 successive weeks. Non-PCN regimens have not been well studied. In patients who are allergic to PCN, doxycycline, 100 mg PO bid for 28 days, can be given when CSF examination has excluded neurosyphilis. The best established regimen for the treatment of **neurosyphilis** is aqueous PCN G, 2–4 million units IV q4h for 10–14 days. Procaine PCN G, 2.4 million units IM qd, plus probenecid, 500 mg PO qd for 10–14 days, is an acceptable alternative when compliance can be ensured. Some experts advocate the administration of benzathine PCN, 2.4 million units IM, following either of these regimens to achieve a duration of therapy comparable to that for other forms of late syphilis. Patients with syphilitic eye disease should also be treated with the neurosyphilis regimen. No non-PCN regimen has been shown to be effective in the treatment of neurosyphilis. Therefore, PCN should be used after desensitization if necessary.

3. **Syphilis during pregnancy** can be managed with one of the preceding PCN regimens. The optimal treatment for PCN-allergic patients is controversial. Doxycycline should be avoided because of its potential adverse effects on both the mother and fetus. PCN skin testing and, if necessary, desensitization are therefore recommended for such patients (see Chap. 12).

4. **Syphilis in HIV-infected patients.** In the majority of patients with HIV infection, serologic tests for syphilis are accurate, although there are reports of false-negative tests and delayed seroconversion. Anecdotal evidence suggests that HIV-infected patients are at increased risk of developing neurosyphilis and have higher treatment failure rates. Current CDC guidelines recommend that primary and secondary syphilis in HIV-infected patients be treated as described above, although some experts advocate more prolonged therapy and a CSF examination prior to treatment for all HIV-infected patients with syphilis, regardless of stage. Careful clinical and serologic follow-up at 1, 2, 3, 6, 9, and 12 months is recommended in either case. All HIV-infected patients with latent syphilis, regardless of duration, should undergo CSF examination. Such patients with normal CSF can be treated with 3 weekly doses of benzathine PCN G.

II. Gonorrhea usually presents as purulent urethritis in men and as urethritis or cervicitis in women after an incubation period of 2–8 days. Humans are the only reservoir. Both sexes, but women in particular, may be asymptomatic carriers.

A. Diagnosis. Gram's stain of a urethral discharge showing gram-negative intracellular diplococci is the best immediate diagnostic aid in men. In women, cervical and urethral smears may be falsely positive due to saprophytic *Neisseria* spp and hence are less specific than smears in symptomatic men. Cultures for *N. gonorrhoeae* should be obtained with noninhibitory swabs (e.g., calcium alginate) of the urethral discharge in men, and of the cervix and rectum of women; **specimens should be plated immediately on warm chocolate agar** (preferably inhibitory media such as the Thayer-Martin medium) and incubated in a carbon dioxide incubator. DNA probes are both sensitive and specific means of diagnosing *N. gonorrhoeae* from urethral and cervical specimens; however, antimicrobial sensitivity data cannot be obtained by this method.

B. Resistance has appeared in increasing numbers of isolates since the mid-1970s. In 1991, 32.4% of isolates of *N. gonorrhoeae* were resistant to PCN or tetracycline (*MMWR* 42[No. SS-3]:29, 1993). Currently, *N. gonorrhoeae* with **plasmid-mediated penicillinase production** accounts for the majority of clinically significant resistant isolates, although **plasmid-mediated high-level tetracycline resistance (TRNG)** also occurs. Other strains may have **chromosomally mediated antimicrobial resistance (CMRNG)** to PCN and other commonly used antimicrobials. Ceftriaxone resistance has not been reported, but resistance to fluoroquinolones has been detected (*MMWR* 43:325, 1994). Ideally, all *N. gonorrhoeae* isolates should be tested for penicillinase production. In addition, all "posttreatment" isolates and isolates from patients with disseminated gonococcal infections (DGIs) or gonococcal ophthalmia should be tested for TRNG and CMRNG.

C. Treatment

1. **Uncomplicated urethral and endocervical gonorrhea.** Several regimens have been shown to be safe and effective for the treatment of *N. gonorrhoeae*. These include **ceftriaxone,** 125 mg IM; **cefixime,** 400 mg PO; **ciprofloxacin,** 500 mg PO; or **ofloxacin,** 400 mg PO. PCN-sensitive isolates can be treated with a single dose of (1) amoxicillin, 3.0 g PO, (2) ampicillin, 3.5 g PO, or (3) procaine PCN G, 4.8 million units IM distributed to two injection sites. Probenecid, 1 g PO, should accompany each of these regimens. Symptoms present after therapy usually represent reinfection rather than treatment failure. Cultures for *N. gonorrhoeae* should be obtained and isolates tested for antimicrobial susceptibility. Because coexistent *Chlamydia trachomatis* occurs in up to 40% of women and 25% of heterosexual men with gonorrhea, regimens that will treat both infections are recommended. All these regimens should be followed by **doxycycline,** 100 mg PO bid for 7 days; **azithromycin,** 1 g PO in a single dose; or, for pregnant patients or those unable to tolerate tetracyclines, **erythromycin,** 500 mg PO qid for 7 days.

2. **Anorectal disease** can be treated with any of the above regimens.

3. **Pharyngitis.** Patients with pharyngitis should be treated with either ceftriaxone or ciprofloxacin.

4. **Acute salpingitis.** Gonococcal and nongonococcal salpingitis are clinically indistinguishable. Although first episodes are usually due to *N. gonorrhoeae* or *C. trachomatis*, subsequent infections often involve other pathogens, including gram-negative bacilli and anaerobes. The treatment of choice is not established. The USPHS currently recommends several potential antimicrobial combinations; however, data to assess the relative efficacy of these combinations are not available.

    a. **Inpatient antimicrobial therapy** is recommended when (1) the diagnosis is unclear, (2) potential surgical emergencies (e.g., appendicitis) cannot be excluded, (3) a pelvic abscess is suspected, or when the patient (4) is pregnant, (5) is severely ill, (6) has HIV infection, (7) is unwilling or unable to follow an outpatient regimen, (8) is a prepubertal child, (9) has not responded to outpatient therapy, or (10) cannot return for follow-up within 72 hours. Treatment should be given IV for at least 4 days, including at least 2 days after fever resolves. This course should be followed by oral therapy for a total of 10–14 days. Suggested regimens include (1) doxycycline, 100 mg IV q12h, plus cefoxitin, 2 g IV q6h, or cefotetan, 2 g IV q12h, followed by doxycycline, 100 mg PO bid; or (2) clindamycin, 900 mg IV q8h, plus gentamicin, 2.0 mg/kg IV followed by 1.5 mg/kg IV q8h, followed by doxycycline, 100 mg PO bid, or clindamycin, 450 mg PO qid.

    b. **Outpatient treatment** can be attempted in reliable patients with none of the indications for hospitalization listed previously. The therapy of choice is ceftriaxone, 250 mg IM, followed by doxycycline, 100 mg PO bid for 14 days.

5. **Disseminated gonococcal infections (DGIs).** Gonococcal bacteremia is often associated with fever, characteristic skin lesions, polyarthralgias, and tenosynovitis. Purulent monoarticular or occasionally polyarticular arthritis may follow and often requires joint aspiration (see Chap. 24). Patients with DGI should receive IV therapy for at least 3 days or until improvement occurs, followed by oral antimicrobials to complete a minimum of 7 days of therapy.

Ceftriaxone, 1 g IV qd for 7 days, is the treatment of choice. For patients who respond rapidly, therapy can be completed with cefixime, 400 mg PO bid, or ciprofloxacin, 500 mg PO bid. Patients with DGI should also be treated for concomitant chlamydial infection with doxycycline, azithromycin, or erythromycin (see sec. **II.C.1**).

6. **Meningitis and endocarditis** may occur in patients with DGI. Therapy with ceftriaxone, 2 g IV q12h, or, for susceptible isolates, with PCN G, at least 10 million units/day, is effective and should be continued for 10–14 days for meningitis and at least 4 weeks for endocarditis.

III. **Nongonococcal urethritis (NGU)** refers to urethral inflammation in men that is not attributable to *N. gonorrhoeae*. It cannot be differentiated from gonorrhea on the basis of symptoms. *C. trachomatis* is responsible for up to 40% of NGU seen in the United States and Western Europe. *Ureaplasma urealyticum* causes 20–40% of cases, with less than 5% due to *Trichomonas vaginalis*. The cause of the remaining cases is unclear. Persistent urethritis in a patient treated for gonorrhea (postgonococcal urethritis) may represent coinfection with these organisms.

A. **Diagnosis.** NGU should be diagnosed if Gram's stain for *N. gonorrhoeae* and subsequent culture are negative in a man with urethritis, or if urethritis persists despite treatment for gonorrhea. A specific chlamydial diagnosis can be made by direct testing of urethral secretions for chlamydia or chlamydial antigens (culture requires special techniques) or a DNA probe for chlamydia. Therapy of NGU is usually initiated on the basis of negative Gram's stain and a compatible history without waiting for a negative *N. gonorrhoeae* culture.

B. **Treatment** of nongonococcal and postgonococcal urethritis is doxycycline, 100 mg PO bid for at least 7 days; erythromycin, 500 mg PO qid for 7 days, is an alternative. Azithromycin, 1 g in a single dose, may be effective as well. Routine treatment of sexual partners of men with NGU is recommended.

IV. **Lymphogranuloma venereum (LGV)** is due to strains of *C. trachomatis* antigenically distinct from those causing NGU. The primary lesion is an often trivial genital ulceration followed 1–2 weeks later by inguinal adenopathy and constitutional symptoms. In women and homosexual males, symptoms in the anal and rectal areas are common. LGV is treated with the same drugs as NGU, but for 21 days. Fluctuant nodes should be aspirated to decrease the chance of spontaneous drainage with scarring.

V. **Chancroid** is due to *Haemophilus ducreyi*. The typical lesion, which is painful, nonindurated, and ulcerative, is often associated with tender inguinal adenopathy. Recommended regimens include (1) azithromycin, 1 g PO in a single dose; (2) ceftriaxone, 250 mg IM as a single dose; and (3) erythromycin base, 500 mg PO qid for 7 days. Amoxicillin, 500 mg, plus clavulanic acid, 125 mg PO tid for 7 days, and ciprofloxacin, 500 mg PO bid for 3 days, are alternatives. As with LGV, aspiration of fluctuant nodes is recommended. HIV-infected patients may not respond as well to the 1- to 3-day regimens.

VI. **Genital herpes simplex infection** (primarily type II) usually presents with painful vesicles or shallow ulcerations (unroofed vesicles) involving the vulva, labia, or cervix in women, or the penis in men. Primary infection (first episode) may be associated with fever and inguinal adenopathy, whereas recurrent disease rarely produces constitutional symptoms. **Acyclovir,** 200 mg PO 5 times/day for 7–10 days, or, for severely ill patients, 5 mg/kg IV q8h, is effective treatment for primary disease. Patients with more than 6 recurrences/year may have a marked decrease in the rate of recurrence when given prophylactic acyclovir, 400 mg PO bid. Prophylaxis should be stopped after 1 year to determine if disease continues to recur frequently. Less frequent recurrences are usually treated symptomatically. Pain can be treated with analgesics and topical anesthetics (e.g., benzocaine spray); sitting in a warm bath to urinate may relieve the severe dysuria frequent in women. Pregnant women with active genital lesions at the time of delivery should deliver by cesarean section to reduce the likelihood of neonatal transmission.

VII. **Vaginitis** presents as a vaginal discharge, often with a musty or foul odor, and associated dysuria, burning, or pruritus. The most common etiologic organisms are

Trichomonas vaginalis and *Candida albicans. Gardnerella* (formerly *Haemophilus*) *vaginalis,* in combination with anaerobic organisms, is responsible for bacterial vaginosis, previously known as nonspecific vaginitis. Trichomoniasis is usually venereally transmitted, but nonvenereal transmission has been described. *Candida* vaginitis and bacterial vaginosis are not venereally transmitted, and therefore treatment of sexual partners is not indicated.

A. **Diagnosis.** Although gross appearance of the discharge may be characteristic, diagnosis requires microscopic verification. Wet-mount examination of a drop of discharge mixed in a few drops of isotonic saline under high-dry magnification should demonstrate pear-shaped, motile *T. vaginalis.* A drop of 10% potassium hydroxide (KOH), added to lyse epithelial cells, may enhance visualization of *Candida* budding yeast forms, with or without *Candida* pseudohyphae. A diagnosis of bacterial vaginosis is usually based on three of the following four criteria: (1) a vaginal discharge; (2) malodor, often intensified after the addition of 10% KOH to a wet-mount slide; (3) clue cells (vaginal epithelial cells with overlying clumps of bacteria); or (4) a vaginal pH more than 4.5.

B. **Therapy**
   1. *Trichomonas vaginalis* **infection** in nonpregnant women is treated with single-dose metronidazole, 2 g PO. Sexual partners should also be treated. Pregnant women may obtain symptomatic relief and are sometimes cured with clotrimazole, 100 mg intravaginally qhs for 7 nights.
   2. *Candida albicans* **vaginitis** responds to local therapy with miconazole or clotrimazole vaginal cream or suppositories, 100 mg intravaginally qhs for 7 days or 200 mg qhs for 3 days. The response may be better with longer regimens or a higher total dose. Nystatin vaginal suppositories, 100,000 units qhs for 14 days, are also effective. In patients who do not respond to topical therapy, ketoconazole, 200 mg PO, or fluconazole, 100 mg PO qd for 5–10 days, may be effective. Severe or refractory disease should prompt evaluation for HIV infection.
   3. **Bacterial vaginosis** is treated with metronidazole, 500 mg PO bid for 7 days. Clindamycin 2% cream, 5 g intravaginally qhs for 5 days, is an alternative for **pregnant women** and those who are unable to tolerate metronidazole.

Mycobacterial Infections

I. **Tuberculosis (TB)** is a systemic disease caused by *M. tuberculosis.* Pulmonary disease is the most frequent clinical presentation. Lymphatic involvement, genito-urinary disease, osteomyelitis, and miliary dissemination may occur, as well as meningitis, peritonitis, and pericarditis. Most cases of active TB in the United States are the result of reactivation rather than primary infection. Patients with an increased likelihood of reactivation include those with medical risk factors such as HIV infection, silicosis, diabetes mellitus, chronic renal insufficiency, malignancy, malnutrition, and other forms of immunosuppression. The prevalence of TB is increased among immigrants from Southeast Asia, the Indian subcontinent, and Central America. Mycobacteria resistant to primary agents are also more common in these patients.

A. **Diagnosis** of TB is established by culturing the organism. Positive fluorochrome or acid-fast smears are presumptive evidence of active TB, although nontuber-culous mycobacteria and some *Nocardia* spp may give positive results with these techniques. Use of radiometric culture systems and species-specific DNA probes to rapidly group organisms can provide valuable information much faster than traditional methods. Drug susceptibility testing should be performed on all initial isolates from patients with TB.

B. **Treatment** of TB does not require hospitalization to initiate therapy but does provide an opportunity for intensive patient education. **Respiratory isolation** for hospitalized patients with pulmonary disease in negative-pressure rooms is essential. **The local health department should be notified of all cases of TB** so that contacts can be identified, compliance with therapy ensured, and follow-up provided.

1. **Chemotherapy.** Antituberculous therapy is based on two principles: (1) At least two drugs to which the organism is susceptible must be used because of the high incidence of primary drug resistance to a single drug, and (2) extended therapy is necessary because of the prolonged generation time of mycobacteria. Compliance with multidrug regimens for prolonged periods is difficult, so directly observed therapy (DOT) should be considered for all patients. The following treatment recommendations follow those of the American Thoracic Society and the CDC (*Am J Respir Crit Care Med* 149:1359, 1994).

   a. **Initial therapy of uncomplicated pulmonary TB (including cavitary disease) should include four drugs** unless the likelihood of drug resistance is very small. Only when the rate of primary resistance to isoniazid (INH) in the community is clearly documented to be less than 4%, the patient has not received prior therapy for TB, has not been exposed to any contacts with drug-resistant TB, and is not from an area where drug-resistant TB is prevalent should initial therapy include only 3 drugs. **INH**, 300 mg, **rifampin** (RIF), 600 mg, **pyrazinamide** (PZA), 1.5–2.0 g, and **ethambutol** (EMB), 15 mg/kg, or **streptomycin**, 15 mg/kg IM, should be administered daily initially. If the isolate proves to be fully susceptible to INH and RIF, EMB (or streptomycin) may be dropped, and INH, RIF, and PZA continued for 8 weeks, followed by 16 weeks of INH and RIF daily. Several effective options also exist for intermittent DOT (*MMWR* 42[No. RR-7]:1, 1993).

   b. **Drug resistance.** Organisms resistant only to INH can be effectively treated with the 6-month regimen consisting of initial therapy with INH, RIF, PZA, and EMB. INH should be discontinued, and the remaining 3 drugs should be continued for the duration of therapy.

      Therapy of multidrug-resistant TB has been less well studied, and consultation with an expert in the therapy of TB should be considered. Therapy should include at least 3 drugs to which the organism is susceptible. Careful documentation of bacteriologic sputum culture conversion is important, and therapy should be continued for at least 12 months, and possibly as long as 24 months after cultures convert to negative. Surgery should be considered for patients in whom the bulk of the disease is resectable.

   c. **Extrapulmonary disease** in adults can be treated in the same manner as pulmonary disease, with 6- to 9-month short-course regimens.

   d. **Pregnant patients** should be treated with INH, RIF, and EMB for 9 months. PZA and streptomycin should be avoided.

2. **Monitoring response to therapy. Patients with pulmonary TB should have weekly sputum smears and cultures for the first 6 weeks after initiation of therapy.** Smears and cultures should then be obtained monthly until negative cultures are documented. Continued symptoms or persistently positive smears or cultures after 3 months of treatment should raise the suspicion of drug resistance or noncompliance and should prompt referral to an expert in the treatment of TB.

3. **Monitoring for adverse reactions.** Patients should have a baseline laboratory evaluation at the initiation of therapy that includes hepatic enzymes, bilirubin, CBC, and serum creatinine. Routine laboratory monitoring for patients with normal baseline values is unnecessary. However, monthly clinical evaluations with specific inquiries about symptoms of drug toxicity should take place. Patients who are taking EMB should be tested for visual acuity and red-green color perception.

4. **Glucocorticoid administration** in TB is controversial. Prednisone, 1 mg/kg PO qd initially, has been used in combination with primary antituberculous drugs for life-threatening complications such as meningitis and pericarditis.

C. **Chemoprophylaxis.** In up to 5% of individuals whose intermediate-strength tuberculin skin test (TST) converts from negative to positive, active disease will develop within 1 year of conversion if left untreated. Adequate prophylaxis will substantially reduce this risk. Criteria for a positive TST are (1) **5-mm induration** for patients with HIV infection or other defect in cell-mediated immunity, contacts of a known case, and patients with chest radiographs typical for TB; (2) **10-mm induration** for immigrants from high-prevalence areas (Asia, Africa, and Latin America), prisoners, the homeless, parenteral drug abusers, nursing home residents, the medically underserved, low-income populations (including high-risk minorities such as African Americans, Hispanics, and Native Americans), and patients with chronic medical illnesses; and (3) **15-mm induration** for individuals who are not in a high-prevalence group (*MMWR* 38:313, 1989). Prophylactic INH, 300 mg PO qd (adult dosage) for 6–12 months, should be administered for (1) persons in whom a TST conversion develops within 2 years of a previously negative TST regardless of their age; (2) persons with a history of untreated TB or chest radiographic evidence of previous infection; (3) all TST reactors younger than 35 years of age, regardless of the duration of the positive skin test; (4) persons with a positive TST, regardless of age, who are at high risk for development of active disease, including patients with AIDS, diabetes mellitus, end-stage renal disease, hematologic or lymphoreticular malignancy, conditions associated with rapid weight loss or chronic malnutrition, silicosis, and patients receiving immunosuppressive therapy; and (5) household members and other close contacts of patients with active disease with a reactive TST. Immunosuppressed persons, including those with HIV infection, should receive 12 months of prophylactic treatment. Close contacts who have a negative TST but who are at high risk for TB should also be treated. Treatment may then be stopped if a repeat TST at 3 months is negative. Untreated contacts with a nonreactive TST should have a repeat TST after 3 months. RIF, 600 mg PO qd for 6 months, may be used as an alternative prophylactic agent in patients who are intolerant of INH.

II. **Nontuberculous mycobacteria (NTM)** have become more frequent causes of disease over the past 15 years (*Clin Infect Dis* 15:1, 1992). The most common presentations are pulmonary infection, lymphadenitis, disseminated disease, and skin and soft-tissue involvement. Many NTM are more resistant to chemotherapy than *M. tuberculosis,* and multiple drug combinations are frequently used. Susceptibility testing should always be obtained to guide treatment.

A. **Pulmonary disease** ranges in severity from self-limited infection to progressive, destructive lung disease. The majority of cases occur in patients with preexisting lung disease. *Mycobacterium avium* complex (MAC) and *M. kansasii* are the most common NTM in this setting, although *M. xenopi* is common in some locations. All may be cultured from the sputum of patients with underlying chronic pulmonary disease, and the distinction between colonization and infection can be difficult. Clinical criteria for the diagnosis of pulmonary disease caused by NTM have therefore been developed (*Am Rev Respir Dis* 142:940, 1990). The optimal treatment for MAC infection remains unclear. Experience with HIV-infected patients suggests that regimens containing clarithromycin or azithromycin, EMB, and RIF may be the most effective (*N Engl J Med* 329:898, 1993). *M. kansasii* is typically susceptible to RIF, EMB, and INH; therapy should be for 18 months. PZA is ineffective against *M. kansasii.*

B. **Lymphadenitis** of the cervical, submandibular, and submaxillary lymph nodes occurs almost exclusively in young children. After an asymptomatic period, involved nodes may suppurate and drain. MAC is the most common NTM isolated, with most of the remaining cases due to *M. scrofulaceum.* Surgical excision prior to suppuration is the most reliable therapy. More than 90% of lymphadenitis at any site in adults is due to *M. tuberculosis.*

C. **Skin and soft-tissue infections** have been reported with virtually all of the NTM, but are most commonly due to *M. marinum, M. fortuitum, M. chelonae,* and *M. ulcerans. M. marinum* is the most common organism when there has been exposure to water. Limited disease may be treated with a single agent such as doxycycline, ciprofloxacin, or TMP/SMX. Disease due to the rapidly growing mycobacteria, *M. fortuitum* and *M. chelonei,* results from inoculation of contaminated material following trauma, injections, and surgery. Dissemination may occur in immunosuppressed individuals. Clarithromycin has become the drug of choice for initial treatment (*Ann Intern Med* 119:482, 1993), but therapy should also be guided by susceptibility data. Surgical debridement may be a useful adjunct to pharmacotherapy.

D. **Disseminated disease** typically occurs in immunosuppressed patients and may be caused by MAC, *M. kansasii,* and *M. fortuitum.* Treatment is as described above.

Actinomycotic Infections

I. **Actinomycosis.** PCN is the drug of choice for actinomycosis. PCN G, 1.5–3.0 million units IV q4h, should be given for at least 6 weeks, followed by 6–12 months of oral PCN VK, 2–4 g/day, to prevent relapse. Tetracycline is an alternative in the PCN-allergic patient. Surgical drainage of localized lesions may be helpful.

II. **Nocardiosis.** Most infections require a prolonged course of therapy. Sulfadiazine or sulfisoxazole, given in amounts sufficient to produce peak serum levels of 120–150 μg/ml (e.g., 2 g PO q6h), is the therapy of choice. IV therapy can be used, but TMP/SMX is currently the only drug available in the United States by this route. Alternatives for patients with sulfonamide sensitivity include minocycline or the combination of ampicillin plus erythromycin. Therapy should be given for a minimum of 6 weeks.

Systemic Mycoses

The major fungal pathogens of North America are *Histoplasma capsulatum, Coccidioides immitis, Blastomyces dermatitidis,* and *Sporothrix schenckii.* The most common opportunistic fungal pathogens are *Cryptococcus neoformans, Candida* spp, *Torulopsis glabrata, Aspergillus* spp, and *Rhizopus* spp. Treatment schedules for most mycoses are based on clinical experience. Therefore, the recommendations that follow are general guidelines.

I. **Cryptococcosis.** Pulmonary cryptococcosis in a normal host is generally a self-limited disease that requires no specific treatment. **Meningeal infection** should always be excluded by a lumbar puncture; CSF should be examined for the presence of organisms (India ink preparation) and for the presence of cryptococcal antigen. Localized disease in an immunocompromised patient or disseminated disease, including meningitis, always requires therapy. The treatment of choice for meningitis in patients without AIDS is amphotericin B, 0.7 mg/kg/day IV, and flucytosine, 37.5 mg/kg PO q6h, for a total duration of 6 weeks in most patients. Flucytosine levels should be monitored to minimize toxicity. Selected patients without underlying disease or immunosuppression can be treated with 4 weeks of therapy if (1) meningitis is diagnosed early and is not complicated by neurologic abnormalities; (2) the pretreatment CSF has greater than 20 leukocytes/mm^3; (3) the pretreatment serum cryptococcal antigen titer is less than 1 : 32; and, (4) after 4 weeks of therapy, a CSF India ink preparation reveals no yeast and the CSF and serum cryptococcal antigen titers are less than 1 : 8 (*N Engl J Med* 317:334, 1987). Pulmonary disease in immunocompromised patients can be treated with the same regimen. Fluconazole, 200–400 mg PO qd, is effective against *Cryptococcus neoformans,* but its role in patients without AIDS has not been evaluated.

II. **Blastomycosis** causes both acute and chronic pulmonary infections and may disseminate to the skin, bone, genitourinary tract, and uncommonly, to the CNS. Although some acute pulmonary infections remit without therapy, progressive blastomycosis develops in most patients in whom the diagnosis is made. Therefore, treatment is indicated. Amphotericin B, 0.3–0.6 mg/kg/day (1.5–2.5 g total dose), should be given to patients with life-threatening disease or CNS involvement, and to patients who are immunocompromised. Itraconazole, 200–400 mg PO qd for a minimum of 6 months, has become the treatment of choice for non–life-threatening, nonmeningeal disease.

III. **Histoplasmosis.** Infection with *Histoplasma capsulatum* is asymptomatic in the vast majority of individuals. Symptomatic infections are unusual and are typically self-limited. A subset of patients, however, will develop chronic, progressive pulmonary histoplasmosis or occasionally disseminated infection. Treatment is indicated for chronic fibronodular and cavitary pulmonary disease, disseminated disease, and infection in immunocompromised hosts. The treatment of choice for moderately severe to severe disease and for immunocompromised hosts is amphotericin B, usually with a 1.5–2.5 g total dose. Itraconazole, 200 mg PO tid for 3 days, then 200–400 mg daily for 6–12 months, is effective therapy in mild disease in nonimmunocompromised patients (*Clin Infect Dis* 19[Suppl 1]:S19, 1994).

IV. **Coccidioidomycosis.** The majority of primary infections with *Coccidioides immitis* resolve without specific treatment. Black, Asian, pregnant, debilitated, and immunocompromised patients are at increased risk for dissemination, as are those with severe primary infections (e.g., complement fixation titers >1:32, progressive pulmonary disease, persistent symptoms >6 weeks in duration, negative skin test, or persisting serum precipitins). Patients with severe or rapidly progressive disease or disseminated disease should be treated with amphotericin B, with a total dose of 1–3 g depending on the clinical response. A lumbar puncture should always be performed to rule out meningeal involvement. The role of the azole antifungal agents itraconazole and fluconazole in coccidioidomycosis is under study. Disease of mild to moderate severity has been successfully treated with fluconazole, 400 mg PO qd initially. Higher doses of fluconazole are being studied for the treatment of meningitis (*Clin Infect Dis* 16:349, 1993).

V. **Invasive aspergillosis** usually presents with pulmonary infiltrates, sinusitis, or skin nodules in granulocytopenic or otherwise severely immunocompromised patients. Treatment of this life-threatening infection requires amphotericin B, 1 mg/kg/day, with a 2.0–2.5 g total dose. Itraconazole has activity against aspergillus, but its role in therapy has not been established.

VI. *Candida* **spp and** *T. glabrata.* Oropharyngeal candidiasis occurs in both normal and immunocompromised hosts, including patients using oral contraceptives or being treated with inhaled or systemic steroids, antimicrobials, or chemotherapeutic agents, and patients with AIDS. Systemic infections with these organisms are occurring with increased frequency. They usually occur in immunocompromised patients, patients receiving broad-spectrum antimicrobials or parenteral hyperalimentation, postoperative patients, and patients with indwelling central venous access.

A. **Oral and esophageal candidiasis. Oral disease** can be treated with nystatin or clotrimazole (e.g., clotrimazole troches, 10 mg dissolved slowly in the mouth 5 times/day). Esophageal disease responds to ketoconazole, 200–400 mg PO qd; fluconazole, 100–200 mg PO or IV qd; or low-dose amphotericin B, 10–20 mg IV qd for 7–14 days.

B. **Catheter-related fungemia** with these organisms is a common nosocomial infection. Serious complications, including endophthalmitis, osteomyelitis, and other visceral involvement may develop, and the mortality of untreated fungemia is high. Treatment is therefore recommended for all patients, even though some infections may clear spontaneously with removal of the catheter and modification of other risk factors. In nonimmunocompromised patients without evidence of dissemination, a brief course of 200 mg amphotericin B may be adequate provided that fungemia resolves promptly with removal of the catheter. Other patients should receive therapy for disseminated disease.

C. **Disseminated disease** is treated with amphotericin B, 0.5 mg/kg/day, with a 0.5–1.5 g total dose. Fluconazole, 200–400 mg IV or PO, is an alternative for nonneutropenic patients who are unable to tolerate amphotericin B, although non-*albicans* species of *Candida* tend to be less susceptible to azoles.

VII. Sporotrichosis. Lymphocutaneous or cutaneous sporotrichosis may be treated with a saturated solution of potassium iodide (SSKI), although it is often poorly tolerated. Extracutaneous disease should not be treated with SSKI. SSKI is begun at 5 drops tid in milk or juice and is increased slowly until a maximum of 40 drops tid is attained or drug intolerance develops. Treatment should be continued for 1–2 months after all lesions have cleared. Toxicities include increased lacrimation and salivation, an unpleasant taste, gastric irritation, and diarrhea. Itraconazole is effective and better tolerated than SSKI for the treatment of cutaneous and lymphocutaneous disease. It is administered at a dose of 200 mg PO qd for 3–6 months. Extracutaneous disease other than meningitis can be treated with itraconazole, 200 mg PO bid, for up to 1–2 years. Severely ill patients and those with meningeal disease should be treated with amphotericin B, with a 1.5- to 2.5-g total dose.

Malaria

Malaria is caused by protozoa of the genus *Plasmodium*. It is endemic to most of the tropical and subtropical world. Malaria begins as a nonspecific illness characterized by fever and chills, headache, myalgias, arthralgia, nausea, vomiting, or diarrhea. Left untreated, the illness may result in severe anemia, thrombocytopenia, pulmonary edema, hypoglycemia, encephalopathy, and death. Most cases of malaria in travelers would be preventable with better pretravel advice and appropriate chemoprophylaxis (*N Engl J Med* 329:31, 1993). Malaria should be suspected when illness occurs in a patient who has recently visited an endemic area. **Diagnosis** is made by identification of the parasites in a blood smear stained with Giemsa stain. Current information on the incidence of resistance in various regions of the world, prophylaxis, and treatment issues can be obtained from the CDC: (404) 332-4555.

I. Prevention. The risk of infection depends on the traveler's destination, route and mode of travel, season, and planned activities. No chemoprophylaxis regimen is 100% effective, so mosquito avoidance measures are important. Such measures include wearing long-sleeved shirts and trousers, using mosquito repellents containing diethyltoluamide (DEET), sleeping in protected quarters, and using insecticide-impregnated mosquito netting. **Chemoprophylaxis** for travelers to areas of the world where chloroquine-resistant *Plasmodium falciparum* is not present should consist of chloroquine, 300 mg base (or 500 mg salt) PO once/week, beginning 2 weeks before departure, and continuing for 4 weeks after leaving the malarious area. Mefloquine, 250 mg PO once/week is the drug of choice for prevention of chloroquine-resistant *P. falciparum* malaria. Mefloquine resistance has been reported in areas of Thailand and Cambodia, however. Doxycycline, 100 mg PO qd, is an effective alternative for travel to these areas and for patients who are unable to take mefloquine (pregnant women; patients with a history of seizures, psychiatric disorders, or cardiac conduction abnormalities; patients taking beta-adrenergic antagonists or quinidine; or patients whose activities require fine-motor coordination). Prophylaxis with primaquine phosphate, 26.3 mg salt PO qd for 14 days, is recommended to prevent relapses for individuals with significant exposure to *P. vivax* and *P. ovale*, as these protozoa have an extra erythrocytic stage. Normal glucose-6-phosphate dehydrogenase (G6PD) levels should be documented prior to administration of primaquine.

II. Treatment

   A. *Plasmodium falciparum* malaria, the most severe form of the disease, is a potential medical emergency. Chloroquine resistance is widespread. To date the only areas of the world where there has been no documented chloroquine resistance are Central America west of the Panama Canal, Haiti, the Dominican Republic, Egypt, and most countries in the Middle East. Sulfadoxine and pyrimethamine (Fansidar) resistance occurs in Southeast Asia and the Amazon (CDC, *Health Information for International Travel*, 1994). **Chloroquine resis-**

tance should be presumed in patients in whom *P. falciparum* malaria develops
unless a careful history reveals travel only to areas where resistance does not
occur. Chloroquine resistance should also be presumed in patients with
severe infections (i.e., parasitemia >5% or mental status changes) and those
in whom malaria develops despite chloroquine prophylaxis.

1. *Plasmodium falciparum* malaria, which is presumed to be **chloroquine
   resistant,** should be treated with two drugs: quinine sulfate, 650 mg PO tid
   for 3 days, and doxycycline, 100 mg PO bid for 7 days. Fansidar, 3 tablets PO
   as a single dose, can be substituted for tetracycline, unless the patient
   acquired the disease in an area with Fansidar resistance. Patients who
   acquire *P. falciparum* in Thailand or surrounding countries should receive a
   7-day course of quinine and doxycycline. **Severe *P. falciparum* infection
   requires parenteral therapy** with quinidine gluconate, 10 mg/kg IV over 1–2
   hours, followed by 0.02 mg/kg/minute as a continuous infusion (*N Engl J Med*
   321:65, 1989) and doxycycline, 100 mg IV q12h or 100 mg PO bid. Patients
   who require IV quinidine should be monitored for hypotension and arrhythmias in an intensive care setting (see Chap. 7). When the level of parasitemia
   falls to less than 1% and the patient is able to take oral medication, quinine
   sulfate can be substituted to complete a total of 3 days of quinidine/quinine.
   Doxycycline should be given orally to complete a 7-day course of therapy. For
   parasitemias greater than 10%, exchange transfusion should be considered.

2. *Plasmodium falciparum* malaria acquired in areas where chloroquine resistance does not occur can be treated with **chloroquine base,** 600 mg (1,000 mg
   chloroquine phosphate) PO, followed in 6 hours by 300 mg PO and an
   additional 300 mg PO qd for 2 days. Severe infections should be treated as in
   sec. **II.A.1**.

B. **Nonfalciparum malaria** is less severe and usually responds to oral chloroquine
   (see sec. **II.A.2**). Patients with *P. vivax* or *P. ovale* infection may relapse several
   months after their initial illness because of the persistence of dormant forms
   (hypnozoites) in the liver. Therefore, after screening for G6PD deficiency,
   patients should also be treated with primaquine, 26.3 mg salt (15 mg of base) PO
   qd for 14 days. Relapses should be treated with chloroquine and primaquine.

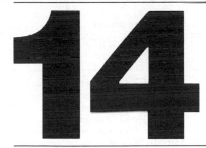

The Immunocompromised Host

William Powderly and
Thomas Bailey

Human Immunodeficiency Virus Infection and AIDS

Human immunodeficiency virus–type 1 (HIV-1) is a human retrovirus that infects lymphocytes and other cells bearing the CD4 surface marker. Infection leads to lymphopenia, CD4 lymphocyte deficiency and dysfunction, impaired cell-mediated immune response, and polyclonal B-cell activation with impaired B-cell response to new antigens. This immune derangement gives rise to **AIDS,** which is characterized by opportunistic infections and unusual malignancies. The time from infection with HIV to the onset of AIDS ranges from months to many years, with a median incubation period of about 10 years in adults. The virus is transmitted primarily by sexual and parenteral routes. **Major risk groups** therefore include sexual contacts of infected persons (in the United States, 50% of patients with AIDS are male homosexuals), IV drug users, recipients of infected blood products, and children born to HIV-infected mothers; however, infection is becoming more prevalent outside these traditional risk groups, and AIDS is now the leading cause of death for men between 25 and 44 years of age in the United States. Treatment of AIDS includes specific antiretroviral therapy and treatment of infectious and neoplastic complications.

I. **Management of the HIV-positive patient.** Patients with HIV infection may present acutely near the time of seroconversion, at a late stage with an AIDS-defining complication, or at any time in between. Initial assessment of patients should be targeted at the determination of the degree of immunodeficiency, with particular attention to the need for initiation of antiretroviral therapy and prophylactic therapy against opportunistic pathogens.

   A. **Primary HIV infection.** Initial infection with HIV-1 is usually asymptomatic but may be associated with a mononucleosis-like syndrome; treatment is supportive. Primary HIV infection is also associated with aseptic meningitis, spinal vacuolar myelopathy, peripheral neuropathy, and subacute encephalitis.

   B. **Initial assessment.** Most patients are asymptomatic initially. Some may develop recurrent oral candidiasis, lymphadenopathy, weight loss, fevers, night sweats, and chronic diarrhea (**AIDS-related complex [ARC]**). History and physical examination should focus on such complications. Abnormal laboratory findings may include anemia, thrombocytopenia, and leukopenia. The most important initial laboratory test is measurement of the CD4 (T4) lymphocyte count. The normal range for adults is 600–1,500 cells/mm^3. Counts less than 500 cells/mm^3 usually indicate HIV-associated immunodeficiency. The recommended frequency of measurement of the CD4 count in HIV-positive patients is shown in Table 14-1.

   C. **Antiretroviral therapy.** All available agents act by inhibition of the viral enzyme reverse transcriptase, with consequent interference with viral replication. However, inhibition of replication is incomplete, and emergence of resistance is almost inevitable. The rate of appearance of resistant strains of HIV-1 correlates with the degree of immunodeficiency and is much greater in patients with advanced disease.

      1. **Zidovudine (ZDV; azidothymidine, AZT)**

         a. **Indications.** ZDV is indicated for therapy of **symptomatic** HIV infection in patients with CD4 lymphocyte counts less than 500 cells/mm^3, for patients

Table 14-1. Immunologic monitoring of the HIV-positive patient

CD4 lymphocyte count (cells/mm³)	Recommendation
>600	Repeat CD4 count every 6 mos
500–600	Repeat CD4 count every 3 mos
<500	Repeat CD4 count in 1 week: if <500, consider ZDV therapy
300–500	Repeat CD4 count every 6 mos
	Initiate ZDV therapy in symptomatic patients; consider ZDV therapy in asymptomatic patients
200–300	Repeat CD4 count every 2–3 mos
<200 or <14% of total lymphocytes	Institute PCP prophylaxis
	Initiate ZDV therapy in all patients if not previously instituted
<100	Consider rifabutin for MAC prophylaxis

ZDV = zidovudine; PCP = *Pneumocystis carinii* pneumonia; MAC = *Mycobacterium avium* complex.

with AIDS, and for all HIV-infected persons with CD4 counts less than 200 cells/mm³ (see Table 14-1). In general, patients can expect improvement in symptoms and stabilization of the CD4 count. The duration of response varies with the stage of disease and is shorter in patients with advanced disease. **Asymptomatic** patients with CD4 counts between 200 and 500 cells/mm³ may experience a slowing of progression of their disease or a delay in the onset of disease, but a survival benefit has not been demonstrated. ZDV therapy in such patients should be initiated only after a careful discussion between the physician and patient of its benefits and risks.

   b. Administration. The recommended dosage of ZDV is 100 mg PO 5 times daily, although dosages of 200 mg q8h are widely used. ZDV, 100 mg q8h, has also been shown to have antiviral activity, but the long-term clinical efficacy of this dosage remains unproved (*N Engl J Med* 323:1009, 1990).

   c. Adverse effects. Nausea, myalgias, insomnia, and severe headaches are common side effects but are usually temporary. A mild macrocytic anemia is common. More severe marrow hypoplasia with anemia or neutropenia can also occur, especially in patients with advanced HIV disease. The anemia may respond to erythropoietin in patients with low levels of endogenous erythropoietin. In patients with recurrent bone marrow suppression, lower dosages of ZDV (100 mg PO q8h) may be effective and less toxic. Proximal myopathy with muscle wasting or myositis may occur with long-term (>1 year) use of ZDV. A rare syndrome of hepatic failure, preceded by hepatic steatosis, has been described with long-term ZDV use.

  2. Dideoxyinosine (ddI) is a nucleoside analog indicated for treatment of AIDS and symptomatic HIV infection in patients who cannot tolerate or are deteriorating on ZDV, and for patients with CD4 counts less than 300 cells/mm³ who have received more than 4 months of ZDV therapy. The dosage is 200 mg PO bid (125 mg PO bid for individuals weighing <60 kg). The most important side effect is pancreatitis, and the drug should not be used in patients with a previous history of pancreatic disease. Other side effects include peripheral neuropathy and GI intolerance. This drug appears to be minimally toxic to bone marrow.

  3. Dideoxycytidine (ddC; zalcitabine) is a nucleoside analog indicated for treatment of advanced HIV disease in patients who cannot tolerate or are deteriorating on ZDV. The recommended dosage is 0.75 mg PO tid. A distal sensory peripheral neuropathy, characterized by paresthesias and pain, is the most important dose-limiting toxicity; it occurs in up to 25% of patients. The neuropathy is reversible if the drug is discontinued; some patients may tolerate a lower dose (0.375 mg PO tid).

4. **Use of antiretroviral agents.** Most available evidence suggests that ZDV should be the initial choice among the available nucleoside agents. Many patients experience nausea and headache during initiation of ZDV therapy, and it is important to counsel patients that these effects are temporary. The duration of benefit with ZDV is variable, and the decision to initiate alternative therapies needs to be based on the individual patient's clinical and immunologic response. When a decision to change is made, many physicians combine ddI or ddC with ZDV rather than initiate monotherapy with an alternate agent. However, **no clinical trials have yet demonstrated the superiority of combination nucleoside therapy in advanced HIV disease.** Patients with very advanced disease may have exhausted all available options and may have experienced deterioration despite several years of nucleoside treatment. In such patients, the toxicities of the drugs may outweigh any clinical benefit, and consideration should be given to discontinuing all antiretroviral therapy with continuation of agents only to prevent opportunistic infections.

D. **Prophylactic measures.** Because **tuberculosis** (TB) is an important complication of HIV infection, screening by skin testing should be performed at the time of initial assessment. However, patients are often anergic, and in such patients, chest radiography should be performed. Prophylaxis is indicated in patients whose chest radiographs are consistent with healed TB, patients with a prior positive purified protein derivative (PPD) skin test, or populations where the prevalence of TB infection is estimated to be more than 10%. Immunizations such as annual influenza vaccine, pneumococcal vaccine, and hepatitis B vaccine (in hepatitis B–seronegative patients) may also be offered. Prophylaxis against *Pneumocystis carinii* pneumonia (PCP) (see sec. **II.E**) is indicated when the CD4 count is less than 200 cells/mm^3, or when the percentage of CD4 lymphocytes is less than 14% of the total lymphocyte count. Prophylaxis for *Mycobacterium avium* infection and *Toxoplasma gondii* (in seropositive patients) should be considered when the CD4 count is less than 100 cells/mm^3.

II. **Treatment of HIV-associated opportunistic infections**
   A. **Viral infections**
      1. **Cytomegalovirus (CMV) infection** is common in patients with AIDS. Manifestations include viremia with fever and constitutional symptoms, chorioretinitis, esophagitis, gastritis, enterocolitis, pancreatitis, acalculous cholecystitis, bone marrow suppression, necrotizing adrenalitis, and lower respiratory tract infections. Therapies include **ganciclovir (DHPG)**, 5 mg/kg q12h IV for 14 days, or **foscarnet**, 60 mg/kg q8h IV for 14–21 days. Relapse after discontinuation of the drug is common, necessitating maintenance therapy with DHPG, 5 mg/kg/day, or foscarnet, 90–120 mg/kg/day. Both agents are associated with significant toxicity. The major side effect of DHPG is **myelosuppression.** It is **usually necessary to discontinue ZDV when systemic DHPG is given.** Concomitant granulocyte macrophage colony-stimulating factor (**GM-CSF**) can be used as a means of ameliorating DHPG myelotoxicity (see Chap. 18). Foscarnet is associated with significant **nephrotoxicity,** and 250–500 ml of isotonic saline should be administered prior to foscarnet infusion. Significant metabolic abnormalities, notably **hypocalcemia,** occur with foscarnet infusion, and the use of an infusion pump is recommended. Foscarnet has been shown to be as effective as DHPG in treating CMV retinitis and may be associated with a longer overall survival, possibly related to its antiretroviral activity (*N Engl J Med* 326:213, 1992). The optimum therapy for other invasive CMV syndromes has not been established.
      2. **Other Herpesviridae. Herpes simplex virus (HSV)** infection has been associated with esophagitis, proctitis, pulmonary disease, and large, atypical,

persistent, cutaneous ulcerations. **Acyclovir,** 400 mg PO 3 times daily or 5 mg/kg IV q8h, is usually effective, but relapses are frequent. **Foscarnet** should be used for acyclovir-resistant HSV. **Varicella zoster virus** may cause typical dermatomal lesions or may be disseminated. Recurrent disease, meningoencephalitis, and cranial neuritis have been reported. Acyclovir, 10 mg/kg q8h IV, is the treatment of choice for serious infections. Evidence of Epstein-Barr virus infection is common in patients with AIDS, particularly hairy leukoplakia. Oral acyclovir may be effective, but should be reserved for symptomatic cases.

3. **JC virus** is a papovavirus associated with **progressive multifocal leukoencephalopathy,** which is characterized by altered mental status, visual loss, weakness, and abnormalities of gait. Nonenhancing, hypodense lesions are seen on CT of the head, but MRI is probably more sensitive. No effective therapy has been identified.

B. **Bacterial infections** are common in patients with AIDS and often recur or follow an atypical or aggressive course despite adequate therapy. Therapy must be individualized but, in general, intense initial therapy followed by prolonged suppression is often necessary.

1. **Nontyphoidal salmonellae** (especially *S. typhimurium*) are associated with invasive disease that often recurs or persists despite appropriate antimicrobials. Initial IV therapy with ampicillin, ceftriaxone, or trimethoprim and sulfamethoxazole (TMP/SMX) should be followed by long-term oral suppressive therapy based on susceptibility testing (e.g., amoxicillin, 500 mg PO tid). However, relapse may occur as soon as IV therapy is discontinued.

2. **Syphilis.** The natural history of syphilis may be altered by HIV infection. Reactivation of previously treated disease, active disease with negative serology, asymptomatic neurosyphilis, and relapse after standard therapy have all been reported. The optimal management of syphilis in this setting remains unclear. Lumbar puncture of seropositive patients, IV penicillin G (see Chap. 13) for suspected infections, and long-term maintenance therapy are all potentially necessary measures.

3. **Bacterial pneumonias** occur with increased frequency and are usually due to *Streptococcus pneumoniae, Haemophilus influenzae,* or group B *Streptococcus.* Recurrent bacterial pneumonias are now included in the Centers for Disease Control case definition of AIDS. Pneumonia due to gram-negative enteric organisms occurs in advanced HIV disease. Chest radiographs may reveal typical lobar pneumonia, but diffuse interstitial infiltrates similar to those in PCP have been reported. These infections usually respond to specific antimicrobial therapy, but relapses are common (see Chap. 13).

C. **Mycobacterial infections**

1. *Mycobacterium tuberculosis.* **TB** occurs with increased frequency in patients with AIDS, particularly among IV drug users. Both primary and reactivation infection occur. The pattern of disease observed may vary according to the stage of HIV illness. Apical cavitary disease is rare in patients with advanced HIV disease but is commonly seen in patients with early HIV infection. TB in patients with advanced HIV disease more commonly resembles a progressive primary infection, with localized or diffuse pulmonary infiltrates, hilar adenopathy, and a high likelihood of extrapulmonary dissemination. Sputum smears are often negative, so that delayed diagnosis is common. Antituberculous therapy should be initiated whenever acid-fast bacilli are discovered in any specimen from a patient with AIDS. The American Thoracic Society recommends standard isoniazid (INH) and rifampin (RIF) therapy plus ethambutol (EMB) and pyrazinamide (PZA) for the first 2 months of treatment pending the results of susceptibility testing, which should be obtained in all cases (see Chap. 13). Treatment should be continued for a total of 6 months and for at least 3 months after the last positive culture. If INH resistance or intolerance is documented, INH can be discontinued and PZA continued for the entire 6-month duration of therapy. Clinical and bacteriologic response should be closely monitored. Prophylaxis with INH for 12

months should be considered in any HIV-positive patient with a reactive (5-mm induration) PPD skin test (see Chap. 13).

Several outbreaks of TB have been described in which the isolate of *M. tuberculosis* is resistant to both INH and RIF (multidrug-resistant [MDR] TB). The prevalence of MDR-TB is particularly high in the urban areas of the northeastern United States. The possibility of MDR-TB should be considered in individuals from an endemic area, particularly those who are homeless or who have a history of substance abuse, and in individuals with a history of irregular or incomplete prior therapy for TB. The possibility of resistant TB should also be considered in patients whose disease progresses despite adequate therapy, smear remains positive after 2 months of treatment, or culture remains positive after 4 months. Resistant TB in AIDS is associated with a high mortality rate. Therapy should include at least three drugs (to which the organism is sensitive) that have not been used previously.

2. *M. avium* **complex (MAC)** infection is one of the most frequent opportunistic problems in patients with AIDS. Generalized infection with fever of unknown origin, weight loss, and GI disease are the most common manifestations. The new macrolide antimicrobial, clarithromycin 500–1,000 mg PO bid, in combination with EMB, 15 mg/kg/day PO, is the best available therapy. Rifabutin, 300 mg/day, prevents MAC bacteremia in patients with CD4 lymphocyte counts less than 100 cells/mm^3.

D. **Fungal infections**
   1. **Candidiasis**. Persistent oral, esophageal, and vaginal infections are common, but disseminated infections are rare in the absence of other risk factors such as IV catheters. The severity and frequency of mucocutaneous candidiasis increase with declining immune function. Several therapeutic options, both local and systemic, are available for oral candidiasis and are equally efficacious. **Fluconazole**, 200 mg PO qd for 14–28 days, is the therapy of choice for esophageal infection, but fluconazole-resistant candidiasis is increasingly recognized as a complication of advanced HIV infection. **Itraconazole** is occasionally effective but many patients require IV **amphotericin B** therapy (see Chap. 12).
   2. *Cryptococcus neoformans* is the most common cause of fungal CNS disease in patients with AIDS. Patients usually present with headache and fever and may have mental status changes. Symptoms may be mild, so the **threshold for performing a lumbar puncture should be low.** Initial treatment is with amphotericin B, 0.7 mg/kg/day, and flucytosine, 25 mg/kg PO q6h for 2–3 weeks, followed by fluconazole, 400 mg PO qd for 8–10 weeks. Following acute treatment, lifelong maintenance therapy is required with fluconazole, 200 mg PO qd. Response is usually monitored clinically and is usually slow. Repeat lumbar puncture is indicated for clinical deterioration. In addition to routine CSF chemistries, cell count, and cryptococcal antigen and culture, the **CSF opening pressure should always be measured** to assess the possibility of intracranial hypertension as a potential complication.
   3. *Histoplasma capsulatum* is an important pathogen in AIDS patients from endemic areas and may cause disseminated disease and septicemia. Patients typically present with fever of unknown origin, hepatosplenomegaly, and weight loss. Pancytopenia may result from bone marrow involvement. Amphotericin B, 0.5–1.0 g total dose IV, should be used as initial therapy. Maintenance therapy with daily itraconazole, 400 mg PO qd, should be given routinely.
   4. *Coccidioides immitis* also occurs in AIDS patients from endemic areas. Extensive pulmonary disease with extrapulmonary spread is common. Amphotericin B therapy is appropriate, and, as with histoplasmosis, lifetime maintenance therapy with either itraconazole or fluconazole is indicated. Coccidioidal meningitis requires intracisternal or intraventricular therapy with amphotericin B. Fluconazole, 400 mg qd, is a promising agent for the treatment of coccidioidal meningitis and may alleviate the need for intraventricular therapy.

Table 14-2. Treatment of *Pneumocystis carinii* pneumonia

Mild disease (A-a gradient <35 at $F_{1}O_2$ = 21%)

1. TMP/SMX	2 double-strength tablets PO tid for 21 days[a]

Alternatives (if patient does not tolerate TMP/SMX)

2. Atovaquone	750 mg PO tid for 21 days
3. Dapsone	100 mg PO for 21 days
plus Trimethoprim	300 mg PO q8h for 21 days
4. Clindamycin	600 mg PO q8h for 21 days
plus Primaquine	30 mg PO qd for 21 days

Moderate to severe disease (A-a gradient >35 at $F_{1}O_2$ = 21%)

1. TMP/SMX	5 mg TMP and 25 mg SMX/kg IV q8h for 21 days[b]

Alternatives (if patient does not tolerate TMP/SMX)

2. Pentamidine	4 mg/kg IV over 2 hrs qd for 21 days
3. Trimetrexate	45 mg/m² IV qd for 21 days
plus Leucovorin	20 mg/m² IV or PO q6h for 21 days

Glucocorticoid therapy (well-documented PCP and PaO_2 <75 mm Hg at $F_{1}O_2$ = 21%)

1. Prednisone[c]	40 mg PO bid for 5 days followed by 40 mg PO qd for 5 days followed by 20 mg PO qd for duration of anti-PCP therapy

$F_{1}O_2$ = fraction of inspired oxygen; TMP/SMX = trimethoprim/sulfamethoxazole; PCP = *Pneumocystis carinii* pneumonia; PaO_2 = arterial oxygen pressure.
[a]Serum levels of SMX or TMP should be measured to document absorption.
[b]Peak serum levels of 100–150 µg/ml SMX may be required.
[c]Equivalent dose of methylprednisolone may be used IV if necessary.

   E. *Pneumocystis carinii* **pneumonia (PCP)** remains the most common opportunistic infection in patients with AIDS and a leading cause of mortality. Extrapulmonary disease has also been described, almost always in patients receiving aerosolized pentamidine for prophylaxis.
   1. The treatment of choice for PCP is TMP/SMX (Table 14-2). If oral therapy is used, serum levels of SMX or TMP should be measured to document adequate GI absorption. Peak serum levels of 100–150 µg/ml of SMX may be necessary for therapeutic efficacy. Rashes are common in patients with AIDS who are treated with TMP/SMX, but do not usually require a change in therapy (*Ann Intern Med* 109:280, 1988) and can be managed with antihistamines and nonsteroidal antiinflammatory drugs. Alternatives for patients with moderate to severe PCP who cannot tolerate TMP/SMX or fail to respond during the first 5–7 days of TMP/SMX therapy include **pentamidine** or **trimetrexate** (see Table 14-2). Alternatives for mild disease in patients who cannot tolerate TMP/SMX include **atovaquone, dapsone plus TMP,** or **clindamycin plus primaquine** (see Table 14-2). In patients with well-documented PCP and moderate to severe disease, prevention of respiratory failure and a survival benefit have been demonstrated with **adjunctive administration of glucocorticoids** (*N Engl J Med* 323:1451, 1990) (see Table 14-2).
   2. Prophylactic therapy is indicated for patients who recover from PCP and for HIV-infected patients with CD4 lymphocyte counts less than 200 cells/mm³, or whose CD4 lymphocyte percentage is less than 14% of the total lymphocyte count. Prophylaxis should also be considered in patients with higher CD4 counts who have symptomatic HIV disease (e.g., oral candidiasis, unexplained fevers, or weight loss). **TMP/SMX,** 160 mg/800 mg (1 double-strength tablet) PO qd, is the preferred prophylactic regimen. **Dapsone,** 100 mg PO daily, or **pentamidine,** 300 mg each month by aerosol, are alternatives for patients who are intolerant of TMP/SMX.

F. Protozoal infections

   1. *Toxoplasma gondii* typically causes multiple CNS lesions with encephalopathy and focal neurologic findings. Treatment with sulfadiazine, 25 mg/kg PO q6h, plus pyrimethamine, 100–150 mg PO on day 1, then 50–75 mg PO qd, often results in improvement, but indefinite therapy is needed to prevent relapse. Folinic acid, 5–10 mg PO qd, may be added to minimize hematologic toxicity. For patients who are intolerant of sulfonamides, clindamycin, 600 mg PO qid, may be substituted for sulfadiazine. Glucocorticoid therapy may also be useful for treating increased intracranial pressure. Prophylactic therapy is indicated for seropositive patients with CD4 lymphocyte counts less than 100 cells/mm³. TMP/SMX, 160 mg/800 mg (1 double-strength tablet) PO qd, is effective in the prevention of both PCP and toxoplasmosis. For patients who are intolerant of TMP/SMX, the combination of dapsone, 100 mg PO qd, plus weekly pyrimethamine, 50 mg PO, and folinic acid, 5 mg PO, has been shown to provide prophylaxis for both PCP and toxoplasmosis.

   2. *Cryptosporidium* and *Isospora belli* may cause protozoal enteric infections in patients with AIDS. *I. belli* infection can be treated with TMP/SMX, 160 mg/800 mg PO qid for 10 days and then bid for 3 weeks (*N Engl J Med* 315:87, 1986). Relapses are common. Shorter courses of TMP/SMX therapy followed by prophylaxis with pyrimethamine/sulfadoxine may also be effective (*J Infect Dis* 157:225, 1988). No therapy has proved to be effective for cryptosporidiosis, although there has been some limited success with paromomycin, 500 mg qid.

   3. Microsporidia infection has been associated with diarrhea and weight loss. Diagnosis may be difficult as the organism is usually only demonstrable on small-bowel biopsies. Albendazole, 400 mg PO bid for 4 weeks, may be effective.

G. Neoplasms associated with AIDS include non-Hodgkin's lymphomas and Kaposi's sarcoma. Primary CNS lymphomas are common and may be multicentric.

Other Immunocompromised Hosts

The principal components of the immune system that may be disordered and predispose patients to infection include the phagocytic cells (particularly neutrophilic granulocytes), cellular immunity, and humoral immunity. Defects in these lines of defense may arise alone or in combination as primary immune defects, or secondary to malignancy and antineoplastic therapy, secondary to systemic infection (e.g., CMV), or as the result of immunosuppressive therapy.

I. The neutropenic patient. Neutropenia, usually defined as an **absolute neutrophil count (ANC)** of less than 500 cells/mm³, is common following myelosuppressive chemotherapy. Risk of infection is associated with the degree and duration of neutropenia and the rapidity of decline. Severe, prolonged neutropenia (ANC <100 cells/mm³) places patients at risk from a variety of pathogens, including bacteria, fungi, and certain viruses (particularly HSV). Primary portals of entry to infectious agents include the respiratory tree, damaged alimentary tract mucosa, the perineum, and indwelling venous catheters.

A. Prevention of infection

   1. Bacterial infection. A number of strategies have been attempted to prevent bacterial infections in neutropenic patients, including strict isolation and both systemic and nonabsorbable antimicrobials. However, none of these approaches has proved more effective than careful hand washing prior to contact with the patient. When prolonged neutropenia is expected, it is also prudent for patients to avoid exogenous acquisition of aerobic gram-negative bacteria from fresh fruits, vegetables, and uncooked dairy products. In patients with solid organ tumors who are neutropenic following intensive chemotherapy, consideration can be given to acceleration of granulocyte recovery through the use of granulocyte and granulocyte macrophage colony-stimulating factors (e.g., G-CSF, GM-CSF).

2. **Fungal infection.** Several studies have shown that antifungal agents, such as amphotericin B and the azoles, can decrease fungal colonization in the setting of prolonged neutropenia (particularly with *Candida albicans*), and in some instances decrease the incidence of invasive infection. However, this decrease is often at the expense of a shift toward infection with more resistant fungi, and a mortality benefit has not been proved. Therefore, **routine antifungal prophylaxis is not widely recommended**.

3. **Viral infection.** Herpes simplex stomatitis can be prevented in patients who are undergoing intensive chemotherapy (e.g., bone marrow transplantation or induction therapy for acute leukemia) with acyclovir, 5 mg/kg IV bid or 400 mg PO tid.

B. **Evaluation and empiric treatment of the neutropenic, febrile patient.** All febrile (one temperature >38.5°C, or more than one temperature >38°C), neutropenic patients should be carefully evaluated and empiric antimicrobial therapy initiated.

1. **Evaluation.** Most patients with initial febrile episodes will have no localizing symptoms or signs of infection. However, any clues to the site of infection should be aggressively sought. A careful physical examination should be directed toward the common portals of infection (e.g., chest, mucosal surfaces, catheter sites, perineum), as well as sites of discomfort. Signs of inflammation with neutropenia may be minimal or absent, even when significant infection is present. All patients should have blood cultures, both peripherally and from an indwelling catheter, if one is present. A chest radiograph and urinalysis should also be performed. Further diagnostic measures may be required based on this initial evaluation and the patient's response to therapy.

2. **Empiric antibacterial regimens.** An etiologic agent is not identified in the majority of febrile neutropenic episodes. However, most are believed to result from invasion of the host's endogenous flora. Because both gram-negative and gram-positive bacteria may be involved, the initial regimen should be broad in spectrum. Many centers consider the combination of choice to be an extended-spectrum beta-lactam (e.g., ceftazidime, mezlocillin, or piperacillin) plus an aminoglycoside (e.g., gentamicin, tobramycin, or amikacin) (see Chap. 12). The addition of vancomycin to cover staphylococci should be considered if the patient has an indwelling venous catheter. The combination of vancomycin and ceftazidime can be considered for initial therapy in centers where ceftazidime-resistant organisms are not prevalent. Monotherapy with imipenem-cilastatin is also an option.

3. **Empiric antifungal therapy.** Systemic amphotericin B (0.5–0.7 mg/kg/day) is indicated for patients who remain febrile or who have recurrent fever despite 4–7 days of broad-spectrum antimicrobial therapy. Antifungal therapy should be continued until resolution of neutropenia. For patients with suspected or proved *Aspergillus* pneumonia, daily doses of amphotericin B of up to 1.5 mg/kg/day may be given.

4. **Duration of empiric antimicrobial therapy.** Antibacterial antimicrobials should be continued until WBC count recovery (ANC >500 cells/mm³). If antifungal therapy is given empirically, it may be discontinued after neutrophil count recovery if no definite site of fungal infection is identified. Patients with established deep-seated fungal infection require longer courses of therapy.

C. **Treatment of specific infections in the neutropenic patient.** See Chap. 13.

II. **Patients with impaired cellular immunity** include transplant recipients, patients receiving immunosuppressive therapy, and patients with lymphoreticular malignancies. This is the immune defect that leads to opportunistic infection in AIDS, and the pathogens involved most commonly are delineated in HIV Infection and AIDS, sec. II. Some notable differences in pathogens or approach are discussed below.

A. Prevention of infection
  1. **Bacterial infection.** Major intracellular pathogens to which patients with impaired cellular immunity are predisposed include *Listeria*, mycobacteria, *Nocardia*, *Legionella*, and *Salmonella*. All patients with a positive PPD skin test (≥5-mm induration) or whose chest radiographs show upper lobe fibrosis suggestive of healed TB should be evaluated for preventive therapy with INH. The remainder of these organisms are sufficiently uncommon that specific prophylaxis is not given, but it is likely that TMP/SMX, which most transplant recipients receive for the prevention of *Pneumocystis*, also reduces the risk from these agents.
  2. **Fungal infection.** Major opportunistic organisms in this category include *Cryptococcus neoformans*, *Histoplasma capsulatum*, and *Coccidioides immitis*. Preventive therapy is generally not indicated, except in the case of transplant patients with prior infection with *Coccidioides*, as indicated by a positive serologic test (complement fixation or immunodiffusion). Such patients should receive prophylactic **fluconazole** or **itraconazole** while receiving immunosuppressive therapy; however, these drugs, particularly the latter, **may increase cyclosporine levels.**
  3. **Viral infection**
      a. **Herpes simplex stomatitis** can be prevented in seropositive patients with acyclovir, 400 mg PO bid or 200 mg PO tid.
      b. **Varicella zoster** (shingles) is common in bone marrow transplant patients in the year following the transplant. This infection can be prevented by the use of acyclovir, 800 mg PO bid or 400 mg PO tid.
      c. **CMV** infection and disease are common in transplant patients in the first 3–4 months following transplantation. In allogeneic bone marrow transplant patients, in whom CMV disease can be particularly severe, weekly surveillance cultures of blood and urine for CMV are indicated for the first 3 months following the transplant. If a positive culture is obtained, "preemptive therapy" is indicated with DHPG, 5 mg/kg IV q12h for 2 weeks, followed by 5 mg/kg IV qd until day 100 after the transplant. Other strategies have been attempted in other patient populations, but no clear standard of care has emerged.
      4. **Protozoal infections.** Major opportunistic organisms in this category include *Pneumocystis carinii*, *Toxoplasma gondii*, and *Cryptosporidium*. *Pneumocystis* can be prevented by the use of TMP/SMX, 160 mg/800 mg PO qd. In transplant patients, this drug is usually given for at least the first year following the transplant. It should also be considered in patients who are undergoing aggressive chemotherapy for lymphoreticular malignancy. The other pathogens are sufficiently uncommon that specific prevention is not indicated, but it is possible that toxoplasmosis is prevented by the use of TMP/SMX.
      5. **Helminthic infections.** *Strongyloides stercoralis* may cause disseminated infection in patients with impaired cellular immunity. Patients from endemic areas (e.g., Third World countries), or those with eosinophilia who are being evaluated for transplantation should have stool examinations for this parasite.
B. Treatment of specific infections in the patient with impaired cellular immunity. See Chap. 13.
III. The patient with impaired humoral immunity. Patients in this category include those with agammaglobulinemia, multiple myeloma, and chronic lymphocytic leukemia (CLL). Bone marrow transplant patients may have IgG subclass deficiency following marrow recovery. Patients with impaired humoral immunity are particularly susceptible to encapsulated bacteria, including *Streptococcus pneumoniae* and *Haemophilus influenzae*. Replacement therapy with IV gamma globulin is beneficial for agammaglobulinemia and may be beneficial for patients with CLL who have recurrent infections due to encapsulated organisms or bone marrow recipients with IgG subclass deficiency. Deficient humoral immunity in patients with multiple myeloma is addressed by chemotherapy to reduce the number of malignant plasma cells.

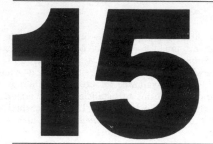

Gastroenterologic Diseases

Michele C. Woodley and
Deborah C. Rubin

Nausea and Vomiting

Nausea and vomiting may result from systemic illnesses, CNS disorders, primary GI diseases, and as side effects of **medications** (e.g., digoxin, theophylline). In otherwise healthy individuals, the most common cause of vomiting is a **viral illness. Intestinal obstruction** can cause nausea and vomiting and can be diagnosed radiographically. **Pregnancy** should be excluded when relevant; treatment of nausea and vomiting during pregnancy should be directed by an obstetrician. Specific therapy can often be initiated once an etiology is established.

I. **Supportive measures.** Oral intake should be withheld or limited to clear liquids if tolerated. Many patients with self-limited illnesses will require no further therapy. Nasogastric (NG) decompression may be beneficial for patients with protracted nausea and vomiting. Parenteral fluid resuscitation is necessary for patients with intravascular volume depletion.

II. **Pharmacotherapy**
   A. **Centrally acting antiemetics** include the phenothiazines and related agents. Prochlorperazine, 5–10 mg PO tid–qid, 10 mg IM q4h (maximum IM dose is 40 mg/day), or 25 mg PR bid; promethazine, 12.5–25.0 mg PO, IM, or PR q4–6h; trimethobenzamide, 250 mg PO tid–qid, 200 mg IM tid–qid, or 200 mg PR tid–qid; and thiethylperazine, 10 mg PO, IM, or PR qd–tid are effective. Drowsiness is a common side effect, and acute dystonic reactions may occur.
   B. **Dopamine antagonists** include **metoclopramide**, 10 mg PO 30 minutes ac and hs, a prokinetic agent used to treat vomiting associated with diabetic gastroparesis. IV metoclopramide is used in nausea and vomiting associated with chemotherapy (see Chap. 19 and Table 19-2). Drowsiness and extrapyramidal reactions may occur.
   C. **Ondansetron**, 32 mg IV infused over 15 minutes beginning 30 minutes before chemotherapy or 0.15 mg/kg IV q4h for 3 doses, is effective in chemotherapy-associated emesis. Constipation may occur.
   D. **Cisapride**, 10–20 mg PO ac and hs, is an effective prokinetic agent. Cisapride enhances gastric emptying and can cause diarrhea.

Diarrhea

The approach to the patient with diarrhea consists of (1) identification and treatment of the specific underlying disease, (2) correction of fluid and electrolyte disturbances (see Chap. 3), and (3) occasional use of nonspecific antidiarrheal agents.

I. **Acute diarrhea.** Infectious agents (viral, bacterial, and parasitic), toxins, poisons, and drugs are the major causes of acute diarrhea. Inflammatory bowel disease may also present as diarrhea. **In hospitalized patients** common causes include lactose intolerance unmasked by hospital diets, antimicrobial-associated diarrhea (including pseudomembranous colitis), drug-induced diarrhea, and fecal impaction.
   A. **Viral and bacterial infections.** The most common causes of diarrhea in the United States include viral enteritis and bacterial infections with organisms

such as enterotoxigenic *Escherichia coli, Shigella, Salmonella, Campylobacter,* and *Yersinia* spp (see Chap. 13). **Evaluation** with stool cultures, methylene blue stain for fecal leukocytes, stool ova and parasite examination, and flexible sigmoidoscopy may be warranted in patients with bloody diarrhea, a prolonged course, or dysenteric symptoms. Most acute diarrheal episodes of viral or bacterial origin are self-limited and do not require antimicrobial therapy.

B. **Parasitic infections**
   1. **Amebiasis** may cause acute diarrhea. It occurs most often in travelers and homosexual men and in areas with poor sanitation. The diagnosis may be confirmed at sigmoidoscopy or by demonstration of trophozoites or cysts of *Entamoeba histolytica* in the stool. **Treatment** for asymptomatic intestinal infection is iodoquinol, 650 mg PO tid for 20 days. Treatment for symptomatic disease is metronidazole, 750 mg PO tid for 10 days, followed by iodoquinol, 650 mg PO tid for 20 days.
   2. **Giardiasis** commonly presents as acute or chronic diarrhea. The diagnosis is confirmed by identification of *Giardia lamblia* trophozoites in the stool, by a duodenal aspirate, or by a small-bowel biopsy. Quinacrine, 100 mg PO tid, or metronidazole, 250 mg PO tid for 7 days is usually effective. More prolonged therapy may be required in the immunocompromised patient.
C. **Drugs** are a frequent cause of diarrhea. Common offending agents include laxatives, antacids, cardiac medications (e.g., digitalis and quinidine), colchicine, and antimicrobial agents. Antimicrobials may produce diarrhea by causing nonspecific alteration of enteric flora or by causing **pseudomembranous colitis secondary to overgrowth of *Clostridium difficile*,** which requires specific therapy (see Chap. 13). Antimicrobial-associated diarrhea without evidence of pseudomembranous colitis usually responds to cessation of the offending agent.

II. **Chronic diarrhea** may be a sign of a serious illness or a functional symptom.
   A. **History.** Frequent small-volume stools associated with urgency and tenesmus suggest the site of the underlying disorder is most likely the distal colon. Stools that are bulky and large in volume often indicate small-bowel disease. Symptoms of steatorrhea suggest small-bowel or pancreatic disease.
   B. **Classification of chronic diarrhea.** In many diarrhea illnesses, there is both an osmotic and a secretory component. Response to feeding and fasting as well as calculation of stool osmolality may help distinguish between them.
   1. **Osmotic diarrhea** is caused by the accumulation of poorly absorbed solutes in the intestine. It usually stops with fasting. Causes include ingestion of lactose (in lactase deficiency) and osmotic laxatives such as milk of magnesia.
   2. **Secretory diarrhea** is caused by abnormal secretion of water and electrolytes into the intestinal lumen. Typically, the diarrhea persists despite fasting. Secretory diarrhea may be caused by bacterial enterotoxins, secretory hormones (e.g., gastrin or vasoactive intestinal peptide), some laxatives, dihydroxy bile acids, and fatty acids.
   3. **Mucosal injury.** Diarrhea with both osmotic and secretory components may result from mucosal diseases such as inflammatory bowel disease, celiac sprue, lymphoma, or ischemic bowel injury.
   4. **Deranged intestinal motility,** which occurs in irritable bowel syndrome, can also cause diarrhea.

III. **Diarrhea in patients with AIDS.** Diarrhea is a common symptom in homosexual men with or without a preexisting diagnosis of AIDS. Often, one or more pathogens can be isolated. In patients with AIDS, **opportunistic agents** including *Cryptosporidium, Isospora,* cytomegalovirus (CMV), and *Mycobacterium avium-intracellulare* (MAI) and tumors such as Kaposi's sarcoma and lymphoma may occur (see Chap. 14). Specific infections include both venereal infections (syphilis, gonorrhea, chlamydiosis, herpes simplex virus [HSV] infection) and nonvenereal infections (amebiasis, giardiasis, salmonellosis, shigellosis).
   A. **Watery diarrhea** is commonly caused by giardiasis, cryptosporidiosis, or MAI infection. Stool examination for ova and parasites as well as acid-fast stains are necessary. Small-bowel biopsy may also be helpful in diagnosis. Giardiasis tends

to be recurrent and difficult to treat (see Chap. 13). No clearly effective treatment is currently available for *Cryptosporidium* or MAI infection (see Chap. 14).

B. Dysenteric symptoms are commonly associated with bacterial pathogens (see Chap. 13), CMV (see Esophageal Disease, sec. **II.D**), and amebiasis (see sec. **I.B.1**).

C. Anorectal symptoms should prompt careful physical examination and proctoscopy with swabs for gonorrhea and HSV culture as well as dark-field examination for syphilis. For treatment of these entities, see Chap. 13.

IV. Nonspecific antidiarrheals are generally overused. In most cases of acute diarrhea, they are unnecessary. In chronic diarrhea, they are not a substitute for treatment of the underlying illness. In *Salmonella* and *Shigella* infections, they may prolong the duration of illness. Antiperistaltic drugs (diphenoxylate, paregoric, loperamide) **may precipitate toxic megacolon** in patients with invasive bacterial infection.

A. Bulk-forming agents (see Constipation, sec. **II.A**).

B. Absorbents (e.g., kaolin plus pectin, 60–120 ml of regular strength or 45–90 ml of concentrate PO after every loose bowel movement).

C. Opioid agents should be used cautiously in patients with asthma, chronic lung disease, benign prostatic hypertrophy, and acute angle-closure glaucoma. Their potential for abuse should be recognized.

1. **Paregoric** (camphorated tincture of opium), 4–8 ml PO qid or 4–8 ml PO after each liquid stool, not to exceed 32 ml/day.

2. **Deodorized tincture of opium,** 0.3–1.0 ml PO qid (maximum 6 ml/day).

3. **Codeine,** 30–60 mg PO bid–qid.

4. **Diphenoxylate hydrochloride** (Lomotil), a meperidine congener, effectively inhibits excessive GI motility. Side effects are uncommon. It is contraindicated in patients with advanced liver disease. Respiratory depression will occur with overdose and may be potentiated by phenothiazine derivatives, barbiturates, and tricyclic antidepressants. Each diphenoxylate tablet or 5 ml of liquid contains 2.5 mg of diphenoxylate hydrochloride and 0.025 mg of atropine sulfate (a subtherapeutic amount added to discourage deliberate overdose). The dosage is 5 mg PO qid until initial control of diarrhea is achieved, followed by the lowest effective dosage.

5. **Loperamide hydrochloride,** 2–4 mg PO after each loose stool, is another effective synthetic opioid antidiarrheal. The maximum dosage is 8 mg/day.

D. Somatostatin may be used in severe refractory diarrhea from metastatic carcinoid syndrome or vasoactive intestinal peptide tumors (VIPomas). This long-acting octreotide is used SC or IV, 100–600 µg/day in 2–4 divided doses.

Constipation

I. Etiology. Constipation is a common problem. Many drugs induce constipation, including narcotics, aluminum hydroxide antacids, anticholinergics, iron supplements, laxatives (long-term use), and some antihypertensive agents. Lack of exercise, disorders that cause pain on defecation (e.g., thrombosed external hemorrhoids and anal fissures or strictures), and systemic diseases such as diabetes, hypothyroidism, and hyperparathyroidism predispose to constipation. Constipation in hospitalized patients may be caused by medications, barium sulfate, or prolonged immobilization. When constipation develops in a middle-aged or elderly person, colon cancer should be considered. In addition, when straining during defecation is especially undesirable (e.g., after recent myocardial infarction [MI] or recent abdominal surgery), avoidance and treatment of constipation are particularly important.

II. Therapy. Treatment of the underlying disease and correction of predisposing factors are the most important aspects of therapy. However, additional therapy may be necessary.

A. Fiber. The addition of 20–30 g/day of dietary fiber is often beneficial for patients with chronic constipation. A fiber supplement such as wheat bran or psyllium with water bid–qid may be used. Fiber therapy may take a few weeks to improve symptoms. Transient bloating often occurs.

B. **Laxatives** may help some patients with constipation that is unresponsive to fiber supplements. Regular use is not advised. Undiagnosed abdominal pain and intestinal obstruction are contraindications to laxative use.

   1. **Emollient laxatives.** Docusate sodium, 50–200 mg PO qd, and docusate calcium USP, 240 mg PO qd, allow water and fat to penetrate the fecal mass. Emollient laxatives promote intestinal absorption of mineral oil; thus, emollient laxatives and mineral oil should not be used concurrently.

   2. **Stimulant cathartics.** Long-term use of these agents is not recommended.

      a. **Castor oil,** 15 ml PO, produces prompt evacuation of the colon.

      b. **Bisacodyl** stimulates colonic peristalsis. It may be administered PO or PR. The dosage is 10–15 mg PO hs; 10-mg rectal suppositories are available and act in 15–60 minutes.

      c. **Extract of cascara and extract of senna** stimulate the colon and usually produce a single bowel evacuation 6–10 hours after administration. The dosage of cascara is 2–6 ml PO qd; 1 tablet of extract of senna is given PO qd–bid. Chronic use of these agents should be avoided because they can cause colonic denervation with atony.

   3. **Osmotic cathartics** are nonabsorbable salts or carbohydrates that cause water retention in the lumen of the colon. Standard preparations and dosages are given below.

      a. **Milk of magnesia,** 15–30 ml PO.

      b. **Magnesium citrate solution,** 200 ml PO of a standard solution.

      c. **Lactulose,** 15–30 ml PO of standard syrup.

      d. **Lavage solutions** containing nonabsorbable sulfate and polyethylene glycol (e.g., GoLYTELY, Colyte) are effective for rapidly clearing the colon in preparation for endoscopic examination or surgery. The dosage is 4–6 liters PO over 3–4 hours.

Esophageal Disease

I. **Reflux esophagitis.** The lower esophageal sphincter (LES) is the major barrier against reflux. **Symptoms** of reflux include heartburn, dysphagia, chest pain, and a variety of ear, nose, and throat symptoms (e.g., hoarseness, sore throat). **Complications** of reflux esophagitis include esophageal stricture, Barrett's esophagus, pulmonary aspiration, and bleeding. Hiatal hernias are often seen on radiographs of patients with reflux esophagitis. However, it is the competency of the sphincter that determines whether acid will enter the esophagus. Medical therapy is aimed at reducing the quantity and acidity of the gastric contents available for reflux or at pharmacologic elevation of LES pressure (*Arch Intern Med* 152:71, 1992).

A. **Life-style modifications** can mitigate mild symptoms.

   1. **Bed blocks.** Placing 6-inch blocks under the head of the patient's bed or a wedge under the mattress or sheet enhances nocturnal acid clearance.

   2. **Diet.** Alcohol, mints, chocolate, fat, and caffeine lower LES pressure and can exacerbate reflux. Weight loss may reduce reflux symptoms.

   3. **Cigarette smoking should be avoided.**

   4. **Medications** that lower LES pressure can increase symptoms. These drugs include theophylline, calcium channel blockers, narcotics, and diazepam.

B. **Medical therapy** is useful in patients with persistent symptoms. A barium swallow or upper endoscopy is indicated in patients who are refractory to medical therapy or who have signs of tissue injury. Such measures are also indicated to exclude infectious esophagitis, esophageal stricture, or tumor.

   1. **Antacids.** For patients with mild or intermittent symptoms, 2 tablespoons of a high-potency liquid antacid after meals or with heartburn may be sufficient (Table 15-1).

Table 15-1. Antacid preparations

Antacid	Buffering capacity (mEq/15 ml)	Buffering capacity (ml/100 mEq)	Sodium content (mEq/15 ml)
$Al(OH)_3$			
Amphojel	30	50	0.30
Basaljel	34.5	43	0.39
Basaljel extra strength	66	23	3.00
$Al(OH)_3 + Mg(OH)_2$			
Maalox TC	82	18	0.09
Maalox Plus[a]	40	37.5	0.18
Mylanta[a]	37.5	40	0.10
Mylanta-II[a]	75	20	0.15
Riopan	45	33	0.04
Gelusil[a]	36	42	0.10
$CaCO_3$			
Tums tablets	19.5[b]	—	0.125[b]
Titralac	33	45	0.00
$Al(OH)_3 + Mg(OH)_2 + CaCO_3$			
Camalox	54	26	0.15

[a]Contains simethicone.
[b]Per 2 tablets.

2. **H_2-receptor antagonists** (Table 15-2) improve symptoms and heal esophageal inflammation. However, prolonged therapy (up to 12 weeks) at doses higher than those used for peptic ulcer disease may be required. Relapse is common when treatment is discontinued; this is true for all medical management of reflux.
3. **Metoclopramide** improves gastric emptying and increases LES pressure. It is most effective when used in combination with H_2-receptor antagonists. Dosages range from 5–15 mg PO qid for up to 4 weeks. Drowsiness, psychiatric symptoms, and extrapyramidal reactions may occur with long-term use.
4. **Omeprazole** blocks parietal cell hydrogen-potassium adenosine triphosphatase (ATPase) and heals severe erosive esophagitis more effectively than H_2-receptor antagonists. It is used for short-term treatment of severe erosive esophagitis (see Table 15-2) (*Gut* 31:509, 968, 1990). **Side effects**, which are uncommon, include diarrhea, nausea, dizziness, and headaches. The risk of carcinoid tumors associated with long-term use still needs to be clarified. An upper endoscopy should be considered before use of omeprazole to exclude other esophageal lesions.
5. **Cisapride**, 10–20 mg PO tid–qid, increases LES pressure and improves esophageal clearance and gastric emptying. It is effective for erosive and nonerosive esophagitis and can be used as an adjunct to antisecretory treatment.
6. **Anticholinergics should not be used** in patients with reflux because these drugs decrease LES pressure.
C. **Surgery** should be considered in patients with aspiration, bleeding, strictures not readily managed with peroral dilatation, or intractable esophagitis despite aggressive medical therapy. Prior to surgery, esophagitis should be confirmed by endoscopy and biopsy, and adequate peristalsis verified by manometry.
II. **Infectious esophagitis** usually presents with odynophagia or dysphagia and is most common in patients with AIDS, malignancy, diabetes, or other causes of impaired immunity. Major pathogens include *Candida albicans*, HSV, and CMV. The presence of typical oral lesions (thrush, herpetic vesicles) may suggest an etiologic agent. Endoscopy with biopsy and brush cytology is often diagnostic.

Table 15-2. Dosing regimens for acid-peptic disease

	Oral therapy				
	DU (acute therapy)	DU (maintenance therapy)	GU	GERD	Parenteral therapy
Cimetidine	300 mg qid 400 mg bid 800 mg hs	400 mg hs	300 mg qid	300 mg qid	300 mg q6h
Ranitidine	150 mg bid 300 mg hs	150 mg hs	150 mg bid	150 mg bid	50 mg q8h
Famotidine	40 mg hs	20 mg hs	40 mg hs	—	20 mg q12h
Nizatidine	300 mg hs 150 mg bid	150 mg hs	—	—	—
Omeprazole	20 mg qd	—	—	20–40 mg qd	—
Cisapride	—	—	—	10–20 mg qid	—

DU = duodenal ulcer; GU = gastric ulcer; GERD = gastroesophageal reflux disease.

A. **General measures.** Transient symptomatic relief can be achieved with viscous lidocaine (2%) swish and swallows, 15 ml PO q3–4h prn. Sucralfate slurry, 1 g PO qid, is also beneficial.

B. ***Candida* esophagitis.** Mild disease can be treated with nystatin oral suspension, 400,000–600,000 units PO qid, or clotrimazole, 10-mg lozenges q6h for 2 weeks. Ketoconazole, 200 mg PO qd–bid or 400 mg PO qd, should be used in more severe disease. For unresponsive disease, a short course of parenteral amphotericin B (0.3–0.5 mg/kg/day) or fluconazole (100 mg PO qd for 7 days) should be considered (see Chap. 13).

C. **HSV esophagitis** in immunocompromised patients may be treated with parenteral acyclovir, 5 mg/kg IV q8h for 7 days or 800 mg PO 5 times/day for 14 days. The dosing interval should be increased in the presence of impaired renal function. In healthy patients, this infection is usually self-limited and treatment is supportive.

D. **CMV esophagitis.** Ganciclovir (DHPG, 5 mg/kg IV q12h) may be effective for a variety of GI CMV infections in immunocompromised hosts.

E. **Discrete ulcers.** Discrete ulcers of the esophagus may be caused by infection (e.g., CMV, HSV), medication (e.g., potassium, quinidine), or malignancy, or may be unexplained, as with AIDS patients. Therapy depends on the specific etiology. Glucocorticoids may be considered for patients with unexplained ulcers and AIDS.

III. **Esophageal motility disorders** may cause noncardiac chest pain or intermittent dysphagia to both liquids and solids. If a barium swallow or upper endoscopy is unrevealing, esophageal manometry studies can be performed to demonstrate spastic disorders and reproduce symptoms. Optimal treatment is not defined, although a variety of agents, including long-acting nitrates, calcium channel blockers, and psychoactive (antidepressant and anxiolytic) agents such as trazodone, 50 mg PO bid–tid, have been used. Gastroenterologic consultation is recommended for advice regarding diagnosis and therapy.

Peptic Ulcer Disease

Peptic ulcer disease (PUD) is ulceration of the gastroduodenal mucosa typically extending through the muscularis mucosa. Approximately 5–10% of the general population will have a peptic ulcer during a lifetime. At least half of these patients will have a recurrence within 5 years. The recent discovery of *Helicobacter pylori*, a spiral, gram-negative urease-producing bacillus, has greatly altered diagnostic and therapeutic considerations in PUD. This organism can be cultured from the stomach of approximately 90% of duodenal ulcer patients and 70–80% of gastric ulcer patients. Eradication of the organism dramatically reduces recurrence of PUD by approximately 75–90% (*Am J Med Sci* 306:381, 1993).

I. **Management considerations.** The goals of ulcer therapy include relief of symptoms and prevention of recurrence and complications.

    A. **H. pylori.** Determination of a duodenal or gastric ulcer by upper endoscopy or radiographic study should be followed by confirmation of *H. pylori* infection. Diagnostic tests for the presence of *H. pylori* vary and include serologic testing, carbon-labeled urea breath tests, rapid urease assay (Clotest), and culture or histologic analysis of endoscopic biopsies. Specific treatment for *H. pylori* in the presence of active duodenal or gastric ulcer disease is described below.

    B. **Gastric ulcers** are malignant in approximately 5% of cases. Therefore, endoscopic biopsy of gastric ulcers at the time of initial diagnosis is recommended. Patients with a gastric ulcer should have an upper gastrointestinal (UGI) series or endoscopy after 6–8 weeks of medical therapy. If the lesion has not changed in size, upper endoscopy with additional biopsies should be performed. If the lesion is smaller but not fully healed, another UGI series or endoscopy should be performed after an additional 6 weeks of therapy. Longer follow-up periods may be necessary to demonstrate healing of large gastric ulcers that are determined to be benign by biopsy (*Arch Intern Med* 143:264, 1983). Surgical therapy should be considered for nonhealing gastric ulcers.

    C. **Duodenal ulcers** are almost never malignant, and demonstration of ulcer healing in the absence of symptoms is unnecessary. Many duodenal ulcers heal even in the absence of therapy. However, H_2-receptor antagonists, sucralfate, and high-dose antacids have been shown to increase the rate of healing and the percentage of ulcers that heal. Each drug is associated with a 70–85% incidence of ulcer healing at 4–6 weeks, compared with 40–50% incidence with placebo. Omeprazole, a proton pump antagonist, can heal duodenal ulcers in 2–4 weeks.

II. **Treatment.** Reduction of stomach acidity and treatment of *H. pylori* are the main goals of therapy in PUD. Gastric acid may be effectively neutralized with antacids, H_2-receptor antagonists, or omeprazole.

    A. **H. pylori regimens.** In patients with PUD and *H. pylori*, treatment should be aimed at healing the ulcer and eradicating the organism. The optimal treatment regimen for *H. pylori* is under active investigation. A standard regimen has included oral antimicrobials (tetracycline, 500 mg qid; metronidazole, 250 mg tid), and bismuth compound (2 tablets qid for 2 weeks). For patients who cannot tolerate this rigorous regimen, antimicrobial-omeprazole and antimicrobial–H_2-receptor antagonist regimens (omeprazole with amoxicillin or clarithromycin, or ranitidine with metronidazole and amoxicillin) have been suggested (*Am J Med Sci* 306:393, 1993).

    B. **H_2-receptor antagonists** (see Table 15-2).

        1. **Duodenal ulcer**

            a. **Acute therapy.** Cimetidine, ranitidine, famotidine, and nizatidine are all effective as short-term therapy for acute duodenal ulcer. Once- or twice-daily dosage regimens may improve patient compliance. Dosage intervals should be prolonged in the presence of renal insufficiency (see Appendix D). Parenteral therapy should be reserved for patients who are unable to tolerate oral medications.

            b. **Therapy to prevent** recurrent ulcer disease includes eradication of *H. pylori* and maintenance H_2-receptor antagonist therapy (see Table 15-2).

        2. **Benign gastric ulcer.** Cimetidine, ranitidine, and famotidine are effective in healing benign gastric ulcer. Gastric ulcers should be followed until completely healed to ensure that they are not malignant (see sec. I.B). Dosage schedules are the same as those for duodenal ulcer.

        3. **Adverse reactions and drug interactions.** Short-term therapy with cimeti-

dine, ranitidine, famotidine, and nizatidine is well tolerated by most patients.
  a. **Cimetidine.** Reversible impotence has been reported with long-term, high-dose cimetidine therapy for Zollinger-Ellison syndrome. Gynecomastia and reduced sperm counts are more common in patients receiving higher than conventional dosages. Elderly patients and patients with impaired hepatic or renal function occasionally develop mental status abnormalities. Leukopenia and thrombocytopenia occur rarely. **Cimetidine impairs metabolism of warfarin anticoagulants, theophylline, and phenytoin** (see Appendix B).
  b. **Ranitidine, famotidine, and nizatidine** have been in use for shorter periods of time than cimetidine, and their toxicity profiles are less well established. Impotence, gynecomastia, and confusion have been reported less frequently with these agents than with cimetidine. In addition, these agents appear to cause little or no interference with the hepatic microsomal enzyme system. Reversible drug-induced hepatitis has been reported with all the H_2 antagonists and may occur more frequently with ranitidine (*Am J Gastroenterol* 82:987, 1987).
C. Omeprazole is a potent inhibitor of the hydrogen-potassium ATPase that profoundly decreases gastric acid secretion (see Esophageal Disease, sec. **I.B.4**). A dosage of 20 mg/day is effective in the acute treatment of duodenal ulcer.
D. Sucralfate, 1 g PO qid (1 hour ac and hs) or 2 g bid, is as effective as H_2-receptor antagonists or high-dose antacids in the healing of duodenal ulcers. Sucralfate does not block acid secretion but appears to act locally at the mucosal surface. The most frequent side effect is constipation in up to 2% of patients. **The absorption of cimetidine, digoxin, fluoroquinolones, phenytoin, and tetracycline may be reduced if given concomitantly with sucralfate.** Sucralfate may also be useful for the treatment of gastric ulcer. Its efficacy in the treatment of peptic esophagitis is not established.
E. Antacids (see Table 15-1). Because alternative therapies require less frequent dosing and are more palatable, antacids are best used as supplemental therapy for pain relief. The choice of antacid is determined by buffering capacity, sodium content, and side effects. In general, liquid antacids are more effective than tablets. Typically, 30 ml of a high-potency liquid antacid provides symptomatic relief. Magnesium hydroxide is a potent antacid, but large or frequent doses can cause severe osmotic diarrhea. Therefore, magnesium hydroxide is combined with aluminum hydroxide in most preparations. For patients who have diarrhea while taking a magnesium hydroxide–aluminum hydroxide mixture, use of a constipating antacid such as pure aluminum hydroxide in alternating doses may be helpful. However, aluminum hydroxide binds phosphate in the intestine and may cause hypophosphatemia. It may also decrease the absorption of tetracycline, thyroxine, and chlorpromazine. Aluminum hydroxide is often used in patients with renal failure because these patients should avoid magnesium-containing antacids. Calcium carbonate is an effective antacid, but high doses may cause hypercalcemia and hypercalciuria.
F. Other therapeutic measures
  1. Diet. There is no evidence that a bland diet improves symptoms or promotes ulcer healing. Patients should be instructed to avoid foods that are reproducibly associated with dyspeptic symptoms. Late evening snacks should also be avoided, since they stimulate gastric acid production when the patient is asleep and unable to take antacids.
  2. Cessation of cigarette smoking should be strongly encouraged because cigarette use is associated with an increased risk of peptic ulcer development, delayed ulcer healing, and an increased rate of ulcer recurrence (*N Engl J Med* 311:689, 1984).
  3. Aspirin and nonsteroidal antiinflammatory drugs (NSAIDs) should be avoided in patients with PUD. High-dose aspirin ingestion is associated with an increased incidence of gastritis and gastric ulcer. Enteric coating or concomitant anti-ulcer therapy may reduce mucosal damage from aspirin. NSAIDs are toxic to the gastric mucosa and are associated with dyspepsia

and mucosal ulcerations. Concomitant therapy with omeprazole, H_2-receptor antagonists, or sucralfate may ameliorate some of these symptoms in patients who have strong indications for continued use of NSAIDs. Misoprostol (a synthetic prostaglandin E derivative), 200 μg PO qid, can help prevent NSAID-associated gastric ulcer and inflammation (*Gastroenterology* 96:675, 1989). Side effects of misoprostol include abdominal pain, self-limited diarrhea, and abortifacient activity.

    4. **Alcohol,** in high concentrations, damages the gastric mucosal barrier and is associated with gastritis. However, there is no evidence that alcohol induces recurrence of PUD.

III. **Complications of peptic ulcer disease**

    A. **GI bleeding** (see Gastrointestinal Bleeding).

    B. **Gastric outlet obstruction** occurs in about 5% of patients with peptic ulcer disease and is more likely to occur with ulcers that are situated close to the pyloric channel. Severe nausea and vomiting suggest obstruction. Plain abdominal radiographs often show a dilated stomach with an air-fluid level. If obstruction is present, nasogastric suction should be maintained for at least 72 hours to decompress the stomach. Dehydration, metabolic alkalosis, and hypokalemia should be corrected. Many patients respond to medical management alone, but the problem tends to recur; endoscopic dilatation or surgical intervention may be required.

    C. **Perforation** occurs in a small percentage of ulcer patients and usually necessitates emergency surgery. In some patients, perforation occurs in the absence of previous symptoms of peptic ulcer disease. A plain upright radiograph of the abdomen may aid diagnosis by showing the presence of free air under the diaphragm.

    D. **Penetration into the pancreas,** when it occurs, is most often associated with ulcers in the posterior wall of the duodenal bulb. The onset of penetration is often characterized by a change in symptoms. The pain becomes severe and continuous, radiates to the back, and is no longer relieved by antacids. Serum amylase is often elevated. These patients frequently require surgery.

    E. **Intractability.** Since the advent of improved medical therapies, the occurrence of operations for intractable ulcer disease has declined dramatically. An active ulcer must be determined radiographically or endoscopically before an operation is performed. The preoperative evaluation of a patient's ulcer should include a fasting gastrin determination and a search for potential reversible factors (e.g., ulcerogenic drugs, cigarette smoking). Significant problems can occur following gastric surgery (see sec. **IV**). Surgical options vary depending on the location of the ulcer (gastric versus duodenal) and the presence of associated complications.

IV. **Morbidity following gastrectomy and vagotomy**

    A. **Abdominal complaints.** The most common complaint after gastric surgery is abdominal discomfort or vomiting after meals. Some patients may have recurrent ulcer, afferent loop obstruction, bile reflux gastritis, gastric outlet obstruction, or stump carcinoma (a late complication). In most postgastrectomy patients with these complaints, however, no surgically correctable lesion exists. Their symptoms are often due to the **dumping syndrome,** which is caused by rapid gastric emptying of a large osmotic load into the upper small intestine. Discomfort and vomiting may be accompanied by vasomotor symptoms (palpitations, sweating, dizziness). Changing the patient's diet to 6 small meals each day that are relatively high in protein and low in refined carbohydrates often decreases these symptoms. Liquids with meals should be avoided. Anticholinergics, fiber in the form of pectin, and ephedrine may also relieve these symptoms. In refractory patients, octreotide, a long-acting somatostatin analog, may be used, but its long-term utility is limited by the need for SC administration.

    B. **Malabsorption.** Mild steatorrhea can occur after gastric surgery and is probably related to decreased intestinal transit time and inadequate mixing of food with bile and pancreatic secretions. Rarely, bacterial overgrowth secondary to afferent loop stasis may lead to steatorrhea. Chronic malabsorption of calcium and vitamin D may cause deficiency of these vitamins. **Metabolic bone disease,** usually osteomalacia, will develop in at least 30% of patients with a Billroth II anastomosis. Calcium and vitamin D supplements should be given (see Chap. 23).

C. **Anemia.** Postgastrectomy anemia typically develops slowly and may be secondary to deficiencies of folate, vitamin B_{12}, or, most commonly, iron. Iron-deficiency anemia is usually a result of dietary iron malabsorption, but blood loss from gastritis or a marginal ulcer may also contribute. When the cause of anemia is identified, an appropriate replacement should be given.

D. **Diarrhea.** Mild diarrhea is a common problem following vagotomy. The patient should be evaluated for treatable conditions (lactase deficiency or fat malabsorption). If none is found, a trial of symptomatic therapy with diphenoxylate or tincture of opium is appropriate (see Diarrhea, sec. **IV.C**).

V. **Zollinger-Ellison syndrome** is caused by a gastrin-secreting, non-beta islet cell tumor of the pancreas or duodenum that results in marked gastric acid hypersecretion (*N Engl J Med* 317:1200, 1987). Approximately two-thirds of Zollinger-Ellison tumors are malignant. Multiple endocrine neoplasia type I (MEN-I) is associated with this syndrome in 25% of patients. **The most common presentation** is a simple duodenal bulb ulcer, but large or multiple ulcers in the distal duodenum or jejunum or recurrent ulceration after an adequate ulcer operation should alert the physician to the possibility of this disease. **Diarrhea** is a common symptom. With currently available H_2-receptor antagonists and omeprazole, the major morbidity and mortality of this syndrome have shifted from the effects of uncontrolled acid hypersecretion to long-term effects of tumor growth. Control of acid hypersecretion with H_2-receptor antagonists and omeprazole (initial dose 60 mg/day) requires much higher doses than those used to treat PUD. Careful dose titration with measurement of acid secretion rates by gastric analysis is necessary. Identification of tumors for possible curative resection and detection of metastases to avoid unnecessary surgery is recommended in many cases.

VI. **Nonulcer dyspepsia** is a common syndrome of persistent ulcer-like symptoms in the absence of radiographic and endoscopic abnormalities. Motor abnormalities, microscopic inflammation, *H. pylori*-associated gastritis, and associated psychiatric disease may explain this syndrome. Therapy remains largely empiric. Treatment to eradicate *H. pylori* is not recommended for these patients (*Am J Med Sci* 306:381, 1993). Although some patients appear to respond to H_2-receptor antagonists, these agents have not been shown to be effective (*N Engl J Med* 314:339, 1986). Some patients may benefit from psychoactive agents such as alprazolam, 0.25–0.50 mg PO bid, or tricyclic antidepressants, including amitriptyline, 25–50 mg PO hs.

Gastroparesis

I. **Etiology.** Delayed gastric emptying occurs in a variety of acute and chronic disorders and metabolic derangements (hypokalemia, hyper- or hypocalcemia, or acute hyperglycemia) or because of the ingestion of medications (e.g., tricyclic antidepressants, narcotics, and anticholinergic agents). **Chronic gastric retention** is frequently associated with diabetes mellitus, scleroderma, and previous gastric surgery but may also be idiopathic. Many other chronic metabolic, endocrine, and collagen vascular diseases can be associated with gastric motor dysfunction. **Mechanical obstruction** should always be excluded. Treatment of chronic gastric emptying disorders is often difficult.

II. **Diagnosis.** Symptoms include nausea, bloating, early satiety, and vomiting. Delayed gastric emptying can be diagnosed by having the patient ingest a radiolabeled solid meal followed by scintigraphic analysis to determine rates of emptying.

III. **Therapy.** Patients should avoid high-fat, high-fiber meals. In severe cases, high-calorie, liquid iso-osmotic meals may be used. Prokinetic agents such as metoclopramide and cisapride have been used with some success. Metoclopramide can be used in dosages of up to 10 mg PO qid. Its efficacy in chronic gastroparesis is variable, and side effects, including dyskinesias and drowsiness, may occur.

Cisapride, 10–20 mg PO ac and hs, may also be effective. Erythromycin, 250 mg PO tid or 200 mg IV, stimulates gastric motility (*N Engl J Med* 322:1028, 1990), but its long-term efficacy remains to be established.

Gastrointestinal Bleeding

Treatment of acute GI bleeding must begin with initial resuscitation and stabilization of the patient. During this time, a history and physical examination can be performed. **Maintaining adequate circulatory volume is essential so that the bleeding site can be localized and definitive therapy can be instituted.** Risk factors for increased morbidity and mortality include (1) age greater than 60 years, (2) more than one comorbid illness, (3) severe blood loss (>5 units), (4) shock (on admission), (5) bright red hematemesis with hypotension, (6) large (>2 cm) ulcers, (7) recurrent hemorrhage (within 72 hours), and (8) emergency surgery.

I. **Evaluation and treatment of the unstable patient**
   A. **Initial evaluation.** A rapid assessment to identify patients requiring urgent intervention should be performed. **Signs of distress** (including confusion, obtundation, diaphoresis, clammy or mottled skin, and hypotension) indicate the need for urgent intervention. **In the hemodynamically compromised patient, resuscitation should be instituted concomitantly with initial assessment.**
      1. **Intravascular volume and hemodynamic status should be assessed immediately. Vital signs** (heart rate, BP, and postural changes) are crucial in the evaluation and management of significant bleeding; they **must be obtained reliably and frequently.** A sudden increase in pulse rate or a change in postural BP is often the only early indication of recurrent bleeding. The physician must also be aware of medications (e.g., beta-adrenergic antagonists) and medical conditions (e.g., autonomic dysfunction) that may alter interpretation of hemodynamic data. **Postural hypotension** (supine to upright fall in systolic BP of >10 mm Hg or increase in heart rate of >20 beats/minute) indicates moderate blood loss (10–20% of circulatory volume). **Supine hypotension** suggests severe blood loss (usually >20% of circulatory volume). Further blood loss results in **shock** with hypotension, tachycardia, peripheral vasoconstriction, diaphoresis, and **ischemic organ damage** (e.g., myocardial ischemia, confusion, or decreased urine output) and requires rapid restoration of circulatory volume and admission to an intensive care unit (ICU) (see Chap. 9). **Evidence of continued blood loss,** including recurrent hematemesis, hematochezia, melena, or changing vital signs, requires rapid initiation of therapy and close monitoring to assess the response to treatment.
      2. **Laboratory evaluation.** Blood specimens for typing and cross-matching, CBC, platelet count, prothrombin time (PT), activated partial thromboplastin time (aPTT), and chemistries should be obtained (see sec. II.C). The hemoglobin and hematocrit are poor indicators of acute blood loss. They may be normal initially despite considerable blood loss and may take hours to equilibrate. BP, pulse, and overt bleeding are better indicators of continued blood loss.
   B. **Therapy** should be instituted as soon as a hemodynamically compromised patient is identified.
      1. **Restoration of intravascular volume** should begin immediately. **Two large-bore IV lines** should be established with 14- to 18-gauge catheters in large peripheral veins. Central venous catheterization offers no advantage over good peripheral access and may delay volume infusion. Isotonic saline, lactated Ringer's solution, or 5% hetastarch (Hespan) can be used until blood products are available. When possible, blood should be used to replace volume in patients with hemorrhagic shock. **Vasopressors are generally not indicated, because hypovolemia is usually the cause of the hypotension** (*Gastro Clin North Am* 22:723, 1993). **The rate of volume infusion** should be guided by the patient's condition and the rate and degree of volume loss

suspected. Patients in shock may require fluids or blood to be "pumped" or hand-infused with large syringes and stopcocks. The blood bank must be notified of the potential demand for blood products. Six units of packed red blood cells (PRBCs) should be available at all times until the patient's condition has stabilized. In some situations, O-negative blood, simultaneous multiple-unit infusions, or transient IV pressor therapy may be necessary (see Chap. 9).

2. **Transfusion therapy** (see Chap. 18). Blood transfusion should be initiated as soon as it is evident that the patient's bleeding is massive, ongoing, or severe enough that colloid replacement alone will not result in adequate circulatory volume and tissue oxygenation. Packed RBC transfusion should be continued until the patient is hemodynamically stable and the hematocrit remains at 25% or greater. **Patients with cardiac or pulmonary disease** may require transfusion to a higher hematocrit ($\geq 30\%$) to prevent ischemia. If active bleeding persists, transfusion therapy must continue to keep pace with ongoing losses until hemostasis is achieved. **Coagulopathy** should be corrected with fresh-frozen plasma (FFP). Initially, 4 units of FFP can be given. Further therapy should be based on clinical assessment. **Thrombocytopenia** with platelet counts of less than 50,000/mm^3 should be corrected with platelet transfusions (see Chap. 18) or with therapy directed at the cause of thrombocytopenia. Patients who require massive transfusions (>3,000 ml) should receive warmed blood to prevent hypothermia. Rarely, hypocalcemia caused by chelating agents in the transfused blood may occur. These complications should be recognized and corrected.

3. **Endotracheal intubation** (see Chap. 9) to prevent aspiration should be considered if diminished mental status from shock or hepatic encephalopathy, massive hematemesis, or active variceal hemorrhage is present. Supplemental oxygen by nasal cannula may be of benefit in selected patients with poor oxygenation.

4. **Central venous monitoring** (see Chap. 9) may be necessary for patients with known or suspected cardiovascular disease. However, this monitoring should not interfere with the primary objective of restoring circulatory volume.

5. **Early consultation** with a gastroenterologist, surgeon, or invasive radiologist is appropriate when significant hemorrhage, continued instability, or active bleeding occurs.

II. **Evaluation and treatment of the stable patient**
A. **History.** Symptoms at presentation may help the physician to differentiate upper from lower GI (LGI) bleeding. **Hematemesis** virtually ensures a UGI source of bleeding. A nasopharyngeal source should be excluded in all patients with hematemesis. Pain may help localize a bleeding source or suggest other diagnostic considerations (e.g., hematobilia, bowel infarction). Medical history should be noted, including (1) prior bleeding episodes, (2) alcohol use, (3) liver disease, (4) coagulation disorders or bleeding tendencies, (5) systemic disease associated with GI lesions, (6) abdominal surgery, (7) trauma, or (8) previous aortic vascular surgery. Medications that may exacerbate or cause GI bleeding, including aspirin-containing preparations, NSAIDs, and glucocorticoids, should also be noted.

B. **Physical examination** may help identify the source of bleeding. Evidence of cirrhosis, cancer, hereditary vascular anomalies, or portal hypertension (e.g., splenomegaly, ascites, and dilated abdominal wall collateral vessels) should be noted. **The digital rectal examination** should include a careful inspection for masses and hemorrhoids, inspection of stool for gross blood, and testing of stool for the presence of occult blood. Often the color and consistency of the stool will help direct further evaluation. **Melena**, a black, sticky stool with a characteristic odor, usually indicates bleeding proximal to the cecum. **Maroon stool** may be seen when the bleeding site is located in the distal small bowel or right colon. **Bright red blood** without a change in vital signs or hematocrit suggests an anorectal or left colonic source. However, brisk upper tract bleeding may present with red blood from the rectum.

C. **Laboratory testing** is appropriate in all patients.
   1. **Complete blood count.** The hemoglobin and hematocrit may not accurately reflect the degree of blood loss in acute bleeding because of the delay in equilibration. It is essential to follow the hematocrit in hospitalized individuals to assess the need for and response to transfusion therapy. In general the hematocrit should increase by approximately 3% for each unit of packed RBCs transfused. Frequent monitoring of the hematocrit (e.g., q6h) is advised in the actively bleeding patient.
   2. **Platelet counts** should be measured in all patients with GI bleeding. Patients with active bleeding and a platelet count of less than 50,000/mm^3 should receive platelet transfusion or other therapy to increase the platelet count (see Chap. 18).
   3. **The prothrombin time and partial thromboplastin time** should be measured in all patients. Patients with active bleeding and a prolonged PT or aPTT should receive FFP (see Chap. 17). In the stable patient, correction of a prolonged PT can be attempted with parenteral aqueous vitamin K (menadiol, 10 mg IV or SC qd, or phytonadione, 10 mg SC qd, for 3 days).
D. **Nasogastric tube placement.** Hematemesis or a bloody aspirate obtained through an NG tube indicates UGI bleeding proximal to the jejunum.
   1. **Gastric aspirate.** A gastric aspirate should be considered positive only if it contains a significant amount of fresh blood or is very dark and strongly positive for occult blood. A bloody gastric aspirate is usually associated with an identifiable UGI tract bleeding site. Testing for occult blood is rarely necessary. **A hemoccult-positive gastric aspirate alone without gross blood or "coffee ground" appearance does not indicate a UGI source of bleeding.** False-negative aspirates may occur if the tube is coiled in the fundus of the stomach, the bleeding is intermittent, or there is a lack of reflux of blood through the pylorus from a duodenal bleeding site. If there is any clinical suspicion of a UGI bleeding source in a patient with hematochezia, an NG tube should be placed.
   2. **Gastric lavage** with an Ewald tube and room-temperature water (or saline) can be used to assess the rate of blood loss in a patient with bright red blood from an NG tube. **The use of iced saline or levarterenol for lavage is of no benefit.** Unless the patient has an obstruction or is suffering from protracted nausea and vomiting, the NG tube can be removed after a diagnostic aspirate is obtained. Recurrent bleeding can be detected by following vital signs, stool appearance, and hematocrit. In addition, an indwelling NG tube can lead to mucosal damage, promote reflux esophagitis, and increase the risk of aspiration.

Upper Gastrointestinal Bleeding

I. **Diagnosis.** Many lesions can lead to UGI tract blood loss (Table 15-3). Hematemesis, melena, a positive NG aspirate, or other history and physical findings may suggest a UGI source of bleeding. The approach to the patient with UGI bleeding depends on the patient's stability, the rate of blood loss, procedural availability, and local expertise. Frequent assessment and treatment of the patient to ensure stability is mandatory during the diagnostic evaluation.
A. **Esophagogastroduodenoscopy (EGD)** is the preferred method of examination of patients with suspected UGI bleeding. This test can be performed at the patient's bedside with high diagnostic accuracy and low morbidity. To effectively diagnose patients, endoscopy should be performed as soon as is reasonably possible (e.g., within 24 hours). Although early diagnostic endoscopy has not been shown to improve mortality, therapeutic endoscopy may reduce transfusion requirements, the length of hospitalization, and the need for emergency surgery (*N Engl J Med* 325:1142, 1991). EGD is indicated for identifying the site of

Table 15-3. Diagnosis at endoscopy for upper gastrointestinal bleeding in 482 patients

Diagnosis*	Patients (no.)	Prevalence (%)
Duodenal ulcer	99	21
Gastric ulcer	96	20
Erosive gastritis	63	13
Esophageal varices	50	10
Angiodysplasia (gastric and duodenal)	34	7
Erosive esophagitis	30	6
Mallory-Weiss tear	26	5
Pyloric channel ulcer	10	2
Gastric tumor	9	2
Erosive duodenitis	7	1
Anastomotic ulcer	4	0.8
Aortoenteric fistula	2	0.4
Metastatic tumor, duodenum	2	0.4
Gastric polyps	1	0.2
Schönlein-Henoch syndrome	1	0.2
Rendu-Osler-Weber syndrome	1	0.2
Blood seen but no lesion identified	15	3
No potential bleeding lesion seen or normal examination findings	50	10

* Some patients had more than one diagnosis.
Source: Reproduced with permission from: GR Zuckerman et al. Upper gastrointestinal bleeding in patients with chronic renal failure. *Ann Intern Med* 102:588, 1985.

bleeding before implementing potentially hazardous therapy such as esophageal balloon tamponade (see sec. II.B.3).

  B. **Arteriography.** When bleeding is so brisk that the GI tract cannot be adequately examined by endoscopy, selective abdominal angiography may localize the site of hemorrhage. However, diagnostic success is likely only when the rate of bleeding is greater than 0.5 ml/minute at the time of the study. Arteriography may be both diagnostic and therapeutic (see sec. II.A.3).

  C. **Upper GI barium radiography** has no role in the initial evaluation of active GI bleeding when endoscopy is available. Barium studies may identify mucosal lesions but cannot localize active bleeding. Furthermore, barium may subsequently interfere with both endoscopic and arteriographic studies.

II. **Therapy of specific lesions.** Although nearly 85% of bleeding episodes resolve with supportive therapy alone, surgical consultation should be obtained early in the management of patients with active GI bleeding.

  A. **Peptic ulcers** are the most common cause of UGI bleeding.

    1. **Therapeutic endoscopy**, when available, offers the advantage of immediate treatment at the time of diagnosis.

    2. **Surgery** is considered the therapy of choice for intractable or recurrent bleeding from peptic ulcer disease. In the patient with exsanguinating hemorrhage, it may be necessary to proceed directly to the operating suite, with resuscitation and endoscopy being completed in this setting. Surgical therapy for PUD should be considered in the situations described below.

      a. **Severe hemorrhage** with significant transfusion requirements (e.g., >5 units in 24 hours) and continued circulatory instability. The overall assessment of the patient and continued hemodynamic instability are of greater concern than exceeding an arbitrary number of transfused units.

      b. **Recurrent bleeding** after nonsurgical management requiring additional transfusion during the same hospitalization.

      c. **Difficulty obtaining sufficient compatible blood.**

    3. **Arterial angiotherapy** can be used to control massive bleeding in those

patients with peptic ulcer disease who are considered at high surgical risk. This therapy requires a skilled interventional radiologist who can perform selective arterial catheterization.

   a. **Arterial vasopressin, 0.15–0.20 units/minute, controls bleeding in some patients with stress ulcers, gastritis, and peptic ulcers.** This therapy requires selective catheterization of the bleeding artery and continuous infusion of vasopressin. The infusion is titrated to control bleeding while minimizing side effects such as bradycardia, myocardial ischemia, and abdominal pain. Patients with known **coronary artery disease** are at **increased risk** for complications from the systemic effects of vasopressin. (see sec. **II.B.2**).

   b. **Arterial embolization,** an alternative to arterial vasopressin, also requires selective arterial catheterization. Absorbable gelatin powder (Gelfoam) particles, metal coil springs, or other agents can be placed in the bleeding vessel to produce immediate occlusion of the vessel. The success rate for hemostasis depends on the location and type of lesion. Most complications occur in patients with previous gastric surgery or diffuse vascular disease.

   4. **H₂ antagonists** are not effective in stopping active UGI bleeding. The efficacy of these agents in reducing the incidence of recurrent hemorrhage during the hospitalization of patients with GI bleeding remains unproved (*Am J Med* 76:361, 1984).

B. **Esophageal variceal hemorrhage** is a medical emergency associated with high morbidity and mortality. As many as one-third of these patients die during initial hospitalization. The etiology and severity of the patient's portal hypertension are the major determinants of long-term survival. **ICU** admission should be considered for all patients with known or suspected varices who have active GI bleeding. **Endotracheal intubation** to protect the airway and prevent aspiration may be necessary. Following stabilization, **early endoscopy** should be performed to confirm the bleeding site. Some patients with suspected variceal bleeding do not have varices or are bleeding from another source (*N Engl J Med* 320:1393, 1989). If the diagnosis of variceal hemorrhage is confirmed and active bleeding persists, several therapeutic options exist (*N Engl J Med* 320:1393, 1989, and 320:1469, 1989).

   1. **Endoscopic sclerotherapy** can be performed at the patient's bedside as soon as the diagnosis of variceal bleeding is confirmed. Sclerotherapy is effective for controlling primary hemorrhage and for the obliteration of varices after the initial bleeding episode but is associated with significant complications (*Am J Gastroenterol* 82:823, 1987). **Recurrent bleeding** occurs in up to 50% of patients who undergo a course of sclerotherapy. Usually, this bleeding is not massive and can be controlled with further sclerotherapy. Bleeding that cannot be controlled with repeat injections should be managed with another form of therapy. **Other complications** include ulcerations, strictures, perforation, and sepsis. **Fever** occurs in up to 40% of patients within the first 48 hours following therapy. Patients with persistent fever after 2 days should be carefully evaluated, as bacteremia may occur during the procedure. **Pulmonary complications** are also common and include abnormal chest radiographs, pleural effusions, and adult respiratory distress syndrome (ARDS). Sclerotherapy of esophageal varices may be most helpful in (1) actively bleeding patients as primary therapy or as a stabilizing measure before shunt or transplant surgery, (2) patients who are not surgical candidates, and (3) patients in whom other forms of therapy have failed. Sclerotherapy is not usually effective for bleeding gastric varices (*Gastrointest Endosc* 32:264, 1986). Early studies using **endoscopic variceal ligation, or banding,** suggest that this type of therapy is as effective as sclerotherapy. It is not available in the United States (*Gastrointest Endosc* 35:431, 1989).

   2. **IV vasopressin** is also used to control variceal hemorrhage, but it is less effective than sclerotherapy. Nevertheless, ready availability, ease of administration, and the potential for success make it a reasonable alternative when

other therapies are not available. **A standard formulation** is 100 units of vasopressin in 250 ml of 5% dextrose in water (0.4 units/ml) delivered by a microdrip infusion pump into a central or peripheral vein on the following schedule: 0.3 units/minute for 30 minutes, followed by increments of 0.3 units/minute every 30 minutes until hemostasis is achieved, side effects develop, or the maximum dosage of 0.9 units/minute is reached (*Hepatology* 6:523, 1986). Once bleeding is controlled, the infusion rate should be gradually reduced. IV vasopressin is as effective as intraarterial vasopressin, with fewer side effects. **Significant complications** include myocardial ischemia and MI, ventricular arrhythmias, cardiac arrest, mesenteric ischemia or infarction, and cutaneous ischemic necrosis. **Vasopressin should be used with extreme caution in patients with vascular disease or coronary artery disease.** All patients should be admitted to an ICU and have cardiac monitoring. The infusion should be reduced or terminated if chest pain, abdominal pain, or arrhythmias develop. **Concomitant IV infusion of nitroglycerin** may reduce undesirable cardiovascular side effects of vasopressin therapy (*Hepatology* 6:406, 1986); its use should be considered in all patients with a history of coronary artery or vascular disease. Nitroglycerin is administered only if the systolic BP is greater than 100 mm Hg. A reasonable dose is 10 µg/minute IV, increased by 10 µg/minute every 10–15 minutes until the systolic BP falls to 100 mm Hg or a maximum dosage of 400 µg/minute is reached (*Hepatology* 6:410, 1986). **IV octreotide acetate (a somatostatin analog)** has been used to reduce portal hypertension in patients with acute variceal hemorrhage and may offer efficacy similar to vasopressin infusion with fewer side effects (*Lancet* 342:637, 1993).

3. **Balloon tamponade** is effective in temporizing variceal bleeding while awaiting more definitive therapy. Several different types of tubes are available: The **Sengstaken-Blakemore tube** and the **Minnesota tube** have both a gastric and esophageal balloon and the **Linton tube** has a large-volume gastric balloon without an esophageal balloon. **These tubes should be used according to the manufacturer's specific directions** for placement, traction, and balloon volume, and with the aid of personnel experienced in the use of such equipment. Balloon tamponade is associated with a high rate of major complications and mortality from tube displacement (*Dig Dis Sci* 34:913, 1989). In patients who are bleeding from gastric varices, the Linton tube may offer better control of hemorrhage than the Sengstaken-Blakemore tube. Guidelines for the use of balloon tamponade are provided below.

   a. **ICU admission** is necessary to ensure careful and frequent monitoring of the patient's condition.

   b. **Prophylactic endotracheal intubation** is often necessary, because aspiration and asphyxiation are major causes of mortality related to balloon tamponade.

   c. **The site of bleeding** should be confirmed by endoscopy, and tube selection should be made with respect to the bleeding site.

   d. **Modification of the Sengstaken-Blakemore tube** by the attachment of an NG tube above the esophageal balloon should be completed before insertion. This NG tube should be connected to high intermittent suction to remove secretions from the patient's posterior pharynx and upper esophagus to help prevent aspiration of oropharyngeal secretions. This tube should be clearly labeled and should not be lavaged.

   e. **Gastric balloon position** should be confirmed by radiography before inflation. Inflating the gastric balloon in the esophagus can result in esophageal rupture.

   f. **All balloon tube outlets** should be clearly labeled, and inflation tubes should be clamped to prevent leakage and migration. Scissors must be kept at the patient's bedside to immediately transect and withdraw the tube if necessary.

   g. **Mucosal ulceration and necrosis** may occur, especially if large balloon volumes, high pressure, or traction are necessary to control bleeding.

Balloon pressure should be reduced intermittently as stated in the manufacturer's instructions and when bleeding has been controlled. The tube, with its balloon deflated, can be left in place so that pressure can be applied again if bleeding resumes.

4. **Surgery** (portacaval or distal splenorenal shunt [DSRS]) controls variceal bleeding in 95% of patients. However, hospital mortality rates are high, and there is a significant incidence of postoperative encephalopathy. The results of surgery for portal hypertension and variceal bleeding depend on the patient's preoperative Child's classification, since the underlying liver disease remains the major factor limiting survival (*Ann Surg* 202:729, 1985). **In patients with good hepatic reserve,** shunts should be considered if the patient (1) fails sclerotherapy, (2) is unable to return for follow-up visits, (3) is at high risk of death from recurrent bleeding because of cardiac disease or difficulty in obtaining blood products, or (4) lives far from medical care. Sclerotherapy with salvage shunt surgery for failures may be superior to DSRS alone (*Ann Intern Med* 112:262, 1990).

5. **Transjugular intrahepatic portosystemic shunt (TIPS)** is a radiologic alternative to a surgical shunt. An expandable metal stent is placed between the hepatic veins and the portal vein. TIPS effectively decompresses the portal vein and is used for patients who fail sclerotherapy, have gastric variceal bleeding, or are poor surgical candidates (*Radiology* 187:413, 1993).

6. **Propranolol and nadolol** in dosages sufficient to reduce the resting heart rate by 25% are effective in preventing variceal bleeding in patients with large varices and in preventing recurrent variceal bleeding, though no benefit in overall survival has been shown (*Ann Intern Med* 117:59, 1992).

7. **Hepatic transplantation** in selected patients can reverse portal hypertension and esophageal and gastric variceal hemorrhage.

8. **Other aggressive surgical procedures,** such as transection of the esophagus, have been used when other attempts to arrest variceal hemorrhage have failed.

C. **Mallory-Weiss tear** is a mucosal tear at the gastroesophageal junction. Patients may have a history of retching or emesis followed by hematemesis. Most patients with a Mallory-Weiss tear stop bleeding spontaneously and seldom have recurrent bleeding. Some patients require therapeutic endoscopic techniques (see sec. **II.A.1**) or arterial angiotherapy (see sec. **II.A.3**) to control the bleeding.

D. **Aortoenteric fistula** is an uncommon but often lethal cause of UGI bleeding. Many patients have a history of prior aortic graft surgery. Patients may present 2 months to 8 years after surgery, with the average onset of symptoms occurring at just over 4 years. The fistula is aortoduodenal in more than 90% of cases. The classic presentation is with a **"herald" bleed** hours to weeks before massive GI hemorrhage. Recognition of this syndrome is essential, as undiagnosed aortoenteric fistulas almost always result in death. In patients at risk, **endoscopy should be performed** immediately, including examination to the fourth portion of the duodenum. If bleeding is massive, the procedure can be performed in the operating suite. Angiography or CT of the abdomen may demonstrate leakage at the graft site or evidence of prosthesis infection, but surgery should not be delayed by such procedures. All patients with prior aortic graft surgery and GI bleeding should be considered to have an aortoenteric fistula until proved otherwise.

E. **Stress ulceration** is a common cause of GI, bleeding in the ICU patient. **Patients at risk** include those with head injuries, burns, major trauma, shock, sepsis, respiratory failure, coagulopathy, and CNS disease requiring intensive care. **Prophylactic therapy** should be provided for all patients at risk. H_2 antagonists, sucralfate, and antacids are effective in preventing severe bleeding (*Ann Intern Med* 106:562, 1987).

F. **Angiodysplasia** of the stomach or small intestine is increasingly recognized as a cause of occult or recurrent GI bleeding and may present with gross bleeding. Renal failure is an important predisposing factor. These mucosal lesions are frequently multiple. Some patients have associated colonic angiodysplasia. The lesions of the UGI tract are most often diagnosed by endoscopy. Actively bleeding lesions can be treated by therapeutic endoscopy. Combined estrogen and progesterone therapy decreases bleeding episodes and transfusion requirements (*Lancet* 335:953, 1990). Although the natural history of this lesion is one of recurrent bleeding and transfusions, the mortality rate is low.

G. **Other causes** of UGI bleeding include gastritis, esophagitis, and malignancy. **Hematobilia** (bleeding into the biliary tree) is a rare cause of GI bleeding that is often associated with jaundice or biliary colic at the time of active bleeding.

Lower Gastrointestinal Bleeding

Common causes of LGI bleeding include diverticulosis, angiodysplasia, neoplasm, inflammatory bowel disease, ischemic colitis, infectious colitis, and anorectal diseases. Brisk UGI or small intestinal bleeding can also mimic LGI bleeding. As with UGI bleeding, LGI hemorrhage will stop spontaneously in many cases. Patients with LGI bleeding should be stabilized and supported while diagnostic studies are performed.

I. **Diagnosis**
   A. **Rectal examination** and anoscopy, proctoscopy, or sigmoidoscopy should be performed to search for a rectal source of bleeding. A rectal source can be diagnosed only if an actively bleeding lesion is seen.
   B. **Technetium-99m labeled red blood cell scanning** (^{99m}Tc RBC scan) should be performed in patients who are thought to have an active LGI bleed, after a UGI bleed has been excluded. Bleeding rates as low as 0.1 ml/minute can be detected and delayed images can be obtained if recurrent bleeding is suspected. If the scan is positive, further localization and therapy with arteriography may be helpful; if the scan is negative, the patient should undergo colonoscopy.
   C. **Arteriography**, which can detect arterial bleeding rates of 0.5 ml/minute, is the best initial test if hemodynamic stability is difficult to maintain because of brisk bleeding. This test allows rapid localization and potential treatment of bleeding lesions.
   D. **Colonoscopy** should be utilized in all patients who can be prepared for endoscopic examination with standard oral lavage. If ^{99m}Tc RBC scanning or arteriography is negative, patients should undergo colonoscopy for definitive evaluation. Colonoscopy allows identification of angiodysplasia, tissue diagnosis of mass lesions, and therapeutic intervention with electrocautery, heater probe, or laser therapy for active bleeding.
   E. **Patients with suspected LGI bleeding** who have no site of blood loss identified on initial studies should be **further evaluated.** Sources of blood loss in the UGI tract and small bowel should be considered. If GI bleeding has ceased and an evaluation, including ^{99m}Tc RBC scan, upper and lower endoscopy, and small-bowel radiographs or endoscopy, does not reveal a potential bleeding site, the patient can be discharged and told to report to the hospital as soon as bleeding recurs. At that time, an immediate ^{99m}Tc RBC scan may localize a bleeding site.
   F. **Hemoccult-positive stool** is often caused by GI blood loss. False-positive results from peroxidase in foods (e.g., broccoli, turnips, radishes, and rare roast beef) can occur. Patients older than age 40 with Hemoccult-positive stool require evaluation of their entire colon with colonoscopy or flexible sigmoidoscopy plus air-contrast barium enema (*Gastroenterology* 92:682, 1987, and 98:855, 1990).
   G. **Idiopathic iron-deficiency anemia** is often caused by GI bleeding (*N Engl J Med* 329:1691, 1993). The initial endoscopic procedure performed should be guided by the patient's symptoms.
II. **Therapy of specific lesions**
   A. **Diverticular hemorrhage** is the most common cause of major LGI bleeding, but it occurs in less than 5% of patients with diverticulosis. Bleeding persists in 20% of patients, and recurrent bleeding is common. In patients with persistent

Table 15-4. Representative dosages for agents used in the management of patients with malabsorption syndromes

Calcium: Normal replacement is 1–2 g/day; calcium carbonate may be given as Titralac (400 mg Ca^{2+}/5 ml) or Os-Cal (250 or 500 mg Ca^{2+}/tablet).

Magnesium: Magnesium gluconate, 500 mg qid (each tablet contains 29 mg of magnesium).

Iron: Ferrous sulfate, one 320-mg tablet qid; each tablet contains 64 mg of iron.

Fat-soluble vitamins

    Vitamin A: 25,000-unit tablets; for severe deficiency, 25,000–100,000 units/day; maintenance is 3,000–5,000 units/day.

    Vitamin D: Initial dosage is 50,000 units 2–3 times weekly; dosage varies considerably based on response as determined by serum and urine calcium.

    Vitamin K: Vitamin K_1 (water-miscible), 10 mg PO or IM qd, or vitamin K_3 water-soluble vitamins (menadione), 10 mg PO qd.

    Folic acid: 1–5 mg PO qd for 4–5 weeks is adequate to replenish stores and correct anemia; maintenance dosage is 1 mg PO qd.

    Vitamin B_{12}: 100–1,000 µg/day IM for 2 weeks as a loading dose (if required); maintenance dosage is 1,000 µg/month.

    Vitamin B complex: Any multivitamin preparation that contains daily requirements (thiamine 1.6 mg, riboflavin 1.8 mg, niacin 20 mg) should be administered twice daily.

---

bleeding, selective arterial vasopressin (see Upper Gastrointestinal Bleeding, sec. **II.A.3**) is often effective. Surgery may be necessary in patients with recurrent or extremely brisk bleeding or patients who fail vasopressin therapy because of continued bleeding or complications (e.g., myocardial ischemia).

B. Angiodysplasia of the colon may cause acute or chronic LGI bleeding. It is a common finding in elderly patients. The colonic lesions are usually found in the cecum and right colon. Bleeding lesions can be treated with intraarterial vasopressin, heater probe, laser therapy, or surgical resection.

Malabsorption and Maldigestion

I. **Diagnosis.** Malabsorption of macronutrients (especially fat) should be considered in patients with unexplained weight loss, steatorrhea, or biochemical abnormalities consistent with malabsorption. Fat malabsorption is suggested by clinical history and qualitative stool fat determination by Sudan black fat staining and is confirmed by quantitative 72-hour fecal fat determination. For an accurate 72-hour fecal fat measurement, the patient should be given a fixed fat (usually 100 g/day) diet beginning 24 hours **before** the stool collection starts. More than 6 g of fat in the stool per day is consistent with malabsorption. The D-xylose absorption and bentiromide (Chymex) tests are screening studies for the presence of diffuse small-bowel mucosal disease (malabsorption) and pancreatic exocrine insufficiency (maldigestion) (see Pancreatitis, sec. **II.B**), respectively. Serum calcium and magnesium levels should be measured. In diseases of the ileum, bile acids and vitamin B_{12} are not absorbed normally. Malabsorption of fat-soluble vitamins may also occur and may require replacement therapy (Table 15-4).

II. **Specific disorders.** Barium radiographs of the small bowel may be abnormal in Crohn's disease, celiac sprue, blind loop syndrome, amyloidosis, and multiple jejunal diverticulosis. **Small-bowel biopsy** is helpful in many kinds of diffuse small intestinal disease, including celiac sprue, giardiasis, Whipple's disease, and lymphangiectasia.

    A. Celiac sprue (gluten-sensitive enteropathy). Patients with celiac disease are sensitive to gluten, a group of proteins present in wheat, barley, rye, and possibly oats. Antigliadin antibodies are found in many patients. Biopsy of the small intestine reveals complete absence of villi; this test is the gold standard for diagnosis. Patients have a clinical and histologic response to a gluten-free diet (see *Gourmet Food on a Wheat-Free Diet.* Springfield, IL: Thomas, 1972). Because of the implications of lifelong therapy, diagnosis should always be confirmed by biopsy. Patients with sprue also commonly have **secondary lactase deficiency** and should eat a lactose-free diet until the small bowel recovers. Patients may require iron, folate, calcium, or vitamin supplements (see Table 15-4). In severely symptomatic or refractory patients, a trial of prednisone, 10–20 mg PO qd, may be effective. The most common cause of continued or worsening symptoms in celiac disease is dietary indiscretion. Sprue is associated with an increased incidence of small-bowel lymphoma; patients who decompensate despite adherence to dietary restriction should be evaluated by barium study or abdominal CT.

B. **Lactose intolerance** is caused by a selective deficiency of lactase. It is present in 70–90% of adult blacks, Asians, and American Indians and in 20% of caucasians. Undigested lactose in the bowel lumen results in osmotic diarrhea. Symptoms consist of abdominal cramps, flatulence, and diarrhea associated with ingestion of dairy products. Temporary lactase deficiency may occur with other small-bowel illnesses such as viral and bacterial enteritis and Crohn's disease. Dietary restriction of milk products is usually sufficient for diagnosis and treatment. Rarely, the diagnosis will need to be confirmed with a hydrogen breath test or lactose tolerance test. Some patients retain enough lactase to tolerate small amounts of dietary lactose (as in highly processed cheese such as cheddar, parmesan, and Roquefort). Yogurt is generally well tolerated. Therapy with enzyme products such as Lactaid liquid or tablets or lactase capsules (2–4 tablets or capsules with each lactose meal) is available.

C. **Bacterial overgrowth** of the small intestine can result from any condition that causes intestinal stasis, including jejunal diverticulosis, scleroderma, afferent loop obstruction of a Billroth II anastomosis, or partial small-bowel obstruction. Deconjugation of bile salts by the excess bacteria causes fat malabsorption. The bacteria may also have a direct toxic effect on the mucosa and can compete for available vitamin B_{12} in the intestine, leading to megaloblastic anemia. The diagnosis of bacterial overgrowth is usually made by history and radiography. **Treatment** with broad-spectrum antimicrobials such as tetracycline, 250 mg PO qid, or amoxicillin/clavulanate, 250–500 mg PO tid (*Adv Intern Med* 38:387, 1993), is helpful. For long-term therapy, antimicrobials usually should be given intermittently (e.g., for 2 weeks out of each month). Surgical correction of the intestinal abnormality may be indicated in certain disorders.

D. **Ileal resection.** Bile salts and vitamin B_{12} are absorbed in the terminal ileum. Loss of more than 50 cm of terminal ileum (as in Crohn's disease) will lead to malabsorption of bile salts; a greater loss may result in malabsorption of vitamin B_{12}. Unabsorbed bile salts pass into the colon and produce a secretory diarrhea in some patients (see Diarrhea, sec. **II.B.2**).

1. **Cholestyramine,** 4 g PO qid, controls diarrhea in these patients by binding bile salts in the intestinal lumen. Loss of more than 100 cm of ileum may result in loss of enough bile salts to produce fat malabsorption. Diarrhea in these patients may be caused by the effects of hydroxy fatty acids on colonic mucosa and may be aggravated by cholestyramine; it will improve with a low-fat diet.

2. **Low-fat diets** (50–75 g/day of fat) will often reduce steatorrhea in patients with ileal resections of greater than 100 cm and will provide a tolerable diet. Diets containing less than 25 g/day of fat, however, are often unpalatable and make it difficult for patients to maintain adequate calories. Medium-chain triglycerides (MCTs), which do not require digestion or solubilization by bile salts, can be used as an additional source of fat in patients with significant fat malabsorption. Although MCT oil is relatively unpalatable, recipe books are available. About 3–4 tablespoons/day (14 g of fat/tablespoon) can be ingested

as MCTs. Larger amounts of MCTs cause diarrhea. Patients with ileal resection and fat malabsorption often require fat-soluble vitamin and calcium supplements in addition to parenteral vitamin B_{12} (see Table 15-4).

E. **Giardiasis** rarely leads to malabsorption in immunocompetent persons but may be present in the intestine of hypogammaglobulinemic patients and is a cause of malabsorption in this group (see Diarrhea, sec. **I.B.2**).

Inflammatory Bowel Disease

I. **Ulcerative colitis** is an idiopathic chronic inflammatory disease of the colon and rectum characterized by remissions and exacerbations. The predominant symptom is **bloody diarrhea.** Proctoscopy is the most important examination for establishing the diagnosis and following the course of therapy, as rectal involvement is essentially universal. Infectious etiologies should be excluded. A barium enema is useful in determining the extent of involvement but can exacerbate the disease and should never be performed during an acute episode. Patients with frequent relapses despite treatment or with fulminant disease will often require surgery. Total proctocolectomy is curative. One of the major risks of long-standing ulcerative colitis is the development of **colon cancer.**

A. **Medical therapy** (*Am J Med* 93:199, 1992) (Table 15-5)

1. **Sulfasalazine** is useful for treatment of mild acute exacerbations and as maintenance therapy for prolonging remission. The intact drug reaches the colon, where it is metabolized to a sulfapyridine moiety (responsible for most of the toxicity) and 5-aminosalicylate (5-ASA), the active component.

a. **Dosage** (see Table 15-5). For patients with active disease, the recommended starting dosage is 0.5 g PO bid, slowly advancing as tolerated to 0.5–1.0 g PO qid. The usual maintenance dosage is 1 g PO bid.

b. **Side effects** include headache, nausea, vomiting, and abdominal pain. These effects are dose-related and are more common in patients treated with 4 g/day or more. Patients who suffer from side effects should have the drug stopped briefly, but it may be restarted at a dosage of 500–1,000 mg/d. **Hypersensitivity reactions** occur less frequently and include skin rash, fever, agranulocytosis, hepatotoxicity, and aplastic anemia. Reintroduction at a very low dose (0.125–0.250 g/day) for a week with increases of 0.125 g/day each week until a dosage of 2 g/day is achieved (*J Clin Gastroenterol* 6:27, 1984) may be considered for patients with rash, but **the drug should be discontinued in patients with more serious hypersensitivity reactions.** Rarely, paradoxic exacerbations of colitis have been reported with sulfasalazine. Sulfasalazine reduces sperm counts in men during therapy.

2. **5-Aminosalicylate (5-ASA)** lacks the sulfa moiety of sulfasalazine and is associated with fewer side effects. It can be used in many patients who are intolerant of sulfasalazine. The most common side effect of this drug is diarrhea. **Mesalamine** is a different 5-ASA preparation that can be given orally, as a suppository, or as an enema. Mesalamine enema is effective in patients with left-sided colitis (see Table 15-5). The major side effect is nephrotoxicity.

3. **Glucocorticoids** are beneficial in patients with moderate or severe colonic disease and may be given in conjunction with sulfasalazine. **Extracolonic manifestations,** such as ocular lesions, skin disease, and peripheral arthritis (the activity of which often parallels that of the colonic disease) also usually respond to glucocorticoids. Disease limited to the rectum (**ulcerative proctitis**) is effectively treated with glucocorticoid enemas. More extensive disease should be treated with oral prednisone, 20–40 mg/day, for several weeks. When symptoms lessen and improvement is noted on proctoscopic examination, prednisone can be tapered over 2–3 months and then discontinued.

Table 15-5. Dosing regimens for patients with mild to moderate inflammatory bowel disease

Drug	Route	Ulcerative colitis (active)	Ulcerative colitis (remission)	Crohn's disease (active)	Crohn's disease (remission)
Sulfasalazine	Oral	0.5–1.0 g PO qid[a]	1 g PO bid	1 g PO qid[a]	—[b]
Olsalazine	Oral	—[c]	500 mg PO bid	—[c]	—[c]
Mesalamine (5-ASA)	Oral released at pH >6	800–1,600 mg PO tid	—[c]	—[c]	—[c]
	Oral time and pH released	1 g PO qid	—[c]	—[c]	—[c]
	Suppository[d]	500 mg PR bid	500 mg PR bid	—[c]	—[c]
	Enema[e]	4 g qhs	1 g hs 3 times/week	—[c]	—[c]
4-Aminosalicylic acid	Enema[e]	2 g qhs	—[c]	—[c]	—[c]
Prednisone	Oral	10–40 mg PO qd		10–40 mg PO qd	—[c]
Hydrocortisone	Suppository	1 PR bid	—[c]	—[c]	—[c]
	Enema	1 qhs	—[c]	—[c]	—[c]
	IV	100 mg IV q6h	—[c]	100 mg IV q6h	—[c]
Methylprednisolone	IV	20 mg IV q12h	—[c]	20 mg IV q12h	—[c]
Metronidazole	Oral	—[c]	—[c]	250 mg PO bid–qid	250 mg PO bid

[a]Starting dosage is 500 mg PO bid.
[b]Efficacy not proved for maintaining remission, though often used 1–2 g PO daily in divided doses.
[c]Either not approved for use, not effective, or still untested for this disease.
[d]For rectal effects only.
[e]For left-sided coloric disease.

Sulfasalazine is then slowly tapered to a maintenance dosage (see Table 15-5). If symptoms persist, the patient should be hospitalized and given initial therapy with hydrocortisone, 50–100 mg IV q6h, methylprednisolone, 20–40 mg IV q12h, or an equivalent dosage of glucocorticoid. Methylprednisolone and dexamethasone have fewer side effects than hydrocortisone. Colectomy should be considered if the patient requires more than 15 mg of prednisone daily over a period of many months. If relapse occurs during sulfasalazine maintenance, glucocorticoids in full doses should again be used and gradually tapered when remission is achieved.

   4. **Immunosuppressive agents** such as azathioprine and 6-mercaptopurine (6–MP) (up to 1.5 mg/kg/day PO) have a limited role in the management of ulcerative colitis but may be used in patients who are unresponsive to conventional medical management and who are not surgical candidates. These agents are most commonly used to reduce the maintenance dosage of glucocorticoids in patients who are not surgical candidates or in whom surgery needs to be delayed. **Immunosuppressive agents should be avoided during pregnancy** if possible.

   5. **Anticholinergic and antidiarrheal drugs** are often beneficial in decreasing abdominal pain and diarrhea. Such drugs include tincture of belladonna, tincture of opium, diphenoxylate, and codeine (see Diarrhea, sec. **IV.C**). They are contraindicated in severe exacerbations of disease.

B. **Diet.** Patients whose disease is in remission have no specific dietary restrictions. Occasionally, lactose intolerance may develop. A low-roughage diet often provides symptomatic relief for patients whose disease is in relapse. Elemental diets may be useful during acute phases of the disease (see Chap. 2).

C. **Fulminant disease and toxic megacolon.** An acute fulminant phase occurs in 5–10% of patients and presents with severe diarrhea, abdominal pain, hemorrhage, hypoalbuminemia, fever, sepsis, electrolyte disturbances, and dehydration. **Toxic megacolon,** in which the colon becomes atonic and partially or segmentally dilates, develops in 1–2% of patients with ulcerative colitis. The diagnosis of toxic megacolon is made when the colon is dilated to a diameter of 6 cm or more (measured radiographically at the midtransverse colon) and systemic toxicity is present. Treatment is described below.

   1. **Nasogastric suction** should be started and the patient should be given nothing by mouth. Total parenteral nutrition (TPN) may be necessary (see Chap. 2).

   2. **Dehydration and electrolyte disturbances** should be vigorously treated. Hypokalemia is common and potassium supplementation may be required.

   3. **Parenteral broad-spectrum antimicrobials** for intraabdominal infection should be administered (see Chap. 13).

   4. **Parenteral glucocorticoids** such as hydrocortisone, 100 mg IV q6h, should be given.

   5. **Total colectomy** must be considered for acutely ill patients who do not respond to intensive medical therapy within 48 hours. Early surgical consultation is necessary for these severely ill patients.

   6. **Anticholinergic and opioid drugs should not be used** because they can precipitate or aggravate toxic megacolon.

D. **Cancer in ulcerative colitis.** Patients with pancolitis have a 10% incidence of colon cancer at 10–20 years with an additional 10% incidence for every decade thereafter. Cancer risk is lower in patients with left-sided disease. Surveillance colonoscopies with multiple biopsies are recommended after approximately 8–10 years, especially in patients with pancolitis.

II. **Crohn's disease,** like ulcerative colitis, is marked by remissions and exacerbations. Common presenting symptoms include nonbloody diarrhea, abdominal pain, and weight loss. In contrast to ulcerative colitis, Crohn's disease can affect any portion of the tubular GI tract and therefore cannot be cured with surgical resection. The clinical course of Crohn's disease is often complicated by fistulas, perianal disease, and strictures.

A. **Therapy of uncomplicated Crohn's disease** (see Table 15-5).

1. **Antidiarrheal agents** may be useful as primary therapy in selected patients with mild exacerbations or postresection diarrhea.
2. **Sulfasalazine,** 0.5 g PO bid, slowly increased as tolerated to 0.5–1.0 g PO qid, is effective in the treatment of mild to moderate acute exacerbations of colonic or ileocolic disease, but not in the treatment of disease confined to the small intestine. Sulfasalazine is not of proved efficacy in maintenance of remission in Crohn's disease.
3. **5-ASA preparations.** There are several 5-ASA preparations that are effective in treating small-intestinal as well as colonic Crohn's disease (see Table 15-5). These have become the therapy of choice for patients with Crohn's disease and can be used by many patients who cannot tolerate sulfasalazine. **Olsalazine** requires bacterial cleavage to release the 5-ASA compound and therefore its use is limited to by patients with colonic disease. **Mesalamine** preparations that allow release of drug in the small intestine treat Crohn's disease of the small intestine more effectively.
4. **Glucocorticoids** such as prednisone, 20–40 mg PO qd, are beneficial in acute exacerbations. In more fulminant disease, glucocorticoids should be given parenterally (methylprednisolone, 20–40 mg IV q6h, or the equivalent dose of another glucocorticoid) (see Table 15-5). Glucocorticoids are not usually required for maintenance of remission in Crohn's disease. As in ulcerative colitis, extraintestinal manifestations (eye, skin, and joint diseases) often parallel colonic activity and respond to glucocorticoids.
5. **Immunosuppressive agents** such as 6-MP and azathioprine have a controversial role in the management of active Crohn's disease. They may be used when glucocorticoids have failed or in an attempt to decrease glucocorticoid requirements. Major side effects include bone marrow suppression and pancreatitis. These drugs should be administered only by persons with experience in taking care of complicated Crohn's disease patients; careful monitoring for toxicity is mandatory. Cyclosporine has been used in severe acute exacerbations of Crohn's disease that are unresponsive to standard intensive therapy, but this treatment remains experimental.
6. **Metronidazole,** 250 mg PO tid, has been shown to be as effective as sulfasalazine in colonic Crohn's disease and may be beneficial in selected patients who are unable to tolerate or are unresponsive to other agents. It is **contraindicated in pregnancy.**
7. **Maintenance of adequate nutrition** is essential. Patients with ileitis frequently need parenteral vitamin B_{12} therapy. Specific oral replacement of calcium, magnesium, folate, iron, vitamin D, and other micronutrients may be necessary. In patients with ileal resection or extensive small-bowel Crohn's disease, oxalate nephrolithiasis may occur; treatment consists of a low-fat, low-oxalate, high-calcium diet. In some cases, elemental formulas or parenteral nutrition are necessary (see Chap. 2).
8. **TPN** (see Chap. 2) and bowel rest may be used as primary medical therapy in conjunction with oral medication or as a bridge to surgery.
B. **Therapy for complications of Crohn's disease**
   1. **Perianal disease.** In conjunction with surgical drainage of obvious abscess collections, metronidazole, 250 mg PO or IV tid, is useful in healing active perianal disease. Significant toxicities include possible teratogenicity and peripheral neuropathy with long-term use (see Chap. 12).
   2. **Fistulas** (enterocutaneous, enterovesicular, enterovaginal). Medical management with parenteral nutrition and bowel rest, metronidazole, or 6-MP may be useful in specific circumstances in conjunction with surgical consultation.
   3. **Intestinal obstruction** may occur as a result of stricture formation. Decompression with a nasoenteral tube, parenteral hydration, and glucocorticoids may allow edema and spasm to subside and eliminate the need for surgery. Patients with intermittent obstructive symptoms should avoid highly indigestible foods such as nuts, popcorn, and hard-skinned fruits, which may precipitate obstruction.
C. **Other therapeutic measures.** Surgery is generally reserved for patients with

fistulas, obstruction, abscess, perforation, or bleeding, and rarely for medically refractory disease. Percutaneous abscess drainage and endoscopic balloon dilatation can be useful in selected patients. Efforts should be made to avoid multiple resections because of the risk of producing short-bowel syndrome.

Common Anorectal Problems

I. **Hemorrhoids**
   A. **External thrombosed hemorrhoids** present with a sudden onset of pain. They appear as tense, bluish lumps covered with skin. If pain is severe, relief can be obtained by excision of the thrombosed vein while the patient is under local anesthesia. If the pain is mild or has already started to resolve, the patient can be given oral analgesics, sitz baths (sitting in a tub of warm water), stool softeners, and topical emollients (see sec. I.B).
   B. **Internal hemorrhoids** commonly present with either bleeding or a prolapsing mass. Pain is not common. Prolapsed internal hemorrhoids appear as masses separated by radial folds. The upper portions are covered with red mucosa. Treatment is described below.
      1. **Bulk-forming agents** such as fiber are useful in preventing straining at defecation.
      2. **Sitz baths** taken for 15 minutes twice daily are useful for relief of inflammation and for hygiene. Tucks Pads (cotton soaked in witch hazel) also give symptomatic relief.
      3. **Ointments and suppositories** containing various analgesics, emollients, astringents, and hydrocortisone (e.g., Anusol-HC Suppositories, 1 PR bid for 7–10 days) may give symptomatic relief. Glucocorticoid-containing suppositories should not be used for long-term therapy.
      4. **Surgery** is indicated if medical management fails.
II. **Anal fissures** present with acute onset of pain during defecation and are often caused by the passage of a hard stool. Anoscopy reveals an elliptical tear in the skin of the anus, usually in the posterior midline. Acute fissures usually heal in 2–3 weeks with stool softeners, analgesics, and sitz baths. Chronic fissures require surgical therapy.
III. **Perirectal abscess** commonly presents as a painful induration in the perianal area. Patients with diabetes or inflammatory bowel disease and immunocompromised patients are at high risk. Because of potentially serious morbidity with delayed treatment, **prompt drainage is essential.** Antimicrobials directed against bowel flora should be administered to patients with significant associated cellulitis or systemic toxicity and to diabetic or immunocompromised patients.

Diverticular Disease

I. **Diverticulosis.** The occurrence of diverticula increases markedly with age. Diverticulosis occurs more often in developed nations than in Third World countries, probably because of a highly refined diet that is low in dietary fiber. Most diverticula are asymptomatic and do not require treatment; however, they can be the cause of profuse **lower GI bleeding,** which in most cases resolves spontaneously.
II. **Diverticulitis** is a complication of diverticular disease in which perforation of a diverticulum occurs. Left lower quadrant pain accompanied by fever and chills, alteration of bowel habits, and laboratory evidence of inflammation are the most common manifestations of acute diverticulitis. Plain abdominal x-ray films should be taken to rule out perforation. Occasionally, a left lower quadrant mass may be present. CT scan is useful in making the diagnosis and ruling out abscess formation. Rarely, fistulas to the bladder, vagina, or skin may form from the diseased colon.

Patients ill enough to require hospitalization should be given nothing by mouth. IV fluid replacement is necessary. NG suction should be instituted if there are signs of bowel obstruction. Outpatients should be given a clear liquid diet until the initial symptoms subside. The choice of antimicrobials depends on the severity of the clinical condition. When the inflammatory response is localized, a course of oral ampicillin, a cephalosporin, or a tetracycline derivative may be used. If the patient is systemically ill, broad-spectrum parenteral antimicrobial coverage appropriate for intraabdominal infection is required (see Chap. 13). Surgical consultation is advisable for hospitalized patients, because operative intervention may be required if complications arise. After the acute episode has subsided, dietary bulk supplementation may help to prevent recurrence.

Irritable Bowel Syndrome

Irritable bowel syndrome (IBS) is the most common GI problem seen by physicians. Typically, patients present with long-standing symptoms of crampy abdominal pain, bloating, excessive flatulence, diarrhea, constipation, or alternating diarrhea and constipation. Lactose intolerance should be excluded, as it may have a similar presentation and the two disorders can coexist (see Malabsorption and Maldigestion, sec. **II.B**). Although IBS is ultimately a diagnosis of exclusion, certain features, including stable weight, chronic GI symptoms, and an unrevealing physical examination often allow a presumptive diagnosis and initiation of treatment without extensive diagnostic testing. Associated psychiatric symptoms are often seen. Patients with new onset symptoms or those who fail an initial therapeutic trial should undergo further evaluation. Some patients respond to dietary bulk supplementation as the sole therapeutic maneuver (see Constipation). Anticholinergics are often prescribed for patients with IBS, although there is no proof of their efficacy. Tincture of belladonna, 5–10 drops PO tid ac; hyoscyamine, 0.125 mg SL prn or 0.375 mg PO bid; and dicyclomine, 20 mg PO qid, are commonly used agents. In patients who are unresponsive to these measures or in those with associated psychiatric symptoms, tricyclic antidepressants in low dosage such as amitriptyline, 10–50 mg PO hs; doxepin, 10–50 mg PO hs; or desipramine, 50 mg PO hs (*Dig Dis Sci* 32:257, 1987), can be helpful.

Pancreatitis

I. **Acute pancreatitis** is commonly associated with excessive alcohol consumption or gallstones. Less common causes include hypercalcemia, hypertriglyceridemia, and a variety of drugs. The **Ranson criteria** provide useful prognostic information. Severe illness and increased mortality are associated with age over 55 years, WBC greater than 16,000/mm^3, glucose greater than 200 mg/dl, serum LDH greater than 350 IU/liter, SGOT greater than 250 IU/liter, hematocrit drop of greater than 10%, rise in BUN greater than 5 mg/dl, arterial PO$_2$ less than 60 mm Hg, base deficit greater than 4 mEq/liter, serum calcium less than 8.0 mg/dl, and estimated fluid sequestration greater than 6 liters. Therapy is largely supportive. Specific therapy is reserved for complications.

A. **Supportive treatment.** Narcotic analgesics are necessary for pain relief. Meperidine is most commonly used, as it has no significant effect on the sphincter of Oddi. Patients should receive nothing by mouth until they are free of pain and nausea. NG suction is needed only in patients with protracted nausea and vomiting. **Aggressive volume repletion** with IV fluids is necessary with careful monitoring of fluid balance and awareness of the potential for significant fluid sequestration within the abdomen. Serum calcium, magnesium, and glucose as well as hematocrit should be monitored, and abnormalities should be corrected as necessary. There is no clear role for prophylactic antimicrobial therapy in acute pancreatitis. Although H_2-receptor antagonists have no proved beneficial effects in the therapy of acute pancreatitis, they may be necessary in severely ill patients with significant risk factors for stress ulcer bleeding (see Gastrointestinal Bleeding).

B. Management of specific complications

1. **Infection.** There are many potential sources of fever in patients with acute pancreatitis, including pancreatic necrosis, abscess, infected pseudocyst, and aspiration pneumonia. In severely ill, febrile patients, culture material should be obtained and broad-spectrum antimicrobials appropriate for bowel flora should be administered (see Chap. 13). The development of fever 2 or more weeks into the course of acute pancreatitis suggests pancreatic abscess formation. CT scan of the abdomen may be helpful in this setting.

2. **Pseudocyst formation.** Persistent pain or hyperamylasemia suggests that a pseudocyst may have formed. Prolonged bowel rest and parenteral nutrition may allow pseudocysts to resolve or develop a mature wall, making surgical or percutaneous drainage safe. Pseudocysts that fail to resolve spontaneously after 4–6 weeks of conservative therapy should be treated definitively because of the risks of infection, hemorrhage, and perforation (*Am J Surg* 137:135, 1979).

3. **Pulmonary complications,** including atelectasis, pleural effusion, pneumonia, and ARDS, can develop in severely ill patients (see Chap. 10).

4. **Acute renal failure** caused by severe intravascular volume depletion or acute tubular necrosis can develop. Occasionally, patients may require acute dialysis (see Chap. 11).

5. **Surgical therapy** may be required for severe hemorrhagic or necrotizing pancreatitis, pancreatic abscess, persistent pseudocyst, and, rarely, common bile duct or duodenal obstruction.

II. Chronic pancreatitis is usually associated with chronic alcoholism. Major complications requiring therapy include chronic pain and exocrine and endocrine insufficiency. The presence of a calcified pancreas on a plain abdominal radiograph is diagnostic of chronic pancreatitis.

A. Pain. Many patients with chronic pancreatitis have severe pain as the major manifestation of their illness. Narcotics are often required for analgesia, and addiction is common. In patients with chronic alcoholic pancreatitis and mild to moderate exocrine insufficiency, oral pancreatic enzyme supplements may be beneficial for pain control (*Gastroenterology* 87:44, 1984). Patients with intractable pain may be candidates for surgical management.

B. Exocrine insufficiency. Weight loss and steatorrhea in a patient with a history of acute pancreatitis suggest pancreatic exocrine insufficiency.

1. **Diagnosis.** The **bentiromide (Chymex) test** is a simple screening study (*Gastroenterology* 89:685, 1985). The more invasive and less widely available secretin test is a direct measure of pancreatic secretion. Alternatively, an empiric trial of pancreatic enzyme replacement may be attempted.

2. **Therapy.** Most patients can be managed with a low-fat diet (<50 g/day) and oral pancreatic enzyme supplements. Supplements should be administered 20–30 minutes before meals and snacks. Non–enteric-coated pancrelipase preparations such as Viokase or Cotazym, 2–4 tablets, can be given in conjunction with H_2-receptor antagonists to prevent degradation by gastric acid. Enteric-coated preparations are stable at acid pH and are released at neutral pH (Pancrease or Creon, 1–2 capsules with meals). In most circumstances, they should not be given with H_2-receptor antagonists since neutralization of gastric pH may lead to dissolution of the enteric coating in the stomach. Fat-soluble vitamin supplementation may be necessary (see Malabsorption and Maldigestion). The use of endoscopic retrograde cholangiopancreatography (ERCP) for drainage of obstructed pancreatic ducts to relieve chronic pain is under investigation.

C. Endocrine insufficiency. Many patients with chronic pancreatitis have abnormalities of glucose tolerance caused by destruction of islet cells and may require supplemental insulin therapy (see Chap. 20).

Gallstones

I. **Cholelithiasis.** Asymptomatic cholelithiasis is a common incidental finding for which no specific therapy is generally necessary. The spectrum of symptomatic cholelithiasis includes a history of prior episodes of biliary colic, the acute onset of right upper quadrant pain, fever, nausea, and vomiting (cholecystitis), or gallstone pancreatitis.

    A. **Cholecystectomy.** The best therapy for symptomatic cholelithiasis remains cholecystectomy. **Laparoscopic techniques** have become increasingly common.

    B. **Medical therapy.** A small, select group of patients with cholesterol stones who have uncomplicated biliary colic or who are at high risk for complications from surgical therapy may qualify for prolonged medical therapy with **chenodeoxycholic acid,** 13–16 mg/kg/day PO in 2 divided doses, or **ursodeoxycholic acid,** 8–10 mg/kg/day PO. Selection criteria include the presence of small (<20 mm in diameter) radiolucent stones in a functioning gallbladder as judged by oral cholecystography. Total dissolution of stones occurs in approximately 30% of patients after 1 year of therapy. **Side effects** include diarrhea and reversible elevations in serum hepatic transaminase levels, although the frequency of such problems appears to be lower with ursodeoxycholic acid.

    C. **Other nonsurgical therapies** include percutaneous instillation of contact solvents such as methyl-tertiary-butyl ether (*N Engl J Med* 320:633, 1989) into the gallbladder and extracorporeal shock wave lithotripsy (*N Engl J Med* 314:818, 1986) alone or in combination. However, experience with these therapies is limited, and neither is necessarily definitive, as the underlying abnormal gallbladder remains in place. Concomitant adjuvant therapy with an oral dissolution agent may be necessary.

II. **Cholecystitis.** Acute cholecystitis is most often caused by obstruction of the cystic duct by gallstones, but acalculous cholecystitis can occur especially in hospitalized patients. Surgical removal of the gallbladder is the mainstay of treatment. IV fluid resuscitation is usually necessary, and broad-spectrum antimicrobial agents may be indicated, especially if sepsis, peritonitis, or abscess is suspected. Severely ill patients who are not surgical candidates can undergo drainage by percutaneous cholecystostomy.

III. **Complications** of cholelithiasis and cholecystitis include choledocholithiasis with common bile duct obstruction and cholangitis, pancreatitis, ileus, gallbladder empyema, and perforation. In patients who have undergone cholecystectomy, **retained common bile duct stones** may complicate the postoperative course. Patients with **ascending cholangitis** due to choledocholithiasis present with right upper quadrant pain, fever, and jaundice (**Charcot's triad**). Therapy consists of parenteral broad-spectrum antimicrobials and drainage of the biliary tree. Ampicillin plus an aminoglycoside usually provides adequate initial therapy, although in severe cases anaerobic coverage may be necessary. ERCP with sphincterotomy and stone removal or placement of a nasobiliary cannula is often performed, as is surgical or radiologic decompression.

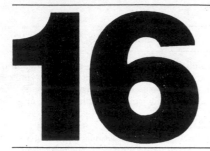

Hepatic Diseases

Heather M. White

Evaluation of Liver Function

Liver disease is frequently classified as acute or chronic. Acute liver disease refers to abnormalities present less than 6 months, and chronic liver disease refers to abnormalities present greater than 6 months. The term *fulminant hepatic failure* specifically implies rapid progression from onset of disease to liver failure over a period of less than 4 weeks and therefore occurs only in acute processes.

I. **Laboratory evaluation** includes several screening tests of liver function. The biochemical profile may include measurement of (1) serum enzymes, including the aminotransferases, alkaline phosphatase, and 5′-nucleotidase; (2) excretory products such as bilirubin, bile acids, and ammonia; and (3) synthetic products such as albumin, coagulation factors, and cholesterol.

A. **Serum enzymes.** Hepatic disorders associated with predominant elevations in AST and ALT are referred to as **hepatocellular**; hepatic disorders with predominant elevations in alkaline phosphatase and 5′-nucleotidase are referred to as cholestatic.

1. **The aminotransferases are aspartate aminotransferase AST (SGOT) and alanine aminotransferase ALT (SGPT).** Markedly elevated levels (>500 units/liter) typically occur with acute hepatocellular injury (e.g., viral, drug-induced, ischemic hepatitis), whereas modest elevation (<300 units/liter) may be seen in a variety of conditions (e.g., acute or chronic hepatocellular injury, infiltrative diseases, biliary obstruction). ALT is generally more sensitive than AST for detecting viral hepatitis. In alcoholic liver disease, AST is elevated in excess of ALT, typically by a factor of 2 or more (*Dig Dis Sci* 24:835, 1979).

2. **Alkaline phosphatase (AP)** is an enzyme present in a variety of body tissues including bone, intestine, and liver. Heat fractionation can be used to distinguish the source of serum AP, but the elevation of other hepatic enzymes is usually most helpful in establishing the hepatic origin of AP. Serum AP levels are most frequently elevated in biliary obstruction, cholestasis, in the setting of space-occupying lesions, or infiltrative diseases of the liver.

3. **5′-nucleotidase** is an enzyme elevated in a similar spectrum of diseases as AP and gamma-glutamyl transpeptidase (see sec. **I.A.4**). 5′-nucleotidase is comparable in sensitivity to AP in detecting biliary obstruction, cholestasis, and infiltrative hepatobiliary diseases.

4. **Gamma-glutamyl transpeptidase (GGT)** is an enzyme present in a variety of tissues. Increases in GGT and AP tend to occur in similar hepatic diseases. The utility of GGT is limited by its high sensitivity and predictable elevation in patients ingesting agents known to stimulate the hepatic microsomal mixed-function oxidase system (e.g., barbiturates, phenytoin, alcohol).

B. **Excretory products**

1. **Bilirubin** is a degradation product of heme. Serum bilirubin concentration represents a balance between bilirubin production and excretion; therefore, levels may be elevated as a consequence of either increased bilirubin production or impaired hepatic excretion. Bilirubin concentration is composed

of both **direct** (conjugated) and **indirect** (unconjugated) fractions. Predominantly indirect bilirubin elevations can occur as a result of excessive bilirubin production (hemolysis or ineffective erythropoiesis), impaired bilirubin conjugation (Gilbert's or Crigler-Najjar syndromes), or reduced hepatic bilirubin uptake (heart failure, portosystemic shunting). Direct bilirubin elevations usually occur as a result of either hepatocellular dysfunction or biliary tract obstruction.

2. **Bile acids** are produced in the liver and are secreted into bile, where they are required for lipid digestion and absorption. Under normal circumstances, bile acids undergo enterohepatic recirculation. Minor degrees of hepatic dysfunction can result in elevations of serum bile acids.

3. **Serum ammonia** may be elevated in hepatic dysfunction due to disturbances in the urea cycle. However, absolute levels do not correlate directly with clinical findings.

C. **Synthetic products**

1. **Serum albumin.** Depressed levels of albumin are most frequently seen with chronic liver disease. However, malnutrition and renal disease may also be associated with hypoalbuminemia. The half-life of albumin is relatively long, so serum levels are frequently preserved in acute liver disease.

2. **Coagulation factors.** All coagulation factors except factor VIII are synthesized by the liver; most have half-lives measured in hours or days. Synthesis of factors II, VII, IX, and X depends on the presence of vitamin K. Therefore, the adequacy of hepatic synthetic function can be estimated by the prothrombin time (PT), which determines the adequate function of factors II, V, VII, and X (see Chap. 17). PT prolongation occurs as a consequence of either impaired coagulation factor synthesis or vitamin K deficiency. Normalization of the PT after administration of vitamin K indicates vitamin K deficiency.

3. **Cholesterol and cholesterol-derived hormones** are synthesized in the liver. Thus, patients with advanced liver disease may have very low cholesterol levels and decreased levels of certain hormones such as testosterone. However, because cholesterol is a major excretory component of bile, disorders of biliary tree obstruction, such as primary biliary cirrhosis, may be associated with marked elevations of serum cholesterol.

II. **Radiographic evaluation**

A. **Ultrasonography (USG)** is best used as a screening tool for biliary tree dilation and gallstone visualization but can also detect parenchymal disease. Color-flow Doppler can assess patency of blood vessels and direction of flow. USG sensitivity and specificity are operator-dependent.

B. **CT with IV contrast** is best used for evaluation of parenchymal liver disease but can assess biliary tree dilation and has the added feature of contrast enhancement to define space-occupying lesions (e.g., abscess, tumor).

C. **MRI** has similar utility to CT but also offers visualization of vessels without IV contrast dye. Limitations of MRI include availability and patient cooperation.

D. **Liver-spleen (LS) scanning** is an older modality used to detect hepatocellular dysfunction by colloid shift.

E. **Percutaneous transhepatic cholangiography (PTC) and endoscopic retrograde cholangiopancreatography (ERCP)** instill contrast dye into the biliary tree and are most useful after preliminary screening by USG, CT, or MRI reveals biliary tree abnormalities.

Hepatotrophic Viruses

I. **Hepatotrophic viruses** include hepatitis A, hepatitis B, hepatitis C, hepatitis D, hepatitis E, and non-A, non-B hepatitis (Tables 16-1 and 16-2).

A. **Hepatitis A (HAV).** Infection with HAV is usually transmitted via the fecal-oral route, and large-scale outbreaks due to contamination of food and drinking water can occur (*Semin Liver Dis* 6:42, 1986). The period of greatest infectivity

Table 16-1. Clinical and epidemiologic features of hepatotrophic viruses

Organism	Hepatitis A	Hepatitis B	Hepatitis C	Hepatitis D	Hepatitis E	NANB
Incubation	2–6 wks	1–6 mos	2 wks–6 mos	3 wks–3 mos	3–6 wks	2 wks–6 mos
Transmission	Fecal/oral Blood Sexual	Blood Sexual Perinatal	Sporadic Blood Sexual Perinatal	Blood Sexual Perinatal	Fecal/oral	Sporadic Blood ?Sexual ?Perinatal
Risk groups	Military personnel Children in day care and their care providers	IVDA Homosexuals Native Asians Health care workers Transfusion recipients	IVDA Health care workers Transfusion recipients	IVDA Anyone with hepatitis B	Travelers to endemic areas	IVDA Health care workers Transfusion recipients
Fever	Common	Uncommon	Uncommon	Uncommon	Common	Uncommon
Nausea/vomiting	Common	Common	Common	Common	Common	Common
Immune complex disease	Uncommon	Common	Common	Common	Common	Unknown
Severity	Mild	Mild to moderate	Mild to Moderate	Moderate to severe	Mild to moderate	Mild to moderate
Diagnosis						
Acute	Anti-HAVIgM	Anti-HBcIgM HBsAG	Clinical	Anti-HDVIgM HDAg	Clinical[a]	Diagnosis of exclusion in appropriate clinical setting
Chronic	NA	Anti-HBcTotal HBsAG	HCVAg RIBA II PCR for HCV RNA	HDAg	NA	Diagnosis of exclusion in appropriate clinical setting

Sequelae						
Fulminant	0.1–0.2%	<5%	<5%	5–20%	1–2%; 10–30% in pregnant women	<5%
Carrier	No	Yes	Yes	Yes	No	Unknown but likely
Chronic hepatitis	No	Yes	Yes	Yes	No	Yes
Prophylaxis						
Adults	ISG[b]	HBIG[c] + vaccine[d]	?ISG	None available[e]	None available	?ISG[b]
Perinatal	ISG[b]	HBIG[f] + vaccine[g]	?ISG[b]	None available[e]	None available	?ISG[b]

NANB = non-A, non-B hepatitis; IVDA = intravenous drug abusers; NA = not applicable; RIBA II = recombinant immunoblot assay II; PCR = polymerase chain reaction; ISG = immune serum globulin.

[a]Testing available from the hepatitis branch of the Centers for Disease Control.

[b]Immune serum globulin. 0.02 ml/kg IM. Use in NANB and HCV unsubstantiated.

[c]Hepatitis B immunoglobulin. 5 ml IM.

[d]Vaccine is either Engerix B, 20 μg IM, or Recombivax, 10 μg IM at 0, 1, and 6 months.

[e]Vaccination against hepatitis B will protect individuals from hepatitis D. No specific vaccine for hepatitis D is available.

[f]Hepatitis B immunoglobulin, 0.5 ml IM within 12 hours of birth.

[g]Vaccine is either Engerix B, 10 μg IM, or Recombivax, 5 μg IM at 0, 1, and 6 months.

Table 16-2. Viral hepatitis serologies

Organism	Acute	Chronic	Recovered	Vaccinated
Hepatitis A	Anti-HAV IgM	Not applicable	Anti-HAV IgG	Anti-HAV IgG[a]
Hepatitis B	Anti-HBcIgM HBsAG HBeAG	Anti-HBcTotal (IgM and IgG) HBsAg HBeAg[b] or HBeAb[b]	Anti-HBcTotal (IgM and IgG) Anti-HBsAg	Anti-HBsAG
Hepatitis C	All tests may be negative Anti-HCV Ab HCV RNA	Anti-HCV Ab RIBA II HCV RNA	Anti-HCV Ab RIBA II	NA
Hepatitis D	Anti-HDVIgM HD Ag[c]	Anti-HDVTotal HD Ag[c]	Anti-HDVTotal[c]	NA[d]
Hepatitis E	Available from CDC only	NA	Available from CDC only	NA
Hepatitis non-A, non-B	All tests negative	All tests negative	All tests negative	NA

RIBA II = recombinant immunoblot assay II; NA = not applicable.

[a] Hepatitis A vaccine is not yet commercially available in the United States.

[b] HBeAg will be present during periods of high replication. HBeAb will be present during periods of low replication.

[c] Markers of hepatitis B infection will also be present because HDV cannot replicate without HBV.

[d] Although no specific vaccine for hepatitis D exists, individuals vaccinated for HBV will be protected from infection with HDV.

is during the 2 weeks prior to the onset of clinical illness; however, due to fecal shedding, enteric precautions are indicated during the first 2–3 weeks of clinical illness. Sexual transmission and parenteral transmission may occur, although the period of viremia is brief.

B. **Hepatitis B (HBV).** The complete HBV agent consists of an outer viral envelope protein (containing the hepatitis B surface antigen [HBsAg]) and the viral nucleocapsid (containing the hepatitis B core antigen [HBcAg]). **HBsAg** is detectable in serum in almost all cases of acute and chronic HBV infection. **HBcAg** does not freely circulate but can be detected within liver cells when there is active viral replication. Hepatitis B e antigen (**HBeAg**) is a component of the HBcAg; it can usually be detected in serum when there is active viral replication. Circulating antibodies against the various viral antigens develop in response to infection, and these antibodies can be detected by serology. Antibody against HBsAg (**anti-HBs**) appears following HBV infection or vaccination; its presence confers immunity (except in rare cases of chronic hepatitis B infection when very low titers of heterotypic anti-HBs are detectable). **Hepatitis B core antibody** can be detected in two fractions—the hepatitis B core immunoglobulin M (IgM) (**anti-HBcIgM**) and the hepatitis B core total (**anti-HBcTotal**). Anti-HBcIgM is usually present in acute infection but occasionally can be detected during periods of high viral replication in chronic disease. Anti-HBcTotal includes IgM and IgG fractions and is positive in acute disease (due to the presence of IgM), in chronic disease (due to predominantly IgG), and in patients who have recovered from infection (due to IgG). Infection with HBV is usually spread via either apparent (e.g., needle-stick, transfusion) or inapparent (e.g., sexual contact) parenteral transmission. Although blood is the most effective vehicle for transmission, HBsAg is present in other body fluids (e.g., saliva, semen, and, rarely, feces and urine), which can also transmit the infection. **Patients with HBV infections should avoid intimate contact (e.g., sharing razors, toothbrushes) with other household members since they are infectious until seroconversion occurs** (*Semin Liver Dis* 6:1, 11, 1986; **or until household contacts have completed vaccination.**

C. **Hepatitis C (HCV)** has a typical incubation period of 6 weeks to 6 months, but it may be as short as 2 weeks. The diagnostic screening test is hepatitis C virus antibody (HCVAb). **The presence of HCVAb suggests prior exposure to HCV, and the antibody does not confer immunity.** HCVAb is often not present in acute infection (60–90% patients), may take up to 12 months to become positive after acute infection, and may be positive in 60–80% with chronic infection (*Science* 244:362, 1989; *N Engl J Med* 321:1494, 1989). Second-generation radioimmunoblot assay (RIBA II) is a confirmatory assay that detects antibodies to 4 components of the HCV genome. No antigen tests for HCV are currently available. Polymerase chain reaction for HCV RNA is currently a research tool to detect viral genomic replication (*Gut* 32:965, 1991). The primary established transmission route is blood exposure (e.g., transfusion, IV drug use); however, up to 60% of patients have no exposure history. Data regarding sexual transmission are conflicting but suggest that HCV may be transmitted sexually, though at a much lower frequency than HBV (*JAMA* 262:1201, 1989; *Ann Intern Med* 112:544, 1990). Sexual transmission appears to occur more frequently when the patient carries both HIV and the HCV viruses (*Ann Intern Med* 115:764, 1991). HCVAb (an IgG antibody) crosses the placenta. and perinatal transmission in nonimmunocompromised patients is rare but may occur (*J Med Virol* 30:178, 1990; *Lancet* 338:17, 1991). As with sexual transmission, the presence of HIV appears to enhance the chances of perinatal transmission. The risk of HCV transmission following a needle-stick injury is estimated at 10% (*Hepatology* 16:1109, 1992). Isolation guidelines are controversial; at a minimum, blood and body fluids should be considered infectious.

D. **Hepatitis D (HDV), or delta agent, requires the presence of HBV for infection and replication to occur.** HDV infection can only occur if an individual with chronic HBV is subsequently exposed to the delta agent (superinfection), or if an individual is simultaneously infected with both HBV and HDV (coinfection). Although HDV is found throughout the world, it is endemic to the Mediterranean basin, the Middle East, and portions of South America; outside these areas, infections occur primarily in multiply transfused individuals and, in the United States, in IV drug abusers. Fulminant disease is more common with HDV, and chronic hepatitis occurs in most patients (*Semin Liver Dis* 6:28, 1986).

E. Hepatitis E (HEV) has an incubation period of 2–6 weeks. Transmission closely resembles that of HAV. HEV has been implicated in epidemics in India, Southeast Asia, Africa, and Mexico. Reported cases in the United States have been in travelers to endemic areas. Diagnostic testing methods are available through the hepatitis branch of the Centers for Disease Control (CDC). HEV is associated with high fatality rates in pregnant women.

F. Non-A, non-B (NANB) is the exclusionary category of hepatotrophic viruses that remains when serologic tests for other viruses are negative. Previously, HCV comprised a significant proportion of this group before reliable serologic tests were available. NANB occurs sporadically and is transmitted via blood exposure. Transmission and isolation recommendations are similar to those of HCV.

II. Management of viral hepatitis includes prophylaxis of close contacts and therapy based on severity and chronicity of disease.

A. Pre-exposure prophylaxis is important but rarely considered. For HAV, pre-exposure prophylaxis should be given to travelers to endemic areas. For trips lasting up to 2 months, immune serum globulin (ISG), 0.02 ml/kg IM, should be administered; for longer travel, ISG, 0.06 ml/kg IM, should be given every 5 months. The Food and Drug Administration (FDA) is currently considering approval of a hepatitis A vaccine. For HBV and HDV, pre-exposure prophylaxis should be considered in patients with multiple anticipated transfusions (e.g., transplant recipients), health care workers, IV drug abusers, household contacts of HBsAg carriers, homosexuals, heterosexual contacts of HBsAg carriers, clients of institutions for the mentally retarded, and Alaskan Eskimos (*Semin Liver Dis* 6:23, 1986). Additionally, the CDC has recommended a universal vaccination program for infants and sexually active adolescents (*MMWR* 40:1, 1991). Prevaccination screening for previous exposure or infection is recommended in the high-risk groups to avoid vaccinating recovered individuals or those with chronic infection. Pre-exposure prophylaxis for HBV consists of recombinant HBV vaccine (10–20 μg IM in the deltoid) given at 0, 1, and 6 months. In patients undergoing hemodialysis and in other immunosuppressed patients, three 40-μg doses of the plasma-derived vaccine are recommended, using the same schedule (*Ann Intern Med* 107:353, 1987). For patients requiring rapid immunity, the dosage schedule may be escalated to 0, 1, and 2 months, but a follow-up booster at 6 months is required for long-lasting immunity. Revaccination is not generally recommended for individuals who fail to respond to the initial series of deltoid-administered vaccinations (*N Engl J Med* 315:209, 1986). The need for and timing of booster doses has not yet been determined. Pre-exposure prophylaxis for HCV, HEV, and NANB is not available.

B. Postexposure prophylaxis (see Table 16-1). Postexposure prophylaxis for HAV should be given to household contacts, sexual partners, or other close contacts of infected patients within 10 days of exposure. Studies indicate this may prevent infection or lessen its severity. Of special importance is the postexposure prophylaxis of HBV in the perinatal period. All infants of infected mothers should receive hepatitis B immune globulin (HBIG) and a series of vaccinations within 12 hours of birth, as this population is at very high risk for chronic infection.

C. Therapy of viral hepatitis is largely supportive. Dietary therapy usually has little role in acute hepatitis. A clear liquid diet may be helpful in those patients with nausea or vomiting. Fat intake should be restricted in individuals with diarrhea, nausea, or vomiting. **Rarely, patients may require hospitalization for IV volume expansion.** Alcohol should be avoided. Multivitamin supplements may be helpful in malnourished or severely anorectic patients. Activity restric-

Table 16-3. Stages of hepatic encephalopathy

Stage	Mental status	Reflexes	EEG
I	Mild confusion Disorientation	Normal No asterixis	Normal
II	Moderate confusion Lethargy	Increased reflexes Asterixis	Abnormal
III	Marked confusion Incoherent speech Arousable	Brisk reflexes/clonus Asterixis	Abnormal
IV	Coma: initially responsive to stimuli, then unresponsive	Absent reflexes No asterixis	Abnormal

tions are recommended if a clinical or biochemical relapse occurs with full ambulation. **Management of acute hepatitis is predominantly performed on an outpatient basis; liver enzymes (AST, ALT) and hepatic synthetic function (bilirubin, albumin, PT) should be monitored to assess recovery.** In a small group of patients (see Table 16-1) fulminant hepatic failure may ensue as reflected by decreasing transaminases, decreasing albumin, increasing bilirubin, and increasing PT.

D. **Fulminant hepatic failure (FHF)** is not restricted to viral hepatitis but may also occur as a result of drugs, ischemia, toxin exposure, acute fatty liver of pregnancy, Wilson's disease, or Reye's syndrome. Viral hepatitis is the most common cause, but the clinical description and medical management applies to all cases of FHF. **Manifestations** are encephalopathy and a prolonged PT. Other features include worsening jaundice, GI bleeding, sepsis, coagulopathy, hypoglycemia, renal failure, and electrolyte abnormalities. **Supportive therapy in the inpatient setting is essential.** Caloric intake should be maintained with dextrose-containing IV solutions. Serum glucose should be monitored every 4 hours, and more often if glucose is less than 60 mg/dl. Vitamin supplements (including vitamin K) should be given. **Antacids or H_2-receptor antagonists,** in a dose sufficient to keep gastric pH greater than 5.0, may prevent upper GI hemorrhage (*Lancet* 1:617, 1989). **Fresh-frozen plasma (FFP)** and blood should be administered when there is evidence of active hemorrhage. However, prophylactic administration of FFP is not recommended, as the administration may lead to volume overload and makes assessment of residual synthetic function difficult. In patients with signs suggestive of elevated intracranial pressure (ICP) (see Chap. 25) or stage III or IV hepatic coma (Table 16-3), an ICP monitor should be placed and IV mannitol (1 g/kg) may be given. Hyperventilation to a pCO_2 less than 30 mm Hg should be reserved for management of acute rises in ICP, as the brain adapts to chronic hyperventilation. Glucocorticoids have little effect on the cerebral edema associated with FHF, and controlled trials have failed to demonstrate their efficacy in this disease (*N Engl J Med* 294:681, 1976; *Gut* 23:625, 1982). In patients with stage IV hepatic coma, mortality exceeds 80% and transplantation should be considered (see Hepatic Transplantation). Death ensues from progressive liver failure, GI bleeding, cerebral edema, sepsis, or arrhythmias.

E. **Chronic viral hepatitis** is defined as the presence of liver inflammation persisting for at least 6 months associated with HBV, HCV, HDV, or NANB infection. Chronic hepatitis is subdivided into (1) the **carrier state,** characterized by normal enzymes and no inflammation on biopsy but persistent circulating viral particles; (2) **chronic persistent hepatitis (CPH),** characterized by the presence of chronic inflammation limited to the portal tracts; (3) **chronic active hepatitis (CAH),** characterized by the presence of chronic inflammation involving the portal tracts and periportal parenchyma; or (4) **cirrhosis,** characterized by severe fibrosis and regenerating nodules. Both CPH and CAH may progress to cirrhosis. A carrier state has long been known in HBV infection, in which patients express the HBsAg in the serum and virus is present on tissue immuno-staining of the liver. HDV can also exist in the carrier state, though by definition the patient must also have HBV. HCV or NANB probably exists in a carrier state, but evaluation for these viral particles is difficult. Although many agents have been tried in viral CPH and CAH, the best results to date are with alpha interferon (α-IFN). In chronic hepatitis B, α-IFN administered over a 4-month period appears to result in a chronic hepatitic sustained loss of viral replication, as well as biochemical and histologic remission in approximately one-third of patients, with loss of HBsAg in approximately 10% (*N Engl J Med* 323:295, 1990). In chronic HCV hepatitis, α-IFN administered over 6–12 months results in a response rate of approximately 50% but is associated with a high rate of relapse (*Semin Liver Dis* 9:259, 1989). Intron A (IFN alpha-2b) is approved for hepatitis C/NANB therapy at a dose of 3 million units (1 ml) SC 3 times/week for 24 weeks. Therapy is appropriate only in selected patients due to significant toxicity and side effects. Intron A is also approved for hepatitis B therapy at a dose of either 10 million units SC 3 times/week or 5 million units qd for 16 weeks. Current FDA guidelines restrict the use of IFN to patients without evidence of decompensated liver disease (e.g., normal synthetic function and no history of variceal bleeding, ascites, or encephalopathy). The success of α-IFN in hepatitis D patients is quite limited, and years of treatment with high doses are required to effect any response (*Semin Liver Dis* 9:264, 1989). Hepatic transplantation may be indicated in advanced disease, but disease recurrence has been documented in HBV, HCV, and HDV.

Toxic and Drug-Related Liver Disease

I. **Intrinsic hepatotoxins** include **direct hepatotoxins** (e.g., carbon tetrachloride, phosphorus), which cause predictable damage to liver cells by direct physicochemical attack, and **indirect hepatotoxins** (e.g., tetracycline, methotrexate, 6-mercaptopurine, acetaminophen, *Amanita phalloides* [mushroom toxin], and alkylated anabolic steroids), which may interfere with hepatocyte metabolic pathways or secretory mechanisms. Oral contraceptives may cause mild abnormalities in liver enzymes, but overt cholestatic jaundice is unusual. Liver disorders associated with oral contraceptives include hepatic adenomas and Budd-Chiari syndrome. Treatment for all intrinsic hepatotoxins includes withdrawal of the offending drug and institution of supportive measures. An attempt to remove the agent from the GI tract should be made in most cases using lavage or cathartics (see Chap. 9). Except for acetaminophen (see Chap. 9) and methotrexate (see Chap. 19) ingestion, no specific therapy is available in most cases.

II. **Idiosyncratic hepatotoxins** may present as either hypersensitivity reactions or idiosyncratic metabolic reactions.

    A. **Hypersensitivity reactions** are characterized by a sensitization period of 1–5 weeks and prompt recurrence of the liver injury in response to a repeat challenge. Associated signs and symptoms include fever, rash, and eosinophilia. Eosinophilic or granulomatous inflammation is a typical histologic finding. Responsible drugs include sulfonamides, nitrofurantoin, paraaminosalicylic acid, phenytoin, and halothane.

    B. **Metabolic idiosyncrasy** occurs in susceptible patients as a result of altered drug clearance or accelerated production of hepatotoxic metabolites (e.g., isoniazid, methyldopa, and perhaps halothane) (*Hepatotoxicity: The Adverse Effects of Drugs and Other Chemicals on the Liver.* New York: Appleton-Century-Crofts, 1978).

III. **Alcohol-induced hepatic injury** is a significant problem in the United States. Although current evidence suggests that alcohol exerts a direct toxic effect on the liver, only 10–20% of chronic alcoholics develop significant liver damage. Thus, additional factors (e.g., genetic, nutritional, environmental) may be important in the pathogenesis of alcoholic liver disease. The spectrum of alcoholic liver disease is broad, and a single patient may be affected by more than one entity.

A. **Fatty liver** is the most common abnormality observed in chronic alcoholics. If fat alone is present, patients are usually asymptomatic. Clinical findings include hepatomegaly and mild liver enzyme abnormalities (usually elevated AP). The disorder is believed to be reversible if alcohol intake is stopped and an adequate nutritious diet is ingested.

B. **Alcoholic hepatitis** may be clinically silent or severe enough to lead to the rapid development of hepatic failure and death. Clinical features include fever, abdominal pain, anorexia, nausea, vomiting, and weight loss. In patients with underlying cirrhosis, manifestations of portal hypertension may predominate. Laboratory features typically demonstrate enzyme elevations in AST, ALT, and AP, with AST characteristically higher than ALT; hyperbilirubinemia and prolonged PT may also be seen. Although clinical presentation is helpful, liver biopsy is required for diagnosis. Features associated with a **poor prognosis** include prolongation of the PT that does not normalize with vitamin K, a markedly elevated total bilirubin, leukocytosis, and an elevated blood urea nitrogen (BUN) or serum creatinine (Cr).

C. **Alcoholic or Laennec's cirrhosis** is the most common cause of cirrhosis in the United States. Diagnosis can only be made by liver biopsy.

D. **Therapy of alcoholic liver disease** includes abstinence from alcohol as well as vitamin and nutrition support. Glucocorticoids, anabolic steroids, and propylthiouracil may improve survival rate and produce biochemical improvement in some patients; however, their use is controversial and their role remains to be determined. In severe cholestatic alcoholic hepatitis, particularly in association with encephalopathy, glucocorticoids may have a role (*Ann Intern Med* 110: 685, 1989).

E. **Drug interactions** between alcohol and a variety of pharmaceuticals may occur. Alcohol may potentiate the effects or alter the metabolism of a number of medications. Potentially dangerous interactions between alcohol and sedative-hypnotics, anticoagulants, and acetaminophen, even in the absence of alcoholic liver disease, may occur in clinical practice due to shared metabolic pathways (*Ann Intern Med* 104:399, 1986).

IV. **Acetaminophen** may cause significant hepatocellular injury in accidental or intentional overdose. Toxic potentiation of alcohol in combination with even therapeutic doses of acetaminophen has been demonstrated to cause significant hepatocellular injury. Management of acetaminophen overdose is a medical emergency (see Chap. 9). Observation for signs of FHF is recommended.

Cholestatic Liver Disease

Cholestatic liver disease is characterized by predominant elevations in AP and bilirubin, although the serum bilirubin may appear normal until late in the course of illness.

I. **Primary biliary cirrhosis (PBC)** is a progressive, cholestatic disorder of unknown etiology resulting in nonsuppurative cholangitis that most often afflicts middle-aged women. The course is highly variable, and patients may be asymptomatic for many years. Pruritus is usually the most troublesome symptom. Typical clinical features include elevated levels of AP, cholesterol, immunoglobulin M, and bile acids associated with the presence of antimitochondrial antibodies, which are present in 95% of patients.

A. **Nutritional deficiencies.** Patients are at risk for malnutrition secondary to fat malabsorption, and a low-fat diet (40–60 g/day) may be helpful in patients with diarrhea. Fat-soluble vitamin deficiency (vitamins A, D, K) is often present in more advanced disease and in those patients with steatorrhea. Vitamin replacement doses include vitamin A, 5,000–25,000 IU PO daily; vitamin D, 50,000 IU

PO 3–5 times/week; and vitamin K_1 (phytonadione), 10 mg SC or IM monthly, or vitamin K tablets, 5–10 mg PO daily. PT and serum levels of vitamin A and 25-cholecalciferol (25-hydroxy vitamin D) should be monitored to assess the adequacy of replacement therapy. Vitamin A deficiency is the least common; large doses of vitamin A can be hepatotoxic and teratogenic, so it should be administered with caution. Zinc deficiency may also occur in some patients, and zinc sulfate, 220 mg PO daily (50 mg elemental zinc) for 4 weeks, will usually correct low serum zinc levels.

  B. **Spontaneous fractures** due to osteoporosis and osteomalacia can occur, and oral calcium supplementation (1.0–1.5 g/day) should be given to all patients with PBC; vitamin D supplementation may also be required (see Chap. 23). Dual-energy radiography or bone densitometry of the spine should be performed in all patients.

  C. **Pruritus** in PBC and other cholestatic diseases is best treated with cholestyramine, a bile acid sequestrant resin. The drug is given as one packet (4 g) mixed with water before the morning meal with additional doses before meals to control symptoms. Cholestyramine should not be given concurrently with vitamins or other medications, since it may impair their absorption. Antihistamines or doxepin (25 mg PO qhs) may provide symptomatic relief. Phenobarbital, 60–120 mg PO daily, can also be added if cholestyramine alone is ineffective in controlling pruritus.

  D. **Therapy for PBC.** No specific therapy has clearly proved effective in altering the course of PBC, but agents currently under investigation include cyclosporine, methotrexate, and ursodeoxycholic acid. Hepatic transplantation may be required in advanced disease.

 II. **Primary sclerosing cholangitis (PSC)** is an idiopathic chronic cholestatic disorder characterized by inflammation, fibrosis, and eventual obliteration of the extrahepatic and intrahepatic bile ducts. Most patients are middle-aged men, and there is a frequent association with inflammatory bowel disease. ERCP or PTC demonstrating strictures or irregularity of the intrahepatic and extrahepatic bile ducts confirms the diagnosis. Clinical manifestations typically include intermittent episodes of jaundice, hepatomegaly, pruritus, weight loss, and fatigue. Episodes of bacterial cholangitis primarily occur in patients who have had surgical biliary drainage procedures. Patients are at a substantially increased risk of developing cholangiocarcinoma. No specific therapy has proved successful; a number of experimental trials with cyclosporine, methotrexate, and ursodeoxycholic acid are ongoing. Supportive therapy is as outlined for PBC. **Cholangitis** episodes should be managed with IV antibiotics (see Chap. 15). Hepatic transplantation should be reserved for patients with advanced disease or recurrent cholangitis.

III. **Granulomatous hepatitis** presents primarily as a cholestatic disorder with many different etiologies. Patients typically present with fever and increased liver enzyme concentrations (particularly AP), and they may have hepatosplenomegaly. The differential diagnosis includes mycobacterial disease, chronic fungal infections, sarcoidosis, drug-induced injury, or idiopathic causes. Specific therapy is directed at the underlying cause. If the clinical suspicion for tuberculosis is high, an empiric trial of antituberculous therapy may be warranted despite negative mycobacterial cultures. Glucocorticoids may be useful in selected noninfectious cases.

Metabolic Liver Disease

A number of treatable metabolic disorders present with hepatocellular dysfunction, including Wilson's disease, hemochromatosis, and alpha$_1$-antitrypsin deficiency. Other rare disorders include glycogen storage disease, phospholipidoses, and Byler's syndrome.

 I. **Wilson's disease** is a recessive inherited disorder of copper overload that may present with FHF but more typically presents with progressive hepatic dysfunction that may be accompanied by neuropsychiatric disorders. The diagnosis is suggested by elevated serum copper levels, low serum ceruloplasmin levels, and elevated

24-hour urinary copper levels, but it is only confirmed by quantitative copper levels on liver biopsy. Treatment is with copper chelating agents (penicillamine or trientine), but hepatic transplantation is necessary in FHF or in patients with progressive dysfunction despite chelation therapy.

II. **Hemochromatosis** is an inherited disorder of iron overload that may present with slate-colored skin, diabetes, cardiomyopathy, arthritis, or hepatic dysfunction and is usually not diagnosed until patients are middle-aged. The diagnosis is suggested by elevated serum iron levels and a high transferrin saturation but is confirmed by quantitative iron levels on liver biopsy. Therapy consists of phlebotomy and genetic counseling. Patients are at increased risk for the development of hepatomas despite therapy.

III. **Alpha$_1$-antitrypsin deficiency** may present with pulmonary, hepatic, or pancreatic manifestations. The diagnosis is suggested by a low serum alpha$_1$-antitrypsin level and can be confirmed by liver biopsy. Liver disease is most often seen with the zz phenotype, but it may rarely occur in heterozygotes. No specific medical therapy for the hepatic disease is available, but transplantation is curative.

Miscellaneous Disorders

I. **Vascular disease of the liver** is due to impaired arterial or venous blood flow.
   A. **Hepatic artery ischemia** may occur as a result of profound hypotension and can result in markedly elevated transaminases, which typically resolve over 24–48 hours if the hypotension is treated. Hepatic artery thrombosis is rare except in liver transplant recipients or after surgery near the porta hepatitis. Systemic arteritis may involve the hepatic artery.
   B. **Hepatic vein thrombosis** (Budd-Chiari syndrome) is the most common hepatic vascular disease. Classically, Budd-Chiari presents with new-onset ascites and tender hepatomegaly. Although there is a strong association with lymphoreticular malignancy or hypercoagulable states, one-third of cases are idiopathic. The use of thrombolytics in the acute setting is controversial. The prognosis is poor, and transplantation is recommended if no malignancy can be identified.
   C. **Veno-occlusive disease (VOD)** is an unusual syndrome of intrahepatic venous obliteration most typically seen after total body irradiation and high-dose chemotherapy in bone marrow transplant recipients. VOD has also been described in renal transplant recipients who have not received irradiation but who have been immunosuppressed with azathioprine. It has also been described in association with ingestion of Jamaican bush teas.
   D. **Portal vein thrombosis** is seen in a variety of clinical settings including cirrhosis (particularly with sudden decompensation), malignancy causing obstruction either by direct invasion of the portal vein or by compression secondary to portal adenopathy, or intraabdominal infections such as Crohn's disease or diverticulitis.

II. **Hepatic abscess** may be either pyogenic or amebic.
   A. **Pyogenic abscess** most often occurs as a complication of either biliary tract disease or malignancy. Clinical features include fever, abdominal pain, and anorexia with tender hepatomegaly. Laboratory studies may demonstrate leukocytosis and elevated AP. The diagnosis is usually confirmed by USG or CT. **Treatment** includes antibiotic therapy and percutaneous drainage; surgical drainage is required in selected cases. Attempts to collect culture material should be performed before initiating antibiotic therapy. Combination therapy with ampicillin (or penicillin), an aminoglycoside, and an antianaerobic drug is recommended when cultures are pending or unavailable. In patients responding to treatment, parenteral therapy is recommended for 10–14 days, followed by 4–6 weeks of oral therapy (*Medicine* 66:472, 1987). Repeat imaging is recommended to document resolution.
   B. **Amebic abscess.** The diagnosis of amebic abscess requires a high index of clinical suspicion and should be considered in patients from endemic areas.

Amebic serology is helpful in establishing the diagnosis. Amebic abscesses should always be treated with metronidazole and/or chloroquine and should never be drained percutaneously or surgically (see Chap. 13).

III. **Sepsis** due to a variety of organisms has been associated with liver function test abnormalities that are typically mild, transient, and of no prognostic significance (*Arch Intern Med* 149:2246, 1989). The most commonly reported abnormality is direct hyperbilirubinemia; however, mild elevations in AST, ALT, and AP have also been noted (usually less than threefold above normal).

IV. **Autoimmune chronic active hepatitis** occurs most often in females and frequently presents with cirrhosis in childhood or young adulthood. Autoimmune hepatitis is characterized by the presence of autoantibodies (antinuclear antibody, anti–smooth muscle antibody, and anti–liver-kidney-microsomal antibody) and hypergammaglobulinemia. Improved life expectancy has been demonstrated in patients treated with glucocorticoids. Therapy is initiated with prednisone, 40–60 mg PO qd, which is then tapered to a maintenance dose of 7.5–10.0 mg PO daily as serum transaminase levels decrease. Combination therapy with azathioprine, 1–2 mg/kg/qd PO, and prednisone may also be used and is associated with fewer glucocorticoid-related side effects. Histologic remission occurs in as many as 80% of patients. Therapy should be discontinued in individuals who fail to demonstrate either a clinical, biochemical, or histologic improvement after 18 months of therapy (*Gastroenterology* 73:1422, 1977). Relapses occur in at least 50% of patients following cessation of therapy. Retreatment is effective in most cases but appears to be associated with more side effects (*N Engl J Med* 304:5, 1981). Many patients require lifelong low-dose therapy. Hepatic transplantation may be offered in end-stage disease.

V. **Hepatoma** is an uncommon cancer but is not an infrequent development in patients with chronic liver disease. Most hepatomas develop in the setting of long-standing liver disease and cirrhosis. Strong associations with viral hepatitis (especially HBV, HCV, and HDV), alcoholic cirrhosis, alpha$_1$-antitrypsin deficiency, and hemochromatosis have been described. Patients with known cirrhosis should be monitored with at least yearly imaging (either USG or CT) and measurement of serum alpha-fetoprotein. More frequent testing may be appropriate in selected cases. Early diagnosis is essential, as the tumors are best managed by surgical resection.

Complications of Hepatic Insufficiency

I. **Portosystemic (or hepatic) encephalopathy (PSE)** is the syndrome of disordered consciousness and altered neuromuscular activity seen in patients with hepatocellular failure or portosystemic shunting. The normal liver protects the systemic circulation from ingested toxic agents and the by-products of intestinal bacterial metabolism. The specific toxins and their mechanisms are unclear, but ammonia, gamma-aminobutyric acid, other amino acids, mercaptans, and short-chain fatty acids have all been implicated.

A. **Precipitating factors** include azotemia from volume contraction, diuretics, or renal failure; use of a tranquilizer, opioid, or sedative-hypnotic medication; GI hemorrhage; hypokalemia and alkalosis; constipation; infection; high-protein diet; progressive hepatocellular dysfunction; and surgery (especially portosystemic shunts).

B. **Treatment** should be initiated promptly. Precipitants should be identified and treated or eliminated whenever possible. Dietary protein should initially be eliminated while adequate calories (25–30 kcal/kg) are administered by either the enteral or parenteral route. Once clinical improvement occurs, a 20- to 40-g/day protein diet may be administered with 10- to 20-g/day increments every 3–5 days. Vegetable-protein diets may be better tolerated by patients with PSE than diets containing meat protein (*Dig Dis Sci* 27:1109, 1982). Branched-chain amino acid enriched formulas are available in both oral and parenteral forms, but their use should be reserved for PSE that is difficult to manage or is unresponsive to usual measures (see Chap. 2).

C. Medical therapies include lactulose, neomycin, and metronidazole.

1. **Lactulose** is a poorly absorbed, synthetic disaccharide. While its mechanism of action is not certain, lactulose appears to produce an osmotic diarrhea and alters intestinal flora, resulting in the production of acidic diarrhea.

   a. **Oral lactulose** can be given in doses of 15–45 ml PO bid–qid. Maintenance dosages should be adjusted to produce 2–3 soft stools per day. Hourly doses of 30–45 ml PO may be used to induce a rapid catharsis during the initial phases of treatment, or in PSE associated with constipation or blood in the GI tract. Oral lactulose should not be given to patients with an ileus or possible bowel obstruction. Overzealous use of lactulose can lead to dehydration, hypernatremia, and patient discomfort due to excessive diarrhea.

   b. **Lactulose enemas**, prepared with 300 ml of lactulose added to 700 ml of tap water, can be administered bid–qid. The enema is administered with the patient on his or her left side and in the Trendelenburg position; during retention, the patient should be rolled onto his or her right side, and the head should be elevated to promote filling of the proximal colon.

2. **Antibiotic preparations** can be effective in treating PSE.

   a. **Neomycin** may be given PO or by nasogastric tube, 1 g q4–6h, or by a retention enema as a 1% solution (1–2 g in 100–200 ml of isotonic saline) bid–qid. Approximately 1–3% of the administered dose of neomycin is absorbed with an attendant risk of ototoxicity and nephrotoxicity. The risk of toxicity is increased in patients with renal insufficiency. Because lactulose is as effective as neomycin in the treatment of PSE and is less toxic, lactulose is preferred for initial as well as chronic therapy (*Gastroenterology* 72:573, 1977). Combination therapy with lactulose plus neomycin should be considered in patients refractory to either agent alone.

   b. **Metronidazole** is useful for short-term therapy when neomycin is unavailable or poorly tolerated; a dose of 250 mg PO q8h is generally effective and well tolerated. Long-term metronidazole is not recommended due to neurotoxicity.

II. **Ascites and edema** occur as a result of avid sodium retention by the kidneys, decreased plasma oncotic pressure, increased splanchnic lymph flow, and elevated hydrostatic pressure in the hepatic sinusoids or portal vein. Treatment of ascites should be performed cautiously and gradually, since ascites itself is rarely life-threatening.

A. **Salt restriction** is the most important initial treatment measure; no more than 1,000 mg Na$^+$/day should be allowed. Rarely, a more rigid restriction may be required; however, most patients find such diets unpalatable and very restricted in protein, so compliance is diminished. A more liberal sodium intake (1,000–2,000 mg/day) can be allowed when a diuresis is effected. Low-sodium liquid formula diets may be useful in some patients.

B. **Bed rest** is occasionally helpful in mobilizing ascites in patients with refractory ascites. After diuresis is initiated, a gradual increase in activity can be allowed.

C. **Diuretics** should be considered in patients who fail to initiate a diuresis with salt restriction and bed rest. Under optimal conditions, the capacity to reabsorb ascitic fluid is no more than 700–900 ml/day; therefore, diuresis should proceed gradually. **Diuretics should not be administered to individuals with an increasing serum creatinine level.** The goal of diuretic therapy should be a daily weight loss of 0.5–1.0 kg in patients with edema and approximately 0.25 kg in patients without edema. The dosage of medication may be increased every 3–5 days to initiate or maintain an adequate diuresis. Spironolactone is the diuretic of choice, starting at a dose of 25 mg PO bid, this may be increased to a maximum of 150 mg PO qid. Amiloride or triamterene is useful in patients who cannot tolerate spironolactone. Loop diuretics may be added when spironolactone fails to initiate a diuresis. Furosemide, 20 mg PO qd, may be used initially, with the dose increased every 3–5 days depending on the response. Such loop diuretic agents are potent and may be associated with serious side effects; patients receiving these drugs should be observed closely for signs of volume contraction, electrolyte disturbances, encephalopathy, and renal insufficiency. In selected situations, other agents such as metolazone or thiazides may be useful.

D. **Water restriction** is not routinely necessary. If dilutional hyponatremia occurs, a fluid restriction of 1,000–1,500 ml/day will usually suffice. A more stringent fluid restriction may be required in patients with severe hyponatremia or those with renal failure and oliguria.

E. **Paracentesis** should be performed for diagnostic purposes (e.g., new-onset ascites, suspicion of malignant ascites, spontaneous peritonitis) or when there is tense ascites causing respiratory compromise or impending peritoneal rupture. Up to 5 liters of ascitic fluid can be safely removed provided that (1) the patient has edema, (2) the fluid is removed slowly (over 30–90 minutes), and (3) a fluid restriction is instituted to avoid hyponatremia (*Hepatology* 5:403, 1985). Rarely, however, paracentesis of as little as 1,000 ml may lead to circulatory collapse, encephalopathy, and renal failure.

F. **Peritoneovenous (LeVeen or Denver) shunts (PVS)** may be useful in the 5–10% of patients with ascites that is refractory to all medical therapy (*Gastroenterology* 82:790, 1982). PVS may be associated with complications such as disseminated intravascular coagulation, shunt closure, and fever. The shunt should be ligated if overt bleeding occurs. PVS should not be used in patients with infected ascites, recent variceal hemorrhage, markedly elevated bilirubin, hepatorenal syndrome, or coagulopathy.

G. **Transjugular intrahepatic portosystemic shunts (TIPS)** have also been used to manage refractory ascites, but experience with these shunts is limited.

H. **Other agents** occasionally helpful in the management of ascites are albumin and dopamine. Albumin is sometimes useful in patients with azotemia and intravascular volume depletion. Unfortunately, albumin rapidly leaves the intravascular space, is expensive, and appears to offer little advantage over the use of crystalloid solutions for volume expansion. Albumin infusion in conjunction with repeated paracentesis appears to be useful and safe in patients with tense ascites (*Gastroenterology* 93:234, 1987). Dopamine in vasodilator doses (1–5 μg/kg/minute) may be administered in an attempt to improve renal blood flow, but its value in ascites management has not been proved.

III. **Spontaneous bacterial peritonitis (SBP)** occurs only in patients with preexisting ascites. The illness is typified by the presence of abdominal pain and distention, fever, decreased bowel sounds, and worsening of hepatic encephalopathy; however, the disease may be present in the absence of specific clinical signs. Studies show that 25% of hospitalized cirrhotic patients have SBP (*Dis Mon* 31:3, 1985). Therefore, cirrhotic patients with ascites and evidence of any clinical deterioration should undergo a diagnostic paracentesis to exclude SBP. The diagnosis is likely when the ascitic fluid contains greater than 250 polymorphonuclear leukocytes (PMNs)/μl. A positive culture confirms the diagnosis. The highest-yield cultures are derived from 10 ml of ascitic fluid inoculated into blood culture bottles at the bedside. The most common organisms are *Escherichia coli*, *Pneumococcus*, and *Streptococcus* (*Hepatology* 8:171, 1988). In suspected cases, empiric antibiotic therapy with a third-generation cephalosporin (e.g., cefotaxime) is appropriate. Aminoglycosides should be avoided as they may precipitate renal failure, do not achieve adequate levels in ascitic fluid, and are inactivated at an acid pH. A repeat paracentesis should be performed 48–72 hours after initiation of therapy if no organism is isolated or clinical deterioration on appropriate therapy is observed. Norfloxacin, 400 mg PO qd, reduces SBP recurrence (*Hepatology* 12:716, 1990), but the causative agent in subsequent SBP episodes in these patients is typically a gram-positive organism, so antibiotic therapy should be adjusted accordingly.

IV. **Portal hypertension** presents with GI bleeding or hypersplenism. GI bleeding is usually due to varices or congested mucosa (see Chap. 15). Splenomegaly is usually associated with thrombocytopenia in advanced cases; occasionally, leukopenia or pancytopenia are seen.

V. **Coagulopathy** occurs as a result of impaired hepatic synthetic function, particularly of vitamin K–dependent coagulation factors. Usually, patients have only a prolonged PT; in very advanced disease, the aPTT may also be prolonged. A syndrome of disseminated intravascular coagulation may occur due to loss of both procoagulant factors and anticoagulant factors such as antithrombin III. The appropriate replacement for vitamin K deficiency is 5–10 mg PO qd or 10 mg SC qd (for patients unable to absorb oral vitamin K or for hospitalized patients). Transfusions of FFP and platelets should be reserved for patients with active bleeding or for those undergoing invasive procedures.

VI. **Impaired drug clearance** can occur in chronic liver disease because the liver and the kidneys are the primary organs involved in drug metabolism and excretion. Drug availability may be increased due to the presence of portosystemic shunts or to decreased levels of drug-binding plasma proteins (e.g., albumin). In most cases, medications can be used safely in patients with liver disease provided that (1) drug dosages are reduced when it is known that a medication undergoes significant hepatic excretion or metabolism; (2) patients are followed closely for signs of toxicity; (3) serum or blood levels are monitored when available; (4) alternative agents that do not undergo significant hepatic excretion or metabolism are used when possible; and (5) drugs associated with the development of chronic liver disease are avoided.

Hepatic Transplantation

Hepatic transplantation is now the accepted therapy for irreversible FHF and for complications of end-stage chronic liver disease. Timing of liver transplantation is a complex issue. Patients with FHF should be considered for transplantation if signs of advanced (stage III or IV) encephalopathy (see Table 16-3), marked coagulopathy (PT >20 seconds), or hypoglycemia are present. Patients with chronic liver disease should be considered for transplantation when complications occur, including refractory ascites, SBP, encephalopathy, variceal bleeding, or severe impairment of synthetic function with coagulopathy or hypoalbuminemia (*Ann Intern Med* 104:377, 1986).

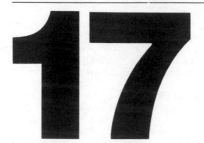

Disorders of Hemostasis

Gregory A. Ewald

Evaluation of Hemostatic Function

I. **Regulation of hemostasis.** The integrity of the vasculature is maintained through a complex series of interactions between the vascular endothelium, subendothelial macromolecules, platelets, and plasma coagulation factors. Disruption of the normal balance between procoagulant and anticoagulant activity can result in hemorrhagic or thrombotic disorders.

A. **Primary hemostasis** in response to vessel injury is achieved as platelets adhere to the subendothelial matrix in a reaction that requires von Willebrand factor (vWF). Platelets are activated and aggregate to form a hemostatic plug, promoting vasoconstriction through the release of thromboxane A_2.

B. **The coagulation cascade.** Formation of a fibrin clot occurs when thrombin is generated from prothrombin as the end-product of both the **intrinsic and extrinsic coagulation pathways** (Fig. 17-1). The coagulation cascade is complex and tightly regulated. It involves multiple proteolytic enzymatic reactions whose products may exert positive or negative feedback. Cofactors (factors Va and VIIIa and tissue factor [TF]), phospholipid surfaces, and calcium are also required for efficient activation of the coagulation cascade. Absence of these proteolytic enzymes or their inhibitors can produce hemorrhagic or thrombotic disorders. In addition to cleaving fibrinogen, thrombin provides positive feedback by activating factors V and VIII, as well as the fibrin cross-linking enzyme, factor XIII. The extrinsic pathway may be initiated by the exposure of blood to TF, a membrane protein present in most extravascular tissues but normally absent from blood cells and intact endothelium. The molecular events that trigger the intrinsic pathway are poorly understood. Although deficiencies of factor XII, prekallikrein, and high-molecular weight kininogen cause prolongation of the activated partial thromboplastin time (aPTT) in vitro, these deficiencies are not associated with clinical bleeding. In contrast, all the other components of the intrinsic, extrinsic, and common pathways are required for normal hemostasis.

C. **Fibrinolysis** (Fig. 17-2). Fibrin is degraded by the proteolytic enzyme plasmin, which is generated selectively from fibrin-bound plasminogen by the action of tissue plasminogen activator (t-PA). Plasminogen may also be activated by the administration of urokinase, a urinary tract enzyme, or streptokinase, a nonenzymatic activator produced by beta-hemolytic streptococci. Circulating alpha$_2$-antiplasmin and plasminogen activator inhibitors (PAI) serve to limit fibrinolysis and prevent systemic fibrinogen degradation. Soluble fibrin degradation products (FDPs) produced by the action of plasmin on fibrin or fibrinogen can bind to fibrin monomers and inhibit coagulation.

D. **Natural anticoagulants** serve to restrict the coagulation process to sites of vascular injury and protect normal vessels from thrombosis.

1. **Prostacyclin (PGI$_2$)** synthesized by endothelial cells inhibits platelet aggregation and promotes vasodilation.

2. **Antithrombin III (ATIII)** inhibits thrombin (IIa) and factors IXa, Xa, and XIa by forming irreversible complexes with these proteases. The inhibitory reaction is accelerated by endothelial surface proteoglycans or by exogenously administered heparin.

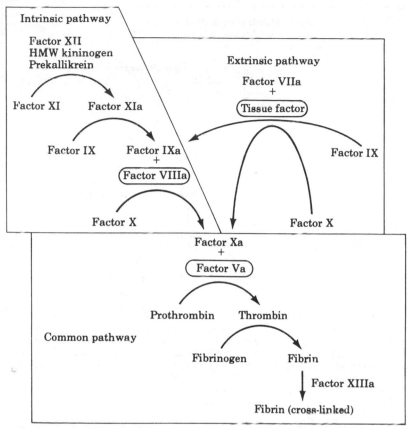

Fig. 17-1. Blood coagulation cascade. Plasma zymogens are sequentially converted to active proteases as depicted by the arrows. Nonenzymatic protein cofactors (*ovals*) are required at several stages of the cascade. Factors IX and X and prothrombin are activated on phospholipid surfaces. Thrombin cleaves fibrinogen, yielding fibrin monomers that polymerize to form a clot. (HMW = high molecular weight.)

3. **Thrombomodulin,** a protein expressed on the luminal surface of endothelial cells, directly inhibits the procoagulant activities of thrombin and accelerates the activation of protein C by thrombin. In the presence of the cofactor **protein S, activated protein C (APC)** specifically degrades factors Va and VIIIa, resulting in further inhibition of coagulation.

II. **History and physical examination.** The cause of abnormal bleeding or thrombosis is often suggested by a careful history. Platelet abnormalities often lead to petechiae, ecchymoses at sites of minor trauma, and prolonged bleeding from superficial lacerations. A coagulation factor deficiency is suggested by the delayed appearance of hemarthroses or deep hematomas. Details of previous bleeding episodes, including **duration and severity** of bleeding, **requirement for blood transfusions,** and **response to hemostatic stress** (e.g., dental extractions, trauma, pregnancy, major and minor surgery) should be obtained. All recent prescription and nonprescription **medications,** including ethanol, aspirin or other nonsteroidal antiinflammatory drugs (NSAIDs), oral contraceptives, and anticoagulants, should be identified. Any

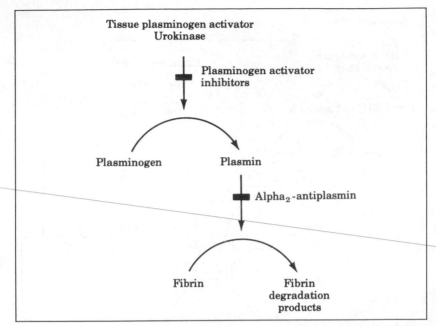

Fig. 17-2. Fibrinolysis. The protease plasmin is generated enzymatically from fibrin-bound plasminogen by tissue plasminogen activator, or independent of fibrin by urokinase. The bacterial cofactor streptokinase forms a nonenzymatic complex with plasminogen, resulting in the conversion of additional plasminogen to plasmin. Plasmin degrades fibrin clots, generating fibrin degradation products. Plasminogen activation and fibrin degradation are inhibited by plasminogen activator inhibitors and alpha$_2$-antiplasmin, respectively.

family history of bleeding or thrombosis should be documented. The **physical examination** should include a careful inspection of the skin, oral mucosa, and joints and a search for evidence of liver disease, uremia, malnutrition, or malignancy.

III. **Laboratory evaluation** can often define the hemostatic disorder responsible for abnormal bleeding. Screening tests, including platelet count, prothrombin time (PT), aPTT, and bleeding time, are useful in evaluating patients with abnormal bleeding, but the results may be normal in cases of mild platelet or coagulation factor disorders. None of these tests detects factor XIII deficiency, which can be established only by fibrin clot solubility assays. Therefore, additional evaluation is important in patients who have significant bleeding but normal screening tests.

A. **The peripheral blood smear** should be examined in all patients with abnormalities of hemostasis. Normally, about 10–20 platelets/oil immersion field can be seen. Quantitative or qualitative abnormalities of leukocytes or erythrocytes may suggest an underlying hematopoietic disorder. Fragmented erythrocytes (schistocytes), suggesting microangiopathy, are seen in thrombotic thrombocytopenic purpura (TTP), hemolytic-uremic syndrome (HUS), and disseminated intravascular coagulation (DIC).

B. **Evaluation of platelet function**

1. **The platelet count,** normally 150,000–400,000/μl, is determined as part of an automated blood count or by manual phase–contrast microscopy. Pseudothrombocytopenia due to ethylenediaminetetraacetic acid (EDTA)-induced platelet clumping is an artifact that can be excluded by examination of the peripheral blood smear and repetition of the platelet count using a blood sample collected in sodium citrate.

2. **The bleeding time** is a **functional** test of primary hemostasis. A normal bleeding time ranges from 2.5–9.5 minutes, but there is considerable individual variability. The bleeding time may be prolonged (greater than 10–15 minutes) in patients with thrombocytopenia (platelet count <100,000/µl), qualitative platelet abnormalities, von Willebrand's disease (vWD), and occasionally vascular disorders (e.g., vasculitis, Cushing's syndrome, connective tissue disorders). **Aspirin** may prolong the bleeding time for up to 1 week following ingestion; other drugs may also have transient effects on the bleeding time (see Platelet Disorders, sec. **III**).

3. **Platelet aggregometry** is used for classification of congenital platelet disorders (e.g., storage pool disease, Glanzmann's thrombasthenia, Bernard-Soulier syndrome) and is rarely useful in the evaluation of acquired bleeding abnormalities.

C. **Evaluation of vWF** is appropriate when the bleeding time is prolonged, the platelet count is normal, and there is no apparent cause of acquired platelet dysfunction (e.g., drugs). vWF is synthesized by endothelial cells and megakaryocytes and forms multimers containing from 2 to more than 40 subunits. vWF is required for normal platelet adhesion and prolongs the half-life of factor VIII.

1. **Ristocetin cofactor activity** is determined by the ability of ristocetin to enable vWF to interact with platelet glycoprotein Ib in vitro. It is reduced in most patients with vWD but may also be reduced when there is an elevated level of plasma protein, such as in the presence of a paraprotein.

2. **Ristocetin-induced platelet agglutination** is decreased in most types of vWD except type 2B, in which agglutination occurs at very low concentrations of ristocetin (see Inherited Bleeding Disorders, sec. **II.A**).

3. **vWF antigen** (factor VIII-related antigen) can be measured by various immunoassays, and the size distribution of vWF multimers can be determined by crossed-immunoelectrophoresis or agarose gel electrophoresis. These tests are useful for the subclassification of vWD.

D. **Evaluation of coagulation factor activity** is accomplished through functional assays that measure the time required for citrate-anticoagulated plasma to clot after the addition of calcium, phospholipids, and an appropriate activating agent. Clotting times can be prolonged by **clotting factor deficiencies, heparin, FDPs, or acquired coagulation factor inhibitors.** The distinction between a coagulation factor deficiency and an acquired inhibitor can often be made by repeating the abnormal coagulation test using a **50 : 50 mixture** of normal plasma with the patient's plasma (see sec. **III.D.7**). Improper collection or delay in processing of a blood sample can adversely affect the results of coagulation factor tests. Polycythemia can result in artifactually prolonged clotting times due to a disproportionately high ratio of anticoagulant to plasma in the sample.

1. **The prothrombin time (PT)** is the clotting time measured after addition of tissue thromboplastin (TF and phospholipids) to recalcified plasma. The normal PT is approximately 11–14 seconds but may vary considerably. Therefore, a control PT using normal plasma should always be performed when determining the patient's PT. Commercial thromboplastin reagents vary considerably in responsiveness to warfarin-induced reduction in clotting factors. Therefore, the **international normalized ratio (INR)** was developed to standardize reporting of the PT ratio obtained with various thromboplastin reagents (see Antithrombotic Therapy, sec. **I.D.1**). The PT measures the activity of the extrinsic and common pathways; it is most sensitive to deficiencies of factors VII and X but may also be prolonged in patients with deficiencies of factor V, prothrombin, or fibrinogen.

2. **The activated partial thromboplastin time (aPTT),** normally 22–36 seconds, is the clotting time measured after addition of phospholipid to recalcified plasma that has been preincubated with particulate material to initiate activation of the contact system (intrinsic pathway). Concentrations of factors VIII, IX, XI, and XII; high-molecular weight kininogen; or prekallikrein below 30% of normal are usually detected by aPTT prolongation.

3. **The thrombin time (TT)** is the time required for plasma to clot after the

addition of thrombin. Normally 11–18 seconds, the TT may be prolonged in DIC, hypofibrinogenemia, or dysfibrinogenemia. Heparin also prolongs the TT but can be neutralized in the lab by the addition of protamine sulfate.

4. **Fibrinogen concentration** is frequently estimated from the clotting time of diluted plasma after addition of excess thrombin (**Clauss** method) but fibrinogen concentration may be underestimated in the presence of FDPs, paraproteins, or heparin. Therefore, hypofibrinogenemia (less than 100 mg/dl) should be confirmed with an end-point turbidometric assay (**Ellis** method), which does not depend on the rate of fibrin polymerization.

5. **Fibrin degradation products (FDPs)** in serum are detected by agglutination of latex beads coated with antibodies to FDPs or fibrinogen. Increased levels of FDPs (>8 μg/ml) occur in DIC and thromboembolic events and in association with fibrinolytic therapy. Severe liver disease may cause mild elevation of FDPs, and a false-positive test may occur in patients with a rheumatoid factor present. Assays for **D-dimer** measure cross-linked FDPs and can help distinguish fibrinogenolytic from fibrinolytic processes.

6. **Specific factor assays** measure the ability of the patient's plasma to correct the clotting time of known factor-deficient plasma. Results are expressed as a percentage of the activity in plasma pooled from normal donors. The normal range for coagulation factor activities is generally 60–160% but should be determined independently by each laboratory.

7. **Assays for acquired anticoagulants.** Prolongation of the PT or aPTT may be due to antibodies that inhibit coagulation factor activity. When an abnormal coagulation test is repeated using a **50:50 mixture** of normal plasma with the patient's plasma, the clotting time will usually remain prolonged if an inhibitor is present but will correct to normal if there is a coagulation factor deficiency. Antibodies that react with specific coagulation factors (e.g., factors VIII or IX) are associated with abnormal bleeding. In contrast, **lupus anticoagulants** often predispose patients to arterial or venous thrombosis, possibly by interfering with the anticoagulant activity of protein C, activation of platelets, or inhibition of PGI_2 production by endothelial cells (*Thrombosis and Hemorrhage*. Boston: Blackwell Scientific, 1994. P. 755). Initially described in patients with systemic lupus erythematosus (SLE), these antibodies interfere with coagulation factor assays in vitro, probably by binding to phospholipids. The presence of a lupus anticoagulant can be confirmed by comparing the clotting time of the patient's plasma to control plasma in the presence of a dilute concentration of phospholipids or by performing a dilute Russell's viper venom clotting time. Assays for antibodies to cardiolipin are positive in some but not all patients with lupus anticoagulants (*Semin Thromb Hemost* 16:182, 1990).

Platelet Disorders

I. **Thrombocytopenia** (Fig. 17-3) is defined as a platelet count less than 140,000/μl. Although hereditary forms exist, most cases are acquired. Thrombocytopenia can result from decreased platelet production, increased peripheral platelet destruction, or sequestration. This distinction is most reliably made by examination of a bone marrow aspirate, which normally contains 3–7 megakaryocytes/low-power field. Normal or increased numbers of megakaryocytes imply increased platelet destruction or sequestration; decreased numbers suggest decreased platelet production. In general, platelet counts in excess of 50,000/μl are not associated with significant bleeding, and severe spontaneous bleeding is unusual in patients with platelet counts higher than 20,000/μl in the absence of coagulation factor abnormalities or concomitant qualitative platelet dysfunction. All patients with thrombocytopenia should be instructed to avoid trauma and to seek early treatment if trauma occurs. **IM injections, rectal examinations and suppositories, and enemas should be avoided** if possible. Phlebotomy should be minimized, and pressure should be

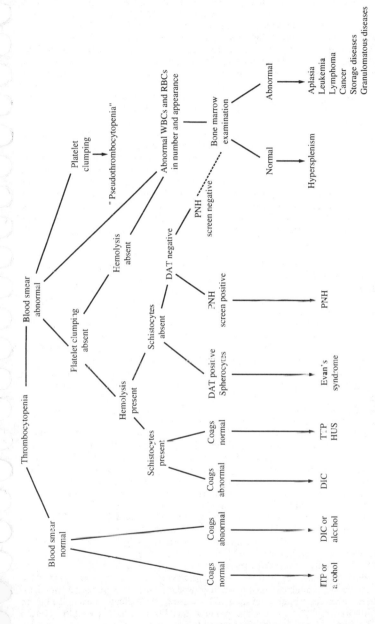

Fig. 17-3. A guide to laboratory evaluation of thrombocytopenia. (Coags = coagulation factors; DAT = direct antiglobulin test; PNH = paroxysmal nocturnal hemoglobinuria; ITP = idiopathic thrombocytopenic purpura; DIC = disseminated intravascular coagulation; TTP = thrombotic thrombocytopenic purpura; HUS = hemolytic-uremic syndrome.) (From C Rutherford, EP Frankel. Thrombocytopenia: Issues in diagnosis and therapy. *Med Clin North Am* 78:557, 1994.)

applied to venipuncture sites for at least 10 minutes. **Drugs known to inhibit platelet function (e.g., aspirin, NSAIDs) should not be given.** Patients should be instructed not to use hard toothbrushes, dental floss, or metal razors. In acute thrombocytopenia, platelet transfusions are generally reserved for patients experiencing hemorrhage or anticipating major surgery. Prophylactic platelet transfusions may be of benefit in patients with chronic thrombocytopenic states such as aplastic anemia or chemotherapy-induced thrombocytopenia (see Chap. 18).

A. **Drug-induced thrombocytopenia** is diagnosed by noting temporal relationships between drug administration and the onset of thrombocytopenia. Decreased platelet production has been associated with thiazide diuretics, amrinone, ethanol, estrogens, trimethoprim/sulfamethoxazole, and chemotherapeutic agents. Increased platelet destruction, presumably through immune mechanisms, can occur in patients receiving quinine, quinidine, heparin, gold salts, rifampin, sulfonamides, penicillin, or valproic acid. Many other drugs have been implicated as rare causes of thrombocytopenia (*Thrombosis and Hemorrhage.* Boston: Blackwell Scientific, 1994. P. 546). **All nonessential drugs should be discontinued in patients with thrombocytopenia of undetermined etiology.** Structurally unrelated drugs may be substituted when necessary. Thrombocytopenia usually resolves within days of discontinuing the offending drug but in some cases can persist for months because of slow excretion of the drug (e.g., gold). Prednisone, 1 mg/kg PO qd, may decrease the duration of thrombocytopenia in some cases. Platelet transfusions are usually ineffective but should be administered in cases of profound drug-induced thrombocytopenia associated with serious hemorrhage.

B. **Autoimmune thrombocytopenia** results from accelerated platelet destruction mediated by antiplatelet antibodies. Most cases arise in previously healthy patients as **idiopathic thrombocytopenic purpura (ITP)**, but similar syndromes occur in association with SLE, chronic lymphocytic leukemia, and lymphoma. Clinical manifestations include severe thrombocytopenia (platelet counts <50,000/µl in most patients), normal erythrocyte and leukocyte morphology, and a normal or increased number of bone marrow megakaryocytes. Platelet-associated IgG can be detected in greater than 90% of patients with ITP but may also be present in other thrombocytopenic states (*Blood* 76:859, 1990). **Acute ITP** usually occurs in children 1–2 weeks after a viral infection and resolves spontaneously within 6 months. Most adult patients with ITP have **chronic ITP**, which is not usually associated with an obvious initiating event. Spontaneous remissions of chronic ITP are rare; however, complete or partial remissions in response to treatment with glucocorticoids or splenectomy occur in approximately 75% of patients. Refractory cases in patients with platelet counts below 20,000/µl have been treated with vinca alkaloids, danazol, cyclophosphamide, or azathioprine with variable success (*Blood* 74:2309, 1989).

1. **Glucocorticoids.** Prednisone, 1–2 mg/kg PO qd, or its equivalent should be administered at the time of diagnosis and as initial therapy in relapsing disease. Selected patients with severe thrombocytopenia and active bleeding may benefit from initial treatment with methylprednisolone, 1 g IV qd for 3 days, followed by prednisone, 1–2 mg/kg PO qd. Two weeks of glucocorticoid therapy may be required before there is an increase in the platelet count. If there is no significant response after 4 weeks of glucocorticoid therapy, a response is unlikely and other treatment should be instituted. The prednisone dosage should be slowly tapered when the platelet count becomes greater than 100,000/µl. A minority of patients (<25%) achieve a complete remission after glucocorticoid therapy alone.

2. **Splenectomy** should be considered in patients who (1) fail to respond to glucocorticoids, (2) develop serious glucocorticoid toxicity, or (3) develop recurrent thrombocytopenia when glucocorticoids are tapered. A rapid increase in the platelet count usually occurs after splenectomy and may be lifesaving if there is serious hemorrhage. **Pneumococcal vaccine should be administered to all patients prior to splenectomy.** Glucocorticoids should be continued following splenectomy until the platelet count returns to normal, followed by a gradual taper. Sixty to 70% of patients with chronic ITP

will achieve sustained remissions following splenectomy. Some patients who relapse more than 6 months following splenectomy have accessory spleens, which may be detected by a variety of radiographic techniques. Accessory splenectomy may produce remission in such patients.

3. **Immunosuppressive therapy** should be considered in patients who remain profoundly thrombocytopenic following splenectomy. **Cyclophosphamide,** 1–2 mg/kg PO qd for 2–3 months, or **azathioprine,** 1–2 mg/kg PO qd for at least 3 months, will improve the platelet count in approximately 60% of patients. **Vincristine,** 1–2 mg IV weekly for 4–6 weeks, may also benefit some patients. However, many patients with chronic thrombocytopenia do not have significant bleeding despite platelet counts below 30,000/μl, and chronic treatment with immunosuppressive agents is usually not justified.

4. **Danazol,** 200 mg PO tid, produces a gradual improvement in the platelet count in some patients with chronic ITP. Several months of therapy may be necessary before improvement occurs, and responses are less frequent in patients less than 45 years of age (*Ann Intern Med* 111:723, 1989).

5. **Platelet transfusions** have limited use in ITP due to rapid destruction of transfused platelets. However, transfusions may be given if there is life-threatening bleeding.

6. **Immune globulin,** 0.4 g/kg IV qd for 5 days, or 1 g/kg IV qd for 2 days, produces a **rapid but temporary increase** in the platelet count in many patients with chronic ITP and may prolong the survival of transfused platelets. Immune globulin should be reserved for patients with severe hemorrhage or those undergoing surgical procedures.

C. **Pregnancy-associated thrombocytopenia** occurs in 5–10% of pregnancies, usually without significant maternal or fetal morbidity. However, infants born to women with chronic ITP may rarely develop severe thrombocytopenia and have an increased risk of intracranial hemorrhage. Studies suggest that thrombocytopenia diagnosed for the first time during pregnancy is not associated with fetal thrombocytopenia and may be treated conservatively (*N Engl J Med* 323:264, 1990). Women with a history of ITP may benefit from glucocorticoids or immune globulin prior to delivery. Cesarean section may be unnecessary if the fetal platelet count is determined to be greater than 50,000/μl.

D. **Human immunodeficiency virus (HIV)-associated thrombocytopenia** is common in patients seropositive for HIV and may be the presenting manifestation of HIV infection. Isolated thrombocytopenia similar to chronic ITP is most frequently observed, but impaired thrombopoiesis, drug-induced thrombocytopenia, or thrombotic thrombocytopenic purpura (TTP) may also occur. Treatment of isolated HIV-associated thrombocytopenia is similar to treatment of chronic ITP (see sec. I.B), with more limited use of glucocorticoids and immunosuppressive therapy because of the underlying immune deficiency. Zidovudine (AZT) therapy (see Chap. 14) may improve the platelet count in some patients.

E. **Transfusion-associated thrombocytopenia.** Acute thrombocytopenia may follow massive transfusion or extracorporeal circulation, due to dilution or mechanical removal of platelets. The thrombocytopenia lasts 3–5 days and may be treated with platelet transfusions. Posttransfusion purpura is a rare type of immune thrombocytopenia that occurs primarily, although not exclusively, in multiparous PI^{A1} antigen–negative women. Onset occurs approximately 7 days after a blood transfusion. The thrombocytopenia is usually severe and may be associated with intracranial hemorrhage. Immune globulin, 0.4 mg/kg IV daily for 5 days, or plasma exchange by plasmapheresis may produce a rapid improvement in the platelet count in some patients. **Platelet transfusions are contraindicated in posttransfusion purpura,** and glucocorticoids are of questionable benefit.

F. **Thrombotic thrombocytopenic purpura (TTP)** is a rare syndrome characterized by thrombocytopenia, microangiopathic hemolytic anemia, and neurologic abnormalities, often accompanied by fever and renal dysfunction. The diagnosis is supported by microangiopathic findings (e.g., schistocytes) on the peripheral blood smear, elevation of the reticulocyte count and serum lactate dehydrogenase, and the absence of laboratory evidence of DIC. The demonstration of characteristic microvascular occlusions in biopsies of skin, gingiva, or other tissues lends further support but is not required to make an initial diagnosis and initiate treatment. The adult **hemolytic-uremic syndrome (HUS)** is a closely related disorder in which renal failure is the predominant manifestation. Thrombotic microangiopathy may also occur in association with pregnancy, SLE, carcinoma, or infection (e.g., HIV, *E. coli* gastroenteritis) or after high-dose chemotherapy or transplantation. **TTP should be viewed as a medical emergency,** and therapy should be instituted promptly because rapid neurologic deterioration and death may ensue. **Platelet transfusions should be avoided** because of the potential for accelerated thrombosis.

1. **Initial therapy** should include daily total plasma exchange by **plasmapheresis** using fresh-frozen plasma (FFP) as the replacement fluid. If plasmapheresis is not available, FFP, 2 units IV q6h, should be given. Plasma therapy should continue until the platelet count has risen to the normal range and then gradually discontinued. Prednisone, 1 mg/kg PO qd, or methylprednisolone, 1 mg/kg IV qd, is usually included in the initial therapy of TTP, although responses to glucocorticoids alone are rare. Aspirin, 325 mg PO qd, and dipyridamole, 75 mg PO q6h, are often administered at the time of diagnosis or added after partial improvement in the platelet count has occurred; however, the effectiveness of these antiplatelet agents in TTP remains uncertain. Because relapses may occur up to several years after an initial episode of TTP, patients should be followed closely and plasma therapy reinstituted promptly if a relapse occurs.

2. **Refractory cases in patients** who do not achieve a prompt hematologic remission or who require prolonged plasma therapy may benefit from **plasmapheresis** using "cryopoor" plasma as the replacement fluid; **vincristine,** 1–2 mg IV at weekly intervals; or **immune globulin,** 0.4 g/kg IV qd for 5 days. Occasional refractory cases have been reported to respond to splenectomy, but this treatment remains controversial.

G. **Hypersplenism** results in inappropriate splenic sequestration and destruction of blood cells. It occurs most often in patients with hepatic cirrhosis and portal hypertension and less frequently in association with splenomegaly of other etiologies. Anemia or leukopenia may be present in addition to thrombocytopenia, which is rarely severe enough to cause serious bleeding. Because of the increased risk of operative mortality in these patients, splenectomy should be considered only if there is unmanageable hemorrhage.

H. **Other causes of thrombocytopenia** include DIC, nutritional deficiencies of folic acid or vitamin B_{12}, bone marrow infiltration due to myelophthisic disease (e.g., tuberculosis, metastatic carcinoma, myelofibrosis), primary hematopoietic disorders (e.g., leukemia, aplastic anemia, myelodysplasia, multiple myeloma, paroxysmal nocturnal hemoglobinuria), and various viral, bacterial, and rickettsial infections. Specific therapy is directed at the underlying disorder.

II. **Thrombocytosis,** defined as a platelet count greater than 400,000/µl, may arise as either a primary or secondary disorder.

A. **Primary thrombocytosis** occurs in myeloproliferative disorders, including polycythemia vera, chronic myelogenous leukemia, and idiopathic myelofibrosis. **Essential thrombocythemia (ET)** is a myeloproliferative disorder in which the platelet count is above 600,000/µl (often >1,000,000/µl) and other myeloproliferative disorders or secondary thrombocytosis (see sec. **II.B**) have been excluded. ET is associated with both thrombotic and hemorrhagic complications. Although the risk of thrombosis or bleeding correlates poorly with platelet count, patients with ET may benefit from treatment with **hydroxyurea,** 15 mg/kg PO qd, to decrease the platelet count below 600,000/µl (*Cancer* 66:549, 1990). **Alpha-interferon** (5,000,000 units SC qd) has also been effective in lowering the platelet count (*Br J Haematol* 79:42, 1991). Intermittent painful erythema and cyanosis of the distal extremities, or erythromelalgia, may respond to aspirin, 325 mg PO qd, or hydroxyurea. Patients with diffuse hemorrhage, extreme thrombocytosis, and no other underlying coagulation abnormalities may benefit from **platelet pheresis** to acutely lower the platelet count.

B. Secondary thrombocytosis may occur in response to splenectomy, iron deficiency, carcinoma, or chronic inflammatory disorders. Platelet counts are occasionally greater than 1,000,000/μl, but there is little risk of thrombosis or hemorrhage, and specific treatment is usually unnecessary.

III. Qualitative platelet disorders. Congenital platelet disorders (e.g., Bernard-Soulier syndrome, Glanzmann's thrombasthenia) may produce a prolonged bleeding time and hemorrhage. However, in most patients, abnormal platelet function results from **acquired disorders**, including uremia, liver disease, paraproteinemia, and myeloproliferative disorders; cardiopulmonary bypass surgery; and drugs, especially aspirin, other NSAIDs, and certain beta-lactam antibiotics (*N Engl J Med* 324:27, 1991). Therapy is primarily directed toward the underlying disease. Patients with uremia may respond to hemodialysis.

A. Platelet transfusions should be administered during episodes of severe bleeding.

B. Desmopressin acetate transiently decreases the bleeding time in many patients with acquired platelet dysfunction. It is administered in a single dose, 0.3 μg/kg IV, prior to surgical procedures.

C. Conjugated estrogens, 0.6 mg/kg IV qd for 5 days, may produce a more durable improvement in the bleeding time in some patients.

D. Cryoprecipitate, 1–2 bags/10 kg IV, may also improve hemostatic function, but its use is associated with the risk of viral transmission (see Inherited Bleeding Disorders, sec. I.A.1.b).

IV. Vascular purpura occurring in a patient with normal platelet function and normal coagulation studies may result from chronic glucocorticoid therapy, purpura simplex, senile purpura, Cushing's syndrome, connective tissue diseases, scurvy, cryoglobulinemia, multiple myeloma, amyloidosis, allergic purpura, certain infections, or factitious purpura. Therapy is directed toward the underlying condition.

Inherited Bleeding Disorders

I. Hemophilia. Inherited deficiencies of factors VIII (hemophilia A) and IX (hemophilia B) are X-linked disorders with similar clinical presentations. Severely affected patients with less than 1% of normal factor VIII or IX activity have frequent spontaneous hemarthroses and other bleeding episodes. In moderate hemophilia (1–5% of normal activity), bleeding is usually associated with known trauma, but occasional spontaneous hemorrhage can occur. Patients with mild hemophilia (5–40% of normal activity) rarely experience hemorrhage in the absence of severe trauma or surgery, and these patients may remain undiagnosed until adulthood. Patients with hemophilia characteristically have a prolonged aPTT, normal PT, and normal bleeding time. Hemorrhagic episodes are generally managed by factor replacement therapy, which should be instituted as early as possible to minimize long-term complications. Treatment of patients with hemophilia is often complicated and may require consultation with a physician experienced in the care of these patients. **Aspirin and NSAID-containing medications should not be administered to patients with hemophilia.**

A. Factor replacement therapy. The specific agent and dosage of replacement therapy is determined by the nature of the bleeding episode and the type of hemophilia. One unit of a coagulation factor is defined as the amount present in 1 ml of fresh plasma pooled from normal donors. Since the plasma volume can be estimated as approximately 50 ml/kg body weight, the following formula can be used to calculate the replacement dose of factor VIII needed to achieve a desired plasma concentration (expressed as % of normal):

Dose (units) = (desired %activity − initial %activity) × (weight in kg)/2

Because **factor IX** appears to have a significant extravascular distribution, the dose required to produce a desired plasma concentration is approximately **twice that predicted by the above formula.** Treatment of hemophilia requires an understanding of the potential infectious complications of factor replacement therapy. Before routine use of viral inactivation procedures in the preparation of coagulation factor concentrates, most patients with severe hemophilia became seropositive for hepatitis viruses B and C and for HIV. Donor screening, heat and chemical treatments, and immunoaffinity purification have markedly reduced, but not completely eliminated, the risks of viral transmission from currently used concentrates (*Semin Thromb Hemost* 19:54, 1993). The development of recombinant coagulation factor concentrates may further reduce these risks.

1. **Low-purity factor replacement products** include FFP and cryoprecipitate (Table 17-1).

   a. **FFP** contains all coagulation factors in approximately normal concentrations. FFP can be used to treat patients with mild factor IX deficiency who require infrequent therapy; however, because FFP is not treated with viral inactivation procedures, factor IX concentrate is the preferred therapy for most patients with hemophilia B.

   b. **Cryoprecipitate** contains factor VIII, vWF, and fibrinogen. The concentration of factor VIII is approximately 100 units/bag; thus, several bags must be pooled to obtain therapeutic levels of factor VIII in patients with hemophilia A. Each bag of cryoprecipitate is derived from one donor and is screened for hepatitis B, hepatitis C, and HIV; it carries a risk of viral transmission similar to 1 unit of packed red blood cells (see Chap. 18).

2. **Factor VIII** concentrate is partially purified from plasma pooled from 2,000–30,000 donors and can be classified as **intermediate** or **high purity** depending on the concentration of factor VIII present (see Table 17-1). In addition to factor VIII, variable amounts of functional vWF are present. All currently available factor VIII concentrates are viral-inactivated. Newer methods of viral inactivation have been successful in eliminating HIV, hepatitis B, and hepatitis C virus transmission (*Semin Thromb Hemost* 19:1, 1993). **Factor VIII concentrate is the preferred therapy for most patients with severe hemophilia A**.

3. **Recombinant (monoclonal) factor VIII** concentrate products are classified as high purity (see Table 17-1). These products are comparable to plasma-derived factor VIII concentrate and have been shown to be efficacious in the treatment of bleeding episodes (*N Engl J Med* 323:1800, 1990). Some reports have suggested that recombinant factor VIII administration results in an increased incidence of factor VIII antibodies compared with plasma-derived concentrates. However, no systematic prospective studies have been performed to date (*Semin Thromb Hemost* 19:62, 1993). Recombinant factor VIII does not carry the risk of viral transmission, but with newer methods of viral inactivation and increased purity in plasma-derived concentrates, the benefits of recombinant factor VIII may not justify its cost. Previously untreated hemophilia A patients and those with documented HIV infection, but without the manifestations of AIDS, may benefit from recombinant factor VIII.

4. **Factor IX concentrates** of high purity are now available (Table 17-2). These are treated with heat or solvent-detergent for viral inactivation and carry little risk of viral transmission. In addition, they carry a much lower risk of causing thromboembolism or DIC, which is occasionally seen with use of prothrombin complex concentrate. Factor IX concentrate is the treatment of choice for patients with hemophilia B.

5. **Prothrombin complex concentrate** contains prothrombin, factor X, and factor IX, as well as variable amounts of factor VII (see Table 17-2). Prothrombin complex concentrates are now heat-treated, and the potential risks of viral transmission are similar to those for factor VIII concentrates. Prothrombin complex concentrates have occasionally been associated with thromboembolism or DIC, presumably due to the presence of activated coagulation factors. Prothrombin complex concentrates should never be given by prolonged continuous infusion, and concurrent use of antifibrinolytic

Table 17-1. Factor VIII products available in the United States

Name	Manufacturer (distributor)	Source	Purity (IU FVIII/mg)	Viral inactivation	Cost/unit*	Comment
Low purity Cryoprecipitate		Plasma	60–125 FVIII units/bag	Screened plasma		
Intermediate purity Humate-P	Behringwerke AG (Armour)	Plasma	15–20	Pasteurized (60°C for 10 hr)	$ 0.95	High titers of vWF
Koäte-HP	Cutter/Miles	Plasma	50–60	Solvent-detergent	$ 0.25	
Factor VIII-SD	NY Blood Center	Plasma		Solvent-detergent	$ 0.16	
Melate	NY Blood Center	Plasma		Solvent-detergent	$ 0.27	
Profilate-SD	Alpha Therapeutic	Plasma	15–30	Solvent-detergent	$ 0.20	
High purity AHF-M	Baxter/Hyland (American Red Cross)	Plasma	2,000–4,000	Solvent-detergent	$ 0.40	
Hemofil M	Baxter	Plasma	2,000–4,000	Solvent-detergent	$ 0.60	
Monoclate-P	Armour	Plasma	2,000–4,000	Pasteurized (60°C for 10 hr)	$ 0.56	
Kogenate	Cutter/Miles	BHK cells	2,000–4,000		$ 0.81	No vWF coexpression Cells express FVIII
Recombinate	Baxter/Hyland	CHO cells	>5,000		$ 0.91	
Heterologous Hyate-C	Speywood Labs	Porcine plasma	≈140			PEG-fractionation

BHK = baby hamster kidney; CHO = Chinese hamster ovary; vWF = von Willibrand factor.
* Price to Department of Health and Human Services, 1993.
Source: Adapted from Recombinant antihemophilic factor. *Medical Letter* 35:78, 1993.

Table 17-2. Factor IX products available in the United States

Name	Manufacturer	Source	Viral inactivation	Comment
Intermediate purity (prothrombin complex concentrate): <2 IU/mg protein				
Konyne 80	Miles	Plasma	Heat-treated (80°C for 3 days)	
Proplex T	Baxter	Plasma	Heat-treated (60°C for 6 days)	
Profilnine Heat-Treated	Alpha Therapeutic	Plasma	Heat/heptane (60°C for 20 hrs)	
High purity (factor IX concentrates): 20–200 IU/mg protein				
Mononine	Armour	Plasma	Sodium thiocyanate/ultrafiltration	
Coagulation Factor IX-SD	Red Cross	Plasma	Solvent-detergent	
AlphaNine-SD	Alpha Therapeutic	Plasma	Solvent-detergent	Low thrombogenicity
Activated products				
Autoplex T	Baxter	Plasma	Heat-treated (60°C for 6 days)	
Feiba VH Immuno	Immuno-US	Plasma	Vapor-heated (60°C for 10 hrs at 1160 mbar)	
rFVIIa*	Novo Nordisk	BHK cells		

BHK = baby hamster kidney.
* Not available in United States.

agents (e.g., epsilon-aminocaproic acid) should be avoided. Prothrombin complex concentrates are used to treat patients with acquired antibodies to factors VIII or IX (see sec. **I.D**). Factor IX concentrates are now the treatment of choice for patients with hemophilia B.

6. **Recombinant factor IX** has been expressed but is not yet commercially available.

B. **Treatment of factor VIII deficiency** is governed by the severity of hemophilia A and the clinical indication.

1. **Minor bleeding,** such as from superficial abrasions and ecchymoses, is managed with local measures and usually does not require factor replacement therapy. **Desmopressin acetate,** 0.3 µg/kg IV, increases the level of factor VIII up to fourfold in many patients with mild or moderate hemophilia A. This dose of desmopressin may be repeated at 12- to 24-hour intervals, although tachyphylaxis may occur (*Blood* 74:1997, 1989). Control of hemorrhagic episodes and preparation for surgery in patients with mild hemophilia A can sometimes be accomplished with this agent alone. Desmopressin cannot substitute for factor replacement therapy in patients with major bleeding or severe factor VIII deficiency.

2. **Major bleeding,** such as from life-threatening hemorrhage, potential airway obstruction, complicated hemarthroses, expanding soft-tissue hematomas, GI hemorrhage, and major surgery, can be treated with a dose of **factor VIII concentrate** calculated to achieve a factor VIII activity of 100% (see sec. **I.A**). The half-life of factor VIII is approximately 12 hours; therefore, one-half of the original dose should be administered q12h for 3–5 days, which should maintain factor VIII activity above 50% (*Blood* 84:3, 1994). Any head trauma serious enough to require medical attention should be treated with a 100% replacement dose of factor VIII, regardless of neurologic findings.

3. **Epsilon-aminocaproic acid (EACA),** an inhibitor of fibrinolysis, can be used to help control mucous membrane bleeding (e.g., from dental surgery) in patients with hemophilia A. EACA, 50–100 mg/kg PO or IV q6h, is administered on the day before surgery and for 3–5 days afterward (maximum dosage 24 g/day) in conjunction with a single 50% replacement dose of factor VIII concentrate immediately before the procedure. **EACA should not be used in patients with hematuria or before infusion of prothrombin complex concentrate.**

C. **Treatment of factor IX deficiency** is similar to that of factor VIII deficiency. The major risks of factor replacement therapy in patients with factor IX deficiency include viral transmission and thrombosis. Improved purification techniques have decreased the risk of both viral infection and thrombosis. Factor IX concentrate has a longer half-life (about 24 hours) than factor VIII (about 12 hours); therefore, the appropriate dosing interval for factor IX is 18–24 hours. Minor bleeding episodes may be treated with **FFP,** often derived from a single donor to minimize viral transmission, but severe bleeding should be treated with high-purity **factor IX concentrate** (not prothrombin complex concentrate). Desmopressin is ineffective in hemophilia B.

D. **Inhibitory antibodies** to factors VIII or IX develop in 5–10% of patients with hemophilia A and in approximately 1% of patients with hemophilia B and are some of the most difficult clinical problems facing the hematologist. Rare patients without a history of hemophilia may also acquire inhibitory antibodies (see Acquired Coagulation Factor Disorders, sec. **IV**). Patients with low inhibitor titers (<10 Bethesda units/ml) can often be treated with factor VIII concentrate or factor IX concentrate but require higher doses. In many patients, the inhibitor titer is initially high or rises dramatically after exposure to exogenous coagulation factors; such patients, called **"high responders," should not be treated with factor concentrates for episodes of minor bleeding.** Hemorrhage in patients with high titers of factor VIII inhibitors is often difficult to treat but may respond to massive doses of factor VIII concentrate, prothrombin complex concentrate, activated prothrombin complex concentrate, or porcine factor VIII. Alternative approaches include extracorporeal immunoabsorption, plasmapheresis, IV immunoglobulin administration, immunosuppressive therapy, and recombinant factor VIIa (*Blood* 75:1069, 1990). Reduction in the inhibitor titer may be achieved in some patients by frequent, regular infusions of small doses of factor VIII (*Prog Hemost Thromb* 9:57, 1989).

E. Hemarthrosis is the most frequently encountered bleeding complication in the adult patient with hemophilia. The duration of an episode and subsequent joint deformity may be minimized by **prompt initiation of factor replacement therapy** and immobilization of the joint for 2–3 days. Arthrocentesis should be considered only if (1) severe pain and swelling are present, (2) a postinfusion factor VIII or IX level is in the desired range, and (3) the affected joint is easily accessible.

II. von Willebrand disease (vWD) is an inherited autosomal disorder characterized by a prolonged bleeding time, decreased ristocetin cofactor activity, and a variable decrease in factor VIII activity that may be associated with prolongation of the aPTT. The clinical manifestations are similar to those of platelet dysfunction, although a patient with markedly decreased factor VIII activity may present with a hematoma or hemarthrosis.

A. Classification. A recent revised classification of the subtypes of vWD based on the phenotype of the vWF protein present in patient plasma and platelets has been proposed (*Blood* 84:3, 1994) (see Evaluation of Hemostatic Function, sec. **III.C**). Patients with type 1 vWD, which accounts for approximately 80–90% of the cases of vWD, typically have mild decreases in ristocetin cofactor and factor VIII activities and a normal vWF multimer pattern. Type 2A vWD results from selective deficiency of the high-molecular weight multimers of vWF, due to qualitative abnormalities in the protein. In type 2B vWD, the interaction between vWF and platelets is enhanced, and accelerated clearance of platelet aggregates may result in thrombocytopenia. Patients with type 3 vWD have severe quantitative deficiencies of vWF, often resulting in clinically significant reduction in factor VIII activity.

B. Treatment. In general, bleeding episodes in patients with vWD are more easily controlled than those in patients with hemophilia. The choice of therapy depends on the type of vWD and the clinical setting.

1. Desmopressin acetate is usually effective in patients with mild or moderate vWD (usually type 1). Dosage and administration of desmopressin in vWD are the same as in factor VIII deficiency (see sec. **I.B.1**). **Desmopressin is contraindicated in patients with type 2B vWD** because of the potential for exacerbating thrombocytopenia. Therefore, the subtype of vWD should be established prior to the administration of desmopressin.

2. Factor VIII concentrates, especially those with high titers of vWF (e.g., Humate-P), are the preferred blood product in all types of vWD when replacement therapy is required. An infusion of 1–2 bags of **cryoprecipitate**/10 kg of body weight will normalize the factor VIII coagulant activity and the bleeding time but carries the risk of viral transmission.

III. Other inherited coagulation factor deficiencies. Patients with hemophilia A, hemophilia B, and vWD constitute more than 90% of all patients with severe inherited bleeding disorders. Deficiencies of other coagulation factors should be considered in patients with abnormal bleeding that is not explained by the more common hereditary or acquired coagulation disorders. In factor XI deficiency, bleeding is usually mild, but extensive postoperative hemorrhage can occur. Treatment with FFP to achieve a factor XI level 30% of normal is adequate for normal hemostasis in most patients.

Acquired Coagulation Factor Disorders

I. Vitamin K deficiency. Vitamin K is a necessary cofactor for the hepatic gamma-carboxylation of certain glutamate residues in coagulation factors VII, IX, and X, prothrombin, protein C, and protein S. The noncarboxylated forms of these proteins are inactive; thus, vitamin K deficiency results in abnormal blood coagulation and bleeding. The PT is usually prolonged but corrects to normal when a 50 : 50 mixture of normal plasma with the patient's plasma is used (see Evaluation of Hemostatic Function, sec. **III.D.7**). Conditions associated with vitamin K deficiency include biliary obstruction, malabsorption syndromes, antibiotic therapy, nutritional deficiency, and warfarin ingestion. Hospitalized patients who are unable to eat and are receiving antibiotics that suppress normal intestinal flora may become vitamin K–deficient in 1–2 weeks without supplementation.

A. **Vitamin K preparations** include vitamin K_1 (phytonadione) and synthetic water-soluble derivatives of vitamin K_3 that require hepatic activation. Hospitalized patients at risk for vitamin K deficiency should receive prophylactic treatment with vitamin K_1, 10 mg PO or SC 3 times/week. Mild deficiency can usually be corrected by administration of vitamin K_1, 10–15 mg SC or IV qd for 1–3 days. Severe deficiency due to overdosage of warfarin or other oral anticoagulants requires treatment with parenteral vitamin K_1, often in large doses (see Antithrombotic Therapy, sec. **I.D.3**). IV administration of vitamin K has rarely been associated with anaphylaxis.

B. **FFP**, 2–4 units IV, should be administered to patients with vitamin K deficiency (PT >1.5 times control) or those receiving oral anticoagulants in the setting of serious hemorrhage. Additional FFP, 2 units IV q8–12h, should be given if bleeding persists and the PT remains prolonged.

II. **Coagulopathies associated with liver disease.** Severe liver disease causes decreased synthesis of fibrinogen, prothrombin, and factors V, VII, IX, X, and XI. Acquired dysfibrinogenemia may result from the synthesis of abnormally glycosylated fibrinogen, and FDPs may be elevated because of reduced hepatic clearance. Thrombocytopenia due to hypersplenism may complicate the hemostatic defect. Bleeding in a patient with liver disease presents a difficult therapeutic problem. Empiric therapy with parenteral vitamin K_1, 10–15 mg SC or IV qd for 3 days, may be administered, although most patients will not respond. Replacement therapy with FFP will often transiently improve hemostatic function, and platelet transfusions may be considered if thrombocytopenia is present.

III. **Disseminated intravascular coagulation (DIC)** is the consequence of intravascular activation of both the coagulation and fibrinolytic systems. Laboratory findings in DIC often include thrombocytopenia, hypofibrinogenemia, increased FDPs, and prolongation of the TT and aPTT. Microangiopathic hemolysis may also occur. DIC varies greatly in clinical severity and may present with a predominance of either bleeding or thrombosis (microvascular or venous). DIC is often associated with malignant neoplasms, infections (e.g., gram-negative sepsis, meningococcemia, Rocky Mountain spotted fever, certain viral infections), acute leukemia (especially promyelocytic leukemia), liver disease, snake bites, spider bites (e.g., brown recluse), obstetric complications, connective tissue diseases, massive trauma, extensive burns, or shock. **Treatment of the underlying condition is the major therapeutic approach to DIC.** Supportive therapy is directed toward preventing hemodynamic compromise and hypoxemia. Both anticoagulant and factor replacement therapy are potentially dangerous in the setting of DIC and should be considered only if serious hemorrhagic or thrombotic complications are present. Platelet transfusions and infusions of FFP or cryoprecipitate may be given if bleeding is the major complication. **Heparin** may be beneficial in some patients; however, its effectiveness remains largely unproved. When given for DIC, heparin should be initiated at a low dosage (e.g., 500 units/hour by continuous IV infusion without a bolus) that may be slowly increased. The desired outcome is cessation of bleeding, increases in the plasma fibrinogen concentration and platelet count, and a decrease in FDPs. The utility of prophylactic heparin therapy during induction chemotherapy for acute promyelocytic (M_3) leukemia is controversial (*Br J Haematol* 68:283, 1988; *Blood* 79:543, 1992).

IV. **Acquired anticoagulants** are substances, usually antibodies, that inhibit the function of specific coagulation factors, frequently factors VIII or IX but occasionally factors V, XI, or XIII or vWF. The presence of an acquired anticoagulant should be suspected when a **prolonged PT or aPTT fails to correct to normal with a 50 : 50**

mixture of the patient's plasma with normal plasma (see Evaluation of Hemostatic Function, sec. **III.D.7**). Inhibitory antibodies may arise in patients with preexisting coagulation factor deficiencies or in association with pregnancy, collagen-vascular diseases, or lymphoproliferative disorders. Inhibitors may develop spontaneously in previously healthy patients or may be induced by certain drugs, such as penicillin, sulfonamides, phenytoin, or isoniazid. Treatment of acute bleeding in patients with inhibitors of factors VIII or IX is discussed under Inherited Bleeding Disorders, sec. **I.D**. Immunosuppressive therapy with cyclophosphamide, vincristine, and prednisone may be effective in patients with refractory cases (*Ann Intern Med* 110:774, 1989). Acquired vWD may result either from the presence of circulating inhibitors of vWF activity or from rapid antibody-induced clearance of vWF. Lupus anticoagulants are antibodies that interfere with phospholipid-dependent coagulation assays but are often associated with thrombosis rather than bleeding.

Thromboembolic Disorders

I. **Predisposing conditions.** Although most cases of thromboembolic disease are idiopathic, several clinical conditions have been associated with an increased risk of thrombosis.
   A. **Inherited deficiencies of antithrombin III, protein C, and protein S** are found more frequently in patients with recurrent thrombosis than in the general population. However, many patients with reduced plasma levels of these proteins do not have a significantly increased risk for thromboembolism (*Semin Thromb Hemost* 16:158, 1990). Recent studies have shown that many patients with venous thrombosis, especially those with a family history of thrombosis, have a genetic defect in the factor V molecule that renders it resistant to the anticoagulant effects of activated protein C (APC) (*N Engl J Med* 330:517, 1994). Laboratory assays for antithrombin III, protein C, and protein S may be unreliable in patients with acute thrombosis, liver disease, or DIC; in pregnancy; and during anticoagulant therapy. In general, the nature and duration of therapy in patients with thromboembolism are primarily determined by the clinical presentation (see sec. **IV.B.2**) and are unlikely to be altered by the identification of an inherited disorder acutely. Therefore, screening for these disorders should probably be limited to patients with recurrent thromboembolism, unusual sites of thrombosis (e.g., axillary, mesenteric, or cerebral veins), or a positive family history of thromboembolism. Patients with antithrombin III deficiency who have a positive personal or family history of thrombosis should receive prophylactic low-dose heparin during pregnancy. Replacement therapy with antithrombin III concentrate may be considered for patients with known inherited antithrombin III deficiency in the setting of acute thrombosis, trauma, or surgery. Asymptomatic individuals with protein C or protein S deficiency are unlikely to benefit from chronic prophylactic antithrombotic therapy.
   B. **Lupus anticoagulants** occur in patients with SLE or other immunologic disorders, in patients with infections (e.g., HIV), or in association with certain drugs (e.g., chlorpromazine, procainamide, hydralazine). A subset of patients with lupus anticoagulants appears to have an increased risk for arterial and venous thrombosis and recurrent spontaneous abortions.
   C. **Other clinical conditions** that may predispose patients to thromboembolism include pregnancy, malignancy, immobilization, congestive heart failure, and cigarette smoking. Thrombosis in patients with nephrotic syndrome may be related in part to acquired antithrombin III deficiency.
II. **Prophylactic therapy** for asymptomatic patients may be effective in preventing thrombosis in certain high-risk situations. Low-dose heparin, 5,000 units SC q12h, has been shown to reduce the incidence of venous thrombosis in patients with acute myocardial infarction or congestive heart failure and may benefit patients undergoing major surgery or prolonged immobilization. Relative contraindications to heparin therapy should be taken into consideration (Table 17-3). Prophylactic

Table 17-3. Relative contraindications to anticoagulant therapy

Active bleeding (e.g., active peptic ulcer disease)
Bleeding tendency (e.g., hemophilia, thrombocytopenia)
Uncontrolled hypertension
Cerebrovascular hemorrhage
Recent surgery or invasive procedures (e.g., arterial or lumbar puncture)
Pericarditis or pericardial effusion
Severe trauma
Pregnancy (contraindications primarily relate to warfarin)
Patients prone to falling (e.g., elderly or debilitated patients)
Inadequate laboratory facilities
Unsatisfactory patient compliance

warfarin therapy is appropriate for all patients with mechanical prosthetic heart valves and certain patients with valvular heart disease or atrial fibrillation (see Chap. 7) (*Chest* 102[Suppl.]:453S, 1992). Intermittent pneumatic leg compression may reduce thrombotic complications associated with certain surgical procedures.

III. **Acute arterial occlusion** is an urgent medical situation that necessitates early recognition and institution of treatment. Arterial occlusions frequently result from embolization of left atrial or ventricular thrombi or from atherosclerotic emboli arising in proximal arteries. Paradoxical arterial embolization from a venous thrombus can occur via an atrial septal defect or patent foramen ovale. Physical findings suggestive of peripheral arterial occlusion include an absent or diminished pulse and coolness or pain in an extremity. In addition to full-dose anticoagulation with **heparin** (see Antithrombotic Therapy, sec. **I.B.1**), most peripheral arterial thrombi require prompt **surgical embolectomy or angioplasty. Fibrinolytic therapy** should be considered in patients with surgically inaccessible peripheral arterial occlusions or early acute myocardial infarction (see Chap. 5).

IV. **Venous thrombosis** occurs frequently in ambulatory and hospitalized patients.
   A. **Superficial thrombophlebitis** poses little risk for embolization and is generally controlled by the supportive measures of local heat, elevation of the affected extremity, and rest. Antiinflammatory agents such as aspirin may also be given.
   B. **Deep venous thrombosis (DVT)** is a more difficult diagnostic and therapeutic problem associated with a significant risk of pulmonary embolism.
      1. **Diagnosis.** Because clinical findings are notoriously unreliable in DVT, the diagnosis should always be established by an objective invasive or noninvasive test. Contrast **venography** remains the most reliable technique for the detection of DVT but is associated with postvenography phlebitis in 5–10% of patients (*Radiology* 165:113, 1987). **Impedance plethysmography** is a non-invasive technique with high sensitivity and specificity in the diagnosis of obstruction of the proximal veins (i.e., iliac, femoral, and popliteal), particularly in ambulatory patients (*Surg Clin North Am* 70:143, 1990). **Real-time (duplex) ultrasonography appears to be the most accurate noninvasive method for the diagnosis of proximal DVT** but is less reliable in detecting isolated calf vein thrombi (*N Engl J Med* 329:1365, 1993). Negative noninvasive studies should either be confirmed by contrast venography or repeated serially during the next 10–14 days. Contrast venography should be performed when the results of noninvasive testing are equivocal.
      2. **Treatment.** Thrombosis confined to the calf veins carries a low risk of embolization, and anticoagulation therapy is usually unnecessary. However, approximately 20% of untreated calf vein thrombi eventually extend into the proximal veins. Therefore, noninvasive testing should be repeated 2–3 days after diagnosis and several additional times during the following 2 weeks if anticoagulation therapy is withheld. In general, patients with proximal DVT detected by either invasive or noninvasive methods should receive supportive measures and anticoagulation with heparin, preferably administered by

continuous IV infusion (see Antithrombotic Therapy, sec. **I.B.1**). Heparin should be continued until 48 hours after oral anticoagulation with warfarin results in an INR of 2–3 (see Antithrombotic Therapy, sec. **I.B.1**) or for a minimum of 5 days (*N Engl J Med* 322:1260, 1990). Oral anticoagulation with warfarin should be started between days 1 and 3 of heparin therapy and continued for 3–6 months, depending on the estimated risks of recurrent thrombosis and hemorrhage in the individual patient. **Low-molecular weight heparin (LMWH)** (see Antithrombotic Therapy, sec. **I.C**) appears to be at least as effective as IV heparin in the treatment of proximal DVT as well as in prevention of DVT in patients undergoing orthopedic surgery, possibly with a decreased incidence of hemorrhage (*N Engl J Med* 326:975, 1992; *Arch Intern Med* 153:1541, 1993; *Ann Intern Med* 121:81, 1994). LMWH may allow patients with proximal DVT to be cared for as outpatients without the need for frequent monitoring of the level of anticoagulation. Adjusted-dose SC heparin is an effective alternative to warfarin for chronic anticoagulation during pregnancy or in situations in which close monitoring is impractical (*Ann Intern Med* 107:441, 1987). Fibrinolytic therapy may accelerate thrombus dissolution, resulting in a reduction in the incidence of postphlebitic syndrome. However, because of uncertain long-term effects and the increased risk of hemorrhagic complications, fibrinolytic agents are not recommended for routine use in patients with acute DVT (*Arch Intern Med* 149:1841, 1989). Patients with recurrent DVT should receive warfarin therapy for an extended period of time, probably indefinitely (*Prog Hemost Thromb* 9:1, 1989). Chronic anticoagulation with adjusted-dose SC heparin is occasionally required to prevent recurrent DVT in patients treated with warfarin. Such patients often have an underlying malignancy or other predisposition to thrombosis.

C. Pulmonary embolism (PE) is a serious complication of DVT. The diagnosis and therapy of PE are discussed in Chap. 10.

Antithrombotic Therapy

I. Anticoagulants. The decision to use an anticoagulant always involves weighing the risk of anticoagulant-induced bleeding against the risk of thrombosis or embolism if therapy is withheld. Before the initiation of anticoagulant therapy, patients must be screened for relative contraindications to therapy (see Table 17-3) because the failure to do so could result in fatal hemorrhage. The final decision to use anticoagulant therapy must always be individualized.

A. Precautions. Patients receiving anticoagulants should be advised to report any signs of bleeding. Invasive procedures and IM injections should be minimized, and antiplatelet medications (e.g., aspirin and NSAIDs) should be avoided. The hematocrit and platelet count should be measured before and periodically after initiating therapy, and the stool should be examined for occult blood. If manifestations of bleeding are present, the PT, aPTT, hematocrit, and platelet count should be promptly determined. Bleeding that occurs in the setting of therapeutic anticoagulation suggests an underlying lesion (e.g., occult carcinoma), which should prompt further diagnostic evaluation and not be attributed to the anticoagulated state.

B. Heparin is a naturally occurring glycosaminoglycan that acts by potentiating the activity of antithrombin III. It is administered parenterally and produces immediate prolongation of the TT, the aPTT, and, to a lesser extent, the PT. The half-life of heparin in the circulation is approximately 60–90 minutes but is prolonged in patients with severe liver disease. Heparin does not cross the placenta.

1. Administration. Heparin therapy is initiated with a loading dose of approximately 5,000 units IV as a bolus injection, followed by 1,000–2,000 units/hour delivered by continuous IV infusion. Heparin dosing based on patient weight (80 units/kg actual body weight by bolus followed by 18 units/kg/ hour infusion) may achieve therapeutic anticoagulation more rapidly without an increased risk of bleeding (*Ann Intern Med* 119:874, 1993). The amount of **heparin should not exceed 25,000 units/bag of IV fluid**, since mechanical pump failure during infusion could lead to massive overdosage. The aPTT should be measured before starting heparin therapy and q6h during adjustment of the infusion rate. An aPTT of 1.5–2.0 times the control value (generally between 50–80 seconds) is considered therapeutic. In most patients, this time can be achieved with infusion rates of 800–1,600 units/hour. When given by adjusted-dose SC administration, the heparin dosage is adjusted to achieve a mid-dose aPTT (measured 6 hours after administration) of 1.5–2.0 times the control value. A dosage of 15,000–17,500 units SC q12h is usually necessary to achieve this degree of anticoagulation.

2. **Heparin-associated thrombocytopenia.** Mild thrombocytopenia commonly occurs in patients 2–10 days after the initiation of heparin therapy; the platelet count usually remains greater than 100,000/µl, and heparin can be continued. Less frequently, severe thrombocytopenia, apparently mediated by an immune mechanism, occurs 6–14 days after starting IV or SC heparin therapy; patients who have been previously treated with heparin may develop severe thrombocytopenia within hours to days of reexposure. Similarly, thrombocytopenia may be observed with LMWHs. Paradoxically, the severe form of heparin-associated thrombocytopenia may be associated with arterial thrombosis. Periodic platelet counts should be obtained in all patients on heparin therapy, and **heparin should be discontinued if severe thrombocytopenia occurs**. Because of the potential for arterial thrombosis, platelet transfusions should be reserved for patients with serious bleeding (*Annu Rev Med* 40:31, 1989).

3. **Reversal of heparin** anticoagulation generally occurs within hours after cessation of heparin infusion. In the rare instances in which anticoagulation must be reversed more rapidly, **protamine sulfate** can be given to neutralize heparin. Protamine sulfate should be administered by slow IV infusion, in doses of no more than 50 mg over a 10-minute period. The dosage is calculated according to the estimated amount of heparin circulating at the time of administration of protamine sulfate. One mg of protamine sulfate will neutralize approximately 100 units of heparin. If given 30–60 minutes after a bolus injection of heparin, approximately 0.5 mg of protamine sulfate will be required for every 100 units of heparin. If heparin is administered by continuous IV infusion, the dose of protamine sulfate should be calculated to neutralize approximately half of the preceding hourly dose of heparin. No more than 250 mg of protamine sulfate should be given except in extreme circumstances. The effect of protamine sulfate should be monitored by determining the aPTT immediately after administration. Rare life-threatening anaphylactic reactions to protamine sulfate may occur, particularly in diabetic patients receiving protamine-insulin preparations (*N Engl J Med* 320:886, 1989).

C. **Low-molecular weight heparins (LMWHs)** are compounds obtained by depolymerization of standard heparin. LMWHs are heterogeneous in size and approximately one-third the size of heparin, with a molecular weight range of 1,000–10,000. They exert anticoagulant effects by binding to antithrombin III, with subsequent antifactor Xa and IIa activity. LMWHs bind less avidly to heparin-binding proteins, which produces a more predictable clinical response, a longer half-life, and less interaction with platelets compared with standard heparin (*Coronary Artery Disease* 3:990, 1992). LMWHs do not cross the placenta. **Dosage** of LMWH varies by the commercial preparation used and is administered SC q12–q24h. Protamine sulfate does not completely neutralize the anticoagulant effect of LMWH but has been shown to reverse anticoagulation associated with LMWH use (*Thromb Haemosta* 63:271, 1990).

D. **Warfarin** interferes with hepatic vitamin K–dependent carboxylation (see Acquired Coagulation Disorders, sec. I). Although the onset of anticoagulation is less rapid than that produced by heparin, warfarin is more convenient for chronic outpatient therapy. After initiation of warfarin therapy, vitamin K–dependent clotting factor activities will decline with approximately the following half-lives: factor VII, 6 hours; factor IX, 24 hours; and factor X and prothrombin, 48 hours. The PT will usually become prolonged in less than 48 hours due to depletion of factor VII, but several more days of therapy may be required before therapeutic anticoagulation occurs. **Warfarin crosses the placenta and may produce significant birth defects or fetal death.**

1. **Administration** is usually initiated with warfarin sodium, 10 mg PO qd for 2 days; subsequent daily doses are adjusted until the PT stabilizes in the therapeutic range. If the indication for anticoagulation is not urgent (not thromboembolic disease), treatment can be initiated with an anticipated maintenance dose of 5 mg, which will reach steady state in approximately 5–7 days. The PT reflects the warfarin dose given 24–48 hours earlier. Because of variability in thromboplastin reagents used to determine the PT, an **international normalized ratio (INR)** has been developed for standardization of warfarin anticoagulation. Calculation of the INR results in the PT ratio (sample/control) that would have been obtained if the World Health Organization thromboplastin standard had been used. For most indications, an INR of 2–3 is considered to be therapeutic. In patients with mechanical prosthetic heart valves, an INR of 2.5–3.5 should be maintained (*Chest* 102 [Suppl.]:453S, 1992). The required maintenance dosage is subject to wide individual variation but usually ranges from 2–15 mg PO qd. Once stabilization of the dosage has been achieved, the INR should be determined approximately every 2 weeks. In the setting of poor patient compliance, the INR should be determined more frequently.

2. **Drug interactions and toxicity.** Maintenance of warfarin anticoagulation may be affected by the dietary intake or absorption of vitamin K or by alterations in warfarin degradation by the liver. Certain drugs displace warfarin from albumin and thus increase its anticoagulant effect; other drugs induce hepatic microsomal enzymes, decreasing warfarin activity (Table 17-4). Any condition that affects liver function or the availability of vitamin K (e.g., alterations in intestinal bacteria or food intake) can affect hemostatic balance and may lead to fatal hemorrhagic or thrombotic complications. Therefore, medication or dietary changes should be accompanied by frequent INR determinations, and the dosage of warfarin should be adjusted accordingly. Warfarin skin necrosis is an extremely rare complication in which a cutaneous microvascular thrombotic process develops 3–10 days after starting warfarin therapy. Several cases have been reported in patients with protein C deficiency (*Semin Thromb Hemost* 16:169, 1990).

3. **Reversal of warfarin anticoagulation.** The PT will gradually return to normal several days following discontinuation of warfarin. This may be hastened by administration of vitamin K_1. If the INR is greater than 6 but less than 10 with no serious bleeding, vitamin K_1, 0.5–1.0 mg IV, may be given. If the INR is above 10 but less than 20, vitamin K_1, 3–5 mg IV, should be effective. If rapid reversal is required (serious bleeding) or the INR is greater than 20, vitamin K_1, 10 mg IV, should be administered and the INR checked every 6 hours (*Chest* 102[Suppl.]:323S, 1992). IV vitamin K_1 should be administered slowly, at a rate not exceeding 1 mg/minute. Patients with severe hemorrhage who require immediate reversal of warfarin anticoagulation should receive FFP, 2–4 units IV.

II. **Fibrinolytic therapy** with urokinase, streptokinase, or t-PA may be indicated in selected patients with acute myocardial infarction, pulmonary embolism, proximal DVT, or peripheral arterial occlusion. Appropriate dosage and administration are determined by the specific indication and fibrinolytic agent used. Contraindications to and use of fibrinolytic therapy in acute myocardial infarction and pulmonary embolism are discussed in Chap. 5 and Chap. 10, respectively.

Table 17-4. Drugs that alter prothrombin time by interacting with warfarin, according to type of interaction

Pharmacokinetic (drugs that change warfarin levels)	Pharmacodynamic (drugs that do not change warfarin levels)	Mechanism unknown (drugs whose effect on warfarin levels is unknown)
Prolongs prothrombin time	**Prolongs prothrombin time**	**Prolongs prothrombin time**
Stereoselective inhibition of clearance of *S* isomer	Inhibits cyclic interconversion of vitamin K	Evidence for interaction convincing
Phenylbutazone	Second- and third-generation cephalosporins	Erythromycin
Metronidazole	Other mechanisms	Anabolic steroids
Sulfinpyrazone	Clofibrate	Evidence for interaction less convincing
Trimethoprim-sulfamethoxazole	Inhibits blood coagulation	Ketoconazole
Disulfiram	Heparin	Fluconazole
Stereoselective inhibition of clearance of *R* isomer	Increases metabolism of coagulation factors	Isoniazid
Cimetidine[a]	Thyroxine	Piroxicam
Omeprazole[a]		Tamoxifen
Nonstereoselective inhibitions of clearance of *R* and *S* isomers	**Inhibits platelet function**	Quinidine
Amiodarone	Aspirin	Vitamin E (megadose)
	Other nonsteroidal antiinflammatory drugs	Phenytoin[c]
Reduces prothrombin time	Ticlopidine	
Reduces absorption	Moxalactam	**Reduces prothrombin time**
Cholestyramine	Carbenicillin and high doses of other penicillins	Penicillins
Increases metabolic clearance		Griseofulvin[b]
Barbiturates		
Rifampin		
Griseofulvin		
Carbamazepine		

[a] Causes minimal prolongation of the prothrombin time.
[b] Has been proposed to cause increased metabolic clearance.
[c] Initial effect due to displacement of warfarin from plasma proteins. Later, antagonizes warfarin by increasing metabolic clearance.
Source: J Hirsch. Oral anticoagulant drugs. *N Engl J Med* 324:1867, 1991.

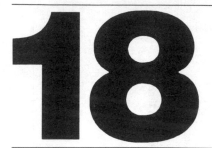

Anemia and Transfusion Therapy

Morey A. Blinder

Approach to the Patient with Anemia

Anemia is a commonly encountered clinical condition that is caused by an acquired or hereditary abnormality of the RBC or its precursors, or may be a manifestation of an underlying nonhematologic disorder. Anemia is defined as a decrease in the circulating RBC mass; the usual criteria are a hemoglobin (Hb) of less than 12 g/dl (hematocrit [Hct] <36%) in women and less than 14 g/dl (Hct <41%) in men.

I. **Clinical manifestations** of anemia vary depending on the etiology, degree, and rapidity of onset. Other underlying disorders such as cardiopulmonary disease may contribute to the severity of symptoms. Severe anemia may be well tolerated if it develops gradually, but generally, patients with a Hb less than 7 g/dl have symptoms of tissue hypoxia (fatigue, headache, dyspnea, light-headedness, angina). Pallor, visual impairment, syncope, and tachycardia may signal anemic hypovolemia, which requires immediate attention.

II. **History and physical examination.** The acute or chronic onset of anemia should be assessed and clues to any underlying systemic process should be sought. One must look for a family history of anemia, drug exposure (including ethanol), or blood loss. Physical findings that aid in diagnosis include lymphadenopathy, hepatic or splenic enlargement, jaundice, bone tenderness, neurologic symptoms, and evidence of blood in the feces.

III. **Laboratory evaluation** is based on the Hb and Hct, reticulocyte count, mean cellular volume, and an examination of the peripheral blood smear.

    A. **The Hb and Hct** serve as an estimate of the RBC mass, but interpretation of them must take into consideration the volume status of the patient. Immediately after acute blood loss, the Hb will be normal because compensatory mechanisms have not had time to restore normal plasma volume.

    B. **The reticulocyte count** reflects the rate of RBC production and is an indicator of the bone marrow response to anemia. The reticulocyte count is usually reported as reticulocytes/100 RBCs (% reticulocytes). The reticulocyte count may also be reported as an absolute number.

Absolute reticulocyte count = % reticulocytes × RBC count

An increase of reticulocytes to greater than 100,000/mm^3 suggests a hyperproliferative bone marrow. The **reticulocyte index (RI)** corrects for the severity of the anemia and assesses the appropriateness of the bone marrow response.

$$RI = \frac{(\text{reticulocyte count} \times \text{patient Hct/normal Hct})}{2}$$

A RI greater than 2–3% indicates increased RBC production, and a value less than 2% indicates that there is a hypoproliferative component to the anemia.

    C. **The mean cellular volume (MCV)** is often used in classifying anemia (microcytic, normocytic, and macrocytic for anemia with low, normal, and high MCV, respectively). Proper use of the MCV in establishing a diagnosis depends on examination of the peripheral smear for the following reasons: (1) small and large cells may be present simultaneously, resulting in a normal MCV; (2)

Table 18-1. Classification of anemia based on red blood cell kinetics

I. Anemias associated with impaired RBC production
   A. Aplastic anemia
   B. Iron-deficiency anemia
   C. Thalassemia
   D. Myelodysplastic syndromes and sideroblastic anemia
   E. Megaloblastic anemia
   F. Anemia of chronic renal insufficiency
   G. Anemia of chronic disease
   H. Zidovudine- and cancer chemotherapy–induced anemia
II. Anemias associated with increased RBC loss or destruction
   A. Bleeding
   B. Hereditary hemolytic anemias
      1. Hemoglobinopathies (e.g., sickle cell disease)
      2. Primary disorders of RBC membrane
      3. RBC enzymopathies (e.g., G6PD deficiency)
   C. Acquired hemolytic anemias
      1. Autoimmune hemolytic anemia
      2. Drug-induced hemolytic anemia
      3. Microangiopathic hemolytic anemia
      4. Traumatic hemolytic anemia
      5. Paroxysmal nocturnal hemoglobinuria

reticulocytes are larger than mature RBCs and will raise the MCV; and (3) abnormal cells may be present in numbers too small to affect the MCV.
   D. **Examination of the peripheral blood smear** is mandatory. The smear must be free of preparative artifact, and RBC morphology is best evaluated in a portion of the smear where the RBCs are nearly touching one another. Heterogeneity in RBC size (anisocytosis) and shape (poikilocytosis) may be seen. Specific morphologic abnormalities (see Anemias Associated with Decreased Red Blood Cell Production and Anemias Associated with Increased Red Blood Cell Loss or Destruction) and any abnormalities in the WBCs or platelets should be sought.
   E. **Special tests** to establish an exact diagnosis should be performed before transfusion of blood if possible.
IV. **Classification of anemias.** Typically, anemia is characterized by the MCV and RI. The RI determines which of the major categories the anemia falls into (Table 18-1). In concert with the RI, examination of the peripheral smear and the MCV often suggests a single diagnosis or a limited number of diagnoses that may be investigated with specific tests. Anemia may be multifactorial in origin (e.g., alcoholism with GI bleeding, nutritional deficiencies, and liver disease). If a patient responds to therapy but then relapses or a patient has a poor response to adequate therapy, additional causes of anemia should be sought.

Anemias Associated with Decreased Red Blood Cell Production

A low RI indicates either an underproduction of RBCs or ineffective erythropoiesis.
I. **Aplastic anemia** is an acquired abnormality of bone marrow stem cells and is associated with anemia, leukopenia, and thrombocytopenia. Most cases are idiopathic, although about 20% are associated with drug or chemical exposure (e.g., benzene, phenylbutazone, gold, D-penicillamine, anticonvulsants, sulfonamides, chloramphenicol) and another 10% are associated with viral illnesses (e.g., viral hepatitis, Epstein-Barr virus, cytomegalovirus [CMV]). Presenting symptoms are

usually related to anemia or thrombocytopenia, although some patients present with fever and leukopenia.

A. Laboratory results. The MCV is normal and there are no unique findings on the peripheral smear. Bone marrow biopsy is necessary for diagnosis and to rule out myelodysplastic syndrome (MDS), leukemia, or infiltration with tumor or granulomas.

B. Therapy is supportive and potentially curative. Any suspected offending drugs should be discontinued.

1. **Early referral** to a center experienced in managing aplastic anemia is recommended. In individuals younger than 50 years of age, bone marrow transplantation (BMT) from an HLA-identical sibling has achieved a long-term survival rate of 60–70%. **Immunosuppressive treatment** with cyclosporine or antilymphocyte (or antithymocyte) globulin should be considered in patients who are not eligible for BMT.

2. **Transfusions** with packed RBCs should be kept to a minimum. Prophylactic platelet transfusions are generally recommended if the platelet count is below 10,000/mm³. Transfusion with blood products from family members should be avoided while BMT is being considered. Blood products should be given through leukocyte-depleting filters to prevent sensitization against HLA antigens.

3. **Infection.** Patients should be instructed to seek medical attention immediately in the event of fever over 38.5°C. Fever with neutropenia requires a physical examination and cultures of potential sites of infection. Empiric antimicrobial treatment similar to that used in patients with chemotherapy-induced myelosuppression is usually necessary (see Chap. 19).

C. Complications that arise after recovery from aplastic anemia include a high risk of subsequent MDS and acute leukemia. Clonal hematopoiesis manifested as paroxysmal nocturnal hemoglobinuria may also occur.

II. **Iron deficiency** is a common disorder worldwide. In the United States, most cases are caused by menstrual blood loss and increased iron requirements of pregnancy. Decreased iron absorption (celiac disease, postgastrectomy) or increased iron requirements (lactation, infancy) may also lead to iron deficiency. In the absence of menstrual bleeding, GI blood loss is the presumed etiology in most patients; appropriate radiographic and endoscopic procedures should be performed to identify a source and to exclude occult malignancy. Complete evaluation of iron deficiency requires identification of the cause.

A. History and physical examination. Evidence of a source of blood loss (melena, menorrhagia) should be sought. In severe iron-deficiency anemia, a history of pica (consumption of substances such as ice, starch, or clay) may be obtained. Splenomegaly is present in 5–10% of patients; koilonychia ("spoon nail") is a rare finding. Iron deficiency may also be associated with glossitis, dysphagia, and esophageal webs (Plummer-Vinson syndrome).

B. Laboratory results. The MCV is usually normal in early iron deficiency. As the Hct falls below 30%, anisocytosis increases and hypochromic microcytic cells appear, followed by a decrease in the MCV. Other findings on the peripheral smear include "pencil cells" and occasional target cells. The platelet count may be increased. Diagnosis requires the documentation of low iron stores, which can usually be accomplished indirectly by measuring serum ferritin.

1. **A serum ferritin level** less than 12 μg/liter (normal 12–300 μg/liter) is indicative of low iron stores. Ferritin is an acute-phase reactant, and normal levels may be seen in inflammatory states, liver disease, or malignancy despite low iron stores. A serum ferritin level of greater than 200 μg/liter generally indicates adequate iron stores regardless of other underlying conditions.

2. **Serum iron** is usually low (<60 μg/dl) and **total iron-binding capacity (TIBC)** is increased (>360 μg/dl) in iron deficiency, but these values may fluctuate in many common clinical conditions and hence are less reliable indicators of iron stores.

3. **A bone marrow biopsy** specimen that shows absent staining for iron is the

definitive test for establishing iron deficiency and is helpful when the serum ferritin fails to confirm the diagnosis.

C. **Therapy** of iron-deficiency anemia requires repleting iron stores with either supplemental oral or parenteral iron; normal dietary intake will only meet daily losses. With therapy, the reticulocyte count will peak in 5–10 days, and the Hb will rise over 1–2 months. The most common cause of poor response to therapy is noncompliance; other causes such as poor absorption, continued blood loss, or a multifactorial anemia must also be considered.

1. **Oral therapy** with ferrous sulfate, 325 mg PO tid (65 mg of elemental iron), taken between meals to maximize absorption, will usually correct the anemia and replete iron stores over 6 months. Approximately 25% of patients will develop GI side effects such as constipation, cramping, diarrhea, and nausea. These side effects can be minimized by initially administering the drug with meals or once daily and increasing the dosage as tolerated. Ferrous gluconate and fumarate are well-tolerated alternative therapies. Sustained-release or enteric-coated preparations dissolve poorly and generally should not be recommended. Concomitant administration of vitamin C has been used to maintain the iron in the reduced state and improve absorption.

2. **Parenteral iron therapy** may be useful in patients with (1) poor absorption (inflammatory bowel disease, malabsorption), (2) very high iron requirements that cannot be met with oral supplementation, or (3) intolerance of oral preparations. The following formula may be used to approximate the amount of iron required to restore the Hb to normal levels and replenish the iron stores:

Iron (mg) = 0.3 × body wt (lb) × (100 − [patient Hb (g/dl) 14.8 × 100])

Iron dextran (Infed) may be administered IM or IV. A typical dosing schedule is 1 ml (50 mg) IM injected deeply into each buttock per day. Extravasation into subcutaneous tissue may cause staining of the skin, which can be minimized by injecting with a Z-track technique. The previously recommended maximal IV dose was 2 ml/day. However, "total dose" (as calculated above) (full therapeutic dose administered as a single IV infusion) IV iron dextran (diluted in 250–500 ml normal saline and infused at 6 mg/minute) has been used with few complications (*J Lab Clin Med* 111:566, 1988). Both IM and IV therapy may rarely be complicated by anaphylaxis, and a 0.5-ml (IM) or 30-mg (IV) test dose should be administered 1 hour before initiating therapy. Delayed reactions such as arthralgia, myalgia, fever, pruritus, and lymphadenopathy may be seen within 3 days of therapy and usually resolve spontaneously or following treatment with nonsteroidal antiinflammatory agents.

3. **Blood transfusion** is not recommended for iron supplementation and should not be used to treat iron-deficiency anemia in the absence of cerebrovascular or cardiopulmonary compromise.

III. **The thalassemias** are a heterogeneous group of inherited disorders characterized by underproduction of either the alpha- or beta globin chains of the Hb molecule. There are four alpha- and two beta-globin genes in a normal cell, and production of the alpha and beta chains is equal. In beta-thalassemia, there is a reduced production of beta-globin chains with normal amounts of alpha-globin. The excess alpha-globin chains form insoluble tetramers in the RBCs, causing membrane damage, ineffective erythropoiesis, and hemolytic anemia. In alpha-thalassemia, the beta tetramers that form are more soluble, and thus the clinical severity is milder.

A. **Alpha-thalassemia** occurs in persons of Mediterranean, African, Middle Eastern, Indian, and Asian descent. Individuals with decreased function of one alpha-globin gene may have only mild microcytosis; the loss of two alpha-globin genes is associated with a mild hypochromic microcytic anemia (Hb >10 g/dl). A deletion or mutation of three of the four alpha-globin genes results in Hb H disease, which is characterized by splenomegaly, chronic hemolytic anemia, and the presence of beta-globin tetramers. A loss of all four alpha-globin genes causes hydrops fetalis.

B. **Beta-thalassemia** occurs worldwide in a distribution similar to that of alpha-thalassemia. Production of beta-globin chains may be diminished or absent from each allele and are described as beta$^+$-thalassemia or beta°-thalassemia, respectively. Beta-thalassemia is commonly classified by the severity of anemia; multiple genotypes exist for each phenotype.

1. **Thalassemia trait** is caused by diminished or absent beta-globin chain synthesis from one gene. Patients are asymptomatic, with a mild hypochromic, microcytic anemia (Hb >10 g/dl).

2. **Thalassemia intermedia** is associated with moderate dysfunction of both beta-globin genes. Clinical severity is intermediate (Hb 7–10 g/dl), and patients are usually not transfusion-dependent.

3. **Thalassemia major** (Cooley's anemia) is caused by severe dysfunction of both beta-globin genes. Anemia is severe, and RBC transfusions are required to sustain life.

C. **History and physical examination.** A family history of microcytosis or microcytic anemia may aid in diagnosis. Splenomegaly and bone abnormalities caused by the expanded marrow are common in Hb H disease and beta-thalassemia major.

D. **Laboratory results.** The MCV is low, and microcytic, hypochromic cells with poikilocytosis, target cells, and nucleated RBCs may be present on the peripheral smear. Hb electrophoresis may aid in the diagnosis.

E. **Treatment** is centered on RBC transfusions adequate to sustain life, improve exercise tolerance, and prevent skeletal abnormalities. In severe forms of thalassemia, the transfusions result in tissue iron overload, which may cause congestive heart failure, hepatic dysfunction, glucose intolerance, and secondary hypogonadism caused by deposition of iron in the hypothalamus. Iron chelation therapy with deferoxamine mesylate may prevent these complications (see sec. III.E.3). **For patients with thalassemia, it is important to avoid the incorrect diagnosis of iron-deficiency anemia and needless and potentially harmful iron supplementation.**

1. **Transfusions.** An Hb of 8 g/dl prevents skeletal deformities and can usually be achieved with 1 unit of **packed RBCs** every 2–3 weeks or 2 units every month. Transfusion-dependent patients should receive packed RBCs through a leukocyte-depleting filter (see Transfusion Therapy).

2. **Splenectomy** removes the primary site of extravascular hemolysis and should be considered if RBC transfusion requirements increase and exceed 1.5 times the previous levels. It should not be performed if the patient is younger than 5–6 years because of the risk of sepsis. Polyvalent pneumococcal vaccine should be administered 1 month before surgery. Postsplenectomy, patients are at risk for overwhelming sepsis (see Chap. 13).

3. **Iron chelation therapy** with deferoxamine mesylate (Desferal), 50–100 mg/kg/day, is usually administered by continuous SC infusion for 10–12 hours/day. If this therapy is started in infants when iron stores are very low, growth failure is possible. However, if this therapy is started before puberty, most patients will achieve normal growth and sexual development. Once clinical organ deterioration has begun, it may not be reversible. Therapy may be complicated by local irritation at the injection site, and pruritus and hypotension may occur if the drug is infused too rapidly. Continuous IV infusion of deferoxamine through an indwelling venous port at the same dosage and schedule may also be used (*Am J Hemat* 41:61, 1992). Patients receiving deferoxamine should be followed at a center where patients with thalassemia are regularly treated. Long-term side effects, particularly with high-dose therapy, include optic neuropathy, sensorineural hearing loss, and increased susceptibility to bacteremia and mucormycosis.

4. **Vitamin C supplementation,** 100 mg PO, given during the infusion of deferoxamine, will increase urinary iron excretion during chelation therapy. **Large doses of vitamin C should be avoided** because they may cause a massive release of iron that may precipitate congestive heart failure. Vitamin C should be taken on an empty stomach to avoid enhanced absorption of dietary iron.

5. **BMT** should be considered in patients with thalassemia major who have HLA-identical related donors.

IV. **Myelodysplastic syndromes (MDSs)** are acquired clonal disorders of hematopoietic stem cells that are classified according to morphologic findings on the peripheral smear and bone marrow biopsy: (1) refractory anemia (RA); (2) RA with ringed sideroblasts (RARS); (3) RA with excess blasts (RAEB); (4) RAEB in transformation; and (5) chronic myelomonocytic leukemia (CMML). MDS may be idiopathic or secondary to radiation, chemotherapy, or toxin exposure. Presentations range from mild cytopenias without symptoms to severe pancytopenia. Progression to marrow failure or acute leukemia commonly occurs. The prognosis for patients with RA and RARS is substantially better than for patients with other forms of the disease. **Sideroblastic anemias** are a heterogeneous group of acquired or hereditary disorders characterized by abnormal RBC iron metabolism. Causes of acquired sideroblastic anemia include drugs (isoniazid, chloramphenicol, ethanol), lead toxicity, malignancy, chronic inflammation, and infection. Acquired idiopathic sideroblastic anemia is considered to be an MDS.

A. **Laboratory results.** The MCV is usually normal or slightly elevated in MDS, but in acquired sideroblastic anemia some cells may be microcytic. Marked anisocytosis and poikilocytosis may be seen in all forms and basophilic stippling is often present. Serum iron and transferrin are normal or elevated. The diagnosis is established by demonstrating abnormal hematopoietic cells in the bone marrow.

B. **Therapy** of MDS is supportive and rarely curative. Myelosuppressive drugs should be stopped, and nutritional deficiencies should be corrected. **Deferoxamine mesylate** (see sec. III.E.3) should be considered for patients with a favorable prognosis after 50–100 units of packed RBCs have been transfused.

1. **Pyridoxine,** 50–200 mg PO qd, may be tried empirically, although the response rate is low and usually occurs in patients with RARS.

2. **Erythropoietin,** 100–300 U/kg SC 3 times/week, may be useful in decreasing RBC transfusion requirements in about 20% of patients and is more likely to be effective when the serum erythropoietin level is below 200 mU/ml.

3. **Chemotherapy** is not usually of benefit for MDS; initiation of treatment after progression to acute leukemia has a low complete response rate. **BMT** should be considered in patients younger than 50 years of age who have an HLA-identical sibling.

V. **The megaloblastic anemias** are a group of disorders associated with altered morphology of hematopoietic cells and other cells that are rapidly dividing because of abnormalities in DNA synthesis. Almost all cases are because of folic acid or vitamin B_{12} deficiency. **Folic acid deficiency** may develop within a few months, and common causes include (1) decreased intake (alcoholism), (2) malabsorption, and (3) increased utilization (hemolytic anemia, pregnancy). In addition, some drugs (ethanol, trimethoprim, pyrimethamine, methotrexate, sulfasalazine, oral contraceptives, and anticonvulsants) may lead to a perturbed folate metabolism. **Vitamin B_{12} deficiency** takes years to develop because very little of the body's store is used each day. Causes of vitamin B_{12} deficiency include (1) pernicious anemia, (2) gastrectomy, (3) pancreatic insufficiency, (4) GI bacterial overgrowth, (5) ileitis or ileal resection, and (6) intestinal parasites.

A. **History and physical examination.** Symptoms are primarily attributable to anemia, although glossitis, jaundice, and splenomegaly may be present. **Vitamin B_{12} deficiency** may cause decreased vibratory and positional sense, ataxia, paresthesias, confusion, and dementia. Neurologic complications may occur in the absence of anemia and may not resolve completely despite adequate treatment. Folic acid deficiency does not result in neurologic disease.

B. **Laboratory results.** The MCV is usually increased and leukopenia and thrombocytopenia may occur. The peripheral smear may show anisocytosis, poikilocytosis, and macro-ovalocytes; hypersegmented neutrophils (containing ≥5 nuclear lobes) are common. Serum lactate dehydrogenase (LDH) and indirect bilirubin may be elevated, reflecting ineffective erythropoiesis and premature destruction of RBCs.

1. **Serum vitamin B_{12} and folate levels** should both be measured. RBC folate may be a more accurate indicator of body folate stores than serum folate,

particularly if it is measured after folate therapy has been initiated. A vitamin B_{12} value (normal 200–900 pg/ml) of less than 100 pg/ml is almost always accompanied by clinical disease. Occasionally, symptomatic patients with vitamin B_{12} values in the normal range respond to therapy.

2. **Serum methylmalonic acid (MMA) and homocysteine** may be useful when the vitamin B_{12} or folate level is equivocal. Both MMA and homocysteine are elevated in vitamin B_{12} deficiency; homocysteine is elevated in folic acid deficiency.

3. **A Schilling test** may be useful in determining the cause of vitamin B_{12} deficiency, but it rarely affects the therapeutic approach.

4. **Bone marrow biopsy** may be necessary to rule out MDS and hematologic malignancy; these disorders may present with findings similar to megaloblastic anemias on the peripheral smear.

C. **Therapy** is directed toward replacing the deficient factor. Blood transfusions are rarely required and may be associated with volume overload when used for these disorders.

1. **Folic acid** may be administered at 1 mg PO qd until the deficiency is corrected. High doses of folic acid (5 mg PO qd) may be needed in patients with malabsorption syndromes.

2. **Vitamin B_{12} deficiency** is corrected by administering cyanocobalamin. A typical schedule is 1 mg IM qd for 7 days, then weekly for 1–2 months or until normalization of the Hb and Hct occurs. Long-term therapy is 1 mg/month. With therapy, the reticulocytosis should rise and peak in 1 week followed by a rising Hb over 6–8 weeks. **Coexisting iron deficiency is present in one-third of patients and is a common cause for an incomplete response to therapy. Empiric therapy of megaloblastic anemia with folic acid alone is not recommended** because the anemia of unrecognized vitamin B_{12} deficiency may partially respond while the neurologic abnormalities progress.

VI. **Anemia of chronic renal insufficiency** is attributed primarily to decreased endogenous erythropoietin production.

A. **Laboratory results.** The Hct is usually 20–30% and the MCV is normal. On peripheral smear the RBCs are normochromic with the occasional presence of echinocytes (burr cells) or acanthocytes (spur cells).

B. **Treatment** of anemia of chronic renal insufficiency has been revolutionized by the availability of recombinant human erythropoietin (Procrit, Epogen). Therapy is indicated in both predialysis and dialysis patients who are symptomatic. Subjective benefits include increased energy, enhanced appetite, better sleep patterns, and improved sexual activity. Objective benefits of reversing the anemia include enhanced exercise tolerance, improved cognitive function, elimination of RBC transfusions, and reduction of iron overload (*Ann Intern Med* 114:402, 1991). Relief of pruritus may occur prior to correction of the anemia (*N Engl J Med* 326:969, 1992).

1. **Administration** of erythropoietin may be IV (for hemodialysis patients) or SC (for predialysis or peritoneal dialysis patients). More than 97% of patients increase their Hct by 10 points or to a level greater than 32% within 12 weeks of therapy. A typical initial dosage is 50–100 units/kg 3 times/week until the Hct reaches 32%; the average maintenance dosage is 75 units/kg 3 times/week. About 10% of patients need more than 200 units/kg 3 times/week. It may be possible to give SC therapy less often than IV to maintain the Hct.

2. **Adverse reactions** to erythropoietin therapy include **hypertension,** which develops or worsens in approximately one-third of patients within 3 months, and **seizures,** which occur in approximately 5% of patients, often in association with uncontrolled hypertension. Use of erythropoietin may cause iron-deficiency anemia.

3. **Suboptimal responses** may occur with coexisting iron deficiency, chronic inflammatory conditions, and acute or chronic bleeding. Hemodialysis patients may also suffer from aluminum intoxication that blunts the response to erythropoietin. Secondary hyperparathyroidism that causes bone marrow

fibrosis and relative erythropoietin resistance may also occur (*N Engl J Med* 328:171, 1993).

VII. Anemia of chronic disease often develops in patients with long-standing inflammatory disease, malignancy, autoimmune disorders, or chronic infection. Abnormalities in mobilizing stored iron, inhibition of erythropoietin production, failure to respond to endogenous erythropoietin, and humoral inhibition of erythropoiesis have all been implicated in the pathogenesis.

    A. Laboratory results. A normocytic normochromic anemia is typical. The peripheral smear is usually normal, although microcytes may be present. Both **serum iron and TIBC** are usually decreased, and transferrin saturation is greater than 10%. **Ferritin** is usually normal but may be elevated, because it is an acute-phase reactant. No test is diagnostic for the anemia of chronic disease.

    B. Treatment is directed at the underlying cause of the disease and at eliminating exacerbating factors such as nutritional deficiencies and marrow-suppressive drugs. Erythropoietin, 12.5–250.0 units/kg SC 3 times/week, can correct the anemia associated with rheumatoid arthritis (*Am J Med* 89:161, 1990).

VIII. Anemia associated with zidovudine or cancer chemotherapy can be treated with erythropoietin, 100–150 units/kg SC 3 times/week, to reduce use of blood products.

Anemias Associated with Increased Red Blood Cell Loss or Destruction

Anemias associated with increased erythropoiesis (i.e., an elevated RI) are caused by bleeding or destruction of RBCs (hemolysis) and may exceed the capacity of normal bone marrow to correct the Hct. Typically the bilirubin and LDH are normal in the bleeding patient and elevated in the patient with hemolysis.

I. Bleeding is much more common than hemolysis. Hidden sites of bleeding (retroperitoneum, fractured hip) may result in laboratory findings that are similar to those seen with a hemolytic process. Treatment of the bleeding patient is discussed in Transfusion Therapy.

II. Hemolytic anemias are classified by the predominant site of hemolysis.

    A. Intravascular hemolysis may present with fever, chills, tachycardia, and backache. Serum haptoglobin levels decrease markedly as this protein binds and removes Hb from the plasma. If hemolysis is severe, free Hb may be measured in the plasma and urine. Renal failure may develop with hemoglobinuria. Hemosiderin may be measured in the urine beginning 7 days after a hemolytic event and is a reliable indicator of chronic intravascular hemolysis.

    B. Extravascular hemolysis is characterized by RBC destruction in the reticuloendothelial system, primarily the spleen. Jaundice and splenomegaly may be present. Haptoglobin levels are normal or slightly reduced.

All patients with suspected hemolysis should have a direct antiglobulin test (DAT, or direct Coombs' test). This test detects the presence of IgG and the third component of complement (C3) on the surface of RBCs and will usually differentiate between immune and nonimmune causes of hemolysis.

III. Sickle cell disease includes sickle cell anemia (HbSS) and other sickling syndromes with double-heterozygous conditions (HbS–beta thalassemia, HbSC). These disorders are associated with structurally abnormal Hb molecules that polymerize under reduced oxygen conditions. The clinical features are a consequence of a chronic hemolytic anemia and vasoocclusive ischemic tissue injury. **Sickle cell trait** occurs in individuals who are heterozygous for Hb S.

    A. Clinical manifestations of sickle cell disease vary widely. Signs of disease usually develop in infancy or childhood. Delayed growth and development and increased susceptibility to infections are common. Treatment is determined by the specific complications that occur. Individuals with sickle cell trait are usually healthy but appear to have an increased risk of sudden death with rigorous exercise.

B. **Laboratory results.** The Hb ranges from 5–10 g/dl in sickle cell anemia, and the MCV may be slightly elevated because of the increased reticulocyte count. Chronic neutrophilia (10,000–20,000/mm^3) is often present, and the platelet count may be increased. The peripheral smear will show the classic distorted sickle-shaped erythrocytes. Howell-Jolly bodies may be seen because of functional asplenism, which usually occurs by the age of 10 years. Target cells may be present, particularly in HbS–beta thalassemia and HbSC. A Hb electrophoresis will distinguish homozygous disease from sickle cell trait and other hemoglobinopathies. Screening tests such as the sickle cell solubility test will not distinguish sickle cell trait from sickle cell disease.

C. **Treatment** must address both the acute and chronic complications of the disease (NIH publication No. 91-2117, 1991).

1. **Prevention and health maintenance**

   a. **Dehydration and hypoxia** should be avoided because they may precipitate or exacerbate sickling. Intense exercise should be strongly discouraged, as well as activities at high altitude and flying in unpressurized aircraft.

   b. **Folic acid,** 1 mg PO qd, should be administered to patients with sickle cell disease because of chronic hemolysis.

   c. **Antimicrobial prophylaxis** with penicillin VK, 125 mg PO bid up to age 3 years, then 250 mg bid, should be given to children between the ages of 2 months and 5 years because of their high risk of pneumococcal infection. Patients who are allergic to penicillin should receive erythromycin, 250 mg PO bid. Antimicrobial prophylaxis has not been proved effective in adults.

   d. **Immunizations** against the usual childhood illnesses should be given to children with sickle cell disease. After 2 years of age, a polyvalent pneumococcal vaccine should be administered. Hepatitis B vaccine is recommended for hepatitis B surface antibody–negative patients. Yearly influenza vaccine is recommended.

   e. **Regular yearly ophthalmologic examinations** are recommended because of a high incidence of proliferative retinopathy leading to vitreous hemorrhage and retinal detachment. Monocular blindness can usually be prevented with laser photocoagulation.

   f. **Surgery and anesthesia.** Local and regional anesthesia may be used without special precautions. With general anesthesia, measures to avoid volume depletion and hypoxia are critical; hypernatremia should be avoided. For major surgery, partial exchange transfusions to decrease the HbS level to less than 50% may be helpful in preventing the acute chest syndrome (see sec. **III.C.3.b**). Partial exchange transfusion is recommended prior to all ophthalmologic surgery.

2. **Complications of chronic hemolysis**

   a. **Aplastic crisis** is characterized by a sudden decrease in Hb and reticulocyte count. This crisis is generally associated with a viral illness, usually parvovirus B19. Transfusion with packed RBCs is the mainstay of therapy, and most patients will recover in 10–14 days. Folic acid deficiency should be excluded.

   b. **Cholelithiasis,** primarily with bilirubin stones, is present in more than 50% of adult patients. Acute cholecystitis should be treated conservatively, and cholecystectomy should be performed when the attack subsides. Elective cholecystectomy for asymptomatic gallstones is controversial.

3. **Complications of vasoocclusive episodes**

   a. **Vasoocclusive pain crises** are the most common manifestations of sickle cell anemia. Pain is typically in the back, ribs, and limbs and lasts for 5–7 days. The pattern of pain is usually consistent in any one patient from crisis to crisis. A deviation from the pattern may suggest another diagnosis such as cholecystitis. Precipitating factors such as an infection should be excluded. Many painful episodes are managed on an outpatient basis with PO or IV fluids, 3–4 liters/day, and analgesia. Codeine or morphine are recommended for moderate or severe pain. Patients who require continued parenteral narcotics, who cannot consume adequate PO fluids, or in whom another complication is suspected (infection, acute chest syndrome) require hospital admission. Supplemental oxygen does not benefit acute pain crisis unless hypoxia is present. **Blood transfusions will not change the immediate course of an acute pain crisis.** Some patients will not require significant amounts of analgesic therapy between crises, although narcotics may be required by others. Patients who suffer from severe recurrent pain crises that require frequent hospitalizations or who are refractory to conventional therapy should be considered for long-term partial exchange transfusions.

   b. **Acute chest syndrome** is associated with chest pain, pulmonary infil-trates, leukocytosis, and hypoxia and is indistinguishable from pneumo-nia. Initial management should include hospitalization, administration of supplemental oxygen to correct hypoxia, and empiric therapy with anti-microbials. Transfusion of RBCs is recommended with multiple-lobe involvement, worsening disease, or hypoxemia (PaO_2 <60 mm Hg).

   c. **Sequestration crisis** is a consequence of blood sequestration in the spleen and is associated with sudden splenomegaly, hypotension, and shock. Hemodynamic support and RBC transfusions are usually required. This event usually occurs in patients with an intact spleen such as infants with HbSS or adults with HbSC or HbS–beta thalassemia disease.

   d. **Infection in children** may be caused by *Streptococcus pneumoniae, Hae-mophilus influenzae*, or other encapsulated organisms. Children who present with fever can be treated empirically on an outpatient basis with ceftriaxone, 50 mg/kg IV daily for 2 days (*N Engl J Med* 329:492, 1993). **Infections in adults** typically occur in tissues that are susceptible to vasoocclusive infarcts (bone, kidney, lung). Treatment of osteomyelitis should be directed by culture of biopsied tissue. *Staphylococcus, Salmo-nella*, and enteric organisms are the most common causes. Urinary tract infections should be treated based on the culture data. Pneumonia is most likely to be *Mycoplasma, Staphylococcus aureus*, or *H. influenzae* and must be distinguished from acute chest syndrome (see sec. III.C.3.b).

4. **Chronic organ damage**
   a. **Osteonecrosis** of the femoral and humeral heads may cause considerable morbidity in approximately 10% of patients. Treatment consists of local heat, analgesics, and avoidance of weight bearing. Hip arthroplasty may be effective in decreasing symptoms and improving function but is associated with a high risk of complications.

   b. **Stroke** occurs most commonly in children younger than 10 years. Without treatment, approximately two-thirds of patients will experience recurrent stroke. Long-term transfusions to maintain the HbS concentration at less than 50% for 5 years reduces the incidence of recurrence (*Blood* 79:1657, 1992).

   c. **Leg ulcers** should be treated with rest, leg elevation, and intensive local care. Wet-to-dry dressings should be applied every 3 hours to debride the ulcer, and topical antimicrobials should be applied. Unna's boot (zinc oxide–impregnated bandage), changed weekly for 3–4 weeks, may be used for nonhealing ulcers. Otherwise, long-term transfusions and split-thickness skin grafts may be necessary.

   d. **Priapism** may respond to hydration and analgesics; however, exchange transfusions are recommended for acute events lasting longer than several hours. Permanent impotence can occur.

   e. **Renal tubular defects** caused by sickling in the anoxic hyperosmolar environment of the renal medulla may lead to isosthenuria (inability to concentrate urine) and hematuria in sickle cell disease and sickle cell trait. These conditions predispose patients to dehydration, which increases the risk of vasoocclusive events.

5. **Pregnancy** in sickle cell disease is associated with an increased incidence of premature delivery and fetal death. RBC transfusions decrease the number of

Table 18-2. Medications for glucose-6-phosphate dehydrogenase deficiency

Safe	Unsafe
Acetaminophen	Acetanilid
Ascorbic acid	Dapsone
Aspirin	Doxorubicin
Chloramphenicol	Furazolidone
Chloroquine	Methylene blue
Colchicine	Nalidixic acid
Diphenhydramine	Niridazole
Isoniazid	Nitrofurantoin
Menadione sodium bisulfite	Phenazopyridine
Phenacetin	Primaquine
Phenylbutazone	Sulfamethoxazole
Phenytoin	Sulfapyridine
Probenecid	Sulfacetamide
Procainamide	
Pyrimethamine	
Quinidine	
Streptomycin	
Sulfamethoxypyridazine	
Sulfisoxazole	
Trimethoprim	
Tripelennamine	
Vitamin K	

Source: Adapted from E Beutler. Glucose-6-phosphate-dehydrogenase deficiency. *N Engl J Med* 324:169, 1991.

vasoocclusive episodes during pregnancy (*N Engl J Med* 319:1447, 1988). In asymptomatic patients, transfusions do not appear to change the outcome of the pregnancy.

6. **Experimental therapy** with hydroxyurea has been shown to increase levels of fetal Hb and decrease hemolysis in patients with sickle cell anemia (*Blood* 79:2555, 1992). BMT has been used in selected patients. These therapies are considered experimental and should be reserved for ongoing clinical trials.

IV. **Hereditary RBC structural protein abnormalities** result in membrane defects that precipitate extravascular hemolysis. The classic example is **hereditary spherocytosis (HS),** which may be autosomal dominant or recessive. HS is associated with a microcytic anemia, splenomegaly, jaundice, cholelithiasis, and spherocytes on the peripheral smear. The **osmotic fragility test** is positive, and the DAT is negative. If therapy is required, splenectomy will correct the anemia. Folic acid should be administered as long-term therapy.

V. **Glucose-6-phosphate dehydrogenase (G6PD) deficiency** is the most common of the hereditary RBC enzyme deficiencies. It is a sex-linked disorder that affects men and is rarely seen in women. The enzyme deficiency results in RBCs that are more susceptible to oxidant stress than normal RBCs and is associated with chronic or episodic hemolysis. Other enzyme deficiencies such as pyruvate kinase deficiency may cause hemolysis. Family history and measurement of enzyme levels will confirm the diagnosis.

A. **Classification.** A mild form of the deficiency occurs in approximately 10% of African-American men and is characterized by hemolytic episodes that are triggered by infections or drug exposure (Table 18-2). A more severe enzyme deficiency, such as the Mediterranean variety, results in hemolysis when susceptible individuals are exposed to fava beans. The most severe type causes hereditary nonspherocytic hemolytic anemia with hemolysis in the absence of a secondary cause.

B. **Laboratory results.** The peripheral smear shows "bite cells"; RBC inclusions **(Heinz bodies)** are seen with special stains. The diagnosis is based on determination of the enzyme level. However, senescent RBCs contain less G6PD and are more easily destroyed than younger cells so that after a hemolytic episode, the G6PD level may be normal, reflecting the younger population of cells in the circulation.

C. **Treatment** consists of adequate hydration to protect renal function during hemolysis, avoidance of precipitating factors, and, if necessary, RBC transfusion.

VI. **Autoimmune hemolytic anemia (AIHA)** is caused by antibodies to RBCs. In warm AIHA, antibodies interact best, with RBCs at 37°C, whereas in cold AIHA, antibodies are most active at lower temperatures. The DAT is often positive in both forms of AIHA.

A. **Warm antibody autoimmune hemolytic anemia** is usually caused by an IgG autoantibody. It may be idiopathic or associated with an underlying malignancy (lymphoma, chronic lymphocytic leukemia), collagen vascular disorder, or drug use.

1. **Clinical presentation** may include weakness, jaundice, and moderate splenomegaly. Severe hemolysis may be associated with fever, chest pain, syncope, and hemoglobinuria.

2. **Laboratory findings** are extravascular hemolysis and usually a decreased serum haptoglobin. The peripheral smear shows spherocytes.

3. **Therapy** should be directed at identifying and treating any underlying cause. In most cases the hemolysis should be treated with glucocorticoids or splenectomy, or both. The approach to treatment is similar to that of idiopathic thrombocytopenic purpura (ITP) (see Chap. 17). **Transfusions** may occasionally be necessary in severe cases, but the transfused RBCs may also be at risk of hemolysis. Treatment with folic acid is also recommended.

B. **Cold antibody autoimmune hemolytic anemia** is associated with episodic cold-induced hemolysis and vasoocclusive events resulting in cyanosis of the ears, nose, fingers, and toes. The two general syndromes are described below.

1. **Cold agglutinin disease** may be chronic and caused by a paraprotein (lymphoma, Waldenström's macroglobulinemia), or acute and transient, secondary to an infection (*Mycoplasma*, mononucleosis). IgM and C3 are found on the RBCs (the DAT identifies only the presence of C3). Hemolysis is extravascular. Treatment is directed at the underlying disease; the acute form requires only supportive measures. Transfusions are best done at 37°C.

2. **Paroxysmal cold hemoglobinuria** is a rare disease that may be idiopathic or associated with acute viral infections (mumps, measles) or tertiary syphilis. Hemolysis is intravascular and the DAT is negative. Avoidance of cold temperatures is important, and any transfused blood should be heated to 37°C to prevent exacerbation of hemolysis.

VII. **Drug-induced hemolytic anemia** may be caused by any of three distinct mechanisms. In all cases, treatment consists of discontinuation of the offending agent.

A. **Drug-induced immune hemolytic anemia** presents similarly to warm-antibody AIHA. Methyldopa is the classic example, but many agents have been implicated. Up to 20% of patients taking this drug have a positive DAT, and 1% have hemolytic anemia indistinguishable from AIHA. Anemia and the positive DAT gradually resolve after discontinuation of the drug.

B. **Haptens** occur when penicillin (or other related antimicrobials) coats RBC membranes, forming a new antigenic determinant. If antibodies against penicillin are present and the patient receives the drug (particularly with high doses), a DAT-positive hemolytic anemia may result.

C. **Immune complexes.** IgM (occasionally IgG) antibodies may develop against drugs such as quinine, isoniazid, and sulfonamides, forming drug-antibody complexes that adhere to RBCs. Since the antibody involved is usually an IgM, the DAT will be positive only for C3.

VIII. **Microangiopathic hemolytic anemia** is a syndrome of traumatic intravascular hemolysis that is thought to be caused by deposition of fibrin strands in the lumen of small blood vessels. It may be seen in disseminated intravascular coagulation

(DIC), thrombotic thrombocytopenic purpura (TTP), hemolytic-uremic syndrome (HUS), severe hypertension, vasculitis, eclampsia, and some disseminated malignancies. The peripheral smear shows schistocytes (fragmented RBCs) and frequently thrombocytopenia. Management of DIC, TTP, and HUS is described in Chap. 17.

IX. **Traumatic hemolytic anemia** refers to intravascular hemolysis that is usually associated with a malfunctioning prosthetic aortic valve. Porcine valves or valves in the mitral position are not as likely to cause significant hemolysis. This phenomenon has also been associated with synthetic arterial bypass grafts. The peripheral smear will show schistocytes and other RBC fragments (these findings may be present to a lesser degree in properly functioning valve replacements). Therapy involves correction of the mechanical abnormality.

X. **Paroxysmal nocturnal hemoglobinuria** is a rare acquired disease of bone marrow stem cells characterized by episodes of intravascular hemolysis. Venous thromboses, particularly of the mesenteric, portal, and cerebral veins, may occur and require anticoagulation. Diagnosis is made by a positive acid-hemolysis test (Ham test) or by finding hematopoietic cells that lack decay-accelerating factor. Androgens (to stimulate erythropoiesis) and glucocorticoids (to decrease lysis) have been used. Iron replacement may be necessary to cover loss in the urine but may precipitate hemolysis. Transfusion of 2 units of packed RBCs prior to iron therapy may prevent hemolysis.

Transfusion Therapy

Advances in collection, preparation, and administration have allowed blood component transfusion to become useful in a wide variety of clinical situations. The administration of blood products exposes the patient to the risk of many adverse effects, some of which are life-threatening. **The benefits and risks of transfusion therapy must be carefully weighed in each situation.** In each case, the indications for transfusion should be recorded in the medical record. It is generally agreed that, if possible, informed consent should be obtained for the administration of all blood products. In elective surgery, the patient may need to be informed several weeks in advance of the procedure so that the options of autologous donation and directed donation may be explored.

I. **Indications for blood product transfusion** are primarily determined by the clinician. The responsible physician also has options regarding the preparation and administration of blood (e.g., types of filter, flow rates), and these should be detailed in the medical orders.

A. **RBC transfusion** is indicated to increase the oxygen-carrying capacity of blood in anemic patients when the anemia is responsible for poor tissue oxygenation. Adequate tissue oxygenation can usually be attained with a Hb of 7–8 g/dl in a normovolemic patient. One unit of packed RBCs will increase the Hb by 1 g/dl (Hct 3%) in the average adult. Patient age, cause and severity of anemia, and coexisting disorders such as cardiopulmonary disease must be considered when determining the need for transfusion. If the cause of anemia is easily treatable (e.g., iron or folic acid deficiency), it is preferable to avoid transfusion. RBCs should not be used as volume expanders, to enhance wound healing, or to improve general "well-being" if symptoms are not related to anemia.

1. **The type and screen procedure** tests the recipient's RBCs for the A, B, and D (Rh) antigen and also screens the recipient's serum for antibodies against other RBC antigens. **Cross-matching** tests the patient's serum for antibodies against antigens in the donor's RBCs and is performed before dispensing a specific unit of blood for a patient.

2. **Preparation.** Most patients should receive packed RBCs that have not been washed or frozen, because these units have the greatest RBC volume. In chronically transfused patients, blood should be administered through a leukocyte-depleting filter to decrease the incidence of alloimmunization and

nonhemolytic febrile transfusion reactions (*Ann Intern Med* 117:151, 1992). For immunocompromised patients or patients receiving directed donations from first-degree relatives, irradiation of blood products is generally recommended. Washed RBCs are rarely indicated.

3. **Administration.** Patient and blood product identification procedures must be carefully followed to avoid mishandling errors. The IV catheter should be at least 18-gauge to allow adequate flow. All blood products that are not leukocyte-depleted should be administered through a 170- to 260-μm "standard" filter to prevent infusion of macroaggregates, fibrin, and debris. Only 0.9% NaCl should be used with blood components to prevent cell lysis. Patients should be observed for the first 5–10 minutes of the transfusion for adverse side effects and at regular intervals thereafter. Each unit of blood should be administered within 4 hours.

B. **Platelet transfusion** is indicated to control or prevent bleeding caused by thrombocytopenia or platelet dysfunction. Platelets isolated from 1 unit of blood should raise the platelet count at least 5,000/mm^3. Transfusion for chronic thrombocytopenia is generally not necessary in the absence of bleeding or other coagulation defects. Patients with temporary severe thrombocytopenia but normal platelet function (e.g., acute leukemia) may benefit from prophylactic transfusion to maintain the platelet count above 5,000–10,000/mm^3. In general, if platelet function is normal and the platelet count is 50,000/mm^3 or greater, it is unlikely that prophylactic transfusion will be beneficial for most invasive procedures. Higher platelet counts may be necessary for major surgery or in situations in which there are additional coagulation defects, sepsis, or platelet dysfunction related to disease or medication. Random donor platelets are generally sufficient, but single-donor platelets are indicated in patients who are refractory.

C. **Fresh-frozen plasma (FFP) transfusion** is indicated to increase the level of clotting factors in patients with a documented deficiency. Specific indications are covered in Chap. 17. One unit of FFP, measuring 200–250 ml, will increase each clotting factor activity by 2–3%. Empiric administration of FFP is generally not necessary if the prothrombin time (PT) and activated partial thromboplastin time (aPTT) are less than 1.5 times normal. FFP should not be used for volume expansion, as a nutritional supplement, or prophylactically following coronary artery bypass surgery. Leukocyte-depleting filters are not needed for FFP transfusions.

II. **Complications of transfusion therapy**
A. **Risks are incurred with all blood component therapy.** Patient concerns are primarily focused on transfusion-associated viral infections.
   1. **Infection.** Testing for viral infections includes HIV-1, HIV-2, human T-cell lymphotropic virus-1 (HTLV-1), hepatitis B virus (HBV), and hepatitis C virus (HCV). The risk of transfusion-associated transmission of HIV-1 from screened blood is estimated to be 1 : 200,000; no cases of HIV-2 have yet been reported from blood products. The incidence of HTLV-1 infection is low and varies with geographic location. Estimates of HBV transmission are similar to HIV-1. By far the most frequently transmitted agent is HCV. Since 1985, the risk of transmission of this virus has decreased markedly as improved testing has been developed. The incidence of HCV transmission was estimated in 1992 to be 1 : 3,300 units and continues to decline. CMV transmission from RBC and platelet transfusion is an important risk in immunocompromised patients. Leukocyte-depleting filters appear to be effective in decreasing the risk. Bacterial transmission may occur and the risk increases with prolonged storage time; offending organisms vary with the blood component. Many parasitic infections, including malaria and trypanosomiasis, have also been transmitted by transfusions.
   2. **Hemolytic transfusion reactions**
      a. **Acute hemolytic reactions** are usually caused by preformed antibodies in the recipient and are characterized by intravascular hemolysis of the transfused RBCs soon after the administration of the incompatible blood. Fever,

chills, back pain, chest pain, nausea, vomiting, and symptoms related to hypotension may develop. Acute renal failure with hemoglobinuria may occur. In the unconscious patient, hypotension or increased bleeding may be the only manifestation. If a hemolytic transfusion reaction is suspected, the transfusion should be stopped immediately and all IV tubing should be replaced. Clotted and EDTA–treated samples of the patient's blood should be delivered to the blood bank along with the remainder of the suspected unit for repeat of the cross-match. Serum bilirubin and tests for DIC should be performed, and the plasma and freshly voided urine should be examined for free Hb. Management includes preservation of intravascular volume and protection of renal function. Urine output should be maintained at 100 ml/hour or greater with the use of IV fluids, diuretics, or mannitol, if necessary. The excretion of free Hb may be improved by alkalinization of the urine. Sodium bicarbonate may be added to IV fluids to increase the urinary pH to 7.5 or greater.

   b. Delayed hemolytic transfusion reactions may occur from 1–25 days after a transfusion and are caused by either an anamnestic response or a primary antibody response to RBC antigens. Many of these patients probably were sensitized to RBC antigens prior to the transfusion, but titers were too low to be detected by the screening procedures. Usually there is a fall in the Hb and Hct and the bilirubin rises. The DAT may be positive, resulting in confusion with autoimmune hemolytic anemia. Delayed hemolytic transfusion reactions may at times be severe; these cases should be treated similarly to acute transfusion reactions.

3. **Nonhemolytic febrile transfusion reactions** are characterized by fevers, chills, urticaria, pruritus, and respiratory distress and are usually seen in previously transfused patients or multiparous women. Antibodies against donor plasma proteins or leukocyte antigens are thought to be the cause. Treatment of symptoms with acetaminophen and diphenhydramine, 25–50 mg PO or IV, is usually sufficient. Rarely, epinephrine or glucocorticoids are required. Some patients may require premedication with acetaminophen, diphenhydramine, or steroids to prevent recurrence of symptoms with subsequent transfusions. Meperidine, 25–50 mg IV, is effective in preventing shaking chills. Leukocyte-depleting filters will prevent reactions caused by sensitivity to donor WBCs. **Anaphylactic reactions** may be seen in patients with IgA deficiency (1 in 1,000 individuals) who receive IgA-containing blood products and develop anti-IgA antibodies.

4. **Volume overload** with signs of congestive heart failure may be seen when patients with cardiovascular compromise are transfused with RBCs. Slowing the rate of transfusion and judicious use of diuretics help prevent this complication.

5. **Noncardiogenic pulmonary edema** is caused by antileukocyte antibodies present in the donor's plasma. The donors are usually multiparous women and should not give further blood donations. The effect is usually transient and therapy is supportive.

6. **Transfusion-associated graft-versus-host disease** is usually seen in immunocompromised patients and is thought to result from the infusion of immunocompetent T lymphocytes (*N Engl J Med* 323:315, 1990). This entity has been reported in immunocompetent patients who share an HLA haplotype with HLA-homozygous blood donors (usually a relative or members of inbred populations). Rash, elevated liver function tests, and severe pancytopenia are seen. The mortality rate is greater than 80%. Direct-donated blood from first-degree relatives should be irradiated to avoid this complication. The chance of receiving blood with shared HLA haplotypes from a random blood donor is extremely low, so irradiation of nonrelated blood products is not indicated for the immunocompetent patient.

B. **Adverse effects from massive transfusion.** Administration of a volume of RBCs or plasma in excess of the normal blood volume of the patient in a 24-hour period **(massive transfusion)** is associated with several additional complications.

1. **Hypothermia** caused by rapid infusion of chilled blood may cause cardiac dysrhythmias. A blood-warming device can prevent this problem.
2. **Citrate intoxication** occurs in patients with hepatic dysfunction and can cause hypocalcemia resulting in paresthesias, tetany, hypotension, and decreased cardiac output. On rare occasions the patient may require calcium gluconate, 10 ml of a 10% solution IV. Calcium should never be added directly to the transfusion product because it may cause the blood to clot.
3. **Acidemia and hyperkalemia** may occur. Hyperkalemia is not usually significant unless the patient was hyperkalemic prior to the transfusion (e.g., because of renal failure or muscle injury). Twenty-four hours after massive transfusion, hypokalemia may occur as RBCs become more metabolically active and take up potassium from the plasma.
4. **Bleeding complications** from dilution of platelets and plasma coagulation factors may be seen during massive transfusion. Correction of platelet and coagulation factor deficiencies should be based on clinical findings and laboratory monitoring rather than an empiric formula. Administration of FFP is usually not necessary if the PT and PTT are less than 1.5 times normal.

C. **Complications associated with platelet transfusions**
1. **Alloimmunization.** Fifty to 75% of patients who receive platelets on a regular basis will develop antibodies against platelet antigens. Clinically, this disorder is diagnosed when platelet transfusion produces little increase in the platelet count. Inadequate platelet count response may also be caused by fever, increased platelet destruction (e.g., ITP), splenomegaly, and increased consumption (e.g., DIC). Patients who do not respond to random-donor platelets may benefit from single-donor products. In situations in which multiple transfusions are foreseen (e.g., BMT), HLA typing will allow HLA-matched single-donor platelets to be used.
2. **Posttransfusion purpura** is a rare syndrome associated with thrombocytopenia, purpura, and bleeding that starts 7–10 days after exposure to blood products containing platelets. It is usually seen in previously transfused individuals or multiparous women who have antibodies against platelet antigen PI^{A1}. The process usually resolves within 10–20 days; however, bleeding may prove fatal during this period. Plasmapheresis (up to three treatments) on alternate days is usually effective in raising the platelet count. Intravenous immunoglobulin has been recommended as an alternative to plasmapheresis. Responses to glucocorticoids are rare. Platelet transfusions are ineffective in this syndrome.

III. **Emergency blood transfusions** should be used only in situations in which massive blood loss has resulted in cardiovascular compromise. Volume expansion with normal saline should be attempted initially. Blood typing can be performed in 10 minutes and cross-matching within 30 minutes in emergency situations. If unmatched blood must be used, it should be group O/Rh-negative type that has been previously screened for reactive antibodies. At the first sign of a transfusion reaction the infusion should be stopped.

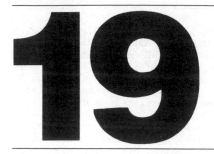

Medical Management of Malignant Disease

Joanne E. Mortimer,
Morey A. Blinder, and
Matthew A. Arquette

Approach to the Cancer Patient

I. **General.** Before initiating chemotherapy or radiation therapy, all patients should have a diagnosis of cancer based on tissue pathology, and if possible, a clinical, biochemical, or radiographic marker of disease should be identified to assess the results of therapy.

A. **Stage and grade of tumor. Stage** is a clinical or pathologic assessment of tumor spread. The major roles of staging are to determine local and regional disease amenable to surgical and radiation therapy, and to define the optimal therapy and prognosis in subsets of patients. The **grade** of a tumor defines its retention of characteristics compared to the cell of origin and is designated as low, moderate, or high as the tissue loses its normal appearance.

B. **Therapy. Induction** is the chemotherapy used to achieve a complete remission. **Consolidation chemotherapy** is administered to patients who initially respond to treatment. **Maintenance therapy** refers to low-dose, outpatient treatment used to prolong remissions; its use has proved effective in a few malignancies. **Adjuvant chemotherapy** is given after complete eradication of a primary malignancy to eliminate any presumed but unmeasurable metastatic disease.

C. **Response to treatment** may be defined by either clinical or pathologic criteria. **A complete response** (or remission) is achieved when all evidence of malignancy is eradicated. **A partial response** is defined as a decrease in tumor mass by more than 50%.

D. **Palliative care and pain therapy.** Pain is present at diagnosis in 5–10% of patients with localized cancer and 60–90% of patients with metastases. Improved oral analgesics, use of indwelling venous access devices, development of home nursing care agencies, and public acceptance of the hospice philosophy now allow patients to receive a large portion of their palliative treatment out of the hospital. Successful treatment of the underlying disease usually provides relief of pain. Painful foci of disease refractory to systemic intervention may be controlled with local radiation therapy, regional nerve block, or an ablative surgical procedure. In many situations, however, analgesics are necessary (see Chap. 1). Nonopioid analgesics should be used initially, followed by opioid analgesics as needed. Medication administered on a prescribed schedule is more effective in maintaining analgesia than that taken intermittently once pain has developed. **Sustained-release morphine,** 30–60 mg PO q8–12h, is particularly efficacious in the management of chronic pain. Occasionally, infusions of morphine, 3–5 mg/hour IV, increased by 2–4 mg/hour as needed, are necessary. When using a morphine drip, the patient must be monitored for respiratory depression, and **naloxone,** 2 ampules IV (0.4 mg/ampule), should be available at the patient's bedside. Under supervision, morphine drips may be used in the home setting. Although tolerance and physical dependency can develop with long-term narcotic administration, drug abuse and psychological dependency seldom occur in the setting of chronic pain from cancer. **These concerns should not compromise the patient's ability to achieve adequate analgesia.**

II. Therapy of selected solid tumors. Recommendations regarding specific chemothcr-apeutic regimens are beyond the scope of this chapter. This section defines guidelines for a treatment plan, but consultation with an oncologist should be obtained prior to drug and dosage selection.

A. Breast cancer

1. **Approach to an undiagnosed lump in the breast.** Approximately 11% of women in the United States will develop breast cancer. A breast lump in a premenopausal woman is less likely to be cancerous than a breast lump in a postmenopausal woman. In a younger woman, a mass should be observed for 1 month to identify any cyclic changes suggesting benign disease. When a mass is found, bilateral mammography should be performed. The accuracy of mammography to diagnose cancer in pre- and postmenopausal women is approximately 90%. Estrogen receptor and progesterone receptor levels should be measured with all newly diagnosed breast cancers.

2. **Surgical options.** Treatment is focused on local control and the risk of systemic spread. Local control with **tylectomy** (lumpectomy and axillary lymph node dissection) is as effective as a modified radical mastectomy. An axillary lymph node dissection should be included because it provides prognostic information and is of therapeutic value.

3. **Adjuvant chemotherapy.** The presence or absence of axillary lymph node metastases is the most important prognostic factor in breast cancer. **Premenopausal women** with axillary lymph node involvement should receive 4–6 cycles of adjuvant chemotherapy. In the absence of axillary lymph node involvement, chemotherapy is often recommended because it has been shown to improve disease-free survival. In **postmenopausal women**, adjuvant therapy is administered according to estrogen receptor status. Tamoxifen increases disease-free survival in both axillary lymph node–negative and –positive patients with estrogen receptor–positive disease. However, improved overall survival has been demonstrated only in lymph node–positive patients. In estrogen receptor–negative postmenopausal women with axillary nodal involvement, chemotherapy may be of benefit (*Cancer* 67:1744, 1991).

4. **Metastatic disease.** Initial treatment is dictated by menopausal status, hormone receptor status, and sites of metastatic disease. Estrogen receptor–negative breast cancer, lymphangitic lung disease, or liver metastasis seldom respond to hormonal manipulation and should be treated with chemotherapy. In other metastatic sites, estrogen receptor–positive disease is treated with hormonal manipulation. Premenopausal women are treated with bilateral oophorectomy or hormonal agents; postmenopausal women are treated with hormonal agents. The various hormonal therapies produce similar response rates, but tamoxifen is most often used as initial treatment because it has few side effects. If the disease responds to hormonal therapy, subsequent progression may respond to further manipulation with other hormonal agents. Chemotherapy should be considered if there is no response to initial hormonal therapy or if there is progression during subsequent hormonal manipulations.

5. **Inflammatory and unresectable cancers.** Inflammatory breast cancer manifests as "peau d'orange" changes or erythema involving more than one-third of the chest wall. Because of the high likelihood of metastases at diagnosis, these patients and patients with inoperable primary breast cancers are initially treated with chemotherapy. Subsequently, surgery and radiation therapy are used for maximal local control.

6. **Radiation therapy** is indicated for patients treated with tylectomy and for some patients with multiple positive axillary lymph nodes. It is also used for palliation of painful or obstructing metastatic lesions.

B. GI malignancies commonly present with vague symptoms and are often advanced at the time of diagnosis.

1. **Esophageal cancers** are either squamous cell (associated with cigarette smoking and alcohol use) or adenocarcinoma (arising in Barrett's esophagus). Surgical resection of the esophagus is recommended when feasible. Local control of unresectable cancers can be achieved with combined chemo-

therapy and radiation therapy. Palliation of obstructive symptoms may be accomplished by radiation therapy, dilatation, prosthetic tube placement, or laser therapy.

2. **Gastric cancer** is usually adenocarcinoma and may be cured with surgery in the rare patient with localized disease. Chemotherapy has been ineffective as adjuvant therapy. Locally advanced but unresectable cancers may benefit from concomitant chemotherapy and radiation therapy. Chemotherapy may offer palliation for metastatic disease.

3. **Colon and rectal adenocarcinomas** are primarily treated by surgical resection. Data have shown prolonged survival in patients with colon cancer and regional lymph node involvement who receive adjuvant 5-fluorouracil (FU) and levamisole for 12 months (*N Engl J Med* 322:352, 1990). Rectal cancer arising below the peritoneal reflection commonly recurs locally after surgery alone; postoperative radiation therapy and FU are recommended. FU is the mainstay of treatment for metastatic colon or rectal cancer, with a response rate of 20%. The addition of leucovorin results in higher response rates but does not clearly prolong survival compared to FU alone. In all patients undergoing surgical resection of colon or rectal cancer, a preoperative carcinoembryonic antigen level should be measured. A persistently elevated or increasing level may indicate residual or recurrent tumor.

4. **Anal cancer.** Chemotherapy with concurrent radiation therapy appears to result in a higher cure rate than surgical resection and usually preserves the anal sphincter and fecal continence (*Am J Med* 78:211, 1985). Surgical resection should be used only as salvage therapy.

C. **Genitourinary malignancies**

1. **Bladder cancer** in the United States is usually a transitional cell carcinoma. A variety of chemical carcinogens, including those in cigarette smoke, have been implicated. Unifocal tumors confined to the mucosa should be managed with cystoscopy and transurethral resection or fulguration, repeated at approximately 3-month intervals; multifocal mucosal disease is treated with intravesicular bacille Calmette-Guérin (BCG), thiotepa, or mitomycin C. Locally invasive cancers should be resected. Adjuvant chemotherapy improves survival when regional lymph node involvement is confirmed in the cystectomy specimen. In metastatic or recurrent disease, the highest response rates are seen with cisplatin-containing regimens.

2. **Prostate cancer.** Local control of the primary lesion may be achieved with either prostatectomy or radiation therapy; the risk of impotence may be lower with radiation therapy. Although not proved as a routine screening test, prostate-specific antigen is useful as a marker for recurrence, bulk of disease, and response to therapy. In patients with metastatic disease, bilateral orchiectomy, luteinizing hormone–releasing hormone (LHRH) analogs, or diethylstilbestrol (DES) relieve bone pain in approximately 85% of cases for a median of 18–24 months. Disease that has relapsed after hormonal therapy seldom responds to further hormonal therapy. The role of chemotherapy is not established. Anemia and bone pain dominate the advanced phases of this disease and are best relieved with transfusions and palliative radiation therapy.

3. **Renal cell cancer** is treated by surgical resection, which may be curative if disease is localized; there is no effective adjuvant therapy. In metastatic disease, progestational agents (e.g., medroxyprogesterone) produce tumor regression in less than 15% of patients. Chemotherapy, alpha-interferon, and interleukin-2 have reported response rates of 15–30%.

4. **Cancer of the testis** is one of the most curable malignancies when treated with chemotherapy. The patient suspected of having cancer of the testis should only have tissue obtained through an inguinal orchiectomy because a transscrotal incision facilitates tumor spread to the inguinal lymph nodes. The initial evaluation should include a serum alpha-fetoprotein (AFP) and beta subunit of human chorionic gonadotropin (beta-HCG), a CT scan of the abdomen and pelvis, and possibly a lymphangiogram. Most patients with seminoma should be treated with radiation therapy. In nonseminomatous germ cell cancer, a

retroperitoneal lymph node dissection should be performed for staging, except
in the instance of bulky abdominal disease or pulmonary metastasis. If microscopic disease is identified at surgery, two alternatives are acceptable: two
cycles of postoperative chemotherapy or observation until relapse occurs followed by institution of chemotherapy. With gross metastatic disease, cisplatin-
based chemotherapy is curative in most germ cell cancers. If tumor markers
normalize after chemotherapy but a radiographic mass persists, exploratory
surgery should be performed. The lesion will prove to be residual cancer in
approximately one-third of the patients. Patients with residual cancer should
receive additional chemotherapy (*J Clin Oncol* 8:1777, 1990).

D. Gynecologic malignancies
  1. **Cervical cancer.** The recognized risk factors are multiparity, multiple sexual
     partners, and human papillomavirus. Carcinoma in situ and superficial
     disease may be treated by endocervical cone biopsy. Microinvasive disease is
     treated with an abdominal hysterectomy. Advanced local disease (invasion of
     the cervix or local extension) is treated with radiation therapy and surgery.
     Inoperable cancer may be controlled with radiation therapy. Metastatic
     disease is treated with cisplatin-based chemotherapy.
  2. **Ovarian cancer** is primarily a disease of postmenopausal women. Because
     symptoms are uncommon with localized disease, most patients present with
     advanced local disease, malignant ascites, or peritoneal metastases. Surgical
     staging and treatment include an abdominal hysterectomy, bilateral
     oophorectomy, lymph node sampling, omentectomy, peritoneal cytology, and
     removal of all gross tumor. If the tumor is localized to the ovary, the surgery
     may be curative and further treatment is not routinely recommended.
     However, if microscopic foci of cancer are identified, chemotherapy is admin-
     istered postoperatively. The serum marker **CA-125,** though not specific, is
     elevated in more than 80% of women with epithelial ovarian cancer and is a
     sensitive indicator of response. After a response is achieved, a "second-look
     laparotomy" is performed to restage and remove residual tumor. Approxi-
     mately one-third of the patients who are in pathologic complete remission
     after a second-look laparotomy are cured. Those patients who have residual
     cancer should receive additional chemotherapy.
E. Head and neck cancer is usually a squamous cell cancer. It may arise in a variety
   of sites, and each has a different natural history. Early lesions may be cured with
   surgery, radiation therapy, or both. Despite aggressive surgical and radiation
   therapy, approximately 65% of patients with head and neck cancer have uncontrolled local disease. Chemotherapy is used for treatment of disseminated disease
   and produces high response rates with a modest improvement in survival.
F. Lung cancer is the most common cause of cancer death in the United States.
   Because of its relationship to cigarette smoking, it is also the most preventable.
   Treatment is based on the histology and stage of the disease. Small-cell lung
   cancer is defined as either limited (confined to one hemithorax and ipsilateral
   regional lymph nodes) or extensive. Non–small-cell lung cancer includes several
   histologic subtypes that all behave in a similar fashion. Whenever possible,
   surgical resection should be attempted for non–small-cell lung cancer because it
   affords the best chance of cure.
  1. **Small-cell lung cancer** is responsible for many paraneoplastic syndromes
     (see Complications of Cancer, sec. II). In limited disease, combination chemo-
     therapy results in an 85–90% response rate, a median survival of 12–18
     months, and a cure in 5–15% of patients. In extensive disease, the median
     survival is 8–9 months, but cures are rare. For patients who achieve a
     complete remission with chemotherapy, **prophylactic whole-brain radiation
     therapy** may be administered to decrease the risk of CNS relapse. Radiation
     therapy to the chest as consolidation therapy may improve survival in limited
     disease but is not recommended in extensive disease.
  2. **Non–small-cell lung cancer** survival rates after resection are not improved
     with adjuvant chemotherapy or radiation therapy. Radiation therapy is the
     conventional treatment for unresectable disease that is confined to the lung

and regional lymph nodes. The use of chemotherapy before or concurrent with radiation may modestly improve survival in patients with a good performance status. In patients with metastatic disease, cisplatin-based combination chemotherapy may modestly improve survival.

G. **Malignant melanoma** should be considered in any changing or enlarging nevus, and suspicious lesions should be removed by excisional biopsy. Subsequently, a wide local excision is performed to remove possible vertical and radial spread of tumor. The depth of invasion is inversely related to the prognosis. Neither adjuvant radiation therapy nor chemotherapy improves the results of surgery alone. Systemic disease may respond to dacarbazine (DTIC), alpha-interferon, or interleukin-2 in 10–30% of patients.

H. **Sarcomas** are tumors that arise from mesenchymal tissue and occur most commonly in soft tissue or bone. Initial evaluation should include a CT scan of the chest, since hematogenous spread to the lungs is common.

1. **The prognosis for soft-tissue sarcoma** is primarily determined by tumor grade and not by the cell of origin. Surgical resection should be performed when feasible and may be curative. In low-grade tumors, local and regional recurrence is most common, and adjuvant radiation therapy may be of benefit. High-grade tumors often recur systemically, but no advantage to the routine use of adjuvant chemotherapy has been consistently demonstrated. In metastatic disease, doxorubicin, ifosfamide, and DTIC produce responses in 40–55% of patients.

2. **Osteogenic sarcomas** are treated with surgical resection followed by adjuvant chemotherapy for 1 year. Treatment of isolated pulmonary metastasis by surgical resection is associated with long-term survival.

3. **Kaposi's sarcoma** in an immunocompetent patient is generally a low-grade lesion of the lower extremities that is readily treated with local radiation therapy or vinblastine. When Kaposi's sarcoma complicates organ transplantation or AIDS, it is more aggressive and may arise in visceral sites. Cutaneous disease may be observed or treated with either alpha-interferon or a low-dose vinca alkaloid. Advanced cutaneous or visceral disease, especially pulmonary disease, should be treated with a vinca alkaloid, bleomycin, or etoposide (*Am J Med* 87:57, 1989).

I. **Cancer with an unknown primary site.** Approximately 5% of cancer patients present with symptoms of metastatic disease, but no primary tumor site is identifiable on physical examination, routine laboratory studies, and chest x-ray. A search for the primary lesion should be directed by the histopathologic cell type and the site of the metastasis. Immunohistochemical stains may identify specific tissue antigens that help to define the origin of the tumor and guide subsequent therapy. **In general, systemic therapy is only helpful if the primary site is identified;** chemotherapeutic regimens do not improve survival when compared to palliative therapy. Two potentially curative circumstances are described below.

1. **Cervical adenopathy** suggests cancer of the lung, breast, head and neck, or lymphoma. In this case, initial evaluation usually includes panendoscopy (nasendoscopy, laryngopharyngoscopy, bronchoscopy, and esophagoscopy) and biopsy of any suspicious lesion prior to excision of the lymph node. If squamous cell carcinoma is identified, the patient is presumed to have primary head and neck cancer, and radiation therapy may be curative.

2. **Midline mass in the mediastinum or retroperitoneum.** In both sexes, a midline mass in the mediastinum or retroperitoneum may be an extragonadal germ cell cancer. Elevations in AFP or beta-HCG further suggest this diagnosis. This neoplasm is potentially curable (see sec. **II.C.4**).

III. **Therapy of hematologic tumors**

A. **Lymphoma** is usually diagnosed by biopsy of an enlarged lymph node.

1. **Staging** of Hodgkin's disease and non-Hodgkin's lymphoma.

a. **Stage I**—disease localized to a single lymph node or group.

b. **Stage II**—more than one lymph node group involved but confined to one side of the diaphragm.

    c. Stage III—disease in the lymph nodes or the spleen and occurring on both sides of the diaphragm.

    d. Stage IV—liver or bone marrow involvement.

    e. B symptoms include fever above 38.5°C, night sweats requiring a change in clothes, or a 10% weight loss over 6 months. These symptoms suggest bulky disease and a worse prognosis.

  2. Hodgkin's disease usually presents with cervical adenopathy and spreads in a predictable manner along lymph node groups. Treatment is based on the presenting stage of the disease; the cell type is relatively unimportant in the natural history and prognosis. Initial evaluation includes a CT scan of the abdomen and pelvis, bilateral bone marrow biopsies, and lymphangiogram to determine the clinical stage of the disease. Exploratory laparotomy with splenectomy and liver biopsy is performed if the findings will change the disease stage and treatment. **Stage IA and IIA** disease are treated with radiation therapy unless a mediastinal mass exceeding one-third of the chest width is present, in which case chemotherapy is included. **Stage IIIA** disease may be treated by either radiation therapy or chemotherapy, whereas all **stage IV** patients should receive combination chemotherapy. When **B symptoms** are present, chemotherapy is recommended regardless of the stage.

  3. Non-Hodgkin's lymphoma is classified as low-, intermediate-, or high-grade based on the histologic type. Staging evaluation is the same as for Hodgkin's disease, but non-Hodgkin's lymphoma has a less predictable pattern of spread. Advanced stage disease (stage III or IV) is usually apparent, and exploratory laparotomy and lymphangiogram are rarely necessary.

    a. Low-grade lymphoma often involves the bone marrow at diagnosis, but the disease has an indolent course. Since this tumor is rarely eradicated, immediate treatment has no impact on survival. Radiation therapy or an alkylating agent (e.g., cyclophosphamide) are used to ameliorate symptoms. Radiation therapy may produce a long-term complete remission in stage I or II disease.

    b. Intermediate-grade lymphoma has a more aggressive course, seldom involves the bone marrow at diagnosis, and may be cured with chemotherapy. Complete response rates exceed 80%. Bulky disease, defined by a tumor mass greater than 10 cm in diameter or a serum lactate dehydrogenase above 500 IU/liter, is less likely to be cured.

    c. High-grade lymphoma (Burkitt's, lymphoblastic, and immunoblastic lymphomas) includes the most aggressive subtypes and has a high frequency of CNS and bone marrow involvement. CSF cytology should be included as part of the initial evaluation. Combination chemotherapy is the mainstay of treatment and should include CNS prophylaxis if the CSF is cytologically free of tumor. If tumor cells are seen in the CSF, additional therapy may be indicated (see Complications of Cancer, sec. **I.B**). Prophylaxis to prevent **tumor lysis syndrome** (see Complications of Treatment, sec. **I.F**) should be performed before induction chemotherapy.

B. Leukemia presents with cytopenias, lymphadenopathy, splenomegaly, or leukostasis. The peripheral blood smear usually distinguishes between acute and chronic leukemia, but a bone marrow aspirate should be performed to confirm the diagnosis and further classify the disease by immunophenotype and cytogenetics.

  1. Acute nonlymphocytic leukemia (ANL) constitutes approximately 80% of acute leukemia in adults. Cytosine arabinoside (ara-C) is the cornerstone of induction therapy and is usually administered with daunorubicin or idarubicin to induce remission. After complete remission, at least one additional cycle of chemotherapy is given as consolidation. Alternatively, allogeneic bone marrow transplantation (BMT) may be used for consolidation.

  2. Acute lymphocytic leukemia (ALL) in adults is considerably more difficult to cure than ALL in children. CNS prophylaxis is necessary. After achieving a complete remission, consolidation chemotherapy is followed by maintenance chemotherapy for at least 1 year.

3. **Chronic lymphocytic leukemia (CLL)** usually presents with lymphocytosis, but lymphadenopathy, splenomegaly, anemia, and thrombocytopenia may occur during the course of the disease. Treatment is similar to that for **low-grade lymphoma** (see sec. **III.A.3.a**) and should be given for control of symptoms. Lymphocytosis alone is not an indication for therapy. Immune hemolytic anemia or immune thrombocytopenia may develop as a complication of CLL and is treated with glucocorticoids (e.g., prednisone, 1 mg/kg PO qd). CLL does not evolve into acute leukemia, but transformation to an intermediate- or high-grade lymphoma may occur (Richter's syndrome).

4. **Chronic myelogenous leukemia (CML)** is diagnosed when the **Philadelphia chromosome** t(9;22) is identified. Leukocytosis and thrombocytosis may be controlled with hydroxyurea for several years before transformation into a **blast crisis** occurs that mimics acute leukemia. Myeloblast transformation responds poorly to therapy, but in lymphoblastic crisis, treatment with vincristine and prednisone is warranted. In either case, the blast phase of CML is seldom cured with chemotherapy. Allogeneic BMT for CML in the chronic phase has been associated with prolonged remissions.

5. **Hairy-cell leukemia** should be considered for patients with splenomegaly and pancytopenia. Use of 2-chlorodeoxyadenosine (Cladribine) produces a high rate of long-term remission in this disease.

C. **Multiple myeloma** is a malignant plasma cell disorder that may present with hypercalcemia, bone pain, or acute renal failure. The initial evaluation should include a radiographic bone survey, bone marrow aspirate, serum and urine protein electrophoresis, beta-2 microglobulin, sedimentation rate, and quantitative immunoglobulins. Since the bone lesions are predominantly osteolytic, radionuclide bone scans are rarely helpful. Treatment generally includes a combination of an oral alkylating agent, vincristine, and a glucocorticoid. Local radiation therapy should be used to relieve painful bone lesions.

Complications of Cancer

I. **Complications related to tumor mass**

A. **Brain metastasis.** Patients with parenchymal brain metastasis may present with headache, mental status changes, weakness, or focal neurologic deficits. Papilledema is observed in only 25% of patients. In patients with malignancy, a CT scan of the head showing one or more round, contrast-enhancing lesions surrounded by edema is usually sufficient for the diagnosis. If cancer has not been diagnosed previously, tissue should be obtained from the brain lesion or a more accessible site before initiating radiation therapy. Therapy with dexamethasone, 10 mg IV or PO, is initiated to decrease cerebral edema and should be continued at a dosage of 4–6 mg PO q6h throughout the course of radiation therapy, or longer if symptoms related to edema persist. Subsequent therapy depends on the number and location of the brain lesions as well as the prognosis of the underlying cancer. Patients with a chemotherapy-responsive neoplasm and a solitary, accessible lesion should be considered for surgical resection. All patients who have not received prior radiation therapy should receive whole-brain radiation therapy.

B. **Meningeal carcinomatosis** should be suspected in a cancer patient with headache or cranial neuropathies. This pattern of spread is most often seen with lung or breast cancer, melanoma, or lymphoma; the diagnosis is confirmed by cytology of the CSF. In general, a CT scan of the head is performed to rule out parenchymal metastases or hydrocephalus prior to performing a lumbar puncture. Local radiation therapy or intrathecal (IT) chemotherapy may provide temporary relief of symptoms (see Chemotherapy, sec. **II.C**). Meningeal lymphoma may respond to IV ara-C.

C. **Spinal cord compression** is most commonly caused by hematogenous spread of cancer to the vertebral bodies followed by expansion into the spinal canal or ischemia of the spinal cord. The most common malignancies that cause spinal cord compression are breast, lung, and prostate cancer, but the diagnosis should be considered in any patient with cancer who complains of back pain. Evaluation and therapy are discussed in Chap. 25.

D. Superior vena cava (SVC) obstruction is most commonly caused by cancers such as lymphoma or lung cancer that arise in or spread to the mediastinum. The compressed SVC leads to swelling of the face or trunk, chest pain, cough, or shortness of breath. Dilated superficial veins of the chest, neck, or sublingual area suggest an engorged collateral circulation. The presence of a mass determined by chest radiograph or CT scan usually confirms the diagnosis. Collateral veins develop the cerebral circulation is not significantly affected but a mediastinal mass may compromise the airway. If the histologic origin of the obstruction is unknown, tissue may be obtained for diagnosis via bronchoscopy or mediastinoscopy. Therapy is directed at the underlying disease. Chemotherapy should be administered through a vein that is not obstructed by the lesion. Neoplasms that are not responsive to chemotherapy are treated with radiation therapy (*J Clin Oncol* 2:961, 1984).

E. Malignant effusions
  1. **Malignant pericardial effusion** commonly results from cancer of the breast or lung. In some patients, the initial presentation is acute cardiovascular collapse from **cardiac tamponade**, requiring emergency pericardiocentesis. After cardiovascular stabilization, some patients may improve with treatment if the tumor is chemotherapy-sensitive. When the pericardial effusion is a complication of uncontrolled disease, palliation may be achieved by pericardiocentesis with sclerosis; the effusion should be completely drained followed by instillation of 30–60 mg of bleomycin through the drainage catheter, which is subsequently clamped for 10 minutes and then withdrawn (*Int J Cardiol* 16:155, 1987). Subxiphoid pericardotomy may be performed in patients whose effusions fail to respond to other treatment (*JAMA* 257:1088, 1987).
  2. **Malignant pleural effusion** develops as a result of pleural invasion by tumor or obstruction of lymphatic drainage. When systemic control is not feasible and reaccumulation of fluid occurs rapidly after drainage, removal of the fluid followed by instillation of a sclerosing agent into the pleural space is recommended. Resistant effusions may be controlled with pleurectomy.
  3. **Malignant ascites** is most commonly caused by peritoneal carcinomatosis and is best controlled by systemic chemotherapy. Therapeutic paracenteses can provide symptomatic relief. Intraperitoneal instillation of chemotherapy has been used but is not routinely recommended.

II. Paraneoplastic syndromes are complications of malignancy that are not directly caused by a tumor mass effect and are presumed to be mediated by either secreted tumor products or the development of autoantibodies. Paraneoplastic syndromes can affect virtually every organ system, and in most cases, successful treatment of the underlying malignancy will eliminate these effects.

A. Metabolic complications
  1. **Hypercalcemia** is the most common metabolic complication in malignancy and can cause mental status changes, GI discomfort, and constipation. Acute and chronic management of hypercalcemia is discussed in Chap. 23.
  2. **Syndrome of inappropriate antidiuretic hormone (SIADH)** should be considered in a euvolemic cancer patient with unexplained hyponatremia (see Chap. 3). Although a variety of neoplasms have been described in association with SIADH, small-cell lung cancer is most often responsible. If chemotherapy is ineffective, radiation therapy may decrease the tumor mass and relieve symptoms (see Chap. 3 for management).
  3. **Cancer cachexia** refers to the clinical syndrome of anorexia, distortion of taste perception, and loss of muscle mass. The asthenic appearance of patients is more often related to tumor type than to tumor burden. Megestrol acetate, 160 mg PO qd, has been used as an appetite stimulant and results in weight gain in some patients (*Semin Oncol* 14:37, 1986).

B. Neuromuscular complications

1. **Polymyositis (PM) and dermatomyositis (DM).** DM, more often than PM, has been associated with a variety of malignancies, including non–small-cell lung, colon, ovarian, and prostate cancer. In some patients, successful treatment of the underlying malignancy has resulted in resolution of the symptoms. An exhaustive search for a malignancy is not recommended because a primary malignancy will be found in less than 20% of patients (*N Engl J Med* 326:363, 1992).

2. **Lambert-Eaton myasthenic syndrome** is characterized by proximal muscle weakness, decreased or absent deep tendon reflexes, and autonomic dysfunction. Electromyography using high-frequency nerve stimulation may show posttetanic potentiation. Small-cell lung cancer is most often associated with this syndrome, and effective chemotherapy may result in improvement. If cancer therapy is ineffective, diaminopyridine, 10–25 mg PO qid, may be of benefit. Worsening symptoms have been reported with the use of calcium channel antagonists; these agents are contraindicated in this syndrome (*N Engl J Med* 321:1567, 1989).

C. Hematologic complications include anemia, neutropenia, and thrombocytopenia and may be associated with the malignancy or its treatment (see Complications of Treatment, sec. I.B).

1. **Erythrocytosis** is a rare complication of hepatoma, renal cell cancer, and benign tumors of the kidney, uterus, and cerebellum. Debulking the tumor with surgery or radiation therapy generally results in resolution of the erythrocytosis. Occasionally, therapeutic phlebotomy is indicated.

2. **Granulocytosis (leukemoid reaction)**, in the absence of infection, occurs in cancer arising in the stomach, lung, pancreas, brain, and lymphoma. Because the neutrophils are mature and seldom exceed $100,000/mm^3$, complications are rare and intervention is unnecessary.

3. **Thrombocytosis** in patients with cancer may be caused by splenectomy, iron deficiency, acute hemorrhage, or inflammation; treatment is not usually necessary. **Thrombocytopenia** may occur following chemotherapy, with splenomegaly, with malignant infiltration of the bone marrow, or by an immune mechanism (see Chap. 17).

4. **Thromboembolic complications.** Mucin-secreting adenocarcinomas of the GI tract and lung cancer have been associated with a "hypercoagulable state" resulting in recurrent venous and arterial thromboembolism. Nonbacterial thrombotic (marantic) endocarditis, usually involving the mitral valve, may also occur. Heparin anticoagulation should be instituted as well as treatment of the underlying cancer. Heparin, IV or SC, to maintain the partial thromboplastin time at 1.5–2.0 times normal, appears to be more effective than warfarin in the prevention of subsequent thrombi (*Blood* 62:14, 1983). In many patients, biochemical evidence of disseminated intravascular coagulation coexists with thromboemboli (see Chap. 17).

D. Glomerular injury resulting in renal failure has been observed as a paraneoplastic syndrome. Minimal change disease is often associated with lymphoma, especially Hodgkin's disease; membranous glomerulonephritis is more often seen with solid tumors. The process may be reversed with treatment of the underlying cancer.

E. Clubbing of the fingers and **hypertrophic osteoarthropathy** (polyarthritis and periostitis of long bones) are most often observed in non–small-cell lung cancer but are also seen with lesions metastatic to the mediastinum. Some improvement in the osteoarthropathy may be achieved with nonsteroidal antiinflammatory drugs (NSAIDs), but definitive therapy requires treatment of the underlying malignancy.

F. Fever may accompany lymphoma, renal cell cancer, and hepatic metastasis. Once an infectious etiology for the fever has been excluded, NSAIDs (e.g., ibuprofen, 400 mg PO qid, or indomethacin, 25–50 mg PO tid) may provide symptomatic relief.

G. Bone metastases are common and may be identified on radiographs or radionuclide bone scans. Radiation therapy is useful for palliation of painful lesions and to prevent fracture in weight-bearing bones.

Chemotherapy

I. **Administration of chemotherapeutic drugs.** The dosage of chemotherapy is usually based on body surface area (Table 19-1); for some agents, dosage is determined by body weight and should be adjusted when changes in body weight occur. One to two weeks following the first dose of chemotherapy, a CBC should be obtained to determine the degree of myelosuppression. Dosage usually must be adjusted for the following conditions: (1) neutropenia, (2) thrombocytopenia, (3) stomatitis, (4) diarrhea, or (5) limited metabolic capacity for the drug. **The advice of an oncologist and precise adherence to a treatment plan is mandatory because of the low therapeutic index of chemotherapeutic agents.**

II. **Route of administration**

A. **Oral drug administration** may be accompanied by nausea and vomiting and may require antiemetic therapy. For some agents, oral absorption is erratic and parenteral administration is preferred.

B. **IV drug administration** should be performed by experienced personnel. Care should be taken to ensure free flow of fluid to the vein, and adequate blood return should be verified before instillation of chemotherapy. Infusions should be through a large-caliber, upper extremity vein. When possible, veins of the antecubital fossa, wrist, dorsum of the hand, and arm ipsilateral to an axillary lymph node dissection should be avoided. In patients with poor peripheral venous access or those requiring many doses of chemotherapy, **indwelling venous catheter devices** should be considered (*JAMA* 253:1590, 1985).

C. **Intrathecal (IT) chemotherapy** is administered for the treatment of meningeal carcinomatosis or as CNS prophylaxis. Side effects include acute arachnoiditis, subacute motor dysfunction, and progressive neurologic deterioration (leukoencephalopathy). Decreased cognitive function has been found in children. Impaired cognitive function and leukoencephalopathy occur more often when IT chemotherapy is combined with whole-brain radiation. **Methotrexate,** 10–12 mg, is diluted in 5 ml of preservative-free nonbacteriostatic isotonic solution. Prior to administration, 5–10 ml of CSF should be allowed to drain; methotrexate is then injected into the spinal canal over 5–10 minutes. To decrease the risk of arachnoiditis, patients should remain in a supine position for 15 minutes after the infusion is completed. To avoid systemic side effects from methotrexate, leucovorin, 5–10 mg PO q6h, should be administered for 8 doses beginning 12–24 hours after IT treatment. **Cytosine arabinoside,** 50–100 mg in 5–10 ml of diluent, may be administered in a similar manner.

D. **Intracavitary instillation** of chemotherapy may be useful in some circumstances. Thiotepa, 30–60 mg, is commonly instilled in the bladder for the treatment of bladder carcinoma. Doxorubicin and cisplatin have been given through an implanted peritoneal catheter for the treatment of peritoneal metastasis.

E. **Intraarterial chemotherapy** is advocated as a method of achieving high drug concentrations at specific tumor sites. Although it is of theoretic advantage, there are no absolute indications for chemotherapy administered by this route.

III. **Chemotherapeutic agents.** A summary of commonly used chemotherapeutic agents, dosages, and toxicities is given in Table 19-1. Class-specific or unique side effects are described below.

A. **Antimetabolites** exert antitumor activity by acting as pseudosubstrates for essential enzymatic reactions. Their greatest toxicity occurs in tissues that are actively replicating (e.g., GI mucosa, hematopoietic cells).

1. **Ara-C** is an analog of deoxycytidine that is most useful in hematologic neoplasms. In standard doses, myelosuppression and GI toxicity are dose-limiting. In high doses, conjunctivitis is common, and prophylaxis with dexamethasone eyedrops, 2 drops OU tid, should be administered. Cerebellar

Table 19-1. Doses and common toxicities of antineoplastic agents

	Dose range/schedule	N&V	Mucositis	Diarrhea	Days to nadir	Skin	Lung	Neurologic	Dose modification for
Antimetabolites									
Cytosine arabinoside	20 mg/m² IV infusion qd × 14–21 days	0	0		10–14 +++	0	+	0	
	100–200 mg/m² IV qd × 5–7 days	++	+	++	10–14 +++	Alopecia	0	0	
	3–6 g/m² IV qd × 3–6 days	+++	+	++	10–14 +++	Alopecia	0	Cerebellar	
Fludarabine	15–30 mg/m² qd × 5 days	+	+	+	7–14 +++	0	0	0	
5-Fluorouracil	350–450 mg/m² IV × 5 days	0	0	++	7–14 +++	Phlebitis	0	Cerebellar	
	200–1,000 mg/m² infusion × 5 days	0	+	+	7–14 +	Hand-foot syn	+	0	
	20 mg/m² IV qd × 28–56 days with leucovorin	0	+++	+++	7–14 ++	Hand-foot syn	0	Cerebellar	
Methotrexate	10–60 mg/m² IV q1–3wk	+	+++	+++	7–14 +	Dermatitis	+	0	Effusions, renal failure
with leucovorin	>1.5 g IV qd × 1 wk	+++	++	++	None	Dermatitis	0	0	Effusions, renal failure
2-Deoxycoformycin	4 mg/m² IV q2wk	+	++	0	7–14 +++	Erythema	0	Lethargy, coma	Renal failure
6-Mercaptopurine	75–100 mg/m² PO qd	+	+	0	7 +	Rash	0	0	Allopurinol, renal, hepatic
Thioguanine	100 mg/m² PO qd × 1–4 days	+	+	0	7–14 ++	0	0	0	Renal
2-Chlorodeoxyadenosine	0.09 mg/kg/d × 7 days	+	0	0	10–30 ++	0	0	0	
Alkylating agents									
Busulfan	2–4 mg/m² PO qd × 4 days	0	0	0	14–28 ++	Hyperpigmentation	+	0	
Chlorambucil	6–14 mg/m² PO qd × 4 days	0	0	0	10–14 ++	0	0	0	
Cyclophosphamide	60–150 mg/m² PO qd × 14 days	+	+	0	10–12 ++	0	0	0	Barbiturates
	500–1,500 mg/m² IV q21d	+++	0	0	7–14 ++	Alopecia	0	0	
	120–200 mg/kg IV for BMT	+++	+++	0	7–14 +++	Alopecia	+	0	
DTIC	300–1,500 mg/m² IV q21–28d	+++	0	+++	None	Alopecia	+	0	
Ifosfamide	800–1,500 mg/m² IV × 4 days q21–28d	+++	0	0	7–10 +++	Alopecia	0	Encephalopathy	
Mechlorethamine	8 mg/m² q 28d	+++	+	+	7–14 ++	Alopecia, rash	0	0	
Melphalan	4–8 mg/m² PO qd × 4 days	0	0	0	10–14 ++	0	0	0	

	Dose	N&V			Nadir (days)	Skin			Organ toxicity
Nitrosoureas									
Carmustine (BCNU)	60–100 mg/m² IV qd × 3 days	+++	0	0	28–35 ++	0	+	0	
Lomustine (CCNU)	100–300 mg/m² PO × 1 day	+	0	0	21–42 ++	0	0	0	
Streptozocin	500–1,500 mg/m² IV qd × 5 days	+++	0	0	None	0	0	0	Renal
Thiotepa	Up to 1.25 g/m² IV with BMT	++	+	+++	7–14 +++	Alopecia, rash	0	0	
Tumor antimicrobials									
Bleomycin	10–20 mg/m² SC × qwk	0	0	0	None	Erythema	+	0	Renal
Dactinomycin	0.4–1.0 mg/m² IV qwk	++	+	0	14–21 ++	Alopecia, rash	0	0	
Daunorubicin	45–60 mg/m² IV qd × 3 days	++	+	+	7–14 +++	Alopecia, vesicant	0	0	Renal, hepatic
Doxorubicin	10–60 mg/m² IV q7–28d	++	+	+	7–14 +++	Alopecia, vesicant	0	0	Renal, hepatic
Idarubicin	10–15 mg/m² IV qd × 3 days	++	+	+	7–14 +++	Alopecia, vesicant	0	0	Renal, hepatic
Mitomycin C	10–15 mg/m² IV q4–6wk	+	+	0	21–28 ++	Vesicant	+	0	Renal, hepatic
Mitoxantrone	10–30 mg/m² IV q21–28d	+	+	+	7–14 ++	Alopecia, vesicant	0	0	
Plant alkaloids									
Etoposide	50–200 mg/m² PO/IV qd × 5 days	0	0	0	10–14 ++	Alopecia, vesicant	0	0	
Vinblastine	5–10 mg/m² IV q1–4wk	+	−	0	4–10 ++	Alopecia, vesicant	0	++ Neuropathy	Hepatic
Vincristine	1–2 mg IV q1–4wk	0	0	0	None	Vesicant	0	++ Neuropathy	Hepatic
Taxol	135–250 mg/m² q21d	+	0	0	10–14 ++	Alopecia	0	Neuropathy	Hepatic
Other agents									
Carboplatin	200–360 mg/m² IV q21–28d	++	0	0	14–28 ++	0	0	0	Renal
Cisplatin	20–120 mg/m² IV × 1–5 days	+++	0	0	None	0	+	0	Renal
Hydroxyurea	500–2,000 mg PO qd	0	0	0	7–10 ++	Skin atrophy	0	0	
L-Asparaginase	1,000–10,000 IU SC qd × 3 days	0	0	0	None	0	0	Encephalopathy	
Procarbazine	100–200 mg/m² PO qd × 7–14 days	+	0	0	7–10 ++	Rash	0	Encephalopathy	

0 = none; + = mild; ++ = moderate; +++ = severe; BMT = bone marrow transplant; N&V = nausea and vomiting.

ataxia, pancreatitis, and hepatitis may also develop. If cerebellar dysfunction occurs during treatment, the ara-C must be discontinued.

2. **5-Fluorouracil (FU)** is a pyrimidine analog that is administered as an injection or as a continuous infusion. When administered as a bolus injection, myelosuppression is dose-limiting; with a 4- to 5-day infusion, stomatitis and diarrhea are dose-limiting. Cerebellar ataxia has been reported with both schedules and requires discontinuation of the drug. Chest pain ascribed to coronary artery vasospasm may occur with infusions and, if suspected, should be treated with a calcium channel antagonist (e.g., nifedipine) or by discontinuing the chemotherapy (*Cancer* 61:36, 1988). FU may be administered over 6–8 weeks and is limited by the development of a palmar-plantar dermatologic toxicity (hand-foot syndrome). Leucovorin may be coadministered with FU to potentiate cytotoxicity; diarrhea is dose-limiting (*J Clin Oncol* 7:1419, 1989).

3. **Methotrexate** is an inhibitor of dihydrofolate reductase and has numerous toxicities. Mucositis is dose-limiting.

   a. **Prolonged reabsorption.** Methotrexate accumulates in effusions and slowly diffuses into the circulation, producing substantial toxicity. Patients with effusions requiring methotrexate should either have the fluid drained before receiving this drug or have the dosage drastically reduced.

   b. **Interstitial pneumonitis,** unrelated to cumulative dose and associated with a peripheral eosinophilia, may occur. It should be treated with glucocorticoids (e.g., prednisone, 1 mg/kg PO qd or equivalent) and precludes additional use of methotrexate.

   c. **Hepatitis** may occur with long-term oral administration but may also occur after a single high dose.

   d. **High-dose methotrexate** may be associated with crystalline nephropathy and renal failure. Urine alkalinization with sodium bicarbonate should be maintained to minimize this risk. Leucovorin is used to "rescue" normal tissue after high-dose methotrexate. The **leucovorin dose** depends on the amount of methotrexate used, but the usual dosage is 5–25 mg IV or PO q6h for 8–12 doses, or until the serum methotrexate concentration is less than 50 nM.

4. **6-Mercaptopurine (6-MP)** is a purine analog that is partially metabolized by xanthine oxidase. To avoid increased toxicity, patients taking allopurinol should receive a 25% dose of 6-MP. Hepatic cholestasis has been observed.

5. **Fludarabine** is an adenosine monophosphate analog that produces myelosuppression (*J Clin Oncol* 9:175, 1991).

6. **2-Chlorodeoxyadenosine** (Cladribine) is a purine substrate analog that is resistant to degradation by adenosine deaminase. Myelosuppression is predictable (*Lancet* 340:952, 1994).

B. **Alkylating agents** are useful in a wide variety of malignancies. These drugs cause DNA cross-linking and strand breaks. Most alkylating agents are cytotoxic to resting and dividing cells. Patients should be counseled that irreversible sterility may develop after treatment with alkylating agents. Chlorambucil, cyclophosphamide, melphalan, and mechlorethamine have been implicated in the development of ANL and myelodysplasia 3–10 years after treatment.

1. **Busulfan (Myleran)** can cause interstitial pneumonitis, gynecomastia, and a reversible syndrome resembling Addison's disease may develop with long-term daily oral administration.

2. **Chlorambucil (Leukeran)** is a well-tolerated orally administered drug. Myelosuppression is dose-limiting and usually readily reversible.

3. **Cyclophosphamide (Cytoxan)** may cause hemorrhagic cystitis (see Complications of Treatment, sec. **I.E**). Adequate hydration to maintain urine output should be achieved while administering the drug. Oral cyclophosphamide should be given early in the day to ensure adequate hydration. High-dose cyclophosphamide is used as a preparative agent before BMT; at these doses a hemorrhagic myocarditis may occur.

4. **DTIC** can produce a flulike syndrome consisting of fever, myalgias, facial flushing, malaise, and marked elevations of hepatic enzymes.

5. **Ifosfamide** is chemically similar to cyclophosphamide, but the incidence of hemorrhagic cystitis is much higher (occurring in 20–30% of treated patients). Administration of 2-mercaptoethanesulfonate (MESNA) (usually infused with ifosfamide at a dosage of at least 0.6 mg of MESNA to 1 mg of ifosfamide) is recommended to lower the incidence of cystitis (see Complications of Treatment, sec. I.E).

6. **Mechlorethamine (nitrogen mustard)** is a skin irritant; protective gloves and eyewear must be used during drug preparation and administration. Development of a drug rash does not prevent further use of this agent.

7. **Melphalan (Alkeran)** is available in oral and injectable forms. An idiosyncratic interstitial pneumonitis may occur, and although usually reversible, it precludes further use of the drug.

8. **Nitrosoureas (carmustine [BCNU] and lomustine [CCNU])** are lipid-soluble and penetrate the blood-brain barrier. BCNU is usually administered in an ethanol solution, and toxicity from the vehicle, including giddiness, flushing, and phlebitis, may occur. Since delayed myelosuppression occurs 6–8 weeks after treatment and may be cumulative, these agents are commonly given at 8-week intervals.

9. **Thiotepa** may be administered IV with bone marrow rescue. When used intravesically, 60–90 mg is administered in 60–100 ml of water and instilled over 2 hours.

C. **Antitumor antibiotics** intercalate adjacent DNA nucleotides, interrupting replication and transcription and causing strand breaks; they are cell cycle–nonspecific.

1. **Anthracycline antibiotics** are associated with a cardiomyopathy consisting of **intractable congestive heart failure** and dysrhythmias. **With doxorubicin,** this complication is seen in approximately 2% of patients receiving 550 mg/m^2, but the incidence increases dramatically at higher cumulative doses. Concomitant cyclophosphamide or previous chest irradiation may potentiate this toxicity. As the cumulative dose approaches 450–550 mg/m^2, serial radionuclide ventriculograms should be performed and the anthracycline should be discontinued if left ventricular function is compromised. Myocardial damage is related to peak serum concentrations and to cumulative dosage; longer (96-hour) infusions have allowed for higher cumulative dosages. These agents may also produce a radiation recall effect consisting of acute toxicity to previous radiation fields, usually to the heart, GI region, or lungs.

   a. **Daunorubicin** is used in the treatment of acute leukemia. Bone marrow suppression is expected, and the dose-limiting toxicity is usually mucositis. Red urine may be caused by the drug and its metabolites.

   b. **Doxorubicin (Adriamycin)** toxicity is similar to daunorubicin, although this drug has a broader spectrum of activity.

   c. **Mitoxantrone** is structurally similar to doxorubicin and daunorubicin but is associated with less cardiac toxicity. Mucositis and myelosuppression are dose-limiting; a bluish discoloration of the urine and sclera may occur.

   d. **Idarubicin** has a more rapid cellular uptake than the other anthracyclines. Toxicity is similar to daunorubicin.

2. **Bleomycin** is useful in combination chemotherapy because it is rarely myelosuppressive. **A test dose,** 1–2 mg SC, should be administered before instituting full doses (especially in patients with lymphoma), because severe allergic reactions with hypotension may occur. Interstitial pneumonitis, which occasionally results in irreversible pulmonary fibrosis, is more common in patients with underlying pulmonary disease or previous lung irradiation or in patients receiving a cumulative dosage of 200 mg/m^2. Pulmonary symptoms and chest radiographs should be monitored.

3. **Mitomycin C** is associated with delayed myelosuppression that worsens with repeated use of the drug. Interstitial pneumonitis has been observed. The **hemolytic-uremic syndrome** has been reported, is exacerbated by RBC transfusions, and should be suspected in patients with sudden onset of a microangiopathic hemolytic anemia and renal failure.

Table 19-2. Recommendations for antiemetic therapy

See Table 19-1 under the column N&V:
0	No medication necessary
+	Phenothiazine or butyrophenone ± antihistamine
+ +	Phenothiazine or butyrophenone ± antihistamine ± anxiolytic ± glucocorticoid
+ + +	Phenothiazine or butyrophenones ± antihistamine ± anxiolytic ± glucocorticoid + high-dose metoclopramide
	or
	Ondansetron or Granisetron ± glucocorticoid

Phenothiazines*
Prochlorperazine, 10–30 mg PO or IV q4–6h
Prochlorperazine, 25 mg PR q4–6h
Chlorpromazine, 10 mg PO q4–6h
Trimethobenzamide, 100 mg PO or IM q4–6h

Serotonin receptor antagonists
Granisetron, 10 µg/kg IV 15 min before chemotherapy
Ondansetron, 0.15 mg/kg IV 30 min before chemotherapy and q4h × 2

Butyrophenone
Droperidol, 5 mg IV q4–6h

Metoclopramide,* 2–3 mg/kg IV before chemotherapy and q2h × 3

Antihistamine
Diphenhydramine, 50 mg PO or IV q4–6h

Anxiolytic
Lorazepam, 1–2 mg PO or IV tid–qid

Glucocorticoid
Dexamethasone, 10–30 mg IV before chemotherapy

* May cause extrapyramidal side effects that can be treated with either diphenhydramine, 50 mg PO or IV q4–6h, or benztropine mesylate, 1–2 mg IV or PO q4–6h.

4. **2-Deoxycoformycin** (Pentostatin) is an inhibitor of adenosine deaminase isolated from *Streptomyces*. Myelosuppression is the chief toxicity.
D. **Plant alkaloids.** Vincristine and vinblastine inhibit the assembly of microtubules and disrupt mitosis. Rapid IV injection of any plant alkaloid can produce hypotension.
   1. **Vincristine** often causes a dose-limiting neuropathy. Paresthesias followed by loss of deep tendon reflexes usually occur. Neuritic pain, jaw pain, diplopia, constipation, abdominal pain, and an adynamic ileus are less likely. Other adverse effects include SIADH and Raynaud's phenomenon.
   2. **Vinblastine** is less neurotoxic than vincristine and is usually limited by myelosuppression. In high doses, myalgias, obstipation, and transient hepatitis may occur.
   3. **Etoposide (VP-16).** The major dose-limiting toxicity is myelosuppression.
   4. **Teniposide (VM-26)** is a semisynthetic derivative of podophyllotoxin. Toxicities include myelosuppression, hypersensitivity reactions, alopecia, and hypotension.
   5. **Taxol** has a unique antitubulin mechanism that disrupts microtubule assembly. Because taxol is dissolved in cremophor, hypersensitivity reactions may occur and are related to the infusion rate. In addition, myelosuppression, arthralgias, neuropathy, and arrhythmias may occur.
E. **Platinum-containing agents** act as intercalators, causing single- and double-strand breaks in DNA.
   1. **Cisplatin** produces severe nausea and vomiting; aggressive antiemetic therapy is mandatory (Table 19-2). The patient should be aggressively volume

expanded with isotonic saline to prevent renal toxicity. One liter of saline should be administered over 4–6 hours before and after chemotherapy. The dosage of cisplatin should be reduced for patients with renal insufficiency and should be withheld if the serum creatinine is greater than 3 mg/dl. Other toxicities include hypomagnesemia and ototoxicity.

2. **Carboplatin** is a cisplatin analog with less neurotoxicity, ototoxicity, and nephrotoxicity than cisplatin; myelosuppression is the dose-limiting toxicity.

F. Other agents

1. **Hydroxyurea,** an oral agent that inhibits ribonucleotide reductase, is used in the management of the chronic phase of CML and other myeloproliferative diseases. The dosage is adjusted according to the peripheral blood neutrophil and platelet count.

2. **L-Asparaginase** hydrolyzes asparagine, depleting cells of an essential substrate in protein synthesis. Allergic or anaphylactic reactions may occur. Other toxicities include hemorrhagic pancreatitis, hepatic failure with depression of clotting factors, and encephalopathy.

3. **Procarbazine** is an oral agent that inhibits DNA, RNA, and protein synthesis. It is a monoamine oxidase inhibitor, and therefore tricyclic antidepressants, sympathomimetic agents, and tyramine-containing foods must be used with caution (see Chap. 1). Procarbazine has a disulfiram-like effect, so ethanol should not be ingested while taking this medication.

G. Hormonal agents lack direct cytotoxicity. In general, they have few serious adverse effects. In disseminated disease, eventual resistance to hormonal agents should be anticipated.

1. **DES** is an estradiol analog used in the treatment of breast and prostate cancer. The usual dosage is 5 mg PO tid in women and 1–3 mg PO qd in men. Adverse effects include nausea, gynecomastia, fluid retention, hypertension, and thrombophlebitis. Thromboembolic and cardiovascular complications limit its usefulness in prostate cancer.

2. **Gonadotropin agonists.** Two LHRH agonists are used in the treatment of metastatic prostate cancer. Leuprolide acetate and goserelin acetate may be given as a monthly SC depot injection, and leuprolide acetate is also available in a daily injection form. The first weeks of treatment may be associated with an initial flare in tumor symptoms, bone pain, fluid retention, hot flashes, sweats, and impotence. Signs of neurologic dysfunction or urinary obstruction should be carefully monitored.

3. **Progestational agents.** Megestrol acetate, 40 mg PO qid, and medroxyprogesterone, 10 mg PO qd, have been used in the treatment of a variety of neoplasms. Principal toxicities include weight gain, fluid retention, hot flashes, and vaginal bleeding with discontinuation of therapy. Both agents have been used in the treatment of cachexia associated with cancer and AIDS (see Complications of Cancer, sec. II.A.3).

4. **Tamoxifen** is an estrogen antagonist. The usual dosage is 10 mg PO bid. After 7–14 days of treatment, a **hormone flare** (increasing bone pain, erythema, and hypercalcemia) occurs in approximately 5% of women with estrogen receptor–positive breast cancer and bone metastases. The symptoms abate over 7–10 days, and 75% of these patients respond to tamoxifen. Palliation of pain, control of hypercalcemia, and continuation of the drug are recommended. The long-term administration of tamoxifen is not associated with a systemic antiestrogen effect (vaginal atrophy, osteoporosis, or increased risk of heart disease).

H. Immunotherapy. In general, the use of immunotherapeutic agents such as interleukin-2, monoclonal antibodies, and gamma-interferon must be regarded as investigational. BCG vaccine, methane-extracted residue, and *Corynebacterium parvum* have not proved effective as immunoadjuvants.

1. **Levamisole** is administered with FU as adjuvant therapy in colon cancer (see Approach to the Cancer Patient, sec. II.B.3). The dosage of 50 mg PO tid for 3 days q2wk is well tolerated and does not appear to add to the toxicity of FU.

2. **Alpha-interferon** is used for hairy-cell leukemia and the chronic phase of CML. Toxicity includes nausea and vomiting, flu-like symptoms, and head-

Table 19-3. Treatment of extravasation of selected chemotherapeutic agents

Drug	Compress	Antidote
Dacarbazine	Hot	Isotonic thiosulfate IV and SC
Daunorubicin	Cold	DMSO applied topically to vein
Doxorubicin	Cold	DMSO applied topically to vein
Etoposide	Hot	Hyaluronidase (150 U/ml) 1–6 ml SC × 1
Mechlorethamine		Isotonic thiosulfate IV and SC
Mitomycin C		Isotonic thiosulfate IV and SC
Vinblastine	Hot	Hyaluronidase (150 U/ml) 1–6 ml SC × 1
Vincristine	Hot	Hyaluronidase (150 U/ml) 1–6 ml SC × 1

DMSO = dimethyl sulfoxide.

aches. Acute toxicity may respond to acetaminophen; with continued administration these symptoms subside.

I. **Retinoids** have been used as therapeutic and chemopreventive agents. 13-*Cis*-retinoic acid, 50–100 mg/m^2 PO qd for 12 months, has been shown to lower the incidence of second primary tumors in patients previously treated for head and neck cancer (*N Engl J Med* 323:795, 1990). All-*trans*-retinoic acid, 45–100 mg/m^2 PO qd, has resulted in remissions in acute promyelocytic leukemia and resolution of associated disseminated intravascular coagulation. Common toxicities include dry skin, headaches, nausea and vomiting, and elevation of transaminases (*Blood* 76:1704, 1990).

Complications of Treatment

I. **Chemotherapy** often causes serious or life-threatening toxicity. The most common and predictable toxicities are to rapidly proliferating cells of hematopoietic and mucosal tissue. Since repair of these tissues cannot be accelerated, palliation during the healing process is the primary goal.

   A. **Extravasation** of certain chemotherapeutic agents from venous infusion sites may lead to severe local tissue injury. Offending agents are identified as vesicants in Table 19-1. Initial symptoms of pain or erythema may appear within hours or may be delayed for up to 1–2 weeks. When extravasation occurs, the steps described below should be taken.

   1. **Stop the chemotherapy infusion.** While the venous catheter is still in place, approximately 5 ml of blood should be aspirated to remove any residual drug.

   2. **Certain drugs require hot or cold compresses** and may be neutralized by instillation of agents locally through the catheter and subcutaneously into the nearby tissue (Table 19-3).

   3. **Observe the area closely** for signs of tissue breakdown; surgical intervention for debridement or skin grafting may be necessary. Extravasation injuries usually result in severe pain, so adequate analgesia should be supplied (*J Clin Oncol* 5:1116, 1987).

   B. **Myelosuppression** from most agents reaches its peak 7–14 days following treatment (see Table 19-1). Prophylactic measures to reduce bleeding are mandatory; however, empiric antimicrobials or antifungal agents are not generally recommended.

1. **Risk of infection** increases dramatically when the neutrophil count is less than 500/mm^3 and is directly related to the duration of the neutropenia. In the absence of neutrophils, signs of infection or inflammation may be muted. A febrile neutropenic patient should be presumed to be infected and must be evaluated and treated promptly. A physical examination must be performed to locate potential sites of infection, with particular attention to indwelling catheter sites, sinuses, and the oral and rectal areas. **Cultures** of blood, urine, stool, sputum, and other foci suspected of bacterial infection should be collected, and a chest radiograph should be obtained. **Empiric antimicrobial treatment** should be initiated immediately after cultures are obtained. In the absence of any obvious source, the antimicrobials should provide broad coverage for gram-negative bacilli and gram-positive cocci. In choosing a regimen, local susceptibility patterns should also be considered. Empiric therapy may consist of an aminoglycoside and semisynthetic penicillin, a double beta-lactam combination, or a single agent such as cefoperazone, 1–2 g IV bid; ceftazidime, 1–2 g IV q8h; or imipenem, 500–1,000 mg IV qid. **Modification of the antimicrobial regimen** according to the culture data or clinical picture may become necessary. Additional agents to treat *Staphylococcus epidermidis*, *Clostridium difficile*, or anaerobic infections are commonly necessary. Persistent fever, in the absence of other data, usually does not warrant an empiric change in the antibacterial therapy. Amphotericin B (0.5–1.0 mg/kg qd) should be added empirically if the fever continues longer than 72 hours (see Chap. 14). Antimicrobials are continued until the neutrophil count is greater than 500/mm^3.

2. **Thrombocytopenia** below 20,000/mm^3 that is the result of chemotherapy should be treated with platelet transfusions to minimize the risk of spontaneous hemorrhage (see Chap. 18). When prolonged thrombocytopenia is anticipated, histocompatibility testing should be performed prior to therapy so that HLA-matched single-donor platelets may be provided when alloimmunization makes the patient refractory to random donor platelets.

3. **Red blood cell transfusions** are indicated for patients who have symptoms of anemia, active bleeding, or a hemoglobin concentration below 7–8 g/dl (see Chap. 18). Because of anecdotal reports of graft-versus-host disease associated with transfusions, radiation of all blood products is generally recommended for immunosuppressed marrow transplant patients.

4. **Growth factors** include many cytokines that may ameliorate the myelosuppression associated with cytotoxic chemotherapy. They act on hematopoietic cells, stimulating proliferation, differentiation, commitment, and some functional activation. Because they can increase myelosuppression, they should not be given within 24 hours of chemotherapy and radiation. They also should be avoided in myeloid malignancies because of the potential stimulation of malignant cells (*N Engl J Med* 327(1):28, (2):99, 1992).

   a. **Granulocyte colony-stimulating factor (G-CSF)**, given at an initial dose of 5 μg/kg SC or IV beginning the day after the last dose of cytotoxic chemotherapy, may reduce the incidence of febrile neutropenic events. Blood counts should be monitored twice weekly during therapy. G-CSF should be stopped when neutrophil counts rise to 5,000–7,000/mm^3. Bone pain is a common toxicity usually managed with nonnarcotic analgesics.

   b. **Granulocyte-macrophage colony-stimulating factor (GM-CSF)**, given at a dose of 250 μg/m^2/day beginning the day after the last dose of cytotoxic chemotherapy, may shorten the period of neutropenia after BMT.

   c. **Erythropoietin** given at a starting dose of 150 units/kg SC 3 times weekly has been shown to improve anemia and decrease transfusion requirements in cancer patients in whom the anemia is predominantly caused by cytotoxic chemotherapy. Hematocrits should be monitored weekly during therapy and the dose should be adjusted accordingly.

C. **Gastrointestinal toxicity**
   1. **Stomatitis** is an unpleasant consequence of many chemotherapeutic agents (see Table 19-1) and is commonly the dose-limiting toxicity of methotrexate and FU. With simultaneous administration of radiation therapy, the toxicity is more severe. Healing generally occurs within 7–10 days of the development of symptoms. The severity of stomatitis ranges from mild (oral discomfort) to severe (ulceration, impaired oral intake, and hemorrhage). In mild cases, oral rinses (chlorhexidine, 15–30 ml swish and spit tid; or the combination of equal parts diphenhydramine elixir, saline, and 3% hydrogen peroxide) may provide relief. In severe cases, IV morphine is appropriate. **IV fluids** should be used to supplement oral intake as needed. Patients with moderate or severe stomatitis may develop aspiration; precautions should include elevation of the head of the bed and availability of a hand-held suction apparatus. In severe or prolonged episodes, superinfection with *Candida* or Herpes simplex requires appropriate diagnosis and antimicrobial intervention.
   2. **Diarrhea** is the result of cytotoxicity to proliferating cells of the intestinal mucosa. In some cases, IV fluids are necessary to avoid intravascular volume depletion. The use of oral opioid agents as antidiarrheals is commonly limited by abdominal cramping. Severe diarrhea associated with FU and leucovorin has been reported to respond to octreotide, 150–500 µg SC tid.
   3. **Nausea and vomiting** may develop in varying degrees and frequency. Suggestions for antiemetic agent(s) are listed in Table 19-2 according to the severity of nausea and vomiting outlined in Table 19-1.
D. **Interstitial pneumonitis** may develop as a dose-related, cumulative toxicity or as an idiosyncratic reaction. The implicated agent should be discontinued, and institution of glucocorticoids (e.g., prednisone, 1 mg/kg PO qd or equivalent) may be of some benefit. The long-term outcome is unpredictable.
E. **Hemorrhagic cystitis** may develop with either cyclophosphamide or ifosfamide. Continuous bladder irrigation with isotonic saline should continue until the hematuria resolves.
F. **Tumor lysis syndrome** occurs in patients with rapidly proliferating neoplasms that are highly sensitive to chemotherapy. Rapid tumor cell death releases intracellular contents and causes hyperkalemia, hyperphosphatemia, and hyperuricemia. Although reported in the treatment of a variety of malignancies, it is usually associated with **high-grade non-Hodgkin's lymphoma** and **acute leukemia**. During induction chemotherapy, prophylactic measures should include allopurinol, 300–600 mg PO qd, and aggressive intravenous volume expansion (e.g., 3,000 ml/m² daily). The addition of sodium bicarbonate, 50 mEq/1,000 ml of IV fluid, to alkalinize the urine above pH 7 may prevent uric acid nephropathy and acute renal failure. When hyperphosphatemia accompanies hyperuricemia, urine alkalinization should be avoided because calcium phosphate precipitation may result in renal failure. Despite these preventive measures, hemodialysis may be needed for hyperkalemia, hyperphosphatemia, acute renal failure, or fluid overload.

II. **Radiation therapy** toxicity is related to the location of the therapy, total dose delivered, and rate of delivery. Larger fractions per dose are associated with more acute normal tissue toxicity than a more protracted delivery.
   A. **Acute toxicity** develops within the first 3 months of therapy and is characterized by an inflammatory reaction. Such toxicity may respond to antiinflammatory agents such as glucocorticoids. Local irritations or burns in the treatment field will generally resolve with time. Close observation and treatment of any infections and palliation of symptoms such as pain, dysphagia, dysuria, or diarrhea (depending on the site of treatment) are the mainstays of supportive care until healing has occurred.
   B. **Subacute toxicities** between 3 and 6 months of therapy and **chronic toxicity** after 6 months are less amenable to therapy, as fibrosis and scarring are present.

Diabetes Mellitus

Matthew J. Orland

Diabetes Mellitus

Diabetes mellitus (DM) refers to a group of disorders manifested by hyperglycemia. Although the pathogeneses of these disorders are diverse, patients with DM ultimately cannot produce insulin in amounts necessary to meet their metabolic needs. They are prone to complications that are related to the severity of their insulin lack and an inability to achieve glycemic control.

I. **Classification**
   A. **Diabetes mellitus** includes three diagnostic types.
   1. **Insulin-dependent (type I) DM** most commonly occurs in children and young adults but may occur at any age. Among individuals with a genetic predisposition to DM, immune-mediated destruction of insulin-producing cells leads to a progressive loss of endogenous insulin. Exogenous insulin is essential to achieve glycemic control, to prevent diabetic ketoacidosis (DKA), and to sustain life.
   2. **Non–insulin-dependent (type II) DM** usually occurs after age 30. A strong genetic predisposition is evident, but the pathogenesis is different from that of type I DM. Most individuals are obese, and resistance to insulin action is prevalent. The production of endogenous insulin is usually adequate to avoid ketoacidosis, but DKA may occur with intense stress. Exogenous insulin may be used to treat hyperglycemia but is not required for survival.
   3. **Other (secondary) DM** associates hyperglycemia with another established cause, including pancreatic disease, pancreatectomy, drugs or chemical agents, Cushing's syndrome, acromegaly, and many uncommon genetic disorders.
   B. **Impaired glucose tolerance** is a classification appropriate for those who manifest abnormal plasma glucose levels but who do not meet the defined diagnostic criteria for DM (see sec. II). Patients with impaired glucose tolerance have an increased risk for development of DM with time and may develop macrovascular complications (see Chronic Complications of Diabetes Mellitus, sec. IV) without manifesting overt DM.
   C. **Gestational DM** refers to patients who develop hyperglycemia during pregnancy. Glucose tolerance in these individuals usually reverts to normal following delivery, but they have an increased risk for development of impaired glucose tolerance and DM later in life.

II. **Diagnosis of diabetes mellitus** can be established when classic symptoms accompany hyperglycemia and when specific diagnostic criteria are met in asymptomatic individuals. Screening is appropriate for patients with a strong family history of DM; significant obesity; recurrent skin, genital, or urinary tract infections; or a pregnancy history complicated by gestational diabetes, prematurity, or birth of an infant larger than 9 lb. In these patients a random plasma glucose (PG) greater than 160 mg/dl or fasting PG greater than 115 mg/dl is an indication for diagnostic testing and close follow-up. Reversible conditions that promote hyperglycemia (Table 20-1) should be identified and corrected, if possible, before the diagnosis of DM is established.
   A. **Symptomatic patients** with polyuria, polydipsia, and weight loss may be diagnosed without further testing when a random PG is greater than 200 mg/dl.

Table 20-1. Conditions that promote hyperglycemia in patients with diabetes mellitus[a]

I. Increased dietary intake (particularly of carbohydrate)
II. Limitation of physical activity
III. Reduction of hypoglycemic therapy
IV. Limitation of endogenous insulin production
    A. Pancreatic diseases (or pancreatectomy)[b]
    B. Drug treatment[b]
        1. Destruction of insulin-producing cells
            a. Streptozotocin
            b. Pentamidine isethionate
        2. Reversible inhibition of insulin secretion
            a. Diazoxide
            b. Thiazide diuretics
            c. Phenytoin
    C. Electrolyte disorders
        1. Hypokalemia
        2. Hypomagnesemia
V. Development of insulin resistance[b]
    A. Infection
    B. Inflammation
    C. Myocardial or other tissue ischemia, or infarction
    D. Trauma
    E. Surgery
    F. Emotional stress
    G. Pregnancy
    H. Drug treatment
        1. Glucocorticoids
        2. Estrogens (including oral contraceptives)
        3. Sympathomimetic agents
        4. Nicotinic acid
    I. Antibodies to insulin
    J. Antibodies to insulin receptors

[a] These conditions (particularly IV and V) should also be investigated in patients with diabetic ketoacidosis or nonketotic hyperosmolar syndrome.
[b] These conditions may also promote transient hyperglycemia among patients without established DM.

When the random PG is less than 200 mg/dl, testing as for asymptomatic patients is usually warranted.

B. Asymptomatic patients. Diagnostic testing should be performed when an abnormal screening result is obtained or when there is a strong clinical suspicion of DM. These **tests should be repeated** and abnormal results should be demonstrated more than once before a diagnosis of DM is made.

    1. Fasting plasma glucose, after an overnight fast, should be greater than 140 mg/dl for a diagnosis of DM.

    2. Oral glucose tolerance testing may be performed when fasting PG does not establish a diagnosis. Results are valid only when patients are not stressed, when physical activity is unrestricted and when daily carbohydrate intake is greater than 150 g. Nonpregnant adults should be given 75 g of glucose in the morning following an overnight fast. PG should be measured at baseline and then at half-hour intervals for 2 hours after glucose administration. A normal test includes (1) a fasting PG less than 115 mg/dl, (2) a 2-hour PG less than 140 mg/dl, and (3) no values greater than 200 mg/dl. A diagnosis of DM can be made if the PG is 200 mg/dl or greater at 2 hours and on at least one of the earlier samples. Intermediate values define impaired glucose tolerance.

C. Modified criteria are defined for pregnant patients (see Diabetes Mellitus in Pregnancy, sec. I).

III. Management of diabetes mellitus. The objectives of diabetes therapy are (1) to avoid the short-term consequences of insulin insufficiency, including symptomatic hyperglycemia (i.e., polyuria, polydipsia, and weight loss), DKA, and nonketotic hyperosmolar syndrome (NKHS), and (2) to ameliorate the complications of long-standing disease. There is evidence that the chronic complications of DM result from metabolic abnormalities, and the Diabetes Control and Complications Trial (DCCT) has demonstrated that intensive efforts to control hyperglycemia can reduce both the incidence and the severity of these afflictions over time (*N Engl J Med* 329:977, 1993). For each patient the physician should devise a treatment plan to yield the best glycemic control possible without promoting frequent or severe hypoglycemia. Clinical practice recommendations are established by the American Diabetes Association (*Diabetes Care* 16[Suppl. 1]:1, 1993).

A. Monitoring of therapy. The objectives of management require careful attention to the status of glucose control and any acute or chronic complications.

   1. Patient assessment should include scrutiny for symptomatic hyperglycemia as may be revealed by nocturia, polyuria, polydipsia, or weight loss, as well as more subtle symptoms such as fatigue or blurred vision. Physical examination should focus on manifestations of complications of DM that affect the eyes, cardiovascular system, kidneys, nerves, and skin. Symptoms of hypoglycemia should also be assessed in patients who are being treated with pharmacologic therapy (see Hypoglycemia).

   2. Glucose measurements are necessary to document efficacy and to guide modification of therapy.

   a. Plasma glucose measurement is appropriate for screening and diagnosis (see sec. II). Falsely low PG values may occur as a result of glycolysis in collection tubes; this can be minimized by routine use of glycolytic inhibitors and rapid processing of samples.

   b. Capillary blood glucose measurement allows a rapid determination of the glucose level in whole blood. Blood glucose monitoring with glucose oxidase reagent strips and portable meters allows a convenient, cost-effective alternative to PG determinations. Errors may occur when a blood sample is inadequate or when timing of the reaction is not measured correctly.

   (1) Self-monitoring of blood glucose (SMBG) using these methods is the preferred means of following glucose control. SMBG is appropriate for all patients with DM. Frequency of monitoring may vary based on the goals for glycemic control and stability of glucose levels. Considerations for frequency of monitoring should include a routine schedule and an intensified program appropriate when therapy is changed or illness occurs (see sec. **III.F**). Measurements should be recorded in an organized fashion by the patient so that they may be reviewed during regular assessment of therapy.

   (2) Reliability of measurement depends on proper instruction and should be periodically reassessed by the physician or diabetes nurse-educator.

   c. Urine glucose measurement can detect the occurrence of blood glucose levels above a variable renal glucose threshold (i.e., 150–300 mg/dl). Glucose oxidase reagent strips or tape provide a semiquantitative measurement of urine glucose that is influenced by both glucose and water excretion; therefore, results correlate poorly with blood glucose levels. Urine assays cannot detect hypoglycemia. Urine glucose measurements may be used when blood glucose monitoring is impractical.

   3. Glycated hemoglobin measurement is an indispensable tool for the assessment of glycemic control and provides the best available standard to estimate relative risk for development of the chronic complications of DM. These assays quantify a nonenzymatic glycation of hemoglobin, which occurs during the life span of RBCs, and can be correlated with mean blood glucose levels over 2–3 months preceding measurement. The percentage of stably glycated hemoglobin in blood (hemoglobin A_{1C}) is usually elevated at the time of diagnosis of DM and falls as glycemic control is attained. Periodic measurements of hemoglobin A_{1C} validate outpatient SMBG data and serve in evaluation of the progress of efforts to achieve treatment goals. Unfortunately, various glycated hemoglobin assays may correlate differently with the status of glycemic control, making knowledge of the lab-specific normal ranges and methods of assay important for proper interpretation. Some hemoglobinopathies may affect glycated hemoglobin levels, and an underestimation of chronic hyperglycemia may result from measurements under circumstances in which RBC survival is reduced (e.g., uremia, hemolytic anemia).

   4. Ketone assays employ the nitroprusside reaction to measure ketones in blood and urine. Ketone overproduction may occur with DKA, prolonged fasting, or alcohol intoxication.

   a. Serum ketone measurement is important to confirm DKA (see Insulin-Dependent [Type I] Diabetes Mellitus). Titration may allow a semiquantitative determination of ketone concentrations, but this is seldom useful.

   b. Urine ketone measurement is a sensitive means of detecting ketones in blood and should be performed by patients prone to DKA when persistent hyperglycemia is noted or when illness or stress is present.

B. Patient education. Optimum treatment of DM requires an informed patient. Management is facilitated when the properly educated patient can make appropriate decisions in daily care.

   1. Early education should emphasize diet planning and techniques for the monitoring of glucose and ketones. The relationships of diet, physical activity, and medications for DM should be conveyed. Specific instructions should be given regarding care in emergencies and for complicating illnesses, including careful SMBG. When insulin or an oral hypoglycemic drug is prescribed, patients must know how to avoid, recognize, and treat hypoglycemia. Basic instructions should also be given to family members and roommates to facilitate care (*Diabetes Forecast* 46:68, 1993).

   2. Team support. Instructions by the physician, a diabetes nurse-educator, and a dietitian are each important to achieve educational goals.

C. Dietary modification is important in all types of DM and may also be beneficial to patients with impaired glucose tolerance. The objectives of dietary management differ according to (1) the diagnostic type of diabetes, (2) the degree of obesity, (3) the coexistence of lipid abnormalities, (4) the presence of diabetic complications, and (5) the concurrent medical therapy. Dietary objectives should be reviewed regularly with the patient and a dietitian. The meal plan should be prepared with consideration of patient preferences, resources, and needs.

   1. Caloric goals should be those required to achieve and to maintain ideal body weight (see Chap. 2). Caloric intake in normal individuals with moderate physical activity is roughly 35 kcal/kg/day; this average estimate may be reduced by 5–15 kcal/kg/day in obese, sedentary patients and should be increased in more active individuals. Reduction of caloric intake is desirable only in overweight patients.

   2. Consistency in composition and timing of meals is important, particularly for patients using fixed insulin regimens or oral hypoglycemic drugs. The optimum plan provides meals of equivalent caloric and carbohydrate content at corresponding times in a daily schedule.

   3. Food composition. The optimum nutrient composition in DM is uncertain (*Diabetes Care* 17:517, 1994). Considerations include the effects of the diet on blood glucose levels and the effect dietary modification might make on a reduction of atherosclerosis and other chronic complications.

   a. Carbohydrate (55–60% of the diet) is essential to maintain caloric intake. Foods with a high refined sugar content should be limited but may be included as part of a balanced meal. Complex carbohydrates are a preferred calorie source. Carbohydrate-containing foods can be classified by a glycemic index related to effects on postprandial blood glucose (*Diabetes Care* 11:149, 1988).

    b. Protein (10–20% of the diet) should be sufficient to maintain nitrogen balance and to promote growth (see Chap. 2). Limitation of protein intake may be appropriate for patients with diabetic nephropathy (see Chap. 11).

    c. Fat (25–30% of the diet) should be restricted. Cholesterol intake should be less than 300 mg/day, and saturated fat intake should be replaced by polyunsaturated fats when possible.

    d. Fiber (25 g/1,000 kcal) in the diet can retard the absorption of sugars and can ameliorate postprandial blood glucose elevation. Fiber-containing foods that aid glucose control include beans, legumes, and guar gum; bran and guar fiber may also help to lower total and low-density lipoprotein (LDL) cholesterol levels.

    e. Artificial sweeteners (e.g., aspartame, saccharin) are available as substitutes for sucrose in soft drinks and many foods.

  4. Alcohol use should be limited. Alcohol inhibits hepatic gluconeogenesis and may promote hypoglycemia in patients using insulin or oral antidiabetic drugs. Sugar-containing alcoholic beverages may also promote hyperglycemia. Alcohol contributes to acute and chronic hypertriglyceridemia (see Chap. 22). Alcohol perturbs sulfonylurea metabolism (see sec. **IV**) and may contribute to the development of lactic acidosis, so caution is warranted for patients taking metformin. A limited consumption of alcohol with meals by patients with DM is acceptable; it should be defined as fat in the meal plan. Patients with neuropathy should avoid alcohol, as functional impairment may be exacerbated.

D. Physical activity offers both benefits and risks for patients with DM. In normal individuals, increased glucose utilization of exercising muscle is balanced by hepatic glucose release; this balance is regulated by insulin and is often disturbed in DM. Marked hyperglycemia and ketosis can occur when DM is poorly controlled. Hypoglycemia may be promoted by excessive exogenous insulin or by the endogenous insulin stimulated by sulfonylureas. Careful planning of meals and insulin dosing is required when insulin-treated patients increase activity or attempt strenuous exercise. Snacks may be used during a period of intense physical activity to balance the effects of fixed exogenous insulin or oral hypoglycemic drug treatment. Exercise may also be detrimental to patients with chronic complications of DM; cardiovascular disease, neuropathy, and retinopathy may yield a functional impairment. Preventive management, including cardiovascular evaluation, proper footwear, and ophthalmologic care, is appropriate, and patient education is essential.

E. Pharmacologic therapy includes treatment with oral antidiabetic drugs or insulin (see secs. **IV** and **V**). Decisions in drug treatment should be based primarily on the type of DM and the goals for glycemic control. Modification of therapy, including any changes in drugs or dosing, should be accompanied by patient education and an intensification of blood glucose monitoring.

F. Hyperglycemic exacerbations. Therapy of DM must address not only the control of glucose in the stable patient but also the management of situations in which routine treatment is inadequate. The stress of illness or trauma increases metabolic demands for insulin, and special attention to diabetes care is required. As treatment is adjusted, the physician should consider (1) the nature of the precipitating stress, (2) the diagnostic type of diabetes, (3) the therapeutic goals established for the patient, (4) the patient's compliance to the usual treatment regimen, and (5) the complications that might result from an adjustment.

  1. Intensification of monitoring should be prompted by changes from the usual glucose profile and should be continued until stability returns and further changes are not anticipated.

  2. Identification of precipitating factors. Correction of an illness or other condition promoting hyperglycemia (see Table 20-1) is the most important aspect of successful treatment. A diagnostic evaluation is warranted when causes of worsening hyperglycemia are not apparent. When possible, a time course of the precipitating stress should be anticipated; resolution usually reverses the increase in insulin demand.

3. **Modification of therapy** is required when symptomatic hyperglycemia is evident or when DKA might occur (see Insulin-Dependent [Type I] Diabetes Mellitus). Dietary modifications are not routinely indicated but may be necessary when a precipitating event has perturbed dietary intake. The initiation of oral antidiabetic drugs or insulin must be accompanied by appropriate patient education (see sec. **III.B**), even when the need is expected to be temporary.

G. **Inability to maintain dietary intake** may occur secondary to GI illness, surgery, trauma, or depression. If insulin or a sulfonylurea is prescribed, management must include meticulous monitoring. Drug dosage reductions and use of oral sugar-containing fluids or IV dextrose are appropriate measures to prevent hypoglycemia (see Hypoglycemia). Metformin use in most cases may be suspended until oral intake is resumed.

H. **Infection** occurs frequently in diabetic patients, and the coexistence of infection and diabetes affects management of both. Patients with uncontrolled DM are often immunocompromised with impaired granulocyte function; improvement in resistance to infection can follow control of blood glucose.

1. **Urinary tract infection** occurs commonly in women with DM. Pathogens include enteric gram-negative bacteria, staphylococci, enterococci, and fungi. Antimicrobial therapy is appropriate. Antimicrobial prophylaxis may be helpful to patients with recurrent infections or neurogenic bladder (see Chronic Complications of Diabetes Mellitus).

2. **Cellulitis** is common in patients with DM. Streptococci and *Staphylococcus aureus* are frequent pathogens; gram-negative and anaerobic infections may also occur when an open ulcer or necrotizing inflammation is present. Treatment of cellulitis may be difficult in extremities compromised by neuropathy or vascular insufficiency.

3. **Skin abscesses** are usually caused by *Staph. aureus*. Large abscesses require drainage; most warrant antimicrobial therapy.

4. **Vulvovaginitis** is commonly caused by *Candida albicans*, and topical antifungal therapy is appropriate (see Chap. 13).

I. **Assessment for chronic complications of diabetes** is important in the routine management of patients with type I DM of 5 or more years' duration, for all patients with type II or other DM, and during diabetic pregnancy. The routine outpatient evaluation should include ophthalmoscopy, cardiovascular assessment, neurologic examination, and examination of the feet. Urinalysis should include an assessment for protein. Screening of selected patients for microalbuminuria may lead to early detection of nephropathy; however, small amounts of urinary albumin also may be present transiently during periods of poor glycemic control. Plasma creatinine and electrolytes should be measured periodically. Monitoring of serum lipid levels is recommended (see Chap. 22). A yearly ECG is advised. Surveillance for retinopathy requires at least yearly screening examinations by an ophthalmologist (see Chronic Complications of Diabetes Mellitus).

J. **Preventive care**. The severity of some diabetic complications may be reduced by specific prophylactic management.

1. **Vaccinations**. Pneumococcal vaccine should be considered for all patients. Yearly influenza vaccination is prudent.

2. **Attention to other risk factors for cardiovascular disease**. Detection and management of hypertension and hyperlipidemia (see Chaps. 4 and 22) and abstinence from cigarette smoking are important health maintenance objectives.

3. **Foot care** is essential for patients with neuropathy (see Chronic Complications of Diabetes Mellitus, sec. **VIII**).

K. **Drug therapy for other conditions** should be chosen with consideration of side effects that may compromise management of hyperglycemia (see Table 20-1) or worsen diabetic complications. In general, therapy should not be withheld if indications for use are sound. Patient education and intensification of glucose monitoring, including SMBG in outpatients, should accompany initial use, change in dosage, or discontinuation of any drug.

Table 20-2. Characteristics of the oral antidiabetic drugs[a]

Generic name	Initial dosage[b]	Maximum dosage	Duration of activity (hrs)[c]
Sulfonylurea			
Glyburide	1.25–5.0 mg PO qd	10 mg PO bid	24–60
Glyburide Prestab[d]	0.75–3.0 mg PO qd	6 mg PO bid	24–60
Glipizide	2.5–5.0 mg PO qd	20 mg PO bid	12–24
Glipizide GITS[e]	5 mg PO qd	20 mg PO qd	24–36
Chlorpropamide	100–250 mg PO qd	250 mg PO bid	60–90
Tolazamide	100–250 mg PO qd	500 mg PO bid	10–24
Acetohexamide	250–500 mg PO qd	750 mg PO bid	12–24
Tolbutamide	250–500 mg PO bid	1,000 mg PO tid	6–12
Biguanide			
Metformin	500 mg PO qd	1,000 mg PO tid	12–24

[a] Sulfonylureas are listed in order of decreasing potency; the only biguanide, metformin, is separated for clarity. Maximum efficacy is similar for all of the drugs at the maximum dosage listed.
[b] The lower dosages are appropriate when initiating treatment in elderly patients, in patients with uncertain meal schedules, or in patients with mild hyperglycemia.
[c] Activity of the sulfonylureas is prolonged in both hepatic and renal failure.
[d] Prestab is a trademark of the Upjohn Corporation.
[e] GITS (Gastrointestinal Therapeutic System) is an extended-release preparation.

IV. Oral antidiabetic drugs. The sulfonylureas lower blood glucose in patients capable of endogenous insulin production. These oral hypoglycemic drugs affect glucose metabolism by the stimulation of insulin secretion and perhaps by some reduction of insulin resistance. Metformin, a biguanide drug, can reduce hyperglycemia in DM through peripheral effects unrelated to insulin secretion.

    A. Sulfonylureas are the most commonly used oral antidiabetic drugs. Sulfonylureas are indicated for nonpregnant adults with type II DM and most secondary DM.

        1. Preparations differ in potency, rates of absorption, durations of action (Table 20-2), and some side effects.

        2. Contraindications. Sulfonylureas should not be used in type I DM, in children, or during pregnancy or lactation. Caution is advised in patients with severe hepatic or renal disease.

        3. Complications of sulfonylurea therapy can occur with any of these drugs. The augmented hypoglycemic potency of glyburide and glipizide may permit their effective usage with fewer drug interactions and dose-related toxic reactions.

            a. Hypoglycemia from sulfonylureas can be severe and prolonged, often warranting observation and therapy well beyond the expected duration of action of the offending drug (see Table 20-2). Alcohol, chloramphenicol, clofibrate, methyldopa, miconazole, monoamine oxidase inhibitors, phenylbutazone, probenecid, salicylates, sulfonamides, and warfarin may potentiate hypoglycemic effects of sulfonylureas, and concurrent use of these drugs requires an intensification of glucose monitoring and dosage adjustment (see Hypoglycemia).

            b. Toxic reactions include skin rash, blood dyscrasias, and cholestatic jaundice. Flushing, tachycardia, nausea, and headache may occur following the consumption of alcohol.

            c. An increased risk of cardiovascular mortality has been shown (*Diabetes* 19[Suppl. 2]:747, 1970) but has not been confirmed by more recent studies and is controversial. This potential risk must be weighed against therapeutic benefits derived from sulfonylurea treatment.

Table 20-3. Pharmacokinetics of insulin after subcutaneous injection*

Insulin type	Onset of action (hrs)	Peak effect (hrs)	Duration of activity (hrs)
Rapid-acting			
Regular	0.25–1.0	2–6	4–12
Semilente	0.5–1.0	3–10	8–18
Intermediate-acting			
NPH	1.5–4.0	6–16	14–28
Lente	1–4	6–16	14–28
Long-acting			
Ultralente (human)	3–8	4–10	9–36
Ultralente (bovine)	3–8	8–28	24–40
PZI	3–8	14–26	24–40

NPH = neutral protamine Hagedorn; PZI = protamine zinc insulin.
* Variations in pharmacokinetics are related to patient differences, species composition, and insulin dose. Human insulins may produce a faster peak effect and a shorter duration of activity than bovine or beef-pork insulins. Larger doses may have a more marked peak effect and a more prolonged duration of activity. Activity may be prolonged in renal failure.

    d. Chlorpropamide may cause hyponatremia and fluid retention.

    e. Glipizide gastrointestinal therapeutic system (GITS) may cause diarrhea not seen with the other glipizide preparations.

  B. Metformin may be used as primary or adjunctive therapy in type II DM and most secondary DM. The precise mechanism of action of metformin is uncertain, but the drug appears to stimulate a nonoxidative metabolism of glucose in peripheral tissues, increasing glucose utilization. A reduction of hepatic glucose production has also been shown. When used alone metformin therapy does not produce hypoglycemia, and this feature may provide an advantage over the sulfonylureas in some patients. Concerns have been expressed regarding stimulation of lactic acidosis, an adverse effect seen with other biguanide drugs, apparently minimized with metformin. Metformin may be particularly beneficial to patients with both DM and hyperlipidemia, as the drug may promote a reduction of triglycerides and LDL cholesterol while increasing high-density lipoprotein (HDL) cholesterol. Metformin is contraindicated in patients with severe liver or renal disease, heart failure, pulmonary insufficiency, pregnancy, and alcoholism. The drug may cause anorexia, which is potentially beneficial to some patients seeking weight reduction, but anorexia may progress to abdominal pain and nausea, particularly during early therapy.

V. Insulin. Exogenous insulin lowers blood glucose in all types of DM. Optimum insulin treatment, however, should approximate physiologic insulin delivery, which at best is difficult with SC injections or even with continuous insulin infusion. A variety of formulations are available to help match release of SC injected insulin to estimated needs.

  A. Insulin formulations differ in type, which is designed to influence the rate of absorption after SC injection (Table 20-3); composition, according to animal or human species; and concentration.

    1. Rapid-acting insulins include regular and semilente types. Only regular insulin is appropriate for IV use; both may be given SC.

      a. IV regular insulin can be given as a bolus or a continuous infusion. An IV insulin bolus produces its maximum effect at 10–30 minutes and may last for 1–2 hours. For most clinical uses, an insulin infusion may be prepared by adding 100 units of insulin to 500 ml of 0.45% saline (i.e., 0.2 units/ml). Like many peptides, insulin adheres to containers and plastic infusion lines; administration should be preceded by flushing lines with approximately 50 ml of the solution to saturate binding sites. Effects of insulin infusions become minimal within 1–2 hours following cessation.

b. **IM regular insulin** produces its maximum effect at 30–60 minutes after injection in patients with normal circulation and lasts for 2–4 hours. The activity is variable and often delayed in hypotensive patients.

c. **SC regular insulin** is prescribed most commonly. Maximum activity occurs 2–6 hours after injection with an insulin syringe (see sec. **V.C**), with activity lasting for 4–12 hours (see Table 20-3). When the dose of insulin is increased, absorption kinetics are affected; a more marked peak effect and a more prolonged duration of activity can be anticipated with larger doses.

2. **Intermediate-acting insulins** include neutral protamine Hagedorn (NPH) and Lente insulins (see Table 20-3), which release insulin from a subcutaneous site during most of a day following injection. This release is not constant; insulin activity reaches a peak 6–16 hours after injection, followed by a slower decline in level and activity. As with regular insulin, pharmacokinetics are dose-dependent.

3. **Long-acting insulins** include Ultralente insulin and protamine zinc insulin (PZI), which are absorbed more slowly than the intermediate-acting insulins. They can be administered to provide a nearly constant level of circulating insulin when given in daily or bid injections.

4. **Species composition.** Insulin from bovine, porcine, and human sources differ in amino acid composition. Human and porcine insulins are less immunogenic than bovine insulin. Pharmacokinetics may also differ; human insulins are often absorbed more rapidly, with earlier peak effects and shorter durations of activity. Care should be taken and monitoring intensified when a change in insulin species composition is prescribed; dosage adjustments may be necessary.

5. **Concentration.** Almost all insulins used in adults are prepared as 100 units/ml, or U-100. Lower concentrations (e.g., U-40) may be used in small children and SC infusion pumps. A U-500 insulin is available for patients with severe insulin resistance.

B. **Mixed insulin therapy** using different insulin types is employed to meet needs for variable insulin delivery while providing a convenient dosing regimen. A combination of rapid-acting and intermediate-acting insulins is most commonly used, mixed in a syringe immediately before administration. When two different insulin types are drawn from the same syringe, care should be taken to avoid cross-contamination of the bottles; when regular insulin is used it should be drawn first. Insulin mixtures may change the pharmacokinetics of component types and yield unexpected results. A delay in the peak activity of regular insulin may be observed when it is mixed with Lente or Ultralente insulins, but when regular insulin is mixed with NPH insulin, the respective activities are not changed. Commercially prepared mixtures of regular and NPH insulins are available, and they may provide a convenient option for patients whose needs match the available formulations. **PZI insulin should not be mixed with other types.**

C. **SC insulin administration.** Methods and timing of insulin administration are at least as important as the insulin doses in treatment of hyperglycemia. The strategy of insulin delivery should be guided by the type of DM and the individual goals for blood glucose control.

1. **Syringe injection.** Disposable syringes with fine (27- to 29-gauge) hypodermic needles are the preferred tools for insulin administration. Bottles of NPH and Ultralente insulins should be agitated gently before an aliquot is removed for injection. Most insulin syringes are calibrated in 1- to 2-unit increments that may be difficult for a visually impaired patient to see. Nondisposable, cartridge-loaded syringe injectors, using replaceable needles, provide an alternative to syringes and may be convenient for patients who use multiple daily insulin injections (MDIIs).

2. **Sites of injection.** Subcutaneous tissue of the anterior abdominal wall, anterior thighs, buttocks, and posterior arms may be used for injection. Sites should be clean, and areas of infection, inflammation, scarring, or lipodys-

trophy should be avoided. The site of injection may affect the kinetics of insulin absorption; absorption is generally fastest from the abdomen and slower from the extremities. It is prudent to alternate (rotate) SC injection sites, but rotation may not be desirable when marked variations in absorption are suspected. Exercise or massage of an injection site may accelerate insulin absorption. Peripheral vasoconstriction may retard insulin absorption.

3. **Portable infusion pumps** that deliver continuous, programmable infusions of insulin provide an alternative to injections. Abdominal sites are the most suitable for placement of an SC infusion catheter; these sites should be rotated and must be inspected regularly for signs of infection.

D. **Complications of insulin therapy**

1. **Hypoglycemia** is the most common and serious complication of insulin treatment. Severity and duration of hypoglycemia can be estimated from the dosages, the methods of injection (e.g., SC, IM, IV), and the pharmacokinetics of the insulins administered (see Table 20-3).

2. **Insulin allergy** may occur, more often in cases when treatment is intermittent. Reactions are often related to insulins of bovine species composition, but allergy can develop with any insulin preparation. Protamine, a component of NPH and PZI formulations, rarely promotes an allergic response. Most reactions are limited and are characterized by erythema, induration, and pruritus at a recent injection site. More generalized manifestations include urticaria and anaphylaxis. Skin tests may aid diagnosis. Uninterrupted treatment with purified human insulins is beneficial for the subsequent prevention of allergic manifestations. When an allergy to human insulin is suspected, a human insulin is still usually continued.

   a. **Treatment of limited reactions** is often unnecessary. Pruritus may respond to antihistamines (see Chap. 1).

   b. **Treatment of systemic reactions** should be guided by the severity of manifestations. Generalized urticaria may respond to antihistamines; however, patients should be observed for more serious reactions. Measures for the management of anaphylaxis are appropriate (see Chap. 9), including treatment with epinephrine and glucocorticoids.

   c. **Desensitization regimens** can be used for patients with significant insulin allergies that require insulin therapy (*Med Clin North Am* 62:663, 1978).

3. **Antibody-mediated insulin resistance** may occur at any time but is most common within the first 6 months of initiation or reinstitution of insulin therapy. Low titers of insulin antibodies are common; however, levels sufficient to raise daily insulin requirements are rare. Hyperglycemia that does not respond to a usual insulin dose is the primary manifestation; other causes of hyperglycemic exacerbations must be excluded (see Table 20-1). A change to human insulin is appropriate. When patients require high doses of insulin, U-500 preparations may be considered.

4. **Lipodystrophy** may occur at sites of insulin injection. **Lipoatrophy** has been related to impure insulin preparations and can be treated with repeated injections of small doses of purified insulin into the periphery of the affected sites. **Lipohypertrophy** occurs when insulin is injected frequently at a single site; if the site is avoided, further treatment is usually unnecessary.

Insulin-Dependent (Type I) Diabetes Mellitus

The absence of endogenous insulin in insulin-dependent DM requires perpetual treatment with exogenous insulin. Analogous to the needs of normal individuals, estimated at 0.6–1.2 units/kg/day (35–50 units/day in adults), daily insulin needs of patients with type I DM may be divided into a **basal requirement** (40–50% of daily insulin need), which is needed to maintain glycemic control between meals and during sleep, and a **dietary requirement** (50–60% of daily insulin need), which is devoted to the control of blood glucose during nutrient intake. The basal requirement should be supplied in an uninterrupted fashion to avoid DKA and death. Successful management respects the basal requirement without compromise and adjusts the dietary requirement as needed to accommodate meal and activity schedules. This balance can be achieved with bid (conventional) insulin treatment but often warrants more frequent insulin dosing. For patients who are motivated to perform frequent SMBG and to make careful decisions to avoid hypoglycemia, an intensive treatment program may allow better glycemic control and a means to reduce the incidence and severity of chronic complications. The DCCT demonstrated that intensively managed patients reduced the early appearance and the progression of retinopathy, nephropathy, and neuropathy by 50–75% when compared to patients treated with conventional therapy (see Diabetes Mellitus, sec. **III**). The regimen of care for patients with insulin-dependent diabetes should be devised to seek a level of control comparable to that achieved by the DCCT as often as possible. Such a regimen may include more frequent insulin injections or use of a SC insulin pump but also includes intensive support in the management of diet and activity (*Medical Management of Insulin-Dependent [Type I] Diabetes* [2nd ed]. American Diabetes Association, 1994).

I. **Management of hyperglycemia** requires an individualized treatment plan. The plan must consider basal needs, dietary intake, physical activity, and preferences in insulin dosing schedules.

   A. **Dietary objectives.** Basic considerations in dietary therapy apply (see Diabetes Mellitus, sec. **III.C**).

   1. **Caloric goals** should be defined to achieve normal growth and development among children and adolescents and to maintain ideal body weight in adults.

   2. **Consistency** must be maintained among patients using fixed daily insulin regimens. A plan that does not allow some flexibility, however, is usually not conducive to long-term compliance. For patients using bid insulin injections, the safest plan includes breakfast, lunch, supper, and a snack at bedtime. Snacks between meals are also appropriate in some patients to balance activities of injected insulins or effects of physical activity.

   B. **Conventional methods of insulin therapy.** Effective management in type I DM warrants at least 2 daily injections and more than 1 insulin type to address both the basal and the dietary requirements. Conventional therapy employs rapid-acting and intermediate-acting insulins, injected bid. Basal and dietary requirements are not met separately, but the basal insulin needs are respected while the peak effects of insulins are adjusted to conform to the meal plan and activity schedule.

   1. **Initiation of insulin therapy.** Although a daily insulin requirement of 35–50 units/day can be defined in most adults, a partial insulin lack is common at the time of diagnosis of type I DM, and lower doses (e.g., 20–40 units/day) often are more appropriate in initial treatment. An empiric algorithm divides the estimated daily insulin requirement into thirds, with two-thirds given before breakfast and one-third given before the evening meal. The morning dose is split into two-thirds intermediate-acting insulin and one-third rapid-acting insulin, and the evening dose is split evenly between the intermediate acting and rapid-acting insulins. Therapy should be carefully monitored, and frequent SMBG should be performed to ensure proper management.

   2. **Timing of insulin administration** must be set with respect to meals and activity. Before insulin is injected, attention must be given to the plan for the following hours; once the dose is given, the plan must be followed to avoid treatment complications. Practical considerations include diagnostic tests and meal distribution procedures in the hospital and fixed work and meal schedules in outpatients.

   3. **Dosage adjustments.** The initial insulin regimen is seldom satisfactory; frequent modification is usually necessary to accommodate changes in diet and activity. Effects of these changes cannot be predicted in the hospital; thus, it is appropriate to provide a conservative regimen that maintains blood glucose in the range of 100–250 mg/dl and is not likely to produce hypogly-

cemia at home. Guided by SMBG, outpatient insulin dosages may later be modified to meet individual goals. Soon after initiation of treatment, many patients with type I DM experience a **"honeymoon period"** with a marked decrease in insulin requirements; this may allow glycemic control with modest amounts of insulin for several months.

   a. Frequent blood glucose measurement is the most satisfactory means to assess therapy. Four measurements daily, preceding meals and at bedtime (qid), usually give ample data for safe and effective insulin adjustment.

   b. Persistent hyperglycemia should be documented before the insulin dosage is adjusted. When hyperglycemia occurs daily during one preprandial period, the timing and distribution of insulin activity may be modified without a substantial change in the total daily insulin dose (see secs. **I.B.3.d** and **e**). When all glucose values are higher than the treatment goals, an increase in the total daily dose is appropriate, and the distribution of insulins should be maintained until a new profile is established.

   c. Hypoglycemia should be avoided by conservative changes in insulin dosing. When glucose values are within 100–250 mg/dl in a stable patient, dose changes of more than 10% are seldom needed, and frequent adjustments should be avoided unless they are motivated by changes in diet or physical activity. Ample communication between the physician and the patient is essential.

   d. Adjustments of intermediate-acting insulin are usually made to control blood glucose (1) before breakfast, with the evening dose, or (2) before supper, with the morning dose. Increases in the evening dose should be made with caution because nocturnal hypoglycemia may result. Optimum management may warrant the administration of the evening dose at bedtime, with rapid-acting insulin given before supper, resulting in a three-injection regimen.

   e. Adjustments of rapid-acting insulin are usually made to control blood glucose (1) before lunch, with the morning dose, or (2) before bedtime, with the evening dose. The administration of regular insulin at bedtime may promote nocturnal hypoglycemia and should be avoided.

   f. Patient variability in insulin absorption should be considered in adjustments of individual insulin doses (see Diabetes Mellitus, sec. **V.A**, and Table 20-3).

   g. Changes in diet and activity warrant careful monitoring of blood glucose and often a modification of insulin dosing. When oral intake is restricted, the basal insulin requirement may be met with intermediate-acting insulin, given in bid injections, totaling one-half (40–50%) of the usual total daily insulin dose.

C. Multiple daily insulin injections (MDII) represent a method of achieving the level of glycemic control attained in the DCCT, and as such are a preferred alternative to conventional insulin treatment in type I DM. Principles of therapy with MDII are based on observations of the plasma insulin levels of normal individuals, and an independent administration is specifically devoted to the basal and the dietary insulin requirements. The basal insulin is provided by daily or twice daily injections of long-acting or intermediate-acting insulins (or both), and the dietary needs are met by doses of regular insulin given before each meal. In addition to its suitability for intensive therapy programs, MDII may also be preferred over bid injections for the management of patients with varied meal schedules (e.g., shift workers, travellers). Ultimately patients prefer MDII regimens because of freedoms gained in meal selection and in timing of meals, which are not as critical as when fixed insulin schedules are prescribed. Initiation of MDII regimens may be difficult for some patients; close contact with an experienced physician is mandatory while educational goals are met.

   1. Initiation of MDII therapy usually follows an interval of conventional treatment during which the patient should show competence in dietary management and both an ability and a willingness to perform frequent SMBG. Initially, 40% of the daily insulin dose should be given as one or two injections of long-acting insulin; one injection may be sufficient when bovine or beef-pork insulin is used and the dose is less than 30 units, but bid dosing is preferable with higher doses or with human insulin (see Diabetes Mellitus, sec. **V.A.4**). The remainder (i.e., 60% of the dose) should be divided among meals, and doses may be varied as indicated by size and composition of each meal; thus, doses are usually different for breakfast, lunch, supper, and snacks, accommodating different meal sizes and carbohydrate contents. Bedtime snacks are often avoided to reduce injections and to allow opportunity for assessment of basal insulin requirements, but a small snack may be eaten when the bedtime blood glucose is less than 100 mg/dl to avoid nocturnal hypoglycemia. The total daily insulin dose with MDII may be less than that with bid insulin treatment because of improved distribution of insulin activity.

2. **Timing of insulin administration.** When long-acting insulin is used, any consistent qd or bid schedule may satisfy basal insulin requirements. Regular insulin doses should be given approximately 30 minutes before meals, allowing time for the absorption of injected insulin to match nutrient delivery from the intestine. Meals may be eaten earlier, however, if the preprandial blood glucose is low. Because the activity of SC regular insulin may persist for longer than a period of postprandial nutrient delivery, caution should be advised in the management of physical activity after meals.

3. **Dosage adjustments** should be guided by at least qid blood glucose monitoring and occasional postprandial and nighttime measurements. Although individual guidelines must be set, an intensive therapy objective of (1) a preprandial glucose of 70–130 mg/dl and (2) a 2-hour postprandial glucose of less than 200 mg/dl is achievable in a closely monitored patient with type I DM. Although this goal can be met, it confers a risk of serious hypoglycemia and demands many management decisions each day.

   a. **Adjustments of long-acting insulin** should be made on the basis of trends occurring in blood glucose (1) in the morning, (2) at night (i.e., 3:00 A.M.), or (3) late postprandial glucoses that are not responsive to changes in the preprandial regular insulin doses. When change from a stable glucose profile is encountered, recommendations for the treatment of hyperglycemic exacerbations apply (see Diabetes Mellitus, sec. **III.F**). Several days should be allowed between dosage changes to verify the response.

   b. **Adjustments of regular insulin** should take into account (1) the size and composition of the ensuing meal, (2) the level of any anticipated physical activity, and (3) the preprandial blood glucose. Although selection of proper preprandial insulin dosages is initially difficult, therapy is ultimately facilitated by supervision and experience.

   c. **Increased morning insulin requirements** may be observed in patients using MDII. These requirements are manifested by hyperglycemia in the morning, increasing from normal at 3:00 A.M. to relative hyperglycemia at 6:00 A.M., despite an otherwise optimum glycemic profile. Management of this "dawn phenomenon" can be achieved with a small dose of intermediate-acting insulin (e.g., 2–3 units) at bedtime, or by a change to alternative methods of insulin delivery.

4. **Complications.** The aim of achieving near-normal glucose with any insulin regimen increases the **risk of hypoglycemia.** MDII should be discontinued or goals for glucose control should be revised if frequent or severe hypoglycemia occurs.

D. **Continuous subcutaneous insulin infusion (CSII)** represents an alternative to insulin injections and provides a method of achieving glucose control analogous to MDII. Principles of treatment with CSII are also modeled from normal insulin levels; the basal insulin requirement is met by a continuous infusion of insulin, and the dietary requirement is addressed by boluses of insulin administered before meals. Sophistication in delivery of basal insulin allows adjustment for regular physical activity schedules and management of the dawn phenomenon. Like MDII, a regimen employing CSII is appropriate for an intensive therapy program, and CSII management is most successful among motivated patients in close communication with an experienced physician.

1. **Initiation of CSII** is best suited to patients experienced in diabetes care and preferably capable of management with MDII. Thus, dosage can be based on previous requirements, similar to those established by an MDII regimen (see sec. **I.C**).

   a. **Catheter placement** and care should be reviewed. The sites should be kept meticulously clean and must be examined regularly.

   b. **Patients should examine pumps before use** and should become adept with their operation to avoid complications.

2. **Timing of insulin administration and dosage adjustments** are managed similarly to MDII regimens (see secs. **I.C.2** and **3**) and must be followed by frequent blood glucose monitoring.

3. **Complications**. Hypoglycemia can occur. Subcutaneous infections, often with *Staph. aureus,* may develop at infusion sites. Severe hyperglycemia or DKA may result from an obstruction or dislodgement of a catheter not noticed by the patient, or by pump failure. If CSII is discontinued, an MDII regimen may be substituted using similar basal and preprandial dosing with careful monitoring.

E. **Hemoglobin A_{1C}** should be measured at 2- to 3-month intervals in patients with type I DM, to validate SMBG data used for daily management, and to prompt revisions of the treatment plan as warranted. Optimum hemoglobin A_{1C} levels are slightly above the normal range; normal levels may indicate frequent hypoglycemia.

II. **Diabetic ketoacidosis (DKA)** occurs as a result of severe insulin insufficiency, usually with a compromise of the basal requirement, and with an excess of counterregulatory hormones (e.g., glucagon). The predisposition to DKA is characteristic of type I DM and may be a presenting manifestation. However, DKA may occur in any patient with diabetes who is sufficiently stressed. The occurrence of DKA requires an explanation, such as an interruption of insulin therapy or a precipitating stress (see Table 20-1), which increases basal insulin needs. The therapy of DKA should include (1) restoration of volume, (2) appropriate electrolyte management, (3) reversal of acidosis and severe ketosis, and (4) control of blood glucose.

A. **Diagnosis**. DKA often presents with weight loss, polyuria, and polydipsia. Common symptoms include vomiting and an abdominal pain that is typically vague and without localizing signs. A severe acidosis promotes hyperventilation. Shock or coma may occur. Laboratory evaluation reveals metabolic acidosis with an elevated anion gap and the presence of serum ketones (see sec. **II.D**). PG is almost always elevated. Other laboratory features may include hyponatremia, hyperkalemia, increased serum urea nitrogen and creatinine, hyperosmolarity, and an elevated level of serum amylase unrelated to abdominal pathology.

B. **Precipitating factors**. Common conditions leading to DKA include insufficient or interrupted insulin therapy and infection or other stress (see Table 20-1). Because an infection is often occult, cultures of blood and urine, careful examination of the skin and feet, and a chest radiograph are indicated. Myocardial infarction (MI) may precipitate DKA, and an ECG is useful both for cardiac assessment and for the evaluation of hyperkalemia. Pregnancy may also precipitate DKA.

C. **Supportive measures**. Stabilization of patients in shock (see Chap. 9) and management of coma (see Chap. 25) should proceed without delay, accompanying specific therapy.

D. **Monitoring of therapy**. Frequent measurements of glucose and electrolytes are essential to assess response to therapy in DKA. A safe approach is to measure blood glucose with glucose oxidase reagent strips q30–60min, and to measure plasma electrolytes q1–2h. Arterial blood gases should be measured to assess the response of pH when bicarbonate therapy is used or when plasma bicarbonate does not respond to 4–6 hours of insulin treatment. Serial measurements of serum ketones are not helpful, because the most prevalent ketone body in DKA is beta-hydroxybutyrate, which is not detected by the nitroprusside reaction; the anion gap is a more reliable parameter of ketoacidosis unless lactic acidosis is also present (see sec. **II.M.1**). Ketonuria can persist following the correction of acidosis, and urine ketones are of only limited utility in following therapy. Pertinent clinical and laboratory data should be recorded in an organized fashion on a flow sheet to facilitate evaluation of therapy.

E. **Fluid management.** Restoration of intravascular volume should be prompt and guided by ongoing considerations of cardiac and renal function. Initial fluids should include isotonic (0.9%) saline or lactated Ringer's solution without additives. Patients with normal cardiac function should receive the first liter of fluid within 1 hour. Shock may warrant more rapid infusion. Volume replacement may then proceed at 1 liter/hour (or more) until the intravascular deficit has been restored.

1. **Monitoring of volume.** Frequent assessment of the heart rate, BP, and urine output is important to guide volume replacement. Bladder catheterization should be avoided as a routine procedure but may be used to assess urine output in hypotensive or comatose patients or when neurogenic bladder is present. Suspected heart failure, MI, or renal failure may warrant the monitoring of central venous pressure or pulmonary artery occlusive pressure (see Chap. 9).

2. **Correction of free water deficit.** A hypotonic solution, such as 0.45% saline, may be used as an alternative to isotonic saline to restore intravascular volume when the serum sodium is greater than 155 mEq/liter.

3. **Maintenance fluids.** When the intravascular volume has been restored, a maintenance infusion containing 0.45% saline is appropriate for all patients. A rate of 150–250 ml/hour is proper for patients with normal cardiac and renal function. Fluid input and output should be monitored.

F. **Bicarbonate therapy** should be considered initially when (1) DKA is accompanied by shock or coma, (2) arterial pH is less than 7.1, or (3) severe hyperkalemia is present (see Chap. 3). Bolus infusion of bicarbonate should be avoided except as an emergency resuscitation measure. A solution of sodium bicarbonate, 88 mEq (two ampules) in a liter of 0.45% saline, can be infused as a substitute for isotonic saline until indications for bicarbonate are no longer present. Sodium bicarbonate may also be used in maintenance fluids (e.g., 44 mEq in a liter of 0.45% saline) regardless of any specific indications for bicarbonate therapy. This measure may reduce hyperchloremia seen with administration of sodium chloride solutions.

G. **Potassium replacement** is a fundamental part of the therapy of DKA. Although hyperkalemia may be observed initially because of metabolic acidosis, patients with DKA are usually deficient in potassium, and **life-threatening hypokalemia can develop during insulin treatment.** Administration of potassium should begin at an initial rate of 10 mEq/hour when the ECG shows no evidence of hyperkalemia and adequate urine output is demonstrated. When plasma potassium is less than 4 mEq/liter at presentation, or when hypokalemia occurs, the infusion of potassium chloride may approach 15–20 mEq/hour (see Chap. 3). Measurements of plasma potassium may be used to guide potassium administration, but delays from the clinical laboratory should not stall therapy. In patients with oliguria or renal failure, potassium levels must be monitored meticulously, and continuous ECG monitoring may be warranted. **Potassium should be administered only in peripheral IV solutions.**

H. **Insulin treatment** in DKA reverses ketogenesis and restores normal nutrient utilization. Although insulin lowers the blood glucose in DKA, the resolution of acidosis and ketone production is the therapeutic objective. A dextrose infusion is necessary (see sec. **II.I**) to avoid hypoglycemia during treatment.

1. **Initial dose.** Therapy should be initiated with regular insulin, 10–15 units (or 0.15 units/kg) IV, as a bolus.

2. **Continuous IV insulin infusion** is the treatment of choice in DKA. Administration of 10 units/hour (or 0.1 units/kg/hour) is appropriate initially (see Diabetes Mellitus, sec. **V.A.1.a**).

3. **IM insulin injections** provide an alternative to IV infusion. The IM route should be avoided in hypotensive patients because absorption is unpredictable. An initial dosage of 10 units (or 0.1 units/kg) IM q1h should be given.

4. **Adjustments of insulin dosage** should be guided initially by blood glucose. After the first hour of treatment the glucose levels should fall by at least 50 mg/dl/hour; a slower response may be indicative of insulin resistance, inadequate fluid administration, or improper insulin delivery. When dextrose is administered, the plasma bicarbonate and anion gap are more appropriate measures of insulin effect. If insulin resistance is suspected, the dosage of IV insulin should be increased by 50–100% in hourly increments. It may be prudent to advance IM insulin more slowly. Insulin can be tapered, with care to maintain the basal requirement (e.g., 1–2 units/hour), when plasma bicarbonate rises to more than 15 mEq/liter and the anion gap resolves. Subsequently, when oral intake is resumed, SC insulin may be given and the IV or IM insulin discontinued (see secs. **II.K** and **L**).

I. **Dextrose administration.** Because the fall in blood glucose caused by insulin treatment is usually more prompt than is the resolution of ketoacidosis, dextrose administration is necessary during therapy. Normalization of blood glucose is not advised during initial therapy of DKA because of a risk of serious hypoglycemia complicating the administration of high doses of rapid-acting insulin. A reasonable goal is to maintain blood glucose at 200–300 mg/dl; IV fluids should contain 5–10% dextrose when glucose levels fall to within this range. When the initial blood glucose is less than 400 mg/dl, dextrose-containing fluids are appropriate as part of the initial fluid regimen.

J. **Phosphate administration.** Insulin treatment promotes cellular uptake of phosphate with a reduction of plasma phosphate levels. Complications of hypophosphatemia in DKA are rare. The use of potassium phosphate in maintenance IV fluids (total dose ≤ 20 mEq K^+) is usually sufficient to mitigate hypophosphatemia until stores can be repleted with oral supplements. When patients are incapable of oral intake for prolonged periods, additional IV phosphate may be given with care to avoid potential complications (see Chap. 23).

K. **Initiation of oral intake.** Nausea, vomiting, and abdominal pain usually resolve during the first few hours of treatment. Patients may eat when they can tolerate food, but ketoacidosis should be corrected before a full diet is resumed.

L. **Prevention of recurrent DKA** should be guaranteed by correction of precipitating factors and by maintenance of uninterrupted insulin therapy with respect for the basal insulin requirement. **Delay in the SC administration of insulin following IV or IM therapy in DKA should be avoided,** and care should be taken to maintain the administration of insulin in doses sufficient to meet metabolic requirements. Rapid-acting insulin should be given SC, alone or in a mixed injection, before the IV insulin is discontinued or concurrently with the last IM injection, so that continuous insulin activity is maintained and the basal needs are met. Measurements of electrolytes should continue at q4h intervals until stability is clearly demonstrated.

M. **Complications of DKA.** Management of shock (see Chap. 9) and coma (see Chap. 25) should accompany specific therapy.

1. **Lactic acidosis** may accompany ketoacidosis, particularly when shock, sepsis, or necrotizing inflammation are also present, or when metformin is used (see Diabetes Mellitus, sec. **IV.B**). Lactic acidosis should be suspected when the pH and anion gap do not respond to insulin therapy. Lactic acidosis may respond to volume replacement, but infusion of bicarbonate may be required (see sec. **II.F**) until the cause is corrected.

2. **Cerebral edema** may occur during therapy of DKA (especially in children) and may be manifested by headache, altered mental status, and papilledema. CT scan of the head can establish the diagnosis. Prompt therapy is warranted for this often fatal complication (see Chap. 25).

3. **Arterial thrombosis** has been recognized as a complication of DKA, which may present as stroke, MI or other organ infarction, or limb ischemia.

Management is specific to the affected area of the body. Thrombectomy and anticoagulation (see Chap. 17) may be appropriate.

Non–Insulin-Dependent (Type II) and Other Diabetes Mellitus

Treatment of non–insulin-dependent and secondary DM is variable, depending most on the extent of endogenous insulin insufficiency observed in each patient. This insufficiency may be related to impaired insulin production, insulin resistance, or both. The absolute deficiency of insulin is usually not severe enough to compromise basal insulin requirements (except in diabetes secondary to severe pancreatic disease or near-total pancreatectomy); thus, patients are resistant to ketoacidosis unless a severe stress is present. Fasting PG is an approximate indicator of the extent of insulin lack. Patients with type II and secondary DM are vulnerable to chronic complications that are related to both the duration and the severity of their hyperglycemia. Management goals are based on the premise that glycemic control is beneficial, and the conclusions of the DCCT have been extrapolated to apply to these patients (*Medical Management of Non–Insulin-Dependent [Type II] Diabetes* [3rd ed]. American Diabetes Association, 1994).

I. **Management of hyperglycemia.** Both short-term and long-term goals should be considered, particularly for obese patients with type II DM. Weight reduction can reduce insulin requirements and improve glucose tolerance; an optimal plan is one that attempts to achieve and maintain ideal body weight.

A. **Dietary objectives.** General principles of dietary management apply (see Diabetes Mellitus, sec. **III.C**).

1. **Caloric reduction** is important for overweight patients with type II DM. Benefits to glucose control may be apparent after only modest weight reduction. Crash dieting for rapid weight loss is seldom beneficial in long-term management, but a hypocaloric diet may be worthwhile in combination with a program of behavior modification to revise long-term eating habits. A goal to reduce weight by roughly 1 pound/week is appropriate and can be achieved in most cases when caloric intake is reduced by 500 kcal/day. Caloric reduction is not desirable for patients already at or near their ideal weight.

2. **Adequate nutrition** should be established, particularly in patients requiring caloric reduction. Vitamin supplements are indicated when daily intake is less than 1,200 kcal.

B. **Physical activity.** A program of regular physical activity is an important adjunct in achieving weight control and also may improve glucose management by enhancing sensitivity to insulin. A graded exercise program should be recommended to untrained patients only after medical evaluation; in patients over age 40 the evaluation should include a resting ECG and consideration of a stress test. Patient education and monitoring may help to avert potential complications (see Diabetes Mellitus, sec. **III.D**).

C. **Oral antidiabetic drugs** may be used in conjunction with dietary modification when indicated (see Diabetes Mellitus, sec. **IV**).

1. **Sulfonylureas** are usually effective in patients with mild to moderate fasting hyperglycemia. Approximately 70% of patients with type II DM initially achieve appropriate reductions of fasting blood glucose (i.e., to <110 mg/dl) with these drugs. Responses may be better among patients with (1) onset of diabetes after age 40, (2) hyperglycemia of less than 5 years' duration, and (3) no previous history of insulin therapy. Among patients using sulfonylureas who initially achieve adequate blood glucose control, secondary failures may occur that usually warrant insulin therapy. Efficacy may also be reduced by concurrent administration of drugs that potentiate hyperglycemia (see Table 20-1).

a. Indications. Hyperglycemia that is unresponsive to diet and physical activity warrants treatment with a sulfonylurea, metformin, or insulin. Decisions regarding these modalities are usually based on clinical criteria (e.g., severity of hyperglycemia, nature of chronic complications, hepatic or renal disease) and on patient acceptance of therapeutic options. Sulfonylureas can be used in the treatment of mild hyperglycemic exacerbations caused by a self-limited or treatable illness, but patients who are severely stressed may not respond to oral antidiabetic therapy.

b. Administration. Sulfonylurea therapy should be initiated with the lowest effective drug dosage (see Table 20-2). The dosage should be increased gradually (e.g., at 1- to 2-week intervals) until treatment goals are achieved or a maximum daily dose is given. Particular care in initial dosage selection and adjustment is appropriate in elderly patients. Blood glucose should be monitored frequently (e.g., bid–qid) to aid adjustments and avert hypoglycemia.

2. Metformin is an oral alternative to the sulfonylureas. It may be useful particularly in the treatment of obese patients with type II DM. An 80% efficacy in primary therapy of mild to moderate fasting hyperglycemia may be expected, and this group may include some patients whose DM is not well controlled with the sulfonylureas. Secondary failures may be anticipated; these failures warrant treatment with a sulfonylurea or insulin.

a. Indications. There are no specific criteria to support metformin therapy over the sulfonylureas, but the lack of complicating hypoglycemia may favor use of metformin for patients with inconsistent diets and activity schedules. Experience in long-term management of DM has exceeded that for treatment of temporary hyperglycemic exacerbations, for which sulfonylureas are preferred. Although hypoglycemic complications may not be a concern, SMBG is still advised to follow the efficacy of metformin therapy.

b. Administration. Metformin should be initiated at a dosage of 500 mg PO qd, which should be continued until initial anorexia and nausea are tolerated. Dosage may be advanced to 500 mg PO bid, then at weekly intervals of 500 mg/day to a total dose of 3,000 mg/day as guided by bid SMBG and avoidance of GI side effects.

3. Combined therapy with a sulfonylurea and metformin may be used as an alternative to insulin. These agents have complementary mechanisms of action, and the combination may be effective for patients who have not achieved desired glycemic control with either drug alone. The newer of the drugs should be started at the lowest initial dosage, with advances guided by qid SMBG, and care should be taken to avoid hypoglycemia. Patients treated with a maximum dosage of a sulfonylurea and manifesting a fasting glucose of greater than 180 mg/dl are not apt to benefit from the addition of metformin; these patients warrant insulin therapy.

D. Insulin therapy. Patients with type II and other DM often need exogenous insulin to manage hyperglycemia. In some patients, insulin may be considered an alternative to oral drug therapy; in others, insulin represents the only effective treatment. Insulin is not a substitute for proper dietary modification. A resistance to insulin action may be severe in some individuals, with exogenous insulin requirements of greater than 100 units daily, implying a total insulin requirement (met by endogenous and exogenous sources) that is far greater and not well estimated by the 0.6–1.2 units/kg/day requirement of normal individuals. An increase in appetite may be perceived and a weight gain may be seen after initiation of insulin treatment; this does not limit the efficacy of insulin in lowering blood glucose levels but underscores the need for ongoing dietary management and strict weight control measures.

1. Indications. Insulin is an alternative in long-term therapy but may be essential to control hyperglycemia during periods of stress (see Table 20-1). Even temporary treatment must be accompanied by patient education and frequent blood glucose monitoring.

2. **Initiation of insulin therapy.** The dosage of insulin required to reduce blood glucose in type II and secondary DM is highly variable. Initially, 10–20 units of an intermediate-acting insulin may be given SC before breakfast; the degree of obesity and severity of hyperglycemia aid in selection of a dose within this range. A lower dose (e.g., 10 units) is appropriate for elderly patients and when switching treatment to insulin from oral antidiabetic drugs.

3. **Dosage adjustments** should be based on results of qid blood glucose monitoring. Measurements before breakfast and supper are often the most useful when treatment is limited to a single injection of intermediate-acting insulin given in the morning; the value before supper usually corresponds to the peak activity of the NPH or Lente insulin. When the lowest of the qid glucose measurements is within the desired range, the insulin activity should be distributed by adding other insulin types (see Table 20-3), additional injections, or both, according to the glucose profile. Gradual adjustments of insulin dosage (i.e., q2–3d) are prudent when measurements are near the therapeutic goals; fluctuations of blood glucose may also be related to diet, physical activity, injection site, and changes in insulin sensitivity occurring during treatment. Only persistent hyperglycemia, recurring 1 or more times of day, should prompt a change of therapy.

   a. **Fasting hyperglycemia** with an otherwise acceptable glucose profile is an indication for (1) distributing or adding 10–25% of the total daily insulin dose to a second injection of intermediate-acting insulin given before bedtime or before supper or (2) considering the use of long-acting insulin.

   b. **Late morning or evening hyperglycemia** may be treated with injections of rapid-acting insulin given before breakfast or supper, respectively. When mixed insulins are given in twice-daily injections, management becomes similar to conventional therapy for type I DM (see Insulin-Dependent [Type I] Diabetes Mellitus, sec. **I.B**).

E. **Therapy with both insulin and oral antidiabetic drugs** has been suggested as an option in the management of type II DM by the results of several research protocols. Combined therapy may be beneficial in some isolated cases, but a general application is not recommended (*Clinical Diabetes* 5:73, 1987). Temporary use of combined therapy may be considered when patients receiving a nearly maximum dosage of oral antidiabetic drugs are faced with an acute indication for improvement in their glycemic control. Decisions for subsequent treatment may be deferred but should eventually be reconciled to one modality.

F. **Hemoglobin A_{1C}** measurements should be used to assess long-term therapy. Measurement at 2- to 6-month intervals is appropriate. Normal hemoglobin A_{1C} levels are an acceptable goal in type II DM and can be achieved without frequent or severe hypoglycemia in many patients using pharmacologic therapy guided by appropriate SMBG.

II. **Nonketotic hyperosmolar syndrome (NKHS)** occurs predominantly in patients with type II and other DM, in whom dehydration and severe hyperglycemia may occur without development of ketoacidosis. NKHS may occur as a sequel to severe stress (see Table 20-1) and may follow stroke or an excessive carbohydrate intake. The pathogenesis of NKHS usually includes impaired renal excretion of glucose; thus, antecedent renal insufficiency or prerenal azotemia are common. As the basal insulin requirement is usually not compromised, excessive ketone production does not occur. Therapy of NKHS should include (1) the restoration of volume and osmolarity and (2) the management of hyperglycemia. Methods of treatment resemble those for DKA (see Insulin-Dependent [Type I] Diabetes Mellitus, sec. **II**).

A. **Diagnosis.** Patients often present with obtundation or coma, severe dehydration, and an underlying illness. Laboratory evaluation should reveal (1) hyperglycemia, often greater than 600 mg/dl; (2) absence of significant ketonemia; and (3) plasma osmolarity of greater than 320 mOsm/liter. Associated findings may include severe azotemia and lactic acidosis.

B. **Recognition of precipitating factors.** Considerations are similar to those for DKA. Insufficiency of insulin is often aggravated by glucocorticoids, and diuretic medications may augment volume depletion. An evaluation for infection and MI may be indicated. Repeated neurologic examination is important, because focal deficits or seizures may become apparent during therapy.

C. **Supportive measures** should include management specific to shock (see Chap. 9) and coma (see Chap. 25). Patients taking glucocorticoids should be given doses appropriate for severe stress (see Chap. 21), but high doses prescribed for treatment of other disease states should be tapered as permitted by their clinical indications.

D. **Monitoring of therapy.** It is appropriate initially to measure electrolytes hourly, and to assess blood glucose at half-hour intervals. Monitoring may be less frequent when improvement is evident, but care should be taken to avoid hypoglycemia.

E. **Fluid replacement. Initial therapy should correct the volume deficit,** and isotonic (0.9%) saline is appropriate. Initial fluids should be given without additives, and a rapid rate of administration is appropriate (e.g., 1 liter/hour or more) until the intravascular volume is restored. When serum sodium or osmolarity measurements become available to guide therapy, 0.45% saline may be given to correct a relative free water deficit. Caution is indicated in treatment of the elderly and of those with MI, heart failure, or renal insufficiency. Frequent clinical assessment is imperative; bladder catheterization and monitoring of CVP or PAOP may be needed. After volume is restored and hyperglycemia has responded to insulin therapy, a 5% dextrose in water (D/W) solution may be given to patients with persistent hyperosmolarity and hypernatremia. Maintenance fluids may be given at 100–250 ml/hour. Prolonged infusion of hypotonic solutions may be warranted, particularly for elderly patients with sustained hyperosmolarity (see Chap. 3).

F. **Electrolyte management.** Potassium deficit should be anticipated during insulin treatment and may be severe in patients taking thiazide or loop diuretics. A lactic acidosis often responds to volume replacement, but bicarbonate administration may be needed (e.g., for pH <7.2) when the lactic acidosis is secondary to necrotizing inflammation or sepsis, or when metformin has been prescribed. Considerations for electrolyte replacement and use of bicarbonate in maintenance IV fluids are similar to those for DKA. Serum phosphate concentration should be monitored.

G. **Insulin treatment** in NKHS restores normal glucose homeostasis; thus, blood glucose is the principal determinant of therapy. Regular insulin, 5–10 units IV, should be given initially when PG is greater than 600 mg/dl at presentation; smaller doses should be given when hyperglycemia is less marked. Insulin can then be given by IV infusion (or IM injection) to lower blood glucose gradually, approximately to 200 mg/dl, prior to initiation of SC insulin treatment.

Diabetes Mellitus in Pregnancy

Maintenance of normal blood glucose levels is particularly important in pregnancy. Patients with preexisting DM who become pregnant are particularly vulnerable to fetal complications, and maternal health can be compromised when diabetic complications occur. The outcome of a diabetic pregnancy can be improved by proper management. Ideal care includes the initiation of an intensive insulin regimen before conception, monitored by meticulous SMBG (i.e., 4–8 times daily) and documented with near-normal hemoglobin A_{1C} levels. The stress of pregnancy also may provoke gestational DM; these patients deserve a prompt diagnosis and specialized management (*Medical Management of Pregnancy Complicated by Diabetes*, American Diabetes Association, 1993).

I. **Diagnosis of gestational DM** may be suggested from symptoms or glycosuria, or from a screening glucose tolerance test revealing a PG of greater than 150 mg/dl 1 hour after a 50-g oral glucose load (recommended at 24–28 weeks in all pregnant women). Normal fasting PG in pregnancy is 60–80 mg/dl; DM may be diagnosed when a fasting PG is greater than 105 mg/dl on more than one occasion. When the fasting PG is equivocal, or when a screening test is positive, gestational DM may be established by a 100 g, 3-hour glucose tolerance test using specific criteria.

II. **Management of hyperglycemia** is facilitated by dietary modification and insulin treatment. Careful monitoring of blood glucose is an essential guide to therapy, because demands for insulin and the renal glucose threshold both change during pregnancy. Preprandial blood glucose values of less than 100 mg/dl are an achievable treatment objective, taking care to avoid hypoglycemia.

   A. **Dietary modification.** Caloric requirements in pregnancy are roughly 5 kcal/kg more than those in nonpregnant adults. Caloric reduction should not be used for glucose control, and some weight gain during pregnancy should be allowed. A limitation of refined carbohydrate is appropriate. Artificial sweeteners should be restricted, because safety in pregnancy has not been established. Protein intake should be sufficient (i.e., 1.5 g/kg). A consistent diet is usually prescribed, including 3 meals and a bedtime snack.

   B. **Insulin treatment** is usually required for pregnant patients with preexisting DM and should be used in gestational DM when dietary modification is inadequate. Insulin requirements vary during pregnancy. In general, requirements are lower in the first trimester, increase after 24 weeks, and drop suddenly in the immediate postpartum period; these changes require close monitoring.

      1. **Patients with preexisting DM** usually require 2 daily insulin injections, and most can benefit from MDII or CSII regimens (see Insulin-Dependent [Type I] Diabetes Mellitus). Human insulin should be used, and variations in pharmacokinetics of human insulins (see Diabetes Mellitus, sec. V) should be considered, particularly with long-acting insulins. The benefit from a bedtime snack may warrant early morning SMBG (e.g., 3:00 A.M.) to help discern fluctuating basal insulin requirements from the glycemic effect of the snack. A labile glycemic profile despite appropriate outpatient management may warrant hospitalization and use of continuous IV insulin therapy, particularly in the peripartum period (see Diabetes Mellitus in Surgical Patients, sec. I.D).

      2. **Patients with gestational diabetes** often do well with less intensive treatment. Management for most patients emulates that for type II DM (see Non–Insulin-Dependent [Type II] and Other Diabetes Mellitus), but hypocaloric diets for weight control should be deferred and oral antidiabetic drugs avoided.

III. **Diabetic ketoacidosis** may occur in pregnant patients and may be deleterious, if not fatal, to the fetus. Management is the same as for nonpregnant adults (see Insulin-Dependent [Type I] Diabetes Mellitus). Urine ketone assays are useful for screening, but morning ketonuria is common even among pregnant patients whose DM is well-controlled.

IV. **Assessment for chronic complications of diabetes** is important in pregnant patients, particularly among those with preexisting DM. Retinopathy and nephropathy may progress rapidly during pregnancy, potentially affecting both maternal and fetal health. Microvascular and macrovascular disease may limit placental circulation and must be considered during the high-risk obstetric assessment.

V. **Lactation** is associated with an increased caloric requirement, roughly 500 kcal/day more than that needed prior to pregnancy. The postpartum period is often a time when patients contemplate weight reduction, however, and this may affect control of DM. Management is facilitated by careful SMBG.

Diabetes Mellitus in
Surgical Patients

Surgery poses a significant stress to diabetic patients and often perturbs dietary management. Careful attention to blood glucose control is necessary to (1) avoid symptomatic hyperglycemia and acute complications (e.g., DKA, hypoglycemia) and (2) allow a normal inflammatory response and wound healing. It is prudent to maintain a blood glucose of 100–250 mg/dl in nonpregnant adults. Elective procedures should be postponed until control is achieved. When possible, minor surgery should be scheduled for early morning to minimize interruption of the usual treatment schedule.

I. **Modification of chronic therapy** should be guided by the patient's usual treatment and by the nature of the surgery. Blood glucose monitoring should be used to guide adjustments. Recommendations for the treatment of hyperglycemic exacerbations apply (see Diabetes Mellitus, sec. **III.F**). It is important to recognize the nutritional needs of surgical patients, and administration of 5% dextrose in IV solutions, enteral tube feedings, or parenteral nutrition should not be withheld because of hyperglycemia (see Chap. 2). It is prudent to consider patient education, including that needed for initiation of insulin therapy for patients not previously treated with insulin, when elective surgery is planned.

A. **Patients whose diabetes is managed with diet alone** often require no additional measures. Human insulin should be prescribed to treat patients with fasting or preprandial glucose greater than 200 mg/dl.

B. **Patients using oral hypoglycemic drugs** should discontinue them on the day preceding major surgery. Insulin should be used when control of hyperglycemia is needed. For a minor procedure not significantly perturbing the meal schedule, oral drugs may be used perioperatively, but they should be held on the morning of surgery and not restarted until reliable oral intake is evident (see Non–Insulin-Dependent [Type II] and Other Diabetes Mellitus, secs. **I.C.2, D.2,** and **E**).

C. **Insulin-treated patients** require dosage adjustments. Decisions about therapy should be related to the diagnostic type of diabetes and the nature of the surgical stress. When insulin is used a dextrose infusion should be available to avert hypoglycemia, and careful monitoring is imperative in the perioperative period.

1. **In insulin-dependent (Type I) diabetes,** maintenance of uninterrupted insulin administration is essential to prevent DKA. Care must be taken so that the basal insulin requirement is not compromised. In general, at least half of the usual daily insulin dose must be administered on the day of surgery and each postoperative day. All or part of the usual dietary insulin requirement may also be given if a diet is prescribed or when IV dextrose is administered. Administration of 5% dextrose in maintenance IV fluids is appropriate to limit lipolysis and ketogenesis in patients with restricted oral intake. Glucose monitoring is mandatory, and periodic measurement of plasma electrolytes and urinary ketones is also advised, as DKA can occur in a stressed, postoperative patient even when blood glucose is not markedly elevated.

a. **For patients using conventional therapy,** a dose of intermediate-acting insulin may be given in the morning before minor surgery, and then bid. Hyperglycemia may be managed with supplements of regular insulin, given q4–6h, and continued until oral intake is resumed. Mixed insulin may then be given, adjusted to dietary intake and blood glucose measurements.

b. **Among patients using MDII or CSII,** the preoperative basal insulin doses should be continued without interruption in the perioperative period. When oral intake is restricted, regular insulin may be given as above (see sec. **I.C.1.a**). When a diet is tolerated, the MDII or CSII regimen should be resumed with adjustments of regular insulin accommodating changes from the usual dietary regimen.

2. **In non–insulin-dependent (Type II) and other DM,** management should reflect the anticipated extent of insulin insufficiency. It may be appropriate to hold insulin in patients scheduled for minor procedures during morning hours, and to give modified therapy based on blood glucose and an anticipated diet after surgery. Patients with large exogenous insulin requirements (i.e., >50 units/day) and those undergoing major surgery should be given insulin preoperatively and in the immediate postoperative period, as guided by blood glucose levels. An appropriate prescription is for one-half to two-thirds of the

usual daily insulin dose as intermediate-acting insulin in anticipation of surgery, then short-acting insulin as needed to control blood glucose postoperatively.

D. **IV insulin infusion therapy** is a desirable alternative to SC insulin in the management of patients undergoing very stressful procedures (e.g., coronary artery bypass, renal transplant). An IV insulin infusion (see Diabetes Mellitus, sec. **V.A.1**) may be started preoperatively and can be continued through the procedure until hemodynamic stability and knowledge of the postoperative insulin requirements permit treatment with SC insulin (or oral antidiabetic drugs). The infusion may be started using half of the patient's usual daily insulin dose, prescribed in units/hour; 0.5–1.0 unit/hour is appropriate initially for patients not previously using insulin. Blood glucose should be measured hourly. For patients with type I DM, care must be taken when IV infusions are discontinued (see Insulin-Dependent [Type I] Diabetes Mellitus, sec. **II.L**).

II. **Emergency surgery** may be needed despite severe hyperglycemia, DKA, or NKHS. Intensive monitoring is indicated, and use of an IV insulin infusion is preferred in perioperative management. When possible, repletion of intravascular volume should precede surgery.

III. **Assessment for chronic complications of diabetes** is important in the perioperative period. Patients with cardiovascular disease and neuropathy are susceptible to asymptomatic MI. Patients with neuropathy are also particularly prone to development of decubitus ulcers, often of the heel, during periods of prolonged immobilization; prophylactic care is warranted. Enteropathy may alter GI responses to surgery and anesthesia.

Chronic Complications
of Diabetes Mellitus

The predisposition to long-term complications is characteristic of all types of DM, and the ability to forestall these complications with control of hyperglycemia suggests strongly that the diabetic state is of pathogenic significance in their evolution. In addition to glycemic control, there are appropriate preventive and palliative therapies (*Therapy for Diabetes Mellitus and Related Disorders* [2nd ed]. American Diabetes Association, 1994).

I. **Ophthalmic complications** of DM include diabetic retinopathy and diseases of the anterior chamber that affect vision. A yearly examination by an ophthalmologist is a minimum requirement for the detection of retinopathy; it is recommended beginning at 5 years after onset in type I DM and at the time of diagnosis in type II DM. Ophthalmologic consultation is also warranted for the management of any acute or progressive visual disturbance.

A. **Diabetic retinopathy** includes **nonproliferative retinopathy**, which is limited to the retina (i.e., microaneurysms, dot or blot hemorrhages, retinal infarcts, hard exudates), and **proliferative retinopathy** (i.e., neovascularization), which extends anterior to the retina and obscures visualization of the underlying retinal details. Diabetic macular edema may limit vision as a result of diabetic retinopathy at any stage. Patients with proliferative retinopathy are especially prone to acute visual loss. Retinal laser photocoagulation can reduce the incidence and retard the progression of visual impairment if employed before irreversible damage occurs. Vitrectomy may be beneficial to patients with an acute vitreous hemorrhage or a traction retinal detachment.

B. **Visual disturbance** may complicate retinopathy or may follow cataract formation, glaucoma, ischemic optic neuropathy, or paresis of the extraocular muscles. Acute monocular visual loss can be caused by hemorrhage, retinal detachment, or embolic retinal infarction. Bilateral visual loss suggests stroke, but may also result from a dominant monocular visual loss when vision in the nondominant eye is insidiously impaired. Blurring of vision may occur because of lens alterations that follow a change in mean PG; often this can take several weeks to resolve. Diplopia may indicate a cranial nerve palsy (i.e., nerves III, IV, VI). "Floaters," "spots," or "webs" may be the presenting descriptions of preretinal or vitreous hemorrhage and mandate prompt ophthalmologic evaluation.

II. **Diabetic neuropathy** may present with sensory symptoms or deficits, motor abnormalities, or autonomic dysfunction.

   A. **Pain** from mononeuropathy may occur in the distribution of a peripheral nerve, often with hyperesthesia. The differential diagnosis includes nerve entrapment and radiculopathy, which warrant specific management. There is no effective, specific therapy for painful diabetic neuropathy, but lowering of blood glucose may help patients with marked hyperglycemia. Success in treatment of chronic pain has been achieved with amitriptyline, 10–150 mg PO qhs. Side effects of amitriptyline may include constipation, postural hypotension, and urinary retention; caution should be used when any of these problems already exists as a manifestation of autonomic neuropathy. Application of capsaicin cream to areas afflicted with painful neuropathy may be helpful to some patients, although benefit may not be apparent until after months of treatment. Potent analgesic drugs may be needed for severe pain (see Chap. 1).

   B. **Sensory deficit** has no specific treatment. Patients must be educated to avoid complications in neuropathic extremities, including trauma, burns, bone injury, and ulcers (see sec. VIII).

   C. **Motor deficit** may result in muscle weakness and atrophy. Physical therapy may be helpful to patients with disability.

   D. **Autonomic neuropathy** may cause postural hypotension, persistent tachycardia, or neurogenic bladder and may contribute to GI complications and impotence. Impaired visceral pain sensation often can obscure symptoms of angina pectoris or MI.

      1. **Postural hypotension** should be treated symptomatically. Supportive measures include rising slowly from the supine or sitting position, particularly from bed in the morning, and limiting supine posturing by elevating the head of the bed at home. Some patients may respond to fludrocortisone, 0.1–0.3 mg PO qd, or sodium chloride, 1–4 g PO qid, or both. Care must be taken to limit supine hypertension, hypokalemia, and volume overload complicating this therapy. Postural changes in BP may interfere with effective treatment of hypertension; caution to avoid disabling symptoms is required when antihypertensive drugs are prescribed (see Chap. 4).

      2. **Neurogenic bladder,** which should be suspected in patients with recurrent urinary tract infection, requires management. Urinary retention is often not noticed by patients with DM and should be considered in treatment for other conditions. Manual pressure or intermittent catheterization (i.e., q3–6h during the day) may be required to promote urination.

      3. **Incontinence** of urine or feces may occur. Fecal incontinence must be distinguished from diarrhea; the latter may be more amenable to treatment (see sec. VI.A).

III. **Diabetic nephropathy** may result in proteinuria, hypertension, and a decline in the glomerular filtration rate (GFR), leading ultimately to renal failure. The course of nephropathy may be favorably altered by early intervention, complementing management of hyperglycemia, including dietary protein restriction, rigorous attention to BP control, and angiotensin-converting enzyme (ACE) inhibition.

   A. **Hypertension** is a manifestation of diabetic nephropathy, and, if untreated, may accelerate renal, retinal, cardiovascular, and cerebrovascular impairment (*Diabetes Care* 16:1394, 1993). The treatment of hypertension should be individualized (see Chap. 4).

   B. **ACE inhibitors** may be particularly beneficial for patients with diabetic nephropathy, reducing proteinuria and retarding progression to end-stage renal disease by means independent from reduction of BP (*N Engl J Med* 329:1456, 1993). These drugs may be of benefit in the management of normotensive, nonpregnant patients with DM who demonstrate microalbuminuria or elevated serum creatinine. Use should be monitored carefully (see sec. III.E and Chap. 11).

   C. **Iodinated IV contrast agents** impair GFR with increased frequency in patients with DM. When possible, diagnostic tests should be chosen to avoid the use of these chemicals. If an IV contrast agent is necessary, liberal hydration should be provided both before and after administration. Fluid balance and serum creatinine should be monitored.

D. **Urinary tract infections** should be treated aggressively (see Diabetes Mellitus, sec. III.H.1 and Chap. 13).

E. **Hyperkalemia** may result from renal failure, hyporeninemic hypoaldosteronism, or, in some patients, from insulin lack. Potassium-sparing diuretics, ACE inhibitors, and, rarely, beta-adrenergic antagonists may promote hyperkalemia; alternative drugs should be chosen when necessary. Acute treatment measures may be necessary (see Chap. 3). When hyperkalemia accompanies a hyperchloremic acidosis, patients may respond to fludrocortisone, 0.05–0.10 mg PO qd. Other patients may respond to insulin therapy.

F. **Management of renal failure** includes dietary modification and the treatment of volume overload, if present (see Chap. 11).

IV. **Macrovascular disease** is accelerated in diabetic patients, promoting increased risk for stroke and MI. Hypertension and hyperlipidemia should be treated as indicated (see Chaps. 4 and 22). Cigarette smoking should be discouraged. Peripheral vascular disease causes limb ischemia and predisposes patients to bacterial infections that are refractory to antimicrobial treatment. Surgical management is often warranted to treat symptomatic peripheral vascular disease (see sec. VIII); pentoxifylline, 400 mg PO tid, may be helpful when surgery is not appropriate.

V. **Coronary artery disease and MI** occur with increased frequency in DM. Heart disease must be considered when dyspnea or unexplained hyperglycemia occurs, even when other symptoms of angina pectoris are atypical or absent. Young age should not preclude the diagnosis of coronary artery disease (see Chap. 5). A yearly ECG should be obtained as part of routine care, and periodic evaluation with a stress test may be appropriate.

VI. **Diabetic enteropathy** is a manifestation of autonomic neuropathy, affecting GI motility.

A. **Diarrhea** in patients with DM warrants diagnostic evaluation (see Chap. 15); symptomatic therapy is appropriate when a correctable cause is not found. Bacterial overgrowth may respond to tetracycline, 250 mg PO qid.

B. **Impaired gastric emptying** may lead to recurrent nausea and vomiting. Patients may respond to cisapride, 10–20 mg PO 30–60 minutes ac and qhs, or metoclopramide, 10–20 mg PO 30–60 minutes ac and qhs. Long-term treatment with these drugs should be avoided when possible. Goals for glycemic control and methods of therapy for hyperglycemia should be reassessed when timing of nutrient delivery is unpredictable.

VII. **Impotence** in men may occur as a result of diabetic neuropathy or vascular disease; a multifactorial etiology is common, including psychological factors related to coping with chronic illness. Some patients will improve with careful glycemic control. For most men with diabetes and impotence, a specialist referral is appropriate for consideration of medical and surgical therapeutic options.

VIII. **The diabetic foot** is a manifestation of chronic neuropathy, aggravated in many cases by vascular insufficiency and infection. Sensory loss allows tolerance of repeated trauma from tight shoes and improper weight bearing, which leads to skin breakdown and ulceration, tissue necrosis, and fracture. Specialized treatment is often necessary to prevent and manage foot disease.

A. **Prophylactic foot care** includes properly fitting shoes, daily examination for injury, and care in the management of calluses and in nail cutting and cleaning.

B. **Patients with foot ulcers** must totally avoid local pressure to allow healing; hospitalization is often required to facilitate management with absence of weight bearing. Infection is common, and osteomyelitis can complicate deep ulcers. The most common pathogens are streptococci and *Staph. aureus*, but gram-negative and anaerobic bacteria (e.g., *Bacteroidies fragilis*) also infect these wounds. Debridement and broad-spectrum antimicrobials or combination antimicrobial regimens with uncompromised gram-positive activity are appropriate in initial therapy of infected ulcers (see Chap. 12). Surgical therapy of peripheral vascular disease may be warranted to allow healing. Amputation may be necessary to prevent recurrent septicemia and death, but a conservative approach to long-term management usually is preferred.

IX. **Depression** is prevalent in patients with DM, both at the time of diagnosis and with long-standing affliction. Treatment may include antidepressant medication, counseling, and involvement in diabetes support groups. Effective treatment of depression may result in an improvement in glycemic control (*J Nerv Ment Dis* 174:736, 1986).

Hypoglycemia

Hypoglycemia complicates therapy with sulfonylureas and insulin and may be a limiting factor of efforts to achieve glycemic control in DM. Management includes prompt treatment and preventive measures. Less commonly, hypoglycemia occurs in nondiabetic patients.

I. **Hypoglycemia in patients with diabetes** usually results from (1) a change in content or timing of meals, (2) an increase in physical activity, or (3) a medication overdosage. Severity is the most important determinant of treatment. Management should include a consideration of the peak effects and durations of action of the insulins or sulfonylureas prescribed (see Tables 20-2 and 20-3). Patients manifesting severe or recurrent hypoglycemia may have an impaired counterregulatory response of glucagon and epinephrine (*Diabetes* 30:260, 1981). The goals for glycemic control should be reassessed when frequent or severe hypoglycemia complicates therapy.

A. **Diagnosis**. Mild hypoglycemic reactions are characterized by irritability, tremulousness, diaphoresis, tachycardia, and confusion. These symptoms result in part from the secretion of epinephrine, a mediator of the counterregulatory response to falling glucose. Insufficient hypoglycemic counterregulation or medication overdose may allow more serious manifestations, such as seizure, stupor, coma, or focal neurologic findings. Plasma or blood glucose measurements, when available, should be used to validate symptomatic hypoglycemia.

B. **Treatment of hypoglycemic episodes** should be guided by (1) the mental status of the patient, (2) the level of blood glucose, and (3) the anticipated clinical course. Prolonged observation is warranted in sulfonylurea overdose. Frequent monitoring of blood glucose (e.g., q15–30min) should verify the efficacy of treatment until the period of vulnerability to recurrent hypoglycemia has passed.

1. **Oral carbohydrate** is sufficient for alert patients when drug overdose is not evident. Oral glucose, sucrose, and potent sugar-containing fluids are effective but can often produce hyperglycemia. One cup (8 oz) of milk, 4 oz of juice without additives, a piece of fruit, a granola bar, or cheese and soda crackers are usually adequate for the treatment of mild hypoglycemia detected by glucose monitoring or from mild adrenergic symptoms. More potent treatments may be considered when the initial response is not sufficient, when gastroparesis is suspected, or when the ability to maintain oral intake is impaired.

2. **IV dextrose** should be given to inpatients when oral intake is restricted, mental function is impaired, medication overdosage is suspected, or a predisposition to prolonged hypoglycemia is anticipated. Initially, 50% dextrose, 25–50 ml, should be given, followed by an infusion of 5–10% D/W to maintain blood glucose greater than 100 mg/dl.

3. **Glucagon**, 1 mg IM (or SC), may be given to treat severe hypoglycemia in outpatients, when complicated by stupor or an inability to tolerate oral treatment, or in inpatients, when oral intake is restricted and there is no IV access available. Glucagon may cause vomiting, and care should be taken to prevent aspiration of gastric contents. Patients who are prone to severe hypoglycemia should have glucagon available for home use; a family member or roommate must be instructed in preparation and injection techniques.

C. **Adjustments of drug therapy** should be aimed at prevention of recurrence of hypoglycemia. Reduction of sulfonylurea dosage is appropriate. A change in the distribution and timing of insulin injections is indicated when hypoglycemia recurs at a particular time of day, but a total daily dose reduction is indicated when hypoglycemia is severe, prolonged, or unpredictable.

D. **Adjustments of diet and physical activity** may be an alternative to changing drug dosage. Carbohydrate intake may be increased or activity reduced at times when recurrent low blood glucose is demonstrated (see Diabetes Mellitus, secs. III.C and III.D).

E. **Hypoglycemia unawareness** is a complication and a potential cause of frequent insulin-induced hypoglycemia. Often with impaired hypoglycemic counterregulation mechanisms, patients afflicted with hypoglycemia unawareness do not develop normal adrenergic symptoms of falling blood glucose levels and are predisposed to insidious development of stupor or coma, heralded by diaphoresis in some cases. Goals for glycemic control among patients with hypoglycemia unawareness must be considered carefully; intensive regimens are not advised when frequent or severe hypoglycemia is threatened. SMBG is a vital management tool for these patients. A patient's recognition of hypoglycemic symptoms may be improved after an interval of less aggressive insulin treatment with a flawless avoidance of hypoglycemia (*Diabetes* 42:1683, 1993). Beta-adrenergic antagonists may contribute to hypoglycemia unawareness; alternative therapy should be chosen when severe or recurrent hypoglycemia occurs in patients taking these drugs.

II. **Spontaneous hypoglycemia** may occur in patients who are not using insulin or oral hypoglycemic drugs. **Fasting hypoglycemia** occurs when hepatic glucose production does not keep up with cellular glucose uptake. Normal adults can maintain blood glucose during 72 hours of fasting. Hypoglycemia may result from an insulinoma, severe liver disease, alcohol intoxication, adrenocortical insufficiency, hypothyroidism, growth hormone deficiency, or malnutrition among patients with renal failure. Presenting symptoms may include dementia, seizures, or bizarre behavior. Therapy should be directed to the specific cause. **Postprandial hypoglycemia** occurs from action of insulin secreted in response to meals. Symptoms are like those of mild insulin-induced hypoglycemia (see sec. I). Postprandial hypoglycemia may occur as a sequel to partial gastrectomy; symptoms appear 1–2 hours after meals. Functional hypoglycemic symptoms, with or without measurable hypoglycemia, may also occur in individuals without antecedent surgery and are often later (e.g., 3–5 hours) in the postprandial period. Some of these patients may manifest impaired glucose tolerance, and dietary management appropriate for diabetes mellitus may be helpful (see Diabetes Mellitus, secs. I.B and III.C).

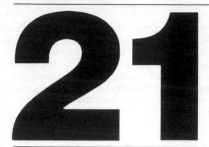

Endocrine Diseases

William E. Clutter

Evaluation of Thyroid Function

The major hormone secreted by the thyroid gland is **thyroxine (T_4)**, which is converted in many tissues to **triiodothyronine (T_3)**, a more potent hormone. This conversion is inhibited by illness, surgery, trauma, and some drugs. Both thyroid hormones are reversibly bound to plasma proteins, primarily **thyroxine-binding globulin (TBG)**. Only the minute unbound fraction enters cells and produces biological effects, and regulatory mechanisms keep this free thyroid hormone concentration within a narrow normal range. Conventional thyroid hormone assays measure total (bound plus unbound) hormone, but total and free hormone concentrations correlate well except in conditions that **increase TBG levels** (e.g., estrogen therapy, pregnancy, acute or chronic active hepatitis, and familial TBG excess) or **decrease TBG levels** (e.g., severe liver disease, malnutrition, nephrotic syndrome, androgen therapy, and familial TBG deficiency). T_4 secretion is stimulated by **thyroid-stimulating hormone (TSH)** produced by the pituitary gland. In turn, TSH secretion is inhibited by T_4, forming an extremely sensitive negative feedback loop. Even small changes in circulating T_4 levels, within the reference range, cause large reciprocal changes in plasma TSH levels.

I. **Diagnostic tests** (*Med Clin North Am* 75:1, 1991). Diagnosis of thyroid disease is based on clinical findings, palpation of the thyroid gland, and measurement of plasma TSH and thyroid hormones. The latter tests cannot be interpreted without clinical information.

   A. **Thyroid gland palpation** should be performed with the patient's neck slightly extended, with the examiner standing behind the patient. The size and consistency of the thyroid are noted, as well as the presence of nodules, tenderness, or a thrill.

   B. **Plasma TSH.** The sensitive negative feedback relationship between thyroid hormone levels and TSH secretion means that **plasma TSH assay is the most useful diagnostic test in patients with suspected thyroid disease**. Currently available tests are **second-generation TSH assays** that are able to measure subnormal TSH levels to a detection limit of 0.1 µU/ml. TSH levels are elevated in **primary hypothyroidism** (due to disease of the thyroid itself) and suppressed to less than 0.1 µU/ml in **hyperthyroidism** (even in the presence of mild or **subclinical hyperthyroidism**—i.e., thyroid hormone excess too mild to cause symptoms). Thus, **a normal plasma TSH level excludes both hyperthyroidism and primary hypothyroidism** with a high degree of certainty.

   1. **Sensitivity of plasma TSH.** TSH levels are usually within the reference range in **secondary hypothyroidism** (due to TSH deficiency) and are not useful to detect this rare form of hypothyroidism. Treatment with dopamine or high doses of glucocorticoids suppresses TSH secretion and may cause falsely normal levels in primary hypothyroidism.

   2. **Specificity of plasma TSH.** Because even very mild changes in thyroid hormone levels affect TSH secretion, **abnormal TSH levels are not specific for clinically important thyroid disease**, which should be confirmed by measurement of plasma thyroid hormone levels (usually plasma T_4).

a. Plasma **TSH may be mildly elevated** (up to 20 μU/ml) in some euthyroid patients with nonthyroidal illness and in subclinical hypothyroidism.

b. **TSH levels may be suppressed** to less than 0.1 μU/ml in nonthyroidal illness, with treatment with dopamine or high doses of glucocorticoids, with subclinical hyperthyroidism, and in some euthyroid elderly patients. Furthermore, TSH levels remain less than 0.1 μU/ml for some time after hyperthyroidism is corrected.

C. **Plasma T$_4$.** The major role of plasma T$_4$ measurements is to confirm the diagnosis of clinical hypothyroidism in patients with an elevated plasma TSH and to confirm the diagnosis and determine the severity of hyperthyroidism when plasma TSH is less than 0.1 μU/ml. Abnormal levels of plasma TBG affect plasma T$_4$ levels without affecting free T$_4$ concentrations, and the extent of plasma hormone binding is usually assessed along with plasma T$_4$. This is most often done with the **T$_3$ resin uptake (T$_3$RU)**, which varies inversely with plasma thyroid hormone–binding capacity. The **T$_4$ index** is the product of plasma T$_4$ and T$_3$RU. It provides an imperfect estimate of free T$_4$ concentration.

D. **Plasma free T$_4$ measured by equilibrium dialysis (free T$_4$-ED)** is the most reliable measure of clinical thyroid status, but results are seldom rapidly available. It is used only in rare cases where the diagnosis is not clear from measurement of plasma TSH and T$_4$. Other types of free T$_4$ assays are not reliable in nonthyroidal illness, which is the major indication for measuring plasma free T$_4$ (*Clin Chem* 37:2002, 1991).

II. **Effect of nonthyroidal illness on thyroid function tests** (*JAMA* 263:1529, 1990). Many illnesses alter thyroid tests, without apparently causing true thyroid dysfunction. It is important to recognize these situations to avoid mistaken diagnosis and therapy.

A. **The low T$_3$ syndrome** occurs in most illness, during starvation, and after trauma or surgery. Conversion of T$_4$ to T$_3$ is decreased and plasma T$_3$ levels are low. It may be an adaptive response to illness; thyroid hormone therapy is not beneficial.

B. **The low T$_4$ syndrome** occurs in severe illness. It may be due to decreased TBG levels, inhibition of T$_4$ binding to TBG, or to suppression of TSH secretion. TSH levels decrease early in severe illness, sometimes to less than 0.1 μU/ml. During recovery they rise, sometimes above the normal range (although rarely higher than 20 μU/ml).

C. **The high T$_4$ syndrome** occurs, though rarely, in acute medical or psychiatric illness. In some cases it is due to increased TBG levels. Plasma TSH levels are not suppressed to less than 0.1 μU/ml, excluding hyperthyroidism.

III. **Effect of drugs on thyroid function tests** (*Med Clin North Am* 75:27, 1991). **Iodine-containing drugs** (such as amiodarone and radiographic contrast agents) may cause hyperthyroidism or hypothyroidism in susceptible patients. Many drugs alter thyroid function tests, especially plasma T$_4$, without causing true thyroid dysfunction. In general, plasma TSH levels are a reliable guide for determining whether true hyper- or hypothyroidism is present.

Hypothyroidism

Hypothyroidism is a common disorder, affecting women most often. Its prevalence increases with age. Subclinical hypothyroidism, in which thyroid function is impaired but normal serum T$_4$ levels are maintained by increased secretion of TSH, is more common than overt clinical hypothyroidism.

I. **Causes. Primary hypothyroidism** accounts for more than 90% of cases. **Chronic lymphocytic thyroiditis (Hashimoto's disease)** is the most common cause of primary hypothyroidism. **Iatrogenic hypothyroidism** due to thyroidectomy or radioactive iodine therapy is also common. Transient hypothyroidism occurs in postpartum and subacute thyroiditis, usually after a period of hyperthyroidism. Drugs (e.g., iodine, lithium, alpha-interferon, and interleukin-2) may cause hy-

Table 21-1. Effects of drugs on thyroid function tests

Effect	Drug
Decreased T$_4$	
True hypothyroidism (TSH elevated)	Iodine (amiodarone, radiographic contrast)
	Lithium
Decreased TBG (TSH normal)	Androgens
Inhibition of T$_4$ binding to TBG (TSH normal)	Furosemide (high doses)
	Salicylates
Inhibition of TSH secretion	Glucocorticoids
	Dopamine
Multiple mechanisms (TSH normal)	Phenytoin
Increased T$_4$	
True hyperthyroidism (TSH <0.1 μU/ml)	Iodine (amiodarone, radiographic contrast)
Increased TBG (TSH normal)	Estrogens, tamoxifen
Inhibited T$_4$ to T$_3$ conversion (TSH normal)	Amiodarone
	Propranolol (high doses)
	Oral cholecystographic agents

pothyroidism. **Secondary hypothyroidism** is uncommon but may occur in any disorder of the pituitary or hypothalamus, including tumors, surgery, or radiation therapy. However, it rarely occurs without other evidence of pituitary disease.

II. **Clinical findings.** Most symptoms of hypothyroidism are nonspecific and develop gradually. They include **cold intolerance**, fatigue, somnolence, poor memory, constipation, menorrhagia, myalgias, and hoarseness. Signs include **slow tendon reflex relaxation**, bradycardia, facial and periorbital edema, dry skin, and nonpitting edema (myxedema). Mild weight gain may occur, but hypothyroidism does not cause marked obesity. Rare manifestations include hypoventilation, pericardial or pleural effusions, deafness, and carpal tunnel syndrome. Laboratory findings may include hyponatremia and elevated plasma levels of cholesterol, triglycerides, and creatine kinase. The ECG may show low voltage and T wave abnormalities.

III. **Diagnosis.** Hypothyroidism is a readily treatable disorder that should be suspected in any patient with compatible symptoms, especially if there is a goiter or a history of radioactive iodine therapy or thyroid surgery.

A. **In suspected primary hypothyroidism, plasma TSH is the best initial diagnostic test.** A normal value excludes primary hypothyroidism, and a markedly elevated value (>20 μU/ml) confirms the diagnosis. If plasma TSH is moderately elevated (<20 μU/ml), the plasma T$_4$ index should be measured. A low T$_4$ index confirms clinical hypothyroidism, while a clearly normal T$_4$ index with an elevated plasma TSH indicates subclinical hypothyroidism, which is unlikely to account for symptoms, especially nonspecific ones such as fatigue and weight gain.

B. **If secondary hypothyroidism is suspected** because of evidence of pituitary disease, the plasma T$_4$ index should be measured, since plasma TSH levels are usually within the reference range and cannot establish this diagnosis (see Anterior Pituitary Gland Disorders, sec. III.B). Patients with secondary hypothyroidism should be evaluated for other pituitary hormone deficits and for a mass lesion of the pituitary or hypothalamus.

C. **In patients with severe nonthyroidal illness,** plasma T$_4$ and T$_4$ index are often low, and it may be difficult to determine whether hypothyroidism is present.
   1. **Plasma TSH is the best initial diagnostic test.** Marked elevation of plasma TSH (>20μU/ml) establishes the diagnosis of primary hypothyroidism. A

normal TSH value is strong evidence that the patient is euthyroid, except in patients with evidence of pituitary or hypothalamic disease or in patients treated with dopamine or high doses of glucocorticoids. Moderate elevations of plasma TSH (<20 μU/ml) may occur in euthyroid patients with nonthyroidal illness and are not specific for hypothyroidism.

2. **Plasma free T_4 by equilibrium dialysis** should be measured in the few cases where it is still unclear whether the patient is hypothyroid. Normal free T_4 levels exclude hypothyroidism, and patients with low plasma free T_4 should be treated for hypothyroidism. Rarely, it may be impossible to determine whether hypothyroidism is present during the illness. In this case, the best approach is to reevaluate thyroid function several weeks after resolution of the illness.

D. **Differential diagnosis.** It is important to distinguish between primary and secondary hypothyroidism since patients with the latter should be evaluated for hypopituitarism. This distinction is easily made with plasma TSH, which is elevated in primary, but not in secondary, hypothyroidism. However, **plasma TSH is seldom below the reference range in secondary hypothyroidism and cannot be used alone to make this diagnosis.**

IV. **Therapy** (*Ann Intern Med* 119:492, 1993; *N Engl J Med* 331:174, 1994). **Thyroxine** is the drug of choice. The usual replacement dose is 100–125 μg PO qd, and most patients require doses between 75 and 150 μg qd. In elderly patients, the replacement dose is somewhat lower. The need for lifelong treatment should be emphasized.

A. **Initiation of therapy.** Young, otherwise healthy adults should be started on 100 μg qd. This produces gradual correction of hypothyroidism, since several weeks of therapy are required to reach steady-state plasma levels of T_4. Symptoms of hypothyroidism begin to improve within a few weeks. In otherwise healthy, **elderly patients**, the initial dose should be 50 μg qd. **Patients with heart disease** should be started on 25 μg qd and monitored carefully for exacerbation of cardiac symptoms.

B. **Dose adjustment**

1. **In primary hypothyroidism, the goal of therapy is to maintain plasma TSH within the normal range.** It may take several months for elevated plasma TSH levels to return to normal with therapy, so there is little value in laboratory monitoring during this time if symptoms improve (*Ann Intern Med* 113:450, 1990). Plasma TSH should be measured after 3–4 months of therapy. The dose of thyroxine is adjusted up or down in 25-μg increments if plasma TSH is abnormal. Further adjustments are made in 12- to 25-μg increments based on testing at 6- to 8-week intervals until plasma TSH is normal. Excessive replacement of thyroxine, indicated by a subnormal TSH, should be avoided since it may accelerate loss of bone density and contribute to osteoporosis (*J Clin Endocrinol Metab* 78:816, 1994).

2. **In secondary hypothyroidism, plasma TSH cannot be used to adjust therapy.** The goal of therapy is to maintain the **plasma T_4 index** near the middle of the reference range. The dose of thyroxine should be adjusted based on T_4 index measurements at 6- to 8-week intervals until this goal is achieved. Thereafter, annual measurement of the T_4 index is adequate to monitor therapy.

3. **Coronary artery disease** may be exacerbated by treatment of hypothyroidism. In patients with coronary artery disease, the initial dose should be 25 μg qd and the dose should be increased slowly, with careful attention for worsening of angina, heart failure, or arrhythmias. In many cases, hypothyroidism can be corrected without difficulty, but if cardiac symptoms worsen despite medical therapy, coronary revascularization should be considered and can be done safely in hypothyroid patients (*Endocr Rev* 6:432, 1985).

4. **Adrenal failure** may be associated with both primary and secondary hypothyroidism and can be exacerbated by thyroid hormone replacement. If nausea, vomiting, or orthostatic hypotension develop after starting therapy, the patient should be tested for adrenal failure (see Adrenal Failure).

C. **Annual follow-up** is warranted in patients with treated hypothyroidism, to ensure continued compliance with thyroxine replacement and allow for adjustment of the dose if necessary. Measurement of plasma TSH alone is sufficient for monitoring therapy.

D. Difficulty in controlling hypothyroidism despite dose adjustment is most often due to **poor compliance** with therapy. Observed therapy may be necessary in some cases. Other causes of increasing thyroxine requirement include (1) **malabsorption** due to intestinal disease or drugs (e.g., cholestyramine, sucralfate, aluminum hydroxide, ferrous sulfate, and lovastatin) that interfere with thyroxine absorption; (2) **other drug interactions** that increase thyroxine clearance (e.g., rifampin, carbamazepine, phenytoin) or block conversion of T_4 to T_3 (e.g., amiodarone); (3) **pregnancy**, in which thyroxine requirement increases in the first trimester; and (4) a gradual decrease in remaining endogenous thyroid function after treatment of hyperthyroidism.

E. Subclinical hypothyroidism, with moderately elevated plasma TSH but normal plasma T_4 levels, is unlikely to be responsible for nonspecific symptoms such as fatigue or weight gain. Some patients experience improvement in symptoms with thyroid hormone replacement, although the possibility of a placebo response should be kept in mind. Such patients are at increased risk of developing overt hypothyroidism, although the rate of progression is usually slow.

F. Surgery. Although patients with hypothyroidism have an increased risk of minor perioperative complications, there is little increase in the risk of serious complications or mortality (*Am J Med* 77:261, 1984). Emergency surgery need not be delayed, but treatment of hypothyroidism should be initiated (see sec. **IV.A**); the initial doses can be given IV. Elective surgery should be postponed until euthyroidism is restored.

G. Emergency therapy of hypothyroidism is rarely necessary. Most patients with hypothyroidism and concomitant illness can be treated in the usual manner (see sec. **IV.A and B**). However, hypothyroidism may impair survival in patients with severe illnesses by contributing to hypoventilation, hypothermia, bradycardia, hypotension, or hyponatremia. There is little evidence to support the contention that severe hypothyroidism alone causes coma or shock.

    1. Confirmatory tests (including serum TSH, T_4 index, and free T_4-ED) should be performed before thyroid hormone therapy is started if hypothyroidism is suspected in a severely ill patient.

    2. Hypoventilation and hypotension should be intensively treated, along with any concomitant illnesses.

    3. Thyroxine, 50–100 µg IV, may be given q6–8h for 24 hours, followed by 75–100 µg IV qd until oral intake is possible. Replacement therapy should be continued in the usual manner if the diagnosis of hypothyroidism is confirmed, and therapy should be discontinued if testing does not support the diagnosis of hypothyroidism. No clinical trials have determined the best method of thyroid hormone replacement in such patients, but this method rapidly alleviates thyroxine deficiency while minimizing the risk of exacerbating underlying coronary disease or heart failure. **Such rapid correction is warranted only in extremely ill patients**; in all others, gradual correction is safer.

    4. Vital signs and cardiac rhythm should be monitored frequently to detect exacerbation of heart disease.

    5. Hydrocortisone, 100 mg IV q8h, is usually recommended during rapid treatment with thyroid hormone on the grounds that such therapy may precipitate adrenal failure.

Hyperthyroidism

I. Causes (Table 21-2). **Graves' disease** causes the majority of cases, especially in young patients. This autoimmune disorder, in which thyroid-stimulating immuno-

Table 21-2. Major causes of hyperthyroidism

Common
    Graves' disease
    Toxic multinodular goiter
Uncommon
    Thyroid adenoma (single nodule)
    Transient
        Postpartum silent thyroiditis
        Subacute thyroiditis
        Iodine-induced
    Factitious

globulins activate the TSH receptor, may also cause two manifestations not found in other causes of hyperthyroidism: proptosis (exophthalmos) and pretibial myxedema. **Toxic multinodular goiter** is a common cause of hyperthyroidism in older patients. Hyperthyroidism may be precipitated by iodine-containing drugs (e.g., amiodarone) or radiographic contrast media, usually in the setting of preexisting nontoxic goiter. **Painless thyroiditis** is common in the postpartum period; it causes transient hyperthyroidism followed by transient hypothyroidism. **Subacute thyroiditis** causes a painful, tender goiter and transient mild hyperthyroidism. TSH-induced hyperthyroidism is extremely rare, and almost all patients with hyperthyroidism have markedly suppressed plasma TSH values.

II. Clinical findings. Symptoms include heat intolerance, weight loss, weakness, palpitations, oligomenorrhea, frequent stools, and anxiety. **Signs** include brisk tendon reflexes, fine tremor, proximal weakness, stare, and lid lag. Cardiac abnormalities may be prominent, including sinus tachycardia, atrial fibrillation, and exacerbation of coronary artery disease or heart failure. In the elderly, hyperthyroidism may cause only nonspecific findings, such as atrial fibrillation, heart failure, weakness, or weight loss, and a high index of suspicion is needed to make the diagnosis.

III. Diagnosis. Hyperthyroidism should be suspected in any patient with compatible symptoms, since it is a readily treatable disorder that may become very debilitating.

  A. Plasma TSH is the best initial diagnostic test. A TSH level greater than 0.1 μU/ml excludes clinical hyperthyroidism. If plasma TSH is less than 0.1 μU/ml, the plasma T_4 index should be measured to determine the severity of hyperthyroidism and a baseline for therapy. If the plasma T_4 or T_4 index is elevated, the diagnosis of clinical hyperthyroidism is established.

  B. If plasma TSH is less than 0.1 μU/ml, but the T_4 index is normal, the patient may have clinical hyperthyroidism, but other diagnoses should be considered.

    1. Elevation of plasma T_3 alone may cause clinical hyperthyroidism, so plasma T_3 should be measured.

    2. Plasma TBG may be low, indicated by a high T_3RU. In this case, plasma free T_4-ED should be measured to determine whether clinical hyperthyroidism is present.

    3. Nonthyroidal illness, therapy with dopamine, or high doses of glucocorticoids may suppress plasma TSH to less than 0.1 μU/ml. This occurs in about 3% of hospitalized patients (*Clin Chem* 33:1391, 1987). A **third-generation TSH assay** with a detection limit of 0.01 μU/ml may be helpful in evaluating patients with suppressed TSH and nonthyroidal illness. Most patients with clinical hyperthyroidism have plasma TSH levels less than 0.01 μU/ml in such assays, while nonthyroidal illness rarely suppresses TSH to this degree (*J Clin Endocr Metab* 70:453, 1990).

    4. Subclinical hyperthyroidism may suppress TSH to less than 0.1 μU/ml. Thus, a suppressed TSH level alone does not confirm that symptoms are due to hyperthyroidism.

Table 21-3. Differential diagnosis of hyperthyroidism

Nature of goiter

Diffuse, nontender: Graves' disease (rarely postpartum silent thyroiditis)
Multiple nodules: Toxic multinodular goiter
Single nodule: Thyroid adenoma
Tender, painful: Subacute thyroiditis
Normal thyroid: Graves' disease (rarely postpartum thyroiditis or factitious)
Proptosis or pretibial myxedema: Graves' disease

C. **Differential diagnosis** (Table 21-3). The cause of hyperthyroidism should be determined to guide therapy. Differential diagnosis is based on the following:

1. The presence of **proptosis** or **pretibial myxedema** indicates Graves' disease (although many patients with Graves' disease lack these signs).

2. Careful **palpation of the thyroid**. A diffuse, nontender goiter is consistent with Graves' disease but may also be due to postpartum silent thyroiditis.

3. History of recent **pregnancy, neck pain,** or **iodine** administration may suggest other possible causes of hyperthyroidism.

4. In most cases, the diagnosis is clear from clinical findings. In a few cases, **24-hour radioactive iodine uptake** (RAIU) is needed to distinguish Graves' disease or toxic multinodular goiter (in which RAIU is elevated) from postpartum thyroiditis, subacute thyroiditis, iodine-induced hyperthyroidism, or factitious hyperthyroidism (in which RAIU is very low). **Thyroid scans are not useful in the diagnosis of hyperthyroidism.**

IV. **Therapy.** Some forms of hyperthyroidism, such as silent thyroiditis or subacute thyroiditis, are transient and require only symptomatic therapy. There are three methods for definitive therapy: radioactive iodine, thionamides, and subtotal thyroidectomy, none of which controls symptoms of hyperthyroidism immediately. During treatment, patients are followed by clinical evaluation and measurement of plasma T_4. Measurement of plasma TSH is useless in assessing the initial response to therapy, since it remains suppressed until after the patient becomes euthyroid. Regardless of which therapy is used, all patients with Graves' disease require lifelong follow-up for recurrent hyperthyroidism or development of hypothyroidism.

A. **Propranolol** or other beta-adrenergic antagonists **relieve symptoms** of hyperthyroidism such as palpitations, tremor, and anxiety. They are used to improve well-being while definitive therapy of hyperthyroidism is being administered, or until transient forms of hyperthyroidism subside. The initial dose of propranolol, 20–40 mg PO qid, is adjusted to alleviate symptoms and tachycardia. Beta-adrenergic antagonist therapy should be gradually reduced, then stopped as hyperthyroidism is controlled. **Verapamil** at an initial dose of 40–80 mg PO tid may be used to control tachycardia in patients with contraindications to beta-adrenergic antagonists (e.g., obstructive lung disease) (*Acta Endocrinol* 128:297, 1993).

B. **Radioactive iodine (RAI, ^{131}I) therapy** is a simple, highly effective treatment for hyperthyroidism. It is concentrated in the thyroid, impairing hormone synthesis and cell replication. A single dose permanently controls hyperthyroidism in about 90% of patients, and further doses can be given if necessary. **RAI therapy is contraindicated in pregnancy,** but it is the treatment of choice for most adults.

1. **Method.** A **pregnancy test** should be performed before therapy in potentially fertile women. Twenty-four-hour RAIU is measured to calculate the dose that is given orally. Antithyroid drugs interfere with RAI therapy and should be discontinued at least 3 days before treatment. If iodine treatment has been administered, it should be stopped at least 2 weeks before RAI therapy. Most patients with Graves' disease are treated with about 8–10 mCi, while treatment of toxic multinodular goiter requires higher doses.

2. **Follow-up.** Several months are usually needed to restore euthyroidism.

Patients should be evaluated at 4- to 6-week intervals, with assessment of clinical findings and plasma T_4, until thyroid function stabilizes within the normal range or symptomatic hypothyroidism develops. The interval between follow-up visits is then gradually increased to annual intervals. **If symptomatic hyperthyroidism persists** after 6 months, a second RAI treatment is given. **If symptomatic hypothyroidism develops,** thyroxine therapy should be initiated (see Hypothyroidism, sec. **IV.A**). Mild hypothyroidism after RAI therapy may be transient and, if the patient is not symptomatic, can be observed for a further 4–6 weeks to determine if it will resolve spontaneously.

3. **Side effects. Hypothyroidism** occurs in 10–30% of patients within the first year following RAI therapy and continues to occur at a rate of about 3%/year thereafter. A slight rise in plasma T_4 may occur in the first 2 weeks after therapy, due to release of stored hormone, but almost never causes clinically evident hyperthyroidism. This increase in T_4 levels is potentially important only in patients with **severe cardiac disease,** who should be treated with thionamides to restore euthyroidism and deplete stored hormone before treatment with RAI. There is no convincing evidence that RAI or any other therapy for Graves' disease affects the course of Graves' ophthalmopathy. RAI therapy does not increase the risk of malignancy in the thyroid or elsewhere, and no increase in the risk of congenital abnormalities has been found in the offspring of women who conceive after RAI therapy. The radiation exposure to the ovaries from RAI therapy is low, comparable to that from many common diagnostic radiographs. Excessive concern for potential teratogenic effects of RAI should not influence physicians' advice to patients.

C. **Thionamides** (*N Engl J Med* 311:1353, 1984). Methimazole and propylthiouracil (PTU) inhibit thyroid hormone synthesis. PTU also inhibits extrathyroidal conversion of T_4 to T_3. Once thyroid hormone stores are depleted (after several weeks to months), T_4 levels decrease. These drugs have no permanent effect on thyroid function, and **in the majority of patients with Graves' disease, hyperthyroidism recurs after therapy is stopped,** usually within 6 months. Spontaneous remission of Graves' disease occurs in about one-third of patients during thionamide therapy, and in this minority, no other treatment may be necessary. Remission is more likely in mild hyperthyroidism of recent onset.

1. **Initiation of therapy.** Before they begin therapy, patients must be warned of the symptoms of life-threatening side effects and the need to promptly stop the drug and contact their physician if these symptoms develop (see sec. **IV.C.2**). Usual starting doses are PTU, 100 mg PO tid, or methimazole, 10–30 mg PO qd; higher initial doses may be used in severe hyperthyroidism.

2. **Side effects** are most likely to occur within the first few months of therapy. **Minor side effects** include rash, urticaria, fever, arthralgias, and transient leukopenia. **Agranulocytosis** occurs in about 0.5% of patients treated with thionamides. Other life-threatening side effects include **hepatitis, vasculitis,** and **drug-induced lupus erythematosus.** These complications usually resolve if the drug is stopped promptly. **Patients must be warned to stop the drug immediately if they develop jaundice or symptoms suggestive of agranulocytosis (e.g., fever, chills, sore throat, bleeding gums)** and to contact their physician promptly for evaluation. Routine monitoring of WBC is not useful for detecting agranulocytosis, which usually develops suddenly.

3. **Follow-up.** Restoration of euthyroidism may take several months. Patients should be evaluated at 4-week intervals, with assessment of clinical findings and plasma T_4. If there is no decrease in plasma T_4 following 4–8 weeks of therapy, the dose should be increased. Doses as high as PTU, 300 mg PO qid, or methimazole, 60 mg PO qd, may be required. Once plasma T_4 falls to normal, the dose is adjusted to maintain plasma T_4 within the normal range. There is no general agreement on the optimal duration of therapy. Some physicians treat patients for an arbitrary period of time after euthyroidism is restored (e.g., 6–12 months); others stop therapy when euthyroidism is restored. Regardless of the duration of therapy, patients must be carefully monitored for recurrence of hyperthyroidism after the drug is stopped.

D. Subtotal thyroidectomy provides long-term control of hyperthyroidism in most patients. Because of the risk of surgical morbidity and mortality, this procedure should be reserved for patients unwilling to be treated with RAI and whose hyperthyroidism cannot be controlled with antithyroid drugs.

1. Surgery may trigger a perioperative exacerbation of hyperthyroidism, and patients should be prepared for surgery by one of two methods.

a. A thionamide is given until the patient is nearly euthyroid (see sec **IV.C**). Supersaturated potassium iodide (SSKI), 40–80 mg (1–2 gtt) PO bid, is then added, and surgery is scheduled 1–2 weeks later. Both drugs are discontinued after surgery.

b. Propranolol, 40 mg PO qid, and SSKI, 1–2 gtt PO bid, are started 1–2 weeks before surgery is scheduled. The dose of propranolol is increased, if necessary, to reduce the resting heart rate below 90 beats/minute. Propranolol, but not SSKI, is continued for 5–7 days postoperatively. Although there is less experience with this method, it usually produces satisfactory results.

2. Follow-up. Patients are evaluated at 4- to 6-week intervals, with assessment of clinical findings and plasma T_4, until thyroid function stabilizes within the normal range or symptomatic hypothyroidism develops. The interval between follow-up visits is then gradually increased to annual intervals. **If symptomatic hypothyroidism develops,** thyroxine therapy should be initiated (see Hypothyroidism, sec. **IV.A**). Mild hypothyroidism after subtotal thyroidectomy may be transient, and, if the patient is not symptomatic, can be observed for 4–6 weeks to determine if it will resolve spontaneously. Hyperthyroidism persists or recurs in 3–7% of patients.

3. Side effects of thyroidectomy include **hypothyroidism** in 30–50% of patients and **hypoparathyroidism** in about 3%. Rare complications include permanent vocal cord paralysis due to recurrent laryngeal nerve injury and perioperative death. The complication rate appears to depend on the experience of the surgeon.

E. Choice of therapy

1. In Graves' disease, the choice of initial therapy is between RAI and thionamides. **RAI therapy** is simple and highly effective and has no life-threatening complications. It is the treatment of choice for most patients but cannot be used in pregnancy and often causes hypothyroidism. **Thionamides** can be used to treat hyperthyroidism in pregnancy but provide long-term control of hyperthyroidism in less than half of patients and carry a small risk of life-threatening side effects (see sec. **IV.C.2**). Thyroidectomy should be used only in patients who refuse RAI therapy and relapse or develop side effects with thionamide therapy.

2. Other causes of hyperthyroidism. Toxic multinodular goiter and toxic adenoma should be treated with RAI (except in pregnancy). Transient forms of hyperthyroidism due to thyroiditis should be treated symptomatically with propranolol. Iodine-induced hyperthyroidism is treated with thionamides and propranolol.

F. Emergency therapy (*Endocrin Metab Clin North Am* 22:263, 1993) is warranted when hyperthyroidism exacerbates heart failure or coronary artery disease, and in rare patients with severe hyperthyroidism complicated by fever and delirium.

1. Serum for confirmatory testing (TSH, T_4 index, free T_4-ED) should be obtained before therapy is initiated if hyperthyroidism is suspected in a severely ill patient.

2. PTU, 300 mg PO q6h, should be given immediately.

3. Iodide (SSKI, 1–2 gtt PO q12h) should be given about 2 hours after the first dose of PTU, to rapidly inhibit thyroid hormone release from the gland.

4. Propranolol, 40 mg PO q6h (or an equivalent dose IV), should be given to patients with **angina or myocardial infarction,** and the dose should be adjusted to prevent tachycardia. Propranolol may benefit some patients with congestive heart failure and marked tachycardia but may also further impair left ventricular function. In patients with heart failure, it should be given only during invasive monitoring of left ventricular filling pressure (see Chap. 9).

5. **Concomitant diseases** should be treated intensively.
6. **Plasma T₄ is measured** every 3–4 days, and the dose of PTU and iodine are gradually decreased as plasma T_4 approaches the normal range. RAI therapy can be performed 2 weeks after iodine has been discontinued.

G. **Hyperthyroidism in pregnancy.** Plasma T_4 increases in the first trimester of pregnancy due to increased levels of TBG but seldom exceeds 15 μg/dl. If hyperthyroidism is suspected, **plasma TSH should be measured initially.** If TSH is less than 0.1 μU/ml, the diagnosis should be confirmed by measurement of plasma free T_4-ED. If the clinical evidence of hyperthyroidism is obvious, marked elevation of the plasma T_4 index is sufficient to confirm the diagnosis. **RAI is contraindicated in pregnancy,** so patients should be treated with thionamides. PTU is usually used because methimazole has been implicated in causing congenital defects.

1. **PTU,** 100 mg PO tid, should be administered and the dose adjusted (see sec. **IV.C**) to maintain the plasma T_4 index near the upper limit of the normal range. The required dose of PTU often decreases in the later stages of pregnancy.
2. **Propranolol,** 10–40 mg PO qid, may be used to relieve symptoms while awaiting the effects of PTU.
3. The fetus and neonate should be carefully monitored for hyperthyroidism.

Euthyroid Goiter

The diagnosis of euthyroid goiter is based on palpation of the thyroid and evaluation of thyroid function. If the thyroid is enlarged, the examiner should determine whether the enlargement is **diffuse** or **multinodular,** or whether a **single nodule** is present. All three forms of euthyroid goiter are common, especially in women. **Imaging studies** such as thyroid scans or ultrasound **provide no useful information** in addition to palpation and should not be performed.

I. **Diffuse goiter.** Almost all euthyroid diffuse goiters in the United States are due to chronic lymphocytic thyroiditis (**Hashimoto's thyroiditis**). The goiter is usually nontender and firm. Since Hashimoto's disease may also cause hypothyroidism, plasma TSH should be measured even in patients who are clinically euthyroid. Small diffuse goiters are usually asymptomatic, and therapy is usually not required. Symptomatic diffuse goiters may shrink with suppression of plasma TSH to the lower limit of the normal range by thyroxine therapy. If treatment is not given, the patient should be monitored regularly for the development of hypothyroidism.

II. **Multinodular goiter (MNG)** is common in older patients, especially women. Most patients are asymptomatic and require no treatment. In a minority of patients, hyperthyroidism (**toxic MNG**) develops (see Hyperthyroidism, sec. I). In rare patients, the gland compresses the trachea or esophagus, causing dyspnea or dysphagia. There is no convincing evidence that thyroxine treatment affects the size of MNGs, and patients with compressive symptoms may require a subtotal thyroidectomy for relief. The risk of malignancy in MNG is low, comparable to the frequency of incidental thyroid carcinoma in clinically normal glands. Evaluation for thyroid carcinoma with needle biopsy is warranted only if one nodule enlarges disproportionately to the rest of the gland.

III. **Single thyroid nodules** (*N Engl J Med* 328:553, 1993) are usually benign, but a small number are thyroid carcinomas. Clinical findings that increase the likelihood of carcinoma include the presence of cervical lymphadenopathy, a history of radiation to the head or neck in childhood, and family history of medullary thyroid carcinoma or multiple endocrine neoplasia syndromes type 2A or 2B. A hard, fixed nodule, recent nodule growth, or hoarseness due to vocal cord paralysis also suggest malignancy. However, most patients with thyroid carcinomas have none of these risk factors, and nearly all single thyroid nodules should be evaluated with **needle aspiration biopsy.** Patients with thyroid carcinoma should be managed in consultation with an endocrinologist. Nodules with benign cytology should be reevaluated periodically. Thyroxine therapy has little or no effect on the size of single thyroid nodules and is not indicated.

Adrenal Failure

Adrenal failure is the syndrome caused by **deficiency of cortisol**, with or without deficiency of aldosterone (*Endocrinol Metab Clin North Am* 22:303, 1993). It may be due to disease of the adrenal glands (**primary adrenal failure, Addison's disease**), with deficiency of both cortisol and aldosterone and elevated plasma adrenocorticotrophic hormone (ACTH), or ACTH deficiency caused by disorders of the pituitary or hypothalamus (**secondary adrenal failure**), with deficiency of cortisol alone.

I. **Causes.** Primary adrenal failure is most often due to **autoimmune adrenalitis**, which may be associated with other endocrine deficits including hypothyroidism and hypoparathyroidism. **Infections** of the adrenal glands such as tuberculosis and histoplasmosis may cause adrenal failure. **Hemorrhagic adrenal infarction** may occur in the postoperative period, coagulation disorders, hypercoagulable states, and sepsis. Adrenal hemorrhage often causes abdominal or flank pain with fever; CT of the abdomen reveals high-density bilateral adrenal masses. Patients with AIDS may develop adrenal failure due to disseminated mycobacterial or fungal infection, adrenal lymphoma, or treatment with ketoconazole, which inhibits steroid hormone synthesis. Secondary adrenal failure is most often due to **glucocorticoid therapy**; ACTH suppression may persist for a year after therapy is stopped. Any disorder of the pituitary or hypothalamus can cause ACTH deficiency, but there is usually other evidence of these disorders.

II. **Clinical findings** are nonspecific, and without a high index of suspicion, the diagnosis of this lethal but readily treatable disease is easily missed. Symptoms include weakness, fatigue, anorexia, nausea, vomiting, and weight loss. Orthostatic hypotension and hyponatremia are common. Symptoms are usually chronic, but patients may suddenly develop shock that is fatal unless promptly treated. This **adrenal crisis** is often triggered by illness, injury, or surgery. All of these symptoms are due to cortisol deficiency and occur in both primary and secondary adrenal failure. Hyperpigmentation (due to marked ACTH excess) and hyperkalemia and volume depletion (due to aldosterone deficiency) occur only in primary adrenal failure.

III. **Diagnosis.** Adrenal failure should be suspected in patients with hypotension, weight loss, hyponatremia, or hyperkalemia.
   A. **The short cosyntropin (Cortrosyn) stimulation test** (250 µg IV or IM, with plasma cortisol measured 30 minutes later) is used for diagnosis. The normal response is a stimulated plasma cortisol greater than 20 µg/dl. This test detects both primary and secondary adrenal failure, except within a few weeks of onset of pituitary dysfunction (*Lancet* 1:1208, 1988).
   B. **The distinction between primary and secondary adrenal failure is** usually clear—hyperkalemia, hyperpigmentation, or other autoimmune endocrine deficits indicate primary adrenal failure, while deficits of other pituitary hormones, symptoms of a pituitary mass (e.g., headache, visual field loss) or known pituitary or hypothalamic disease indicate secondary adrenal failure. If the cause is unclear, the **plasma ACTH** level distinguishes primary adrenal failure (in which it is markedly elevated) from secondary adrenal failure. Most cases of primary adrenal failure are due to autoimmune adrenalitis, but tuberculosis should also be considered, and purified protein derivative testing and chest radiograph should be performed. Radiographic evidence of adrenal enlargement or calcification indicates that the cause is infection or hemorrhage. Patients with secondary adrenal failure should be tested for other pituitary hormone deficiencies and evaluated for a pituitary or hypothalamic tumor.

IV. **Therapy**
   A. **Adrenal crisis** with hypotension must be treated immediately.

1. **If the diagnosis of adrenal failure is known, hydrocortisone, 100 mg IV q8h,** should be administered, and 0.9% saline with 5% dextrose should be rapidly infused until hypotension is corrected. The dose of hydrocortisone is gradually decreased over several days as symptoms and any precipitating illness resolve, then changed to oral maintenance therapy. Mineralocorticoid replacement is not needed until the dose of hydrocortisone is less than 100 mg/day.

2. **If the diagnosis of adrenal failure has not been established,** a single dose of **dexamethasone, 10 mg IV,** should be administered, and a rapid infusion of 0.9% saline with 5% dextrose initiated. A **Cortrosyn stimulation test** should be performed (see sec. **III.A**). After the 30-minute plasma cortisol value has been obtained, hydrocortisone, 100 mg IV q8h, should be administered until the result of the Cortrosyn stimulation test is known. All patients with adrenal crisis should be evaluated for an underlying illness that precipitated the crisis.

B. **Maintenance therapy.** All patients with adrenal failure require cortisol replacement with prednisone; patients with primary adrenal failure also require replacement of aldosterone with fludrocortisone (Florinef).

1. **Prednisone,** 5 mg PO every morning and 2.5 mg PO every evening, should be administered. The dose is adjusted to eliminate symptoms and signs of cortisol deficiency or excess, with most patients requiring between 5 mg PO every morning and 5 mg PO bid. Concomitant therapy with rifampin, phenytoin, or phenobarbital accelerates glucocorticoid metabolism and increases the dose requirement.

2. **During illness, injury, surgery, or the postoperative period, the dose of prednisone must be increased.** For minor illness, the patient should double the dose for 3 days. If the illness resolves, the maintenance dose should be resumed. **Vomiting requires immediate medical attention** with IV glucocorticoid therapy and IV volume expansion. Patients may be given a prefilled syringe of dexamethasone, 4 mg, to be self-administered IM for vomiting or severe illness if medical care is not immediately available. **For severe illness or injury,** hydrocortisone, 100 mg IV q8h, should be given, with the dose tapered as the severity of the illness wanes. The same regimen is used in **patients undergoing surgery,** with the first dose of hydrocortisone given preoperatively. The dose can usually be reduced to maintenance therapy 3–4 days after uncomplicated surgery.

3. **In primary adrenal failure,** fludrocortisone, 0.1 mg PO qd, should be administered in addition to liberal salt intake. The dose is adjusted to maintain BP (both supine and standing) and serum potassium within the normal range; the usual dose is 0.05–0.30 mg PO qd.

4. **Patients should be educated** about management of their disease, including adjustment of the prednisone dose during illness. They should wear a medical identification tag or bracelet.

Cushing's Syndrome

Cushing's syndrome (the clinical effects of glucocorticoid excess) is most often iatrogenic, due to therapy with glucocorticoid drugs. **ACTH-secreting pituitary microadenomas (Cushing's disease)** account for about 80% of cases of endogenous Cushing's syndrome. Adrenal tumors and ectopic ACTH secretion account for a small proportion of cases.

I. **Clinical findings** include truncal obesity, rounded face, fat deposits in the supraclavicular fossae and over the posterior neck, hypertension, hirsutism, amenorrhea, and psychiatric disorders (most often depression). **More specific findings** include thin skin, easy bruising, reddish striae, proximal muscle weakness, and osteoporosis. Mild hyperglycemia is common, but few patients develop diabetes mellitus. Hyperpigmentation or hypokalemic alkalosis suggest Cushing's syndrome due to ectopic ACTH secretion.

II. Diagnosis is based on increased cortisol excretion and lack of normal feedback inhibition of ACTH and cortisol secretion.

   A. The overnight dexamethasone suppression test (1 mg of dexamethasone given PO at 2300 hours; plasma cortisol measured at 0800 hours the next day; normal: plasma cortisol <5 μg/dl) or **24-hour urine cortisol test** may be performed as a **screening test**. Both tests are very sensitive, and a normal value excludes the diagnosis.

   B. An abnormal screening test indicates the need to perform a **low-dose dexamethasone suppression test**. Dexamethasone, 0.5 mg PO, is administered q6h for 48 hours, and urine cortisol is measured during the last 24 hours. Failure to suppress urine cortisol to less than 20 μg/24 hours is diagnostic of Cushing's syndrome. Testing for Cushing's syndrome should not be performed during severe illness or depression, which may result in false-positive results. Phenytoin therapy also causes false-positive dexamethasone suppression tests by accelerating metabolism of dexamethasone. **Random plasma cortisol levels are not useful for diagnosis**, because the wide range of normal values overlaps those seen in Cushing's syndrome. After the diagnosis of Cushing's syndrome is made, further testing to determine the cause is best done in consultation with an endocrinologist.

Anterior Pituitary Gland Dysfunction

The anterior pituitary secretes four **trophic hormones**: adrenocorticotropic hormone (ACTH), thyrotropin (TSH), and the gonadotropins, luteinizing hormone (LH) and follicle-stimulating hormone (FSH); these are secreted along with prolactin and growth hormone. Each trophic hormone stimulates the function of a specific **target gland**. Anterior pituitary function is regulated by hypothalamic hormones that reach the pituitary via portal veins in the pituitary stalk. **The predominant effect of hypothalamic regulation is to stimulate secretion of pituitary hormones, except for prolactin**, which is inhibited by hypothalamic dopamine production. Secretion of trophic hormones is also regulated by **negative feedback** by their target gland hormone, and the normal pituitary response to target hormone deficiency is increased secretion of the appropriate trophic hormone.

I. Causes. Disorders of either the pituitary or hypothalamus can cause anterior pituitary dysfunction.

   A. Pituitary adenomas are the most common pituitary disorder. They are classified by size and function. **Microadenomas** are less than 10 mm in diameter and cause clinical manifestations only by producing hormone excess. Because of their small size, they do not produce hypopituitarism or mass effects. They are common incidental radiographic findings, seen in about 10% of the normal population (*Ann Intern Med* 120:817, 1994). **Macroadenomas** are more than 10 mm in diameter and may produce any combination of pituitary hormone excess, hypopituitarism, and mass effects. **Secretory adenomas** may produce prolactin, growth hormone, or ACTH. **Nonsecretory tumors** may cause hypopituitarism or mass effects.

   B. Other pituitary or hypothalamic disorders. Head trauma, pituitary surgery or radiation, and postpartum pituitary infarction (Sheehan's syndrome) may cause hypopituitarism. Other tumors of the pituitary or hypothalamus (e.g., craniopharyngioma, metastases), inflammatory disorders (e.g., sarcoidosis, histiocytosis X), and infections (e.g., tuberculosis) may cause hypopituitarism or mass effects.

II. Clinical findings. Pituitary and hypothalamic disorders may present in several ways.

   A. Hypopituitarism (deficiency of one or more pituitary hormones). Gonadotropin deficiency is most common, causing amenorrhea in women and androgen deficiency in men. Secondary hypothyroidism or adrenal failure rarely occur alone. Secondary adrenal failure causes deficiency of cortisol but not aldosterone; hypcrkalemia and hyperpigmentation do not occur, although life-threatening adrenal crisis may develop. Deficiency of growth hormone does not produce a distinct clinical syndrome in adults.

B. Hormone excess. Hyperprolactinemia is most common and can be due to a secretory adenoma or to nonsecretory lesions affecting the hypothalamus or pituitary stalk. Growth hormone excess (**acromegaly**) and ACTH and cortisol excess (**Cushing's disease**) are caused by secretory adenomas.

C. Mass effects due to pressure on adjacent structures such as the optic chiasm include headaches and loss of visual fields or acuity. Hyperprolactinemia may also be due to mass effect. **Pituitary apoplexy** is sudden enlargement of a pituitary tumor due to hemorrhagic necrosis. It is an uncommon disorder in which mass effects and hypopituitarism suddenly appear or worsen, and may cause fatal secondary adrenal failure.

D. An incidental finding may be discovered on imaging done for another purpose.

III. Diagnosis of hypopituitarism (*N Engl J Med* 330:1651, 1994). Hypopituitarism may be suspected because of clinical signs of target hormone deficiency (e.g., hypothyroidism), pituitary mass effects (e.g., headaches or visual loss), or evidence of pituitary hormone excess (e.g., acromegaly).

A. Laboratory evaluation for hypopituitarism begins with evaluation of target hormone function, including **serum T₄ index**, and a **Cortrosyn stimulation test**. The Cortrosyn stimulation test is quite sensitive for secondary adrenal failure, except within a few weeks of its onset (e.g., after pituitary surgery or pituitary apoplexy). If recent onset of secondary adrenal failure is suspected, the patient should be treated empirically with glucocorticoids and tested later (see Adrenal Failure, sec. **IV.A.2**). In men, **serum testosterone** should be measured. The best evaluation of gonadal function in women is the **menstrual history**; amenorrhea indicates ovarian dysfunction.

B. If a target hormone is deficient, then its trophic hormone is measured to determine whether target gland dysfunction is primary or secondary to hypopituitarism. An elevated trophic hormone level indicates primary target gland dysfunction. In hypopituitarism, trophic hormone levels are not elevated but are usually not below the reference range. Thus, **pituitary trophic hormone levels can only be interpreted with knowledge of target hormone levels**, and **measurement of pituitary trophic hormone levels alone is useless in diagnosing hypopituitarism**. If pituitary disease is obvious, target hormone deficiencies may be assumed to be secondary, and trophic hormones need not be measured.

IV. Anatomic evaluation of the pituitary and hypothalamus. The pituitary and hypothalamus can be imaged with either CT or MRI. MRI is more sensitive for microadenomas, although hyperprolactinemia and Cushing's syndrome may be caused by tumors too small to be imaged with current techniques. The frequency of occurrence of incidental microadenomas should be kept in mind. **Visual acuity** and **visual fields** should be formally tested in patients with pituitary mass lesions that extend above the sella turcica or hypothalamic tumors.

V. Treatment of hypopituitarism. Deficient target hormones should be replaced. Secondary adrenal failure should be treated immediately, especially if patients are to undergo surgery (see Adrenal Failure, sec. **IV**). Infertility due to gonadotropin deficiency may be correctable, and patients who want to conceive should be referred to an endocrinologist. Treatment of pituitary mass lesions generally requires transsphenoidal surgical resection.

VI. Acromegaly, the syndrome caused by growth hormone excess in adults, is almost always due to a growth hormone–secreting pituitary adenoma.

A. Clinical findings include thickened skin and gradual enlargement of hands, feet, and facial features, especially the jaw and forehead. Old photographs may clarify the change in appearance. Arthritis or carpal tunnel syndrome may develop, and the pituitary adenoma may cause headaches and visual loss. The mortality rates from cardiovascular disease are increased in patients with acromegaly.

B. Diagnosis. Measuring levels of somatomedin C (insulin-like growth factor I [IGF-I]), which mediates the growth-promoting effects of growth hormone, is the

Table 21-4. Major causes of hyperprolactinemia

Pregnancy and lactation
Prolactin-secreting pituitary adenoma (prolactinoma)
Idiopathic hyperprolactinemia
Drugs
 Dopamine antagonists (phenothiazines, metoclopramide, methyldopa)
 Others (verapamil, cimetidine, some antidepressants)
Interference with synthesis or transport of hypothalamic dopamine
 Hypothalamic lesions
 Pituitary macroadenomas
Primary hypothyroidism
Chronic renal failure

best diagnostic test. Marked elevations establish the diagnosis. If somatomedin C levels are only moderately elevated, the diagnosis can be confirmed by giving 75 mg of glucose PO and measuring serum growth hormone every 30 minutes for 2 hours. Failure to suppress growth hormone to less than 2 ng/ml confirms the diagnosis of acromegaly. Once the diagnosis is made, the pituitary gland should be imaged.

C. **Therapy.** The treatment of choice is **transsphenoidal resection** of the pituitary adenoma. Most patients have macroadenomas, and complete tumor resection with cure of acromegaly is often not possible. If somatomedin-C levels remain elevated after surgery, radiation therapy is used to prevent growth of residual tumor and to control acromegaly; the full effect of radiation therapy on growth hormone secretion may take up to 10 years. The somatostatin analog **octreotide,** 100 μg SC tid, can be used to suppress growth hormone secretion while awaiting the full effect of radiation (*Ann Intern Med* 117:711, 1992). Side effects of octreotide include cholelithiasis, diarrhea, and mild abdominal discomfort.

Hyperprolactinemia

Prolactin suppresses gonadotropin secretion, causing hypogonadism, and stimulates milk production by the breast. Unlike other anterior pituitary hormones, prolactin secretion is inhibited by hypothalamic secretion of **dopamine,** and hypothalamic or pituitary lesions that cause deficiency of other pituitary hormones often cause hyperprolactinemia. Stimulation of secretion by suckling and estrogen play roles in regulation.

I. **Causes** (Table 21-4). **In women,** the most common causes of pathologic hyperprolactinemia are prolactin-secreting pituitary **microadenomas** and **idiopathic hyperprolactinemia** (which may be due to undetectable microadenomas or to deficiency of hypothalamic dopamine). **In men,** the most common cause is prolactin-secreting **macroadenoma. Drugs** are an important cause in both sexes. Oral contraceptives have little effect on prolactin levels.

II. **Clinical findings. In women,** hyperprolactinemia causes **amenorrhea** or irregular menses and **infertility**. Only about half of these women have galactorrhea. Prolonged estrogen deficiency reduces bone density and increases the risk of osteoporosis. **In men**, hyperprolactinemia causes **androgen deficiency** and infertility but not gynecomastia; mass effects and hypopituitarism from pituitary macroadenomas are common.

III. **Diagnosis.** Hyperprolactinemia is a **common disorder of young women,** accounting for 15–30% of cases of amenorrhea. Serum prolactin should be measured in women with amenorrhea, whether galactorrhea is present or not; men with secondary hypogonadism; and patients with pituitary macroadenomas. Mild elevations should be confirmed by repeat measurements.

A. **History** should include medications and symptoms of mass effects or hypothyroidism.

B. **Laboratory** evaluation should include **serum TSH** and a **pregnancy test.** The level of **plasma prolactin** is diagnostically helpful, since prolactin levels above 200 ng/ml occur only in prolactinomas, and levels of 100–200 ng/ml strongly suggest this diagnosis. Levels less than 100 ng/ml may be due to any cause except prolactin-secreting macroadenoma, and such levels in a patient with a large pituitary mass do not indicate that it is a prolactinoma.

C. **Pituitary imaging** should be performed in most cases, since large nonfunctional pituitary or hypothalamic tumors occasionally present with hyperprolactinemia. Further tests of pituitary function (see Anterior Pituitary Gland Dysfunction, sec. **III**) and visual field testing are needed only in the minority of patients with a pituitary macroadenoma or hypothalamic lesion.

IV. **Therapy** (*Endocrinol Metab Clin North Am* 21: 877, 1992)

A. **Microadenomas and idiopathic hyperprolactinemia.** Some women may be observed without therapy by periodic follow-up of prolactin levels and symptoms. Hyperprolactinemia usually does not worsen, and in 30–50% of patients, prolactin levels return to normal within 5 years. Enlargement of microadenomas is rare.

1. **Most patients are treated** because of **infertility** or to prevent **estrogen deficiency** and the risk of **osteoporosis.** The treatment of choice is the dopamine agonist **bromocriptine**, which suppresses plasma prolactin and restores normal menses and fertility in most women. The initial dose is 1.25–2.50 mg PO qhs with a snack. The dose is gradually increased at weekly intervals to 2.5 mg bid or tid; then plasma prolactin is measured. The dose is further adjusted at 2- to 4-week intervals, based on prolactin measurements, to the lowest dose that suppresses prolactin to the normal range; doses greater than 10 mg/day are seldom required. It may be possible to maintain normal prolactin levels with a single daily dose. Patients should use mechanical contraception during initial dose titration, since fertility may be restored quickly.

2. **Side effects of bromocriptine** often include nausea and orthostatic hypotension, which can be minimized by gradually increasing the dose, and usually resolve with continued therapy. Nasal congestion, headaches, and constipation may occur. Serious side effects, including Raynaud's phenomenon, pulmonary fibrosis, and psychosis, are rarely seen with doses of less than 10 mg/day.

3. **Women who wish to become pregnant** should stop mechanical contraception after regular menses return. A pregnancy test should be obtained promptly if menses are delayed by more than 2 days. If the test is positive, bromocriptine should be discontinued and routine prenatal care given. The risk of symptomatic pituitary enlargement during pregnancy in patients with microadenomas is about 2%. If headaches or visual loss occur, visual field testing and MRI of the pituitary should be performed. In rare cases where it occurs, pituitary enlargement can usually be controlled by restarting bromocriptine. Extensive experience with bromocriptine has shown increased risk of abortion or congenital defects.

4. **Women who do not wish to become pregnant** should be followed with clinical evaluation and plasma prolactin every 6–12 months. Every 2 years, bromocriptine should be withdrawn for several weeks and prolactin levels measured to determine if the drug is still necessary. Imaging studies are not warranted unless prolactin levels increase substantially.

5. **Transsphenoidal surgery** may be used to resect prolactin-secreting microadenomas but should be restricted to the rare patients who do not respond to or cannot tolerate bromocriptine. Although prolactin levels are restored to normal in most, up to half of patients later relapse. Complications include hypopituitarism, diabetes insipidus, CSF rhinorrhea, meningitis, visual loss, and, rarely, stroke or death.

B. **Prolactin-secreting macroadenomas**

1. Patients should be treated initially with **bromocriptine**, which suppresses prolactin levels to normal in most patients. It **reduces tumor size** and

improves or corrects abnormal visual fields in about 90% of cases. The dose is increased to 7.5 mg/day (see sec. **IV.A.1**) and then plasma prolactin is measured. The dose is adjusted further, at 2- to 4-week intervals, until prolactin levels return to normal or until dose increases produce no further fall in plasma prolactin. MRI or CT (and visual fields, if initially abnormal) should be repeated 2–3 months after beginning therapy. If there is satisfactory tumor shrinkage, with correction of visual abnormalities, bromocriptine therapy may be continued indefinitely, with periodic monitoring of visual fields. In some cases, the full reduction in size does not occur before 6 months. Repeat imaging is probably not warranted unless prolactin levels rise despite therapy.

2. **Transsphenoidal surgery** is indicated to relieve mass effects and prevent further tumor growth if there is little change in tumor size or persistent abnormalities of visual fields. However, the likelihood of surgical cure of hyperprolactinemia due to a macroadenoma is low (10–40%), and most patients require further therapy with bromocriptine to suppress prolactin levels to normal.

3. **Women with prolactin-secreting macroadenomas** should not become pregnant unless the tumor has been surgically resected, since the risk of symptomatic enlargement during pregnancy is 15–35%. Mechanical contraception is essential in such women being treated with bromocriptine. After surgical resection, bromocriptine may be necessary to correct residual hyperprolactinemia and induce fertility.

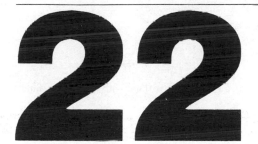

Lipid Disorders

Anne Carol Goldberg

General Considerations

The relationship between the risk of atherosclerotic heart disease and serum lipoprotein levels is well established. Elevated levels of total cholesterol and low-density lipoprotein cholesterol (LDL-C) and low levels of high-density lipoprotein cholesterol (HDL-C) are associated with increased risk. In some situations, such as familial combined hyperlipoproteinemia (FCHL), dysbetalipoproteinemia, and diabetes mellitus, elevated triglyceride levels are also a marker of increased risk of cardiovascular disease. Evidence of the beneficial effects of reduction of serum cholesterol and LDL-C has led to the development of guidelines from the National Cholesterol Education Program for detection, evaluation, and treatment of high blood cholesterol levels in adults (*Arch Intern Med* 148:36, 1988), which were revised in 1993 (*JAMA* 269:3015, 1993). These guidelines place greater emphasis on treatment of patients with preexisting vascular disease than was previously recommended.

Detection and Evaluation

I. **Serum cholesterol** determination is used for screening and initial classification of risk. Cholesterol levels should be obtained in all adults over age 20. Nonlipid cardiac risk factors should also be determined (Table 22-1). **HDL-C** should also be measured when cholesterol is checked. A level of less than 35 mg/dl is considered low. High HDL-C—over 60 mg/dl—may be protective and is treated as a negative risk factor (see Table 22-1). Total cholesterol and HDL-C may be measured in a nonfasting state, but triglycerides and calculated LDL-C must be measured while the patient is fasting. To save time and money, a fasting lipoprotein analysis may be done at the initial visit. Further evaluation depends on the following:

A. **The desirable blood cholesterol level** is less than 200 mg/dl. Individuals in this group who have an HDL-C level over 35 mg/dl should be educated about general dietary and cardiac risk factor modification. Serum cholesterol and HDL-C levels should be remeasured in 5 years. Patients with an initial **HDL-C less than 35 mg/dl** should have a lipoprotein analysis performed on follow-up.

B. **Borderline high blood cholesterol levels** are from 200–239 mg/dl. Further management depends on the presence of coronary heart disease (CHD) or two or more cardiac risk factors (see Table 22-1).

1. **In the absence of CHD or at least two risk factors,** a patient with HDL-C over 35 mg/dl should be given information on diet, physical activity, and risk factor reduction. Serum cholesterol levels should be measured and risk factors assessed annually.

2. **The presence of CHD or two risk factors *or* HDL-C less than 35 mg/dl** requires that lipoprotein analysis be performed. Further decisions are based on the **LDL-C.**

C. **High blood cholesterol** levels are greater than or equal to 240 mg/dl. Lipoprotein analysis should be performed and used for therapeutic decisions.

Table 22-1. Risk factors for coronary artery disease

Positive risk factors
Age
   Male: ≥45 yrs
   Female: ≥55 yrs or premature menopause without estrogen replacement
           therapy
Family history of premature CHD
Current cigarette smoking
Hypertension
Low HDL-cholesterol (<35 mg/dl)
Diabetes mellitus
Negative risk factor: subtract one risk factor if:
High HDL-cholesterol (≥60 mg/dl)

II. **Lipoprotein analysis** is performed on serum obtained after a **12-hour fast.** Total
cholesterol, triglycerides, and HDL-C are measured, and LDL-C is calculated using
the following formula:

LDL-C = total cholesterol − HDL-C − (triglyceride/5)

where triglyceride/5 represents the cholesterol contained in very low density
lipoprotein (VLDL). Because of biologic variability as well as potential measurement error, two or three measurements should be obtained 1–8 weeks apart while
the patient is on his or her usual diet. In patients who are losing weight, are
pregnant, have had major surgery, or are seriously ill (e.g., myocardial infarction
[MI]), cholesterol levels may not be representative, and analysis should be deferred
for at least 6 weeks. In patients who have had an acute MI, lipoprotein levels
measured within the first 24 hours after the MI will provide an approximation of
their usual levels; however, levels may not be stable for up to 12 weeks.

III. **The LDL-C level** along with an assessment of the patient's cardiovascular risk is the
basis for decisions concerning dietary or drug therapy. For patients without
evidence of CHD, the following definitions apply:

   A. **Desirable LDL-C** is less than 130 mg/dl. Patients in this group should be given
general dietary and risk factor information, and total cholesterol and HDL-C
levels should be remeasured in 5 years.

   B. **Borderline high-risk LDL-C** is 130–159 mg/dl. The presence of risk factors
determines further management.

      1. **Absence of two or more risk factors** requires that the patient be given diet
and exercise counseling. Risk factor assessment and lipoprotein analysis
should be performed annually, and dietary counseling should be reinforced.

      2. **Patients with two or more risk factors** are treated similarly to those with
high-risk LDL-C.

   C. **High-risk LDL-C** is greater than 160 mg/dl. Patients should have a clinical
evaluation including history, physical examination, and laboratory tests to
identify secondary causes of hyperlipidemia and familial disorders.

      1. **Secondary causes of hyperlipidemia** include diet, hypothyroidism, diabetes
mellitus, nephrotic syndrome, uremia, and dysproteinemia. Certain **drugs**
can affect lipids. Thiazide diuretics, beta-adrenergic antagonists (particularly
noncardioselective agents; see Chap. 4), glucocorticoids, estrogens, pro-
gestins, retinoids, anabolic steroids, and alcohol have variable effects on
cholesterol, triglycerides, and HDL-C.

      2. **Familial hyperlipoproteinemias** can be associated with severe elevations of
serum lipid levels and often require drug therapy in addition to diet
modifications.

      3. **Treatment** begins with diet therapy and increased physical activity and may
progress to drug therapy. Diet therapy continues even if drug therapy is used.

   4. **Age, sex, state of health, and number of cardiac risk factors** must be considered in making decisions about treatment.
 D. **LDL-C in patients with CHD** or other clinical atherosclerotic disease is classified as optimal or higher than optimal.
   1. **Optimal LDL-C** is less than or equal to 100 mg/dl. These patients should have instruction on diet and physical activity and have levels measured annually.
   2. **Higher than optimal LDL-C** is above 100 mg/dl. Patients should be evaluated similarly to those with LDL-C over 160 mg/dl and should be treated with dietary therapy and possibly drug therapy.
IV. **Serum triglyceride** levels may be found to be elevated in the course of cholesterol evaluation. The National Institutes of Health Consensus Development Panel on Triglycerides, HDL, and Coronary Artery Disease has defined levels of triglycerides to be considered for treatment (*JAMA* 269:505, 1993).
 A. **Normal triglyceride** levels are less than 200 mg/dl.
 B. **Borderline-high hypertriglyceride** levels are 200–400 mg/dl. Nonpharmacologic therapy including diet, exercise, and weight loss is the initial form of therapy for these patients. Drug therapy may be indicated in patients who do not respond adequately to diet and who have coronary artery disease, a positive family history, or the presence of other CHD risk factors.
 C. **High triglyceride** levels are 400–1,000 mg/dl. Nonpharmacologic treatment with diet, exercise, and weight loss is initial therapy, but drug therapy should be considered after an adequate trial of dietary therapy in patients who fail to lower their levels to less than 500 mg/dl because of the risk of pancreatitis.
 D. **Very high triglyceride** levels are over 1,000 mg/dl. These patients are at increased risk for pancreatitis. Nonpharmacologic measures and a search for secondary causes are needed. These patients must be treated aggressively (see Therapy, sec. **VIII.F**).

Diagnosis of Specific Disorders

I. **Hypercholesterolemia** may be due to a primary disorder.
 A. **Familial hypercholesterolemia (FH)** is an autosomal-dominant disorder involving the LDL receptor.
   1. **Heterozygotes** for FH have 50% of the normal number of LDL receptors, elevated LDL-C levels, and cholesterol levels of 350–550 mg/dl. The incidence is approximately 1 in 500 persons. Affected patients often have premature vascular disease and may have tendinous xanthomas. Treatment usually requires drug as well as diet therapy. More severe cases may require the combination of two or more medications.
   2. **Homozygotes** for FH have few or no LDL receptors and thus have markedly elevated LDL-C levels and blood cholesterol levels of 650–1,000 mg/dl. The incidence is 1 in 1 million. Heart disease often begins in early childhood, and many patients die of heart disease in their twenties and thirties. Affected children may have planar and tuberous as well as tendinous xanthomas. They respond poorly to both diet and drug therapy. Plasmapheresis may be effective, and liver transplantation has been done in a few of these patients.
   3. **Familial defective apolipoprotein B-100** is an autosomal-dominant disorder caused by an abnormality in the LDL receptor binding region of apoprotein B-100, the major protein on the surface of LDL particles. It appears to have a frequency, clinical features, and lipoprotein levels similar to the FH heterozygous form.
 B. **Familial combined hyperlipoproteinemia (FCHL)** is associated with an increased risk of vascular disease. Patients may have elevated cholesterol levels, triglyceride levels, or both. The molecular basis of this disorder is unknown; many patients overproduce VLDL. FCHL occurs in 1–2% of the population. The diagnosis is made by the presence of multiple lipoprotein phenotypes within one

family. Family members may have elevated VLDL (type IV), elevated LDL-C (type IIa), or increased levels of both VLDL and LDL-C (type IIb). Diet therapy, weight loss, and exercise are useful initial therapies, but many patients will require drug therapy aimed at correcting specific lipoprotein abnormalities.

    C. Severe polygenic hypercholesterolemia is found in adults whose LDL-C is above 220 mg/dl and who do not clearly demonstrate a monogenic inheritance of hypercholesterolemia. These patients are usually at increased risk for premature CHD. Some will be resistant to diet therapy alone and will require drug therapy.

  II. Hypertriglyceridemia may be secondary to diet, obesity, excess alcohol intake, diabetes mellitus, hypothyroidism, uremia, dysproteinemias, beta-adrenergic antagonists, estrogen, oral contraceptive drugs, and retinoids. Triglyceride levels greater than 400 mg/dl are often associated with an underlying primary disorder. Primary hypertriglyceridemia can be due to FCHL or familial hypertriglyceridemia.

  III. Dysbetalipoproteinemia (type III hyperlipoproteinemia) is a rare (approximately 1 in 5,000) disorder caused by an abnormality of apoprotein E, a protein on the surface of VLDL and other lipoproteins that is important in the uptake of remnant particles by cell surface receptors. Cholesterol-enriched VLDL (beta-VLDL), an atherogenic particle, accumulates. Both cholesterol and triglyceride levels are elevated. Diagnosis is made by a combination of ultracentrifugation and isoelectric focusing, which shows an abnormal apoprotein E pattern. Patients may have planar or tuberoeruptive xanthomas and have an increased risk of vascular disease. Patients with this disorder may respond well to diet modifications and weight loss.

  IV. Hyperchylomicronemia is diagnosed by the presence of a chylomicron layer when plasma is centrifuged or when chylomicrons float to the top of plasma that has been refrigerated overnight. Chylomicrons can be seen when triglyceride levels are in excess of 1,000 mg/dl. The patient may have a rare syndrome involving absence of lipoprotein lipase activity or absent apoprotein CII (a cofactor of lipoprotein lipase). Chylomicrons alone may be increased, as in lipoprotein lipase deficiency, or both VLDL and chylomicrons may be elevated. Total cholesterol levels are often markedly elevated because of the presence of large numbers of VLDL particles that contain cholesterol as well as triglycerides. In patients with primary hypertriglyceridemia, FCHL, or dysbetalipoproteinemia, hyperchylomicronemia may develop in the presence of excessive dietary fat intake, uncontrolled diabetes, alcohol excess, obesity, or other secondary causes of hyperlipidemia. The chylomicronemia syndrome may include abdominal pain, hepatomegaly, splenomegaly, eruptive xanthomas, lipemia retinalis, and pancreatitis. Memory loss, paresthesias, and peripheral neuropathy may also occur.

  V. Low HDL-C levels—less than 35 mg/dl—may be due to a genetic disorder or to secondary causes.

    A. Primary disorders include familial hypoalphalipoproteinemia, primary hypertriglyceridemias, and rare disorders such as fish-eye disease, Tangier disease, and lecithin-cholesterol-acyl transferase (LCAT) deficiency.

    B. Secondary causes of low HDL-C levels include cigarette smoking, obesity, lack of exercise, androgens, some progestational agents, anabolic steroids, beta-adrenergic antagonists, and hypertriglyceridemia.

  VI. Family members of patients with hyperlipidemia should be screened to facilitate diagnosis of primary hyperlipidemias as well as to identify other patients who need treatment.

Therapy

  I. The rationale for therapy of hyperlipidemia is to reduce the risk of atherosclerotic cardiovascular disease. In patients with severe hypertriglyceridemia, the aim is to prevent pancreatitis.

    A. Reduction of cholesterol and LDL-C levels is associated with a reduction of risk of cardiovascular disease. This has been demonstrated by a number of clinical trials involving both primary and secondary prevention (*JAMA* 251:351, 1984; *J Am Coll Cardiol* 8:1245, 1986), as well as angiographic studies of plaque regression (*Circulation* 87:1781, 1993).

B. Hypertriglyceridemia is less clearly associated with cardiovascular disease, but the risk is believed to be increased in FCHL, in diabetic dyslipidemia, or when other risk factors are present. Triglyceride levels above 1,000 mg/dl should be treated to prevent hyperchylomicronemia and pancreatitis.

II. Diet modification is the initial therapy for hyperlipidemia and in most cases should be tried for several months before drug therapy is considered. Weight control and increased physical activity are important aspects of dietary management.

   A. Goals of therapy of hypercholesterolemia should be set. These are minimal goals, and lower levels of LDL-C should be attained whenever possible.

      1. In the absence of risk factors, a target goal LDL-C is less than 160 mg/dl.

      2. The presence of two or more risk factors calls for a target goal LDL-C of less than 130 mg/dl.

      3. In patients with CHD, the goal LDL-C is less than 100 mg/dl.

   B. Monitoring can be performed using total cholesterol levels rather than the more expensive lipoprotein analysis. Total cholesterol levels of 240 mg/dl (in patients without CHD or risk factors), 200 mg/dl (in patients with two or more risk factors), and 160 mg/dl (in patients with CHD) can be used as surrogate goals.

   C. Dietary therapy can be done in a graded fashion.

      1. Step 1 of dietary intervention involves reduction of dietary fat to less than 30% of total calories, decrease of saturated fat intake to less than 10% of calories, and decrease of cholesterol intake to less than 300 mg/day.

         a. Saturated fat intake is reduced by cutting portion sizes of beef, pork, chicken, and fish to 3 oz and limiting total meat consumption to 6 oz/day. Lean cuts of beef and pork should be well trimmed, skin should be removed from chicken and turkey, and fried foods should be avoided. Vegetable oils that are highly saturated, such as coconut oil and palm oil, should be avoided. Low-fat dairy products can be substituted for whole-milk products. Soft margarine, liquid vegetable oils, and low-fat cheese should replace butter, solid vegetable shortening, and high-fat cheese. **Trans-fatty acids,** produced during hydrogenation of liquid oils to make solid fats, raise LDL-C and lower HDL-C (*N Engl J Med* 323:439, 1990). Avoidance of fried foods and use of low-fat baked goods and soft margarines will decrease dietary intake of trans-fatty acids.

         b. Polyunsaturated fats can be obtained from vegetable oils and margarine. Intake of polyunsaturated fat should not exceed 10% of total calories. Very high proportions of polyunsaturated fat in the diet lower HDL-C as well as LDL-C.

         c. Monounsaturated fat should be 10–15% of total calories. These fats are found in vegetable oils, especially olive and canola oil. They also make up some of the fat in meats.

         d. Cholesterol intake can be reduced by restricting egg yolks and organ meats such as liver, kidney, brains, and sweetbreads as well as by keeping portions of beef, poultry, and fish to 5–6 oz/day. A maximum of 4 egg yolks/week (including those used in prepared foods) can be eaten.

         e. Fresh fruits, vegetables, and whole-grain products should be used to increase variety and provide nutrients and fiber. Carbohydrates, especially complex carbohydrates, should make up 55–60% of total calories. A minimum of 2–3 servings of vegetables, 2–3 servings of fruits, and 6 servings of bread, cereal, or other grain products should be included.

      2. If goal cholesterol is not met after 6–12 weeks, referral to a **registered dietitian** for reinforcement of the step 1 diet or instruction in the step 2 diet may be helpful.

      3. The step 2 diet involves further decreases of saturated fat to 7% of calories and of cholesterol intake to less than 200 mg/day.

      4. The duration of diet therapy should be at least 6 months in most patients who do not have preexisting CHD. More intensive dietary therapy will benefit patients with severely elevated LDL-C levels (over 220 mg/dl) and patients with CHD. These patients will often need to proceed to drug therapy within 2–3 months while dietary therapy continues with a step 2 diet. Cholesterol levels should be monitored at 6- to 8-week intervals to provide incentive for change. Gradual initiation of diet changes often works better than drastic alterations.

5. **Adjustments in dietary therapy** need to be made for the elderly, who may have poor nutritional intake, and in pregnant women, who have increased requirements for a number of nutrients. Severely restrictive diets should not be used in young children with the exception of those with primary lipoprotein lipase deficiency, in whom dietary fat restriction is necessary to prevent hyperchylomicronemia.

6. **Improved compliance may be achieved** by setting realistic goals with an emphasis on gradual change; involving the patient, food preparers, and family in making and implementing decisions; and referring patients to registered dietitians who can offer endorsement and encouragement of diet as an effective therapy.

D. **Hypertriglyceridemic patients** usually respond to restriction of dietary fat but may also require decreased intake of simple sugars and alcohol. Some patients who markedly increase the carbohydrate content of their diet will have increases in triglyceride levels. Hypertriglyceridemic patients should generally not be on diets with a fat content of less than 20–25% of calories, except for patients with the chylomicronemia syndrome.

E. **The chylomicronemia syndrome** requires a diet very low in total fat (10–20% of total calories as fat). Primary lipoprotein lipase deficiency is treated with fat restriction and does not respond to drug therapy.

III. **Weight loss** is beneficial if the patient is overweight. Total calories should be adjusted for **gradual** weight loss. Elevated triglycerides often respond well. HDL-C may increase with weight loss and LDL-C may decrease. A general approach is to lower caloric intake by approximately 500 calories/day. Very low-calorie diets are not recommended in most cases.

IV. **Increased physical activity** is an important part of the overall management of patients with hyperlipidemia. It is helpful in lowering triglyceride and cholesterol levels and in raising HDL-C. It can also contribute to weight loss. Regular exercise will also help patients who have lost weight maintain their weight. An exercise program must be designed for the individual depending on his or her state of health, fitness, and cardiac status.

V. **Postmenopausal women** may benefit from hormone replacement therapy as a first-line therapy for hyperlipidemia. Oral estrogens lower LDL-C and raise HDL-C. Triglycerides increase modestly in normotriglyceridemic women. The addition of a progestin such as medroxyprogesterone acetate or micronized progesterone is necessary in women who have a uterus; this may blunt some of estrogen's beneficial effects on lipids.

VI. **Discontinuation of thiazide diuretics and beta-adrenergic antagonists,** if possible, sometimes leads to reduction of triglycerides, cholesterol, and LDL-C and to an increase in HDL-C. Substitution of a cardioselective beta-adrenergic antagonist for a noncardioselective one may be helpful. In postmenopausal women who have triglycerides over 500 mg/dl on estrogen replacement therapy, switching from an oral estrogen preparation to transdermal estrogen will often lead to improvement in triglyceride levels.

VII. **Secondary causes of hyperlipidemia** should be treated. Patients who are hypothyroid should be on adequate replacement dosages of levothyroxine (see Chap. 21). Control of hyperglycemia is critical if diabetic dyslipidemia is to be adequately managed (see Chap. 20).

VIII. **Drug therapy** is considered if maximal diet, weight reduction, and exercise efforts do not reduce serum lipid levels to goal levels after an adequate trial.
A. **Initiation of drug therapy** for hypercholesterolemia should be considered if LDL-C remains greater than 190 mg/dl in patients without CHD or two or more cardiac risk factors. In patients with two or more risk factors, the cutoff point is LDL-C greater than 160 mg/dl. In patients with CHD, drug therapy should be

considered if the LDL-C remains above 130 mg/dl in spite of diet therapy. For patients with CHD who have LDL-C levels of 100–130 mg/dl, use of drug therapy depends on the physician's clinical judgment about the benefits of adding medication. Premenopausal women and men under age 35 who have no other risk factors have a relatively low risk of developing clinical CHD within a few years; drug therapy in this group should be deferred unless the LDL-C is over 220 mg/dl or multiple risk factors are present.

B. **The goals of therapy** are the reduction of LDL-C to less than 100 mg/dl in patients with CHD, less than 130 mg/dl in those with two or more risk factors, and to less than 160 mg/dl in patients without CHD or two or more risk factors.

C. **Diet therapy** is continued even if drug therapy is used.

D. **Drugs that lower LDL-C** are the bile acid sequestrant resins, nicotinic acid, and the HMG-CoA reductase inhibitors. The resins and nicotinic acid have been shown to be both safe and efficacious in reducing cholesterol and the risk of CHD. The HMG-CoA reductase inhibitors are effective in lowering LDL-C. However, their long-term safety has not been established, and they should be used primarily in patients with CHD, more severe hyperlipidemias, or several risk factors.

E. **Second-choice drugs** for lowering LDL-C include gemfibrozil, probucol, and clofibrate.

F. **Hypertriglyceridemia** requiring drug therapy can be treated with nicotinic acid or gemfibrozil.

G. **Dysbetalipoproteinemia** responds well to diet therapy and weight loss. When drugs are needed, nicotinic acid, gemfibrozil, or clofibrate can be used.

H. **In patients with a low level of HDL-C and high LDL-C** level, cholesterol-lowering drugs that also raise HDL-C, such as nicotinic acid, should be given priority (*Arch Intern Med* 149:505, 1989).

I. **Drug combinations** may be useful in certain situations.
   1. **In severe hypercholesterolemia,** it is often necessary to use a combination of diet therapy and two or more drugs to reduce LDL-C to desired levels. Useful combinations include a resin plus nicotinic acid or a resin plus an HMG-CoA reductase inhibitor. Some patients with the heterozygous form of familial hypercholesterolemia respond well to a combination of HMG-CoA reductase inhibitor, resin, and nicotinic acid (*Ann Intern Med* 107:616, 1987).
   2. **Combined LDL-C and triglyceride elevations** may respond to nicotinic acid or HMG-CoA reductase inhibitors as single-drug therapy. A few patients may have adequate control with gemfibrozil alone. Some patients will require the addition of a resin to gemfibrozil or nicotinic acid to have adequate lowering of LDL-C levels.
   3. **Low doses of two drugs** can be combined if higher doses of a single agent are not tolerated by the patient. The combination of an HMG-CoA reductase inhibitor and resin or nicotinic acid and a resin may be quite effective.

J. **The response to therapy should be monitored** by checking cholesterol and triglyceride levels after 4–6 weeks of therapy. If there is no response to a drug after 2–3 months in spite of dosage adjustments, or if there are unacceptable side effects, the drug should be discontinued. If the initial drug produces only a partial response at a tolerated dosage, addition of a second drug with a different mechanism of action may be useful.

IX. **Plasmapheresis and liver transplantation** have been used to treat patients with the homozygous form of familial hypercholesterolemia since these patients respond poorly to drug therapy. Plasmapheresis has also been used for some patients with severe heterozygous FH.

Drugs

I. **Bile acid sequestrant resins** (cholestyramine and colestipol) are insoluble, nonabsorbable, anion-exchange resins that bind bile acids within the intestine, preventing their reabsorption. Since more cholesterol must be used to synthesize bile acids, there is an increase in cell surface receptors for LDL, producing a fall in circulating LDL-C levels. Reduction of LDL-C is dose-dependent; up to 35% reduction can be seen. HDL-C may increase, and VLDL will sometimes increase, usually transiently. The use of resins as single-drug therapy is contraindicated in the presence of elevated triglyceride levels (over 400 mg/dl).

A. Compliance is enhanced and side effects minimized by starting therapy with low dosages and carefully educating the patient about these drugs. The resins are powders that must be mixed with a liquid. The initial dosage of **cholestyramine** is 4 g (1 scoop or packet) PO bid with meals, gradually increasing to 8–16 g PO bid. The initial dosage of **colestipol** is 1 scoop or packet (5 g) PO bid, increasing to a maximum of 15 g PO bid. Lower dosages may be effective in some patients. Increasing the dosage gradually and starting at even lower dosages, such as one-half of 1 packet or 1 packet/day can be helpful. The drug can be mixed in almost any liquid or semiliquid food. Timing close to meals is important. It should be taken within 1 hour of a meal, especially the evening meal if once-a-day dosing is used. Colestipol in **tablet** form are also now available. The tablets contain 1 g of active drug. Dosing is 4–8 tablets once or twice a day with meals. Side effects and efficacy are comparable to powdered resin. Tablets may be more convenient or palatable for patients who dislike the powder.

B. Side effects include constipation, abdominal pain, nausea, vomiting, bloating, heartburn, belching, and flatulence. These effects will often diminish with continued use of the drug. The resins may interfere with absorption of thiazides, digoxin, warfarin, thyroxine, and cyclosporine; these medications should be given at least 1 hour before or 4 hours after the resins.

II. Nicotinic acid is a water-soluble vitamin that can lower levels of VLDL up to 40%, can lower LDL-C by 15–30%, and can raise HDL-C by 10–30%. It is an inexpensive and very useful lipid-modifying drug with a long history of use. Nicotinic acid has been used in several secondary and angiographic trials of lipid lowering (*J Am Coll Cardiol* 8:1245, 1986; *JAMA* 257:3233, 1987; *N Engl J Med* 323:1289, 1990).

A. Dosage should be low initially, with a gradual increase. Initial dosage is 100 mg PO 1–3 times/day **with meals**, increasing slowly (e.g., by 300 mg/day each week) to 2–4 g/day. Maximum daily dose is 6 g/day.

B. Side effects limit the use of high dosages. Cutaneous flushing occurs in most patients, but tolerance usually develops. It is important that nicotinic acid be taken with food to help decrease flushing. Aspirin, 80 mg PO 30 minutes before each dose, can decrease flushing. Other side effects include pruritus, rash, nausea, dyspepsia, anorexia, dizziness, and hypotension. Hyperuricemia, liver function abnormalities, and worsening of glucose intolerance may occur. Baseline liver profiles and uric acid and fasting blood glucose levels should be obtained and monitored monthly while the dosage is being increased to 1–4 g/day and thereafter every 3–4 months. Use of nicotinic acid is contraindicated in patients with gout, peptic ulcer disease, inflammatory bowel disease, and significant arrhythmias. Diabetes mellitus is not an absolute contraindication, especially in patients receiving insulin, but blood sugar levels must be monitored carefully. Use of some generic sustained-release preparations may be associated with increased toxicity, including severe hepatotoxicity (*Ann Intern Med* 111:253, 1989). Severe toxicity is more likely to occur when patients switch abruptly from a nonsustained release to a sustained release preparation without reducing the total dosage. Use of such preparations should be avoided. **Niacinamide has no significant effect** on lipid levels.

III. The HMG-CoA reductase inhibitors are a new class of drugs that inhibit the rate-limiting step in cholesterol biosynthesis. **Lovastatin** is the first drug of this class to be released in the United States. Other drugs in the class are **pravastatin**, **simvastatin**, and **fluvastatin**. All have the same mechanism of action and similar side effects. Fluvastatin is chemically different from the other drugs in the class but acts similarly. Inhibition of enzyme activity leads to a decrease in intracellular cholesterol pools and consequently an increase in LDL receptors; plasma levels of LDL-C are reduced by up to 40% (*N Engl J Med* 318:81, 1988; *Medical Letter* 36:45, 1994). HDL-C increases slightly, and triglyceride levels may also decrease.

A. Initial dosage of lovastatin is 10–20 mg PO with the evening meal. The dosage can be increased to 20 mg PO bid with meals and, if necessary, to 40 mg PO bid. Dosages for pravastatin are 10–40 mg/day; for simvastatin, 5–40 mg/day; and for fluvastatin, 20–40 mg/day. Pravastatin, simvastatin, and fluvastatin do not need to be taken with food and can be given once a day at bedtime.

B. Side effects are usually mild and transient and include bloating, flatulence, dyspepsia, diarrhea, constipation, nausea, abdominal pain, and insomnia. Liver function tests should be followed, preferably at 6-week intervals for the first 3 months, then at 2-month intervals during the first year of therapy, and thereafter every 6 months. Mild elevations of transaminases may occur after starting therapy; these usually decrease with continued therapy. In 1–2% of patients, transaminase elevations to more than 3 times the upper limit of normal have occurred up to 15 months after starting therapy. In such cases, the drug should be discontinued. The HMG CoA reductase inhibitors should be avoided in the presence of active liver disease. Myalgias, myositis, and elevated levels of creatine phosphokinase (CK) have occurred in less than 1% of patients taking lovastatin. Levels of CK should be checked if patients have muscular complaints, and the reductase inhibitor should be discontinued if CK is elevated. The combination of lovastatin with cyclosporine, gemfibrozil, erythromycin, or niacin carries an increased risk of myopathy. Rhabdomyolysis has been reported. The combination of any of the reductase inhibitors with the above medications must be done with great caution because of the risk of myopathy.

IV. Fibric acid derivatives include gemfibrozil, clofibrate, and fenofibrate. They lower levels of VLDL and raise levels of HDL-C. Gemfibrozil and clofibrate are currently available in the United States.

A. Gemfibrozil produces a 0–15% reduction of LDL-C levels in patients with elevated levels. LDL may increase in patients with hypertriglyceridemia. It is useful in patients with hypertriglyceridemia and in combination with resins for combined hyperlipidemia. A primary prevention trial (*N Engl J Med* 317:1237, 1987) showed decreased risk of cardiac disease in hypercholesterolemic and hypertriglyceridemic men treated with gemfibrozil over a 5-year period.

1. Dosage is 600 mg PO bid before meals.

2. Side effects include bloating, abdominal pain, diarrhea, nausea, headaches, and occasional rashes. Liver enzymes should be monitored 2 months after starting the drug. Gemfibrozil potentiates the effects of warfarin and may make bile more lithogenic.

B. Clofibrate is used infrequently because of questions of long-term safety. It is used mostly for severe hypertriglyceridemia and in some patients with dysbetalipoproteinemia.

1. Dosage is 1 g PO bid.

2. Side effects include nausea, diarrhea, liver dysfunction, and rashes. Clofibrate has been reported to cause a myopathic syndrome, especially in patients with renal failure. The incidence of gallstones is increased, and the drug also potentiates the effects of phenytoin, tolbutamide, and warfarin.

V. Probucol reduces levels of LDL-C by 8–15% but also reduces HDL-C by up to 25%. Triglyceride levels are not affected. It may be useful for hypercholesterolemic patients who do not tolerate other drugs.

A. Dosage is 500 mg PO bid with meals.

B. Side effects are uncommon; they include diarrhea, flatulence, nausea, and abdominal pain. Prolongation of the QT interval can also occur. Probucol accumulates in adipose tissue and has a long half-life; it can remain in the body for months after discontinuation.

VI. Neomycin and D-thyroxine have a high potential for serious side effects and are not recommended for general use.

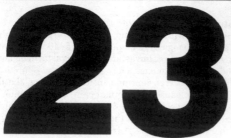

Mineral and Metabolic Bone Disease

Sam Dagogo-Jack and
William E. Clutter

Mineral Disorders

I. **Calcium** is essential for bone formation and neuromuscular function. Approximately 99% of body calcium is in bone; most of the other 1% is in the extracellular fluid (ECF). About 50% of serum calcium is ionized (free) and the remainder is complexed, primarily to albumin. The normal range of serum total calcium is 8.9–10.3 mg/dl (1 mg/dl = 0.25 mM). Changes in serum albumin, especially hypoalbuminemia, alter total serum calcium concentration without affecting the clinically relevant ionized calcium level. Total calcium concentration can be "corrected" for hypoalbuminemia by adding 0.8 mg/dl for every 1.0 g/dl that the serum albumin falls below 4.0 g/dl. However, this correction is imprecise, and if serum albumin is abnormal, clinical decisions should be based on ionized calcium levels, which must lie within a narrow range (4.6–5.1 mg/dl) for normal neuromuscular function. Calcium metabolism is regulated by **parathyroid hormone (PTH)** and metabolites of **vitamin D**. **PTH increases serum calcium** by stimulating bone resorption, increasing renal calcium reabsorption, and promoting renal conversion of vitamin D to its active metabolite calcitriol (1,25-dihydroxyvitamin D [1,25(OH)$_2$D]). PTH also increases renal phosphate excretion. Serum calcium regulates PTH secretion by a negative feedback mechanism; hypocalcemia stimulates and hypercalcemia suppresses PTH release. Secreted PTH is rapidly metabolized, and inactive carboxyterminal fragments constitute most of circulating PTH immunoactivity. **Vitamin D** is absorbed from food and synthesized in skin exposed to sunlight. The liver converts it to 25-hydroxyvitamin D [25(OH)D], which in turn is converted by the kidney to 1,25(OH)$_2$D. The latter metabolite increases serum calcium by promoting intestinal calcium absorption and plays a role in bone formation and resorption. It also enhances phosphate absorption by the intestine. Synthesis of 1,25(OH)$_2$D is stimulated by both PTH and hypophosphatemia and is inhibited by increased serum phosphorus.

A. **Hypercalcemia** (Table 23-1) (*N Engl J Med* 326:1196, 1992) is almost always caused by both increased entry of calcium into the ECF (from bone resorption or intestinal absorption) and decreased renal calcium clearance. More than 90% of cases are due to primary hyperparathyroidism or malignancy.

1. **Primary hyperparathyroidism** causes most cases of hypercalcemia in ambulatory patients. It is a common disorder, especially in elderly women, in whom the annual incidence is about 2/1,000. About 85% of cases are due to an adenoma of a single gland, 15% to hyperplasia of all 4 glands, and 1% to parathyroid carcinoma. Most patients have asymptomatic hypercalcemia found incidentally. Patients may have symptoms of hypercalcemia (see sec. **I.A.4**), nephrolithiasis, osteopenia affecting primarily cortical bone (*Am J Med* 89:327, 1990), or, rarely, a specific bone disorder, **osteitis fibrosa**.

2. **Malignancy** is responsible for most hypercalcemia in hospitalized patients, acting via two major mechanisms. In **local osteolytic hypercalcemia**, tumor cell products, such as cytokines, act locally to stimulate osteoclastic bone resorption. This form of malignant hypercalcemia occurs only with extensive bone involvement by tumor, most often due to breast carcinoma, myeloma, and lymphoma. In **humoral hypercalcemia of malignancy (HHM)**, tumor products act systemically to stimulate bone resorption and, in many cases, to

Table 23-1. Causes of hypercalcemia

Common
  Primary hyperparathyroidism
  Malignancy
Uncommon
  Sarcoidosis, other granulomatous disease
  Vitamin D toxicity
  Hyperthyroidism
  Thiazides
  Lithium
  Milk-alkali syndrome
  Immobilization
  Familial hypocalciuric hypercalcemia
  Associated with renal failure

decrease calcium excretion. **PTH-related peptide**, which acts via PTH receptors but is not detected by PTH immunoassays, is an important mediator of this syndrome. Tumor-derived growth factors may also play a role (*Endocrinol Metab Clin North Am* 20:473, 1991), but PTH itself does not. HHM is most often caused by squamous carcinoma of the lung, head and neck, or esophagus, or by renal, bladder, or ovarian carcinoma. Patients with malignant hypercalcemia almost always have advanced, clinically obvious disease.

3. **Other causes of hypercalcemia** (see Table 23-1) are uncommon and are almost always clinically evident. Thiazide diuretics cause persistent hypercalcemia in patients with increased bone turnover (e.g., mild primary hyperparathyroidism). **Familial hypocalciuric hypercalcemia** (*Endocrinol Metab Clin North Am* 18:723, 1989) is a rare autosomal dominant disorder that causes asymptomatic hypercalcemia from birth.

4. **Clinical manifestations.** Most symptoms of hypercalcemia are present only if serum calcium is above 12 mg/dl and tend to be more severe if hypercalcemia develops rapidly. **Renal** manifestations include polyuria and nephrolithiasis. **GI** symptoms include anorexia, nausea, vomiting, and constipation. **Neurologic** findings include weakness, fatigue, confusion, stupor, and coma. **ECG manifestations** include a shortened QT interval. Patients with hypercalcemia are more susceptible to digoxin toxicity. If serum calcium is above 13 mg/dl, renal failure and ectopic soft-tissue calcification may develop. Polyuria combined with nausea and vomiting may cause marked dehydration, which impairs calcium excretion and may cause rapidly worsening hypercalcemia.

5. **Diagnosis.** Increases in serum albumin can raise the total calcium level slightly, without affecting the clinically relevant ionized calcium concentration. Mildly elevated serum calcium levels should be repeated, and the **serum ionized calcium** should be measured to determine whether hypercalcemia is actually present. The diagnosis of hypercalcemia requires distinction of primary hyperparathyroidism from malignancy.
   a. **The history and physical examination** should focus on (1) the **duration of hypercalcemia** (if present for more than 6 months without obvious cause, primary hyperparathyroidism is almost certain); (2) history of **renal stones** (which are not seen in hypercalcemia of malignancy); (3) clinical evidence of any of the unusual causes of hypercalcemia; and (4) **symptoms and signs of malignancy** (which almost always precede malignant hypercalcemia).
   b. **The serum PTH level** should be measured (*Endocrinol Metab Clin North Am* 18:611, 1989). Current immunoassays measure either the entire PTH molecule (intact PTH assays) or determinants on the carboxyterminal fragment of PTH (midmolecule or C-terminal assays). In most patients,

both assays discriminate between primary hyperparathyroidism and other causes of hypercalcemia (*Clin Chem* 37:162, 1991). However, in renal failure, carboxyterminal fragments accumulate in serum, and an intact PTH assay should be used for diagnosis of hypercalcemia.

c. Other tests should include a CBC and measurement of serum electrolytes. Any evidence of malignancy or other causes of hypercalcemia should be carefully evaluated.

d. Hypercalcemia due to malignancy or the uncommon causes listed in Table 23-1 is almost always evident from the history, physical examination, and routine laboratory tests; serum intact PTH levels are not elevated in these disorders. In a patient with chronic, asymptomatic hypercalcemia, an elevated serum PTH, and no clinical evidence of malignancy, the diagnosis of primary hyperparathyroidism is secure. Malignancy or other causes should be sought if hypercalcemia is severe or develops rapidly and the serum PTH is not elevated.

6. Therapy of hypercalcemia (*Endocrinol Metab Clin North Am* 22:343, 1993) includes measures that increase calcium excretion and decrease resorption of calcium from bone.

a. ECF volume restoration. Severely hypercalcemic patients are almost always dehydrated, and initial therapy is volume expansion with 0.9% saline to restore the glomerular filtration rate (GFR) and promote calcium excretion. The initial infusion rate should be 300–500 ml/hour and should be reduced after the ECF volume deficit has been partially corrected. At least 3–4 liters should be given in the first 24 hours, and a positive fluid balance of at least 2 liters should be achieved.

b. Saline diuresis. After ECF volume is restored, infusion of 0.9% saline (100–200 ml/hour) promotes calcium excretion. Therapy should be monitored with careful records of fluid intake and output, daily weight, and frequent evaluation for evidence of heart failure. **Serum electrolytes,** calcium, and magnesium should be measured q6–12h. Adequate replacement of potassium and magnesium is essential (see sec. **III.B.3** and Chap. 3). Furosemide, 20–40 mg IV bid–qid, adds little to the effect of saline diuresis and may prevent adequate restoration of ECF volume. It should not be given unless clinical evidence of heart failure develops. **Thiazide diuretics must be avoided,** since they impair calcium excretion.

c. Pamidronate is a bisphosphonate that inhibits bone resorption (*Am J Med* 95:297, 1993). A dose of 60–90 mg in 1 liter of 0.9% saline or 5% D/W is infused over 4 hours (*Bone Miner* 9:122, 1990); for severe hypercalcemia (>13.5 mg/dl), 90 mg should be used. Serum calcium should be measured daily. Hypercalcemia abates gradually over several days and remains suppressed for 1–2 weeks. Treatment can be repeated if hypercalcemia recurs. Side effects include asymptomatic hypocalcemia, hypomagnesemia, hypophosphatemia, and transient low-grade fever.

d. Plicamycin (mithramycin) inhibits bone resorption. Because of its toxicity, it is used only in malignant hypercalcemia. A dose of 25 µg/kg in 500 ml 5% D/W, infused IV over 4–6 hours, gradually reduces serum calcium over 2–4 days; its effect persists 5–15 days. Serum calcium should be measured qd and a CBC, prothrombin time, creatinine, and liver enzyme measurements should be obtained every 2–3 days. Treatment can be repeated when hypercalcemia recurs. Plicamycin is less effective and less well tolerated than pamidronate (*Ann Oncol* 3:619, 1992). Side effects include nausea, vomiting, thrombocytopenia, platelet dysfunction, coagulation factor deficiency, renal failure, and hepatic dysfunction. Plicamycin is contraindicated in patients with a bleeding diathesis and should be avoided in patients with renal failure or hepatic dysfunction, or during myelotoxic chemotherapy.

e. Calcitonin inhibits bone resorption and increases renal calcium excretion. Salmon calcitonin, 4–8 IU/kg IM or SC q6–12h, lowers serum calcium 1–3 mg/dl within several hours. The hypocalcemic effect wanes after several days but may be prolonged by concomitant therapy with prednisone, 30–60 mg qd. Side effects include flushing, nausea, and, rarely, allergic reactions. Calcitonin is less consistently effective than other inhibitors of bone resorption but has no serious toxicity and is safe in renal failure. It can be used early in the therapy of severe hypercalcemia to achieve a rapid response but is not useful for long-term therapy.

   f. Glucocorticoids lower serum calcium by inhibiting cytokine release, by direct cytolytic effects on some tumor cells, by inhibiting intestinal calcium absorption, and by increasing urinary calcium excretion. They are effective in hypercalcemia due to myeloma, other hematologic malignancies, sarcoidosis, and vitamin D intoxication. Other tumors rarely respond. The initial dose is prednisone, 20–50 mg PO bid, or its equivalent. It may take 5–10 days for serum calcium to fall. After serum calcium stabilizes, the dose should be gradually reduced to the minimum needed to control symptoms of hypercalcemia. Toxicity (see Chap. 24) limits the usefulness of glucocorticoids for long-term therapy.

   g. Oral phosphate inhibits calcium absorption and promotes calcium deposition in bone and soft tissue. It should be used only if the serum phosphorus level is less than 3 mg/dl and renal function is normal, to minimize the risk of soft-tissue calcification. Doses of 0.5–1.0 g elemental phosphorus PO tid (see sec. **II.B.3**) modestly lower serum calcium in some patients. Serum calcium, phosphorus, and creatinine should be monitored frequently, and the dose should be reduced if serum phosphorus exceeds 4.5 mg/dl or the product of serum calcium and phosphorus (measured in mg/dl) exceeds 60. Side effects include diarrhea, nausea, and soft-tissue calcification. **IV phosphate should never be used to treat hypercalcemia**.

   h. Gallium nitrate inhibits bone resorption. A regimen of 200 mg/m^2 in 1 liter 5% D/W or 0.9% saline infused IV over 24 hours and repeated daily for 5 days, has been used to treat malignant hypercalcemia (*Ann Intern Med* 108:669, 1988). A saline diuresis of at least 2 liters/day should be maintained during treatment. Side effects include hypocalcemia, hypophosphatemia, and impairment of renal function; in a few patients receiving higher doses, optic neuritis has developed. Gallium should not be used if serum creatinine is greater than 2.5 mg/dl. There is relatively little experience with the use of gallium for treatment of hypercalcemia.

7. Acute management is warranted if severe symptoms are present or serum calcium is greater than 12 mg/dl. The goal is alleviation of symptoms, rather than brisk normalization of serum calcium. The first step is **replacement of ECF volume** with 0.9% saline (see sec. **I.A.6.a**). **Saline diuresis** with 0.9% saline, 100–200 ml/hour, should then be continued. An inhibitor of bone resorption should be given early; **pamidronate** is the drug of choice. If pamidronate is not effective, **plicamycin** may be used, but the latter is more toxic and should be used only in malignant hypercalcemia. Calcitonin is rarely necessary but can be used in patients with renal failure or added to another drug to rapidly control severe hypercalcemia. In oliguric renal failure that cannot be treated with IV saline, **hemodialysis** with a calcium-free dialysate lowers serum calcium temporarily.

8. Chronic management of hypercalcemia

   a. Parathyroidectomy is the only effective therapy for primary hyperparathyroidism. The natural history of asymptomatic hyperparathyroidism is not fully known, but in many patients the disorder has a benign course, with little change in clinical findings or serum calcium concentration for years. The possibility of progressive loss of bone mass and increased risk of fracture are the main concerns. The increased risk of fracture may be nonprogressive following the diagnosis of hyperparathyroidism (*Arch Intern Med* 152:2269, 1992). Deterioration of renal function is possible but unlikely in the absence of nephrolithiasis. Currently, it is impossible to predict which patients will develop complications. **Indications for surgery**

include (1) symptoms due to hypercalcemia, (2) nephrolithiasis, (3) reduced bone mass (more than 2 standard deviations below mean for age), (4) serum calcium more than 12 mg/dl, (5) age less than 50, and (6) infeasibility of long-term follow-up. Surgery is a reasonable choice in healthy patients even if they do not meet these criteria, since it has a high success rate, with low morbidity and mortality. However, asymptomatic patients can be followed by assessing clinical status and serum calcium and creatinine levels at 6- to 12-month intervals. Bone mass at the hip should be assessed annually, using dual-energy radiography. Surgery should be recommended if any of the above criteria develop or if there is progressive decline in bone mass or renal function.

Parathyroidectomy performed by a surgeon experienced in the procedure has a success rate of 90–95%. After surgery, Chvostek's and Trousseau's signs and serum calcium levels should be monitored daily for several days. There is often a brief (1–2 days) period of mild, asymptomatic hypocalcemia. In rare patients with overt bone disease, hypocalcemia may be severe and prolonged (the hungry bone syndrome), requiring therapy (see sec. **I.B.3**). Other complications include permanent hypoparathyroidism and injury to the recurrent laryngeal nerve. Reexploration has a lower success rate and a greater risk of complications and should be performed at a referral center. Parathyroid localization procedures are not indicated before initial neck exploration but may be helpful before reexploration (*World J Surg* 15:706, 1991).

Medical therapy has not been shown to affect the clinical outcome of primary hyperparathyroidism. However, in postmenopausal women with primary hyperparathyroidism, ethinyl estradiol, 30 μg PO qd, lowers serum calcium slightly and may help to preserve bone mass (*J Bone Miner Res* 6 S2:S125, 1991). In patients with symptomatic hypercalcemia who refuse or cannot tolerate surgery, physical activity should be encouraged, along with a diet containing at least 2–3 liters of fluid and 8–10 g of salt/day. Dietary calcium should not be restricted, and thiazide diuretics must not be used. Oral phosphate therapy (see sec. **I.A.6.g**) may lower serum calcium but also raises serum PTH levels; its benefits do not clearly outweigh risks, and it should be used only if symptomatic hypercalcemia cannot be surgically corrected.

b. **Therapy of malignant hypercalcemia** may control symptoms while antineoplastic therapy takes effect but rarely succeeds for a long period unless the cancer responds to treatment. Since patients usually have extensive, unresectable disease, with median survival less than 3 months, the initial decision should be whether therapy is warranted. This judgment depends on the prospect for effective treatment of the cancer and the expected quality of life. Treatment of hypercalcemia may palliate symptoms such as anorexia, nausea, and malaise that could be attributed to cancer (*Ann Intern Med* 112:499, 1990). However, in comatose patients with advanced cancer for which no further antineoplastic therapy is planned, hypercalcemia should generally not be treated.

After acute management of hypercalcemia, physical activity and a diet containing at least 2–3 liters of fluid and 8–10 g of salt/day should be encouraged, and nausea should be treated. Restriction of dietary calcium is not helpful. Repeated doses of IV **pamidronate** (see sec. **I.A.6.c**) can be given when hypercalcemia recurs. Plicamycin may be used if pamidronate is ineffective. **Prednisone,** 20–50 mg PO bid, usually controls hypercalcemia in multiple myeloma and other hematologic malignancies. Oral **phosphate** can be tried if the serum phosphorus level is low and renal function is normal.

c. **Hypercalcemia due to other disorders.** Vitamin D toxicity should be treated with prednisone and a low-calcium diet (<400 mg/day). The effects of vitamin D itself may take up to 2 months to abate, but the toxicity of its metabolites is more short-lived. Hypercalcemia due to sarcoidosis responds to prednisone, and a dose of 10–20 mg/day may be sufficient for long-term control.

B. **Hypocalcemia.** The most common cause of low total serum calcium is **hypoalbuminemia.** If serum free (ionized) calcium is normal, then no disorder of calcium metabolism is present. If ionized calcium cannot be measured, the total serum calcium can be corrected by adding 0.8 mg/dl for every 1 g/dl decrease of serum albumin below 4 g/dl to determine if true hypocalcemia is present. **Causes of low serum free calcium** levels include renal failure, hypoparathyroidism (either idiopathic or postsurgical), severe hypomagnesemia, hypermagnesemia, acute pancreatitis, rhabdomyolysis, tumor lysis syndrome, vitamin D deficiency, pseudohypoparathyroidism (PTH resistance), and, rarely, multiple citrated blood transfusions. A low serum free calcium level is common in critically ill patients, sometimes without evident cause. Drugs may cause hypocalcemia, including antineoplastic agents (cisplatin, cytosine arabinoside), antibiotics (pentamidine, ketoconazole, foscarnet), and drugs used to treat hypercalcemia (see sec. **I.A.6**) (*Endocrinol Metab Clin North Am* 22:363, 1993).

1. **Clinical manifestations** vary with the degree and rate of onset; chronic hypocalcemia may be asymptomatic. Alkalosis augments calcium binding to albumin and increases the severity of symptoms. Increased excitability of nerves and muscles causes paresthesias and **tetany,** including carpopedal spasms. **Trousseau's sign** is development of carpal spasm when a BP cuff is inflated above systolic pressure for 3 minutes. **Chvostek's sign** is twitching of facial muscles when the facial nerve is tapped anterior to the ear. The presence of these signs is known as **latent tetany.** Severe hypocalcemia may cause lethargy or confusion, or, rarely, laryngospasm, seizures, or reversible heart failure. The ECG may show a prolonged QT interval. Chronic hypocalcemia may cause cataracts and calcification of the basal ganglia.

2. **Diagnosis.** The **history and physical examination** should focus on (1) previous neck surgery (hypoparathyroidism may develop immediately or gradually over years); (2) disorders associated with idiopathic hypoparathyroidism (e.g., hypothyroidism, adrenal failure, candidiasis, vitiligo); (3) family history of hypocalcemia (which may be present in hypoparathyroidism or pseudohypoparathyroidism); (4) drugs that cause hypocalcemia or hypomagnesemia (see sec. **III.B**); (5) conditions that cause vitamin D deficiency (see Metabolic Bone Disease, sec. **II**); and (6) findings of pseudohypoparathyroidism (short stature, short metacarpals). **Laboratory studies** should include measurement of serum free calcium, phosphorus, magnesium, creatinine, and PTH. Serum phosphorus is elevated in hypocalcemia resulting from most causes, except vitamin D deficiency, in which it is usually low. Serum PTH is elevated in disorders other than hypoparathyroidism and magnesium deficiency.

3. **Acute management.** Symptomatic hypocalcemia should be treated as an emergency with 10% **calcium gluconate** (90 mg elemental calcium/10 ml), 2 ampules (20 ml) IV over 10 minutes, followed by infusion of 60 ml of calcium gluconate in 500 ml 5% D/W (1 mg/ml) at 0.5–2.0 mg/kg/hour. Serum calcium should be measured q4–6h. The infusion rate should be adjusted to avoid recurrent symptomatic hypocalcemia and to maintain the serum calcium between 8 and 9 mg/dl. The underlying cause should be treated or long-term therapy started, and the IV infusion then gradually tapered. **Hypomagnesemia,** if present, must be treated to correct hypocalcemia (see sec. **III.B.3**). In patients taking digoxin, the ECG should be monitored since hypocalcemia potentiates digitalis toxicity. **Calcium and bicarbonate are not compatible IV admixtures.**

4. **Long-term management** of hypoparathyroidism and pseudohypoparathyroidism requires calcium supplements and vitamin D or its active metabolite to increase intestinal calcium absorption. Since PTH cannot limit urinary calcium excretion in these diseases, hypercalciuria and nephrolithiasis are potential side effects. **The objective is to maintain serum calcium levels slightly below the normal range (between 8–9 mg/dl),** which usually prevents manifestations of hypocalcemia and minimizes hypercalciuria. While the

dose of vitamin D is being titrated, serum calcium should be measured twice a week. When a maintenance dose is achieved, serum and 24-hour urine calcium levels should be monitored every 3–6 months, since unexpected fluctuations may occur. If urine calcium exceeds 250 mg/24 hours, the dose of vitamin D should be reduced. **If hypercalcemia develops,** vitamin D and calcium should be stopped until serum calcium falls to a normal concentration, then both should be restarted at lower doses. Hypercalcemia due to calcitriol usually resolves within 1 week, and serum calcium should be monitored q24–48h. Hypercalcemia due to vitamin D itself may take over 2 months to resolve, and that due to calcifediol (25-[OH]D) resolves in 7–30 days. Symptomatic vitamin D–induced hypercalcemia should be treated with prednisone (see sec. **I.A.6.f**). In mild vitamin D toxicity, serum calcium can be monitored at weekly intervals until it returns to normal.

a. **Oral calcium supplements. Calcium carbonate** (Oscal, 250 or 500 mg elemental calcium/tablet; Tums Extra-Strength, 400 mg elemental calcium/5 ml; or various generics) is the least expensive compound. The initial dosage is 1–2 g elemental calcium PO tid during the transition from IV to oral therapy. For long-term therapy, the typical dosage is 0.5–1.0 g PO tid with meals. Calcium carbonate is well absorbed when taken with food, even in patients with achlorhydria. Side effects include dyspepsia and constipation.

b. **Vitamin D.** Dietary deficiency can be corrected by 400–1,000 IU/day, but treatment of other hypocalcemic disorders requires much larger doses of vitamin D or use of an active metabolite. **Calcitriol** or $1,25(OH)_2D$ (Rocaltrol, 0.25- or 0.5-µg/capsule) has a rapid onset of action. The initial dose is 0.25 µg PO qd, and most patients are maintained on 0.5–2.0 µg PO qd. The dose can be increased at 2- to 4-week intervals. **Vitamin D** (50,000 IU or 1.25 mg/capsule) requires weeks to achieve full effect. The initial dose is 50,000 IU PO qd, and usual maintenance doses are 50,000–100,000 IU PO qd. The dose can be increased at 4- to 6-week intervals. Calcitriol is much more expensive than vitamin D, but its lower risk of toxicity makes it the best choice for most patients.

c. **Other measures.** In patients with severe hyperphosphatemia, serum phosphorus should be lowered to less than 6.5 mg/dl with oral phosphate binders (see sec. **II.A.2.b**) before vitamin D is started. If hypercalciuria develops at serum calcium levels less than 8.5 mg/dl, hydrochlorothiazide, 50 mg PO qd, can be used to reduce urinary calcium excretion.

II. **Phosphorus** is critical for bone formation and cellular energy metabolism. About 85% of body phosphorus is in bone, and most of the remainder is within cells; only 1% is in the ECF. Thus, serum phosphorus levels may not reflect total body phosphorus stores. Phosphorus exists in the body as phosphate, but serum concentration is expressed as mass of phosphorus (1 mg/dl phosphorus = 0.32 mM phosphate). The normal range is 3.0–4.5 mg/dl, with somewhat higher values in children and postmenopausal women. Serum phosphorus is best measured in the fasting state, since there is diurnal variation, with a morning nadir, and since carbohydrate ingestion and glucose infusion lower serum phosphorus, while a high-phosphate meal raises it. Major regulatory factors include **PTH,** which lowers serum phosphorus by increasing renal excretion; $1,25(OH)_2D$, which increases serum phosphorus by enhancing intestinal phosphate absorption; **insulin,** which lowers serum levels by shifting phosphate into cells; dietary phosphate intake; and renal function.

A. **Hyperphosphatemia** is most often due to **renal failure** but also occurs in hypoparathyroidism, pseudohypoparathyroidism, rhabdomyolysis, tumor lysis syndrome, and metabolic and respiratory acidosis, and after excess phosphate administration.

1. **Clinical manifestations** are due to hypocalcemia (see sec. **I.B.1**) and ectopic calcification of soft tissues, including blood vessels, cornea, skin, kidney, and periarticular tissue. Chronic hyperphosphatemia contributes to renal osteodystrophy.

Table 23-2. Causes of severe hypophosphatemia (<1 mg/dl)

Alcohol abuse and withdrawal
Respiratory alkalosis
Malabsorption
Oral phosphate binders (aluminum-containing antacids)
Refeeding after malnutrition
Hyperalimentation
Severe burns
Therapy of diabetic ketoacidosis

2. **Management** (*N Engl J Med* 320:1140, 1989) includes the following:
   a. **Restriction of dietary phosphate** to 0.6–0.9 g/day.
   b. **Oral phosphate binders.** In patients with renal failure, **calcium carbonate** (see sec. **I.B.4.a**) is given at an initial dosage of 0.5–1.0 g elemental calcium PO tid with meals. The dosage can be increased at intervals of 2–4 weeks to a maximum of 3 g tid. The goal of therapy is to maintain serum phosphorus levels between 4.5 and 6.0 mg/dl. Serum calcium and phosphorus levels should be measured frequently and the dose adjusted to keep the serum calcium less than 11 mg/dl and the calcium-phosphorus product less than 60, to minimize the risk of ectopic calcification. If hyperphosphatemia persists despite doses of calcium that cause hypercalcemia, small doses of aluminum (Al) gels can be added—for example, **Al hydroxide** (600 mg/tablet or 320 mg/5 ml) or **Al carbonate** (600 mg/tablet or 400 mg/5 ml), 5–10 ml or 1–2 tablets PO tid with meals. Side effects of Al gels include nausea and constipation; **prolonged use in renal failure may cause Al toxicity** (see Chap. 11).
   c. **Saline diuresis** (see sec. **I.A.6.b**) will reduce acute hyperphosphatemia in patients without renal failure.
   d. **Dialysis** may be required to treat hyperphosphatemia in severe renal failure.
B. **Hypophosphatemia** (*Endocrinol Metab Clin North Am* 22:397, 1993) may be caused by impaired intestinal absorption, increased renal excretion, or redistribution of phosphate into cells. **Severe hypophosphatemia** (<1 mg/dl) (Table 23-2) usually indicates total body phosphate depletion. However, during therapy of diabetic ketoacidosis, hypophosphatemia seldom reflects severe phosphate depletion and very rarely causes clinical manifestations. **Moderate hypophosphatemia** (1.0–2.5 mg/dl) is common in hospitalized patients and may not indicate total body phosphate depletion. In addition to the conditions listed in Table 23-2, moderate hypophosphatemia may be caused by (1) infusion of glucose, (2) dietary vitamin D deficiency or malabsorption, and (3) increased renal phosphate loss due to hyperparathyroidism, the diuretic phase of acute tubular necrosis, renal transplantation, familial X-linked hypophosphatemia, Fanconi's syndrome, oncogenic osteomalacia, and ECF volume expansion.
   1. **Clinical manifestations** typically occur only if there is total body phosphate depletion and the serum phosphorus level is less than 1 mg/dl. Muscular abnormalities include weakness, rhabdomyolysis, impaired diaphragmatic function, respiratory failure, and congestive heart failure. Neurologic abnormalities include paresthesias, dysarthria, confusion, stupor, seizures, and coma. Hemolysis, platelet dysfunction, and metabolic acidosis rarely occur. Chronic hypophosphatemia causes rickets in children and osteomalacia in adults (see Metabolic Bone Disease, sec. **II**).
   2. **Diagnosis.** The cause is usually apparent, but if not, measurement of urine phosphorus levels helps define the mechanism. Excretion of more than 100 mg/day during hypophosphatemia indicates excessive renal loss. Family history, serum calcium and PTH, and urine amino acids help distinguish

among renal causes. Low serum 25(OH)D suggests dietary vitamin D deficiency or malabsorption.

3. **Management**
   a. **Moderate hypophosphatemia** (1.0–2.5 mg/dl) is usually asymptomatic and requires no therapy except correction of the cause. Persistent hypophosphatemia should be treated with oral phosphate supplements, 0.5–1.0 g of elemental phosphorus PO bid–tid. Preparations include Neutra-Phos (250 mg elemental phosphorus and 7 mEq each of sodium and potassium/ capsule) and Neutra-Phos K (250 mg elemental phosphorus and 14 mEq potassium/capsule). The contents of capsules should be dissolved in water. Fleet Phospho-Soda (815 mg phosphorus and 33 mEq sodium per 5 ml) can also be used. For patients who require long-term therapy, bulk powder is more economical; a 64-g bottle of Neutra-Phos dissolved in 1 gallon of water provides 250 mg elemental phosphorus/75 ml. Serum phosphorus, calcium, and creatinine should be measured daily as the dose is adjusted. Side effects include diarrhea, which is often dose-limiting, and nausea. Hypocalcemia and ectopic calcification are rare unless hyperphosphatemia occurs.
   b. **Severe hypophosphatemia** (<1 mg/dl) may require IV phosphate therapy when associated with serious clinical manifestations. However, unless there is evidence of preexisting phosphate depletion from another cause, **IV phosphate should not be used in the treatment of diabetic ketoacidosis**. IV preparations include potassium phosphate (1.5 mEq potassium/mM phosphate) and sodium phosphate (1.3 mEq sodium/mM phosphate). An infusion of 0.08–0.16 mM phosphate/kg (2.5–5.0 mg elemental phosphorus/kg) in 500 ml 0.45% saline is given IV over 6 hours. Further doses should be based on symptoms, and the serum calcium, phosphorus, and potassium, which should be measured q6h. IV infusion should be stopped when serum phosphorus is greater than 1.5 mg/dl or when oral therapy is possible. Because of the need to replenish intracellular stores, 24–36 hours of phosphate infusion may be required. **Extreme care must be used to avoid hyperphosphatemia**, which may cause hypocalcemia, ectopic soft-tissue calcification, renal failure, hypotension, and death. In renal failure, IV phosphate should be given only if absolutely necessary. **Hypophosphatemic patients are frequently hypokalemic and hypomagnesemic**, and these disorders must be corrected as well. (Conversion equations for phosphate therapy are: 1 mM phosphate = 31 mg phosphorus, and 1 mg phosphorus = 0.032 mM.)

III. **Magnesium** (*Endocrinol Metab Clin North Am* 22:377, 1993) plays an important role in neuromuscular function. About 60% of body magnesium is in bone, and most of the remainder is within cells. Only 1% is in the ECF, and serum magnesium levels often do not reflect total body magnesium content. Since clinical effects of magnesium disorders are determined primarily by tissue magnesium content, **serum magnesium levels have limited diagnostic value**. Normal serum concentrations are 1.3–2.2 mEq/liter.
   A. **Hypermagnesemia** occurs in **renal failure,** usually after therapy with magnesium-containing antacids or laxatives, and during treatment of preeclampsia with IV magnesium.
      1. **Clinical manifestations** are usually seen only if serum magnesium is greater than 4 mEq/liter. Neuromuscular abnormalities include areflexia, lethargy, weakness, paralysis, and respiratory failure. Cardiac findings include hypotension; bradycardia; prolonged PR, QRS, and QT intervals; complete heart block; and asystole. Hypocalcemia may occur.
      2. **Therapy.** Hypermagnesemia can be prevented by avoiding magnesium preparations in renal failure. Asymptomatic hypermagnesemia requires only withdrawal of this therapy. Severe, symptomatic hypermagnesemia should be treated with **10% calcium gluconate,** 10–20 ml IV over 10 minutes to temporarily antagonize the effects of magnesium. Prompt supportive therapy is critical, including mechanical ventilation for respiratory failure and a

temporary pacemaker for bradyarrhythmias. In severe renal failure, **hemodialysis** is required for definitive therapy. In patients without severe renal failure, 0.9% saline with 20 ml of 10% calcium gluconate/liter can be given at 150–200 ml/hour to promote magnesium excretion.

B. **Magnesium deficiency** may be caused by (1) decreased intestinal absorption due to malnutrition, malabsorption, prolonged diarrhea, or nasogastric aspiration; or (2) increased renal excretion caused by hypercalcemia, osmotic diuresis, and several drugs, including **loop diuretics, aminoglycosides, amphotericin B, cisplatin,** and **cyclosporine.** It often complicates **alcoholism** and **alcohol withdrawal.**

1. **Clinical manifestations.** Magnesium deficiency often causes **hypokalemia** and **hypocalcemia,** which contribute to the clinical picture. Neurologic abnormalities include lethargy, confusion, tremor, fasciculations, ataxia, nystagmus, tetany, and seizures. ECG abnormalities include prolonged PR and QT intervals. Atrial and ventricular arrhythmias may occur, especially in patients treated with digoxin.

2. **Diagnosis.** Magnesium deficiency should be suspected in the clinical situations described above. In these settings, hypomagnesemia is sufficient to establish the diagnosis of magnesium deficiency. However, routine measurement of serum magnesium without clinical suspicion of magnesium deficiency has little diagnostic value. The etiology of hypomagnesemia is usually evident, but if not, measurement of urine magnesium levels helps define the mechanism. Excretion of more than 2 mEq/day during hypomagnesemia indicates excessive renal loss.

3. **Treatment**. In patients with normal renal function, excess magnesium is readily excreted, and there is little risk of causing hypermagnesemia with recommended doses. However, magnesium must be given with extreme care in **renal failure** because of the risk of hypermagnesemia.

a. **Mild or chronic hypomagnesemia** can be treated with 240 mg elemental magnesium PO qd–bid. Magnesium oxide preparations include Mag-Ox 400 (240 mg elemental magnesium/400-mg tablet) and Uro-Mag (84 mg elemental magnesium/140-mg tablet). The major side effect is diarrhea.

b. **Severe, symptomatic hypomagnesemia** can be treated with 50% magnesium sulfate (4 mEq/ml), 2–4 ml IV over 15 minutes, followed by an infusion of 48 mEq in 1 or more liters of IV fluid over 24 hours. Because of the need to replenish intracellular stores, the infusion should be continued for 3–7 days. Serum magnesium should be measured q24h and the infusion rate adjusted to keep serum magnesium less than 2.5 mEq/liter. Tendon reflexes should be tested frequently, since hyporeflexia suggests hypermagnesemia. Reduced doses and more frequent monitoring must be used in even mild renal failure. (Conversion equations for magnesium therapy are: 1 mM = 2 mEq = 24 mg elemental magnesium.)

Metabolic Bone Disease

Metabolic bone diseases decrease the mass and strength of the skeleton, predisposing to fracture. Bone mass increases until about age 30, then gradually declines. In women, after menopause or premature ovarian failure, estrogen deficiency leads to a period of accelerated bone loss lasting 5–10 years. **Osteopenia** (Table 23-3) is a general term for abnormally low bone mass. Its clinical importance is due to the increased risk of fracture, which may occur with minimal trauma. The most common cause of osteopenia is **osteoporosis;** other causes include **osteomalacia** and the bone disease of **hyperparathyroidism.**

I. **Osteoporosis** (see Table 23-3) is defined as low bone mass with a normal ratio of mineral to osteoid (the organic matrix of bone). Primary osteoporosis is the most common form and is classified into two major types. **Postmenopausal osteoporosis** becomes clinically manifest about 10 years after menopause, with a peak incidence

Table 23-3. Causes of osteopenia

Osteoporosis
Primary
Postmenopausal (type I)
Senile (type II)
Idiopathic (in younger men and women)
Secondary
Cushing's syndrome (including glucocorticoid therapy)
Hyperthyroidism
Hypogonadism in men
Immobilization
Chronic heparin administration
Osteogenesis imperfecta and related disorders
Primary hyperparathyroidism
Osteomalacia
Myeloma
Mastocytosis
Renal osteodystrophy

in the 60s and early 70s. Predominantly trabecular bone is lost, leading to vertebral crush fractures and Colles' fractures of the distal forearm. Other symptoms include acute or chronic back pain, kyphosis, and loss of height. **Senile osteoporosis** presents after about age 70 in both sexes. Both cortical and trabecular bone is lost, leading to increased risk of hip and vertebral fractures. Vertebral fractures may cause back pain and kyphosis. Hip fractures are much more serious, causing considerable disability, loss of independence, and mortality. The most important **risk markers for osteoporosis** are female sex, white or Asian race, early menopause (spontaneous or due to oophorectomy), and therapy with glucocorticoids. Other factors including lean body mass, positive family history of osteoporosis, low calcium intake, lack of exercise, smoking, and alcohol abuse may also indicate increased risk.

A. Diagnosis. Osteoporosis may be detected following fractures that occur with minimal trauma, as an incidental finding on an x-ray, or by measurement of bone density. Diagnosis of primary osteoporosis requires exclusion of secondary forms of osteoporosis and other causes of osteopenia (see Table 23-3). The history, physical examination, and a few basic laboratory tests are usually diagnostic. Testing should include a CBC, multichannel chemistry screening, measurement of serum thyroid-stimulating hormone (TSH) levels, urinalysis, and serum protein electrophoresis. Serum calcium and phosphorus levels are normal in osteoporosis, and the alkaline phosphatase level is normal except for brief elevations after a fracture; abnormal values suggest a cause other than primary osteoporosis. Osteomalacia (see sec. II) should be suspected if there is a history of GI disease or if serum calcium, phosphorus, or alkaline phosphatase levels are abnormal. Bone biopsy is not necessary in patients with typical osteoporosis. However, if there are unusual features, it may help to diagnose other causes of osteopenia. **Bone mass measurements** are the most sensitive and specific tests for osteopenia and predict the risk of fracture. **Dual-energy radiography (DER)** measures bone mass of the lumbar spine and proximal femur with high precision. It is widely available at low cost and is the method of choice (*Am J Med* 94:646, 1993). Quantitative CT measures lumbar trabecular bone mass. It is less widely available and more expensive than DER. **Indications for bone mass measurement** are not clearly established (*N Engl J Med* 324:1105, 1991). General screening of perimenopausal women is not recommended. However, since the finding of low bone density influences women's decisions about estrogen replacement therapy and other preventive measures for

Table 23-4. Postmenopausal hormone replacement regimens

Unopposed estrogen Conjugated estrogens, 0.625 mg PO qd* *or* Transdermal estradiol, 0.05-mg patch twice weekly
Estrogen + cyclic progestin Estrogen (as above) *plus* Medroxyprogesterone, 5–10 mg PO qd 10–14 days/month
Estrogen + continuous progestin Estrogen (as above) *plus* Medroxyprogesterone, 2.5 mg PO qd

* Equivalent doses include ethinyl estradiol, 20 μg PO qd, or estradiol, 1 mg PO qd.

osteoporosis (*Ann Intern Med* 116:990, 1992), bone mass measurement is useful in women who want to take long-term estrogen only if their risk for osteoporosis is greater than average. Bone density should also be measured in patients with signs of osteoporosis on conventional x-rays, since these signs are not specific.

B. **Prevention** (*N Engl J Med* 327:620, 1992) is preferable to treatment of osteoporosis, since no therapy fully restores lost bone mass. All perimenopausal women should consider estrogen replacement therapy. **Risk factors** for osteoporosis (see sec. I) should be assessed, and **bone mass** should be measured if additional information about fracture risk will help a woman decide whether to take estrogen. Bone mass more than 1 standard deviation below the mean for premenopausal women strongly supports the need for estrogen replacement. Other data that should be considered in discussing the benefits and risks of estrogen replacement therapy include hysterectomy status, risk factors for coronary artery disease and breast cancer, indications for short-term estrogen therapy (flushing and vaginal atrophy), and the presence of contraindications to estrogen therapy (see sec. I.B.1.d). **Estrogen replacement therapy is indicated for all women with premature menopause in the absence of contraindications.**

1. **Estrogen replacement** after menopause inhibits bone resorption, slows the loss of bone mass, and reduces the risk of hip and vertebral fractures (*Ann Intern Med* 117:1016, 1038, 1992). **There is considerable observational evidence that the benefits of estrogen replacement outweigh the risks in most women** (*N Engl J Med* 330:1062, 1994). Cohort studies show that women receiving estrogen have a lower risk of myocardial infarction, stroke, and cardiovascular death, and a lower death rate from all causes (*N Engl J Med* 325:756, 1991; *Arch Intern Med* 153:1201, 1993). **Estrogen therapy is especially important in women with premature or surgical menopause.** Other people in whom the balance of risk and benefit is particularly likely to be beneficial include women who have had a **hysterectomy**, women at **increased risk of osteoporosis**, and women with **coronary artery disease** or who have increased risk of coronary disease.

   a. **Regimens** (Table 23-4). **Estrogen plus cyclic progestin** is used most often, with progestin given on days 1–14 of each month; estrogen should be given every day to prevent estrogen withdrawal symptoms. Women who have side effects at recommended doses of estrogen may be treated with conjugated estrogen, 0.3 mg PO qd, along with 1,500 mg calcium/day. **Estrogen plus continuous progestin** is much less likely to cause menstrual bleeding and therefore is preferred by some women (*Lancet* 343:250, 1994). **Unopposed estrogen should be used in women who have had a hysterectomy.**

   b. **Duration of therapy.** Estrogen replacement should begin as soon as possible after menopause to delay the rapid phase of bone loss, but estrogen has beneficial effects on bone mass at least until age 75 (*Ann Intern Med* 117:1, 1992). The optimal duration of therapy is not known, but at least 10 years of treatment is needed to augment bone mass at age 75, when most hip fractures occur (*N Engl J Med* 329:1141, 1993).

   c. **Regular evaluation** should include breast examinations, annual mammography, and prompt evaluation of unexpected vaginal bleeding with endometrial biopsy.

   d. **Contraindications** include a history of breast or endometrial cancer, recurrent thromboembolic disease, acute liver disease, and unexplained vaginal bleeding. **Relative contraindications** include fibrocystic breast disease, uterine myomata, endometriosis, or a family history of breast cancer.

   e. **Side effects** include breast tenderness, bloating, and headache, which may be alleviated by a reduction in dose. Menstrual bleeding occurs in most women taking estrogen plus cyclic progestin but is rare after 6 months of treatment with estrogen plus continuous progestin. Unopposed estrogen therapy increases the risk of endometrial carcinoma, but estrogen plus cyclic progestin does not. No consistent increase in risk of breast carcinoma has been found (*JAMA* 268:1900, 1992). Postmenopausal estrogen replacement therapy does not increase the incidence of hypertension or thromboembolism.

2. **Calcium** supplementation slows the rate of bone loss in postmenopausal women with average diets (*Ann Intern Med* 120:97, 1994; *N Engl J Med* 328:460, 1993). The **recommended daily calcium intake** for postmenopausal women is 1,500 mg, and 1,000 mg for premenopausal women (*Am J Med* 94:646, 1993). Most, if not all, postmenopausal women should take calcium supplements to achieve this intake, and calcium supplementation is also reasonable for premenopausal women. **Calcium carbonate**, 500–1,000 mg elemental calcium/day is adequate, together with **vitamin D**, 400–800 IU (available in combined pills). Side effects of calcium include dyspepsia and constipation.

3. **Exercise.** Regular walking or other weight-bearing exercise for 1 hour 3 times a week protects bone mass (*Ann Intern Med* 108:824, 1988).

4. **Prevention of injury** (*N Engl J Med* 320:1055, 1989). Most hip and wrist fractures are caused by falls. Risk factors for falls, including visual and balance disorders, postural hypotension, and home environmental hazards, should be corrected. Use of sedatives, antihypertensives, and alcohol should be minimized. Since vertebral collapse is precipitated by flexion of the spine, lifting should be minimized.

5. **Excessive thyroid hormone replacement** therapy should be avoided (*Ann Intern Med* 113:265, 1990).

C. **Treatment of established osteoporosis** (*N Engl J Med* 327:620, 1992). **Estrogen** therapy (see sec **I.B.1**) increases bone mass and decreases the risk of fracture in women with osteoporosis, at least until age 75 years (*Ann Intern Med* 117:1, 1992). **Calcium** supplements (see sec. **I.B.2**) and vitamin D (800 IU/day) should be given to reduce the risk of hip fracture (*N Engl J Med* 327:1637, 1992). Measures to prevent injury are also important (see sec. **I.B.4**). **Calcitonin** and **etidronate** can be used in (1) women over 75, (2) women for whom estrogen is contraindicated, and (3) men with osteoporosis.

1. **Calcitonin.** In women with osteoporosis, treatment with salmon calcitonin for 1–2 years increases vertebral bone density and decreases the risk of vertebral fracture (*Br Med J* 305:556, 1992). Bone mass does not continue to increase after 2 years, and the value of more prolonged therapy is not clear. The usual dosage is 50 IU SC qd or 3 times/week. Side effects include nausea, flushing, and, rarely, allergic reactions. Other drawbacks include the high cost and need for injections.

2. **Etidronate**, given in 3-month cycles for 3 years, may increase vertebral and hip bone density but has not been shown to decrease the risk of vertebral, hip, or other fractures (*Am J Med* 95:557, 1993). The dosage is 400 mg of etidronate PO qd (taken 2 hours before or after meals to ensure absorption) for the first 2 weeks of each 3-month cycle, followed by 2½ months of

treatment with calcium carbonate, 500 mg PO qd. The optimal duration of therapy is not established. Side effects include nausea and diarrhea.

D. Glucocorticoid-Induced osteoporosis. Pharmacologic doses of glucocorticoid cause bone loss, which is only partially reversible after the drug is stopped (*Ann Intern Med* 119:963, 1993). There are no well-established methods of prevention or treatment of glucocorticoid-induced osteoporosis. The **dose of glucocorticoid** should be reduced to the minimum needed to treat the underlying disease. Weight-bearing **exercise** should be encouraged with physical therapy and adequate analgesia, if needed. **Estrogen replacement** should be prescribed to postmenopausal women without contraindications (see sec. **I.B.1.d**). Calcitonin (see sec. **I.C.1**) may be tried in patients with established glucocorticoid-induced osteoporosis (*N Engl J Med* 328:1781, 1993) but has not been shown to reduce fractures in these patients.

II. Osteomalacia (*Clin Endocrinol Metab* 2:125, 1988) is characterized by defective mineralization of osteoid. Bone biopsy reveals increased thickness of osteoid seams and decreased mineralization rate, assessed by tetracycline labeling. **Causes of osteomalacia** include (1) vitamin D deficiency; (2) **malabsorption** of vitamin D and calcium due to gastrectomy or to intestinal, hepatic, or biliary disease; (3) disorders of vitamin D metabolism (e.g., renal disease, vitamin D–dependent rickets); (4) vitamin D resistance; (5) chronic hypophosphatemia (see Mineral Disorders, sec. **II.B**); (6) renal tubular acidosis; (7) hypophosphatasia; and (8) therapy with anticonvulsants, fluoride, etidronate, or aluminum compounds.

A. Clinical manifestations include diffuse skeletal pain, proximal muscle weakness, waddling gait, and propensity to fractures. X-ray findings include osteopenia and radiolucent bands perpendicular to bone surfaces (pseudofractures or Looser's zones). Serum alkaline phosphatase is elevated, and serum concentrations of phosphorus, calcium, or both are decreased.

B. Diagnosis (*Am J Med* 95:519, 1993). Osteomalacia should be suspected in a patient with osteopenia, elevated serum alkaline phosphatase levels, and either hypophosphatemia or hypocalcemia. **Serum 25(OH)D** levels may be low, establishing the diagnosis of vitamin D deficiency or malabsorption. Radiographs of the chest, pelvis, and hips may reveal characteristic pseudofractures. If neither serum 25(OH)D nor x-rays are diagnostic, a bone biopsy may be required for diagnosis.

1. **Dietary vitamin D deficiency** can initially be treated with vitamin D, 50,000 IU PO weekly for several weeks to replete body stores, followed by long-term therapy with 400–1,000 IU/day. Preparations include calcium supplements containing vitamin D (Os-Cal + D, 125 IU/250- or 500-mg tablet), many multivitamins (400 IU/tablet), and vitamin D drops (200 IU/drop or 8,000 IU/ml).

2. **Malabsorption of vitamin D** may require therapy with high doses, ranging from 50,000 IU PO/week to 50,000 IU PO qd. The dose should be adjusted to maintain serum 25(OH)D levels within the normal range. Calcium supplements, 1 g PO qd–tid, may also be required. Serum 25(OH)D, serum calcium, and 24-hour urine calcium levels should be monitored every 3–6 months to avoid hypercalcemia (see Mineral Disorders, sec. **I.B.4**). If osteomalacia does not respond to high doses of vitamin D, calcifediol (25[OH]D, 20- or 50-μg/capsule), 20–100 μg PO qd, may be better absorbed. If the underlying disease responds to therapy, the dose of vitamin D must be reduced accordingly.

III. Paget's disease of bone (*Endocrinol Metab Clin North Am* 19:177, 1990) is a focal skeletal disorder characterized by rapid, disorganized bone remodeling. It usually occurs after age 40 and most often affects the pelvis, femur, spine, and skull. Clinical manifestations include bone pain and deformity, degenerative arthritis, pathologic fractures, neurologic deficits due to nerve root or cranial nerve compression (including deafness), and, rarely, high-output heart failure and osteogenic sarcoma. Most patients are asymptomatic, with disease discovered incidentally because of an elevated serum alkaline phosphatase level or an x-ray taken for other reasons.

A. Diagnosis. A bone scan can be used to identify involved areas, which are then evaluated with x-rays. The radiographic appearance is usually diagnostic, and biopsy is rarely necessary. The serum alkaline phosphatase level is elevated, reflecting the activity and extent of disease. Serum and urine calcium levels are usually normal but may increase with immobilization.

B. Management. Most patients require no therapy, or analgesics only. Indications for specific therapy include (1) bone pain not relieved by analgesics, (2) nerve compression syndromes, (3) pathologic fracture, (4) elective skeletal surgery, (5) progressive skeletal deformity, (6) immobilization hypercalcemia, (7) hypercalciuria with nephrolithiasis, and (8) high-output heart failure. Serum alkaline phosphatase should be measured during treatment; a 50% reduction, along with symptomatic improvement, indicates an adequate therapeutic response.

    1. Etidronate (Didronel, 200 or 400 mg/tablet) inhibits both bone resorption and formation and is generally the drug of first choice. It is given as a 6-month course, 5 mg/kg PO qd, taken with water at the midpoint of a 4-hour fast. After each course, the drug should be discontinued for at least 6 months, to avoid the osteomalacia seen with longer therapy. After a treatment course, symptoms and serum alkaline phosphatase should be determined; prolonged remissions may occur. Repeated courses can be given for evidence of recurrence. Side effects include nausea and diarrhea; osteomalacia is rare with this regimen. Etidronate should not be used if lytic disease of weight-bearing bones is present.

    2. Calcitonin inhibits bone resorption. The initial dose of **salmon calcitonin** is 100 IU SC or IM qd. When an adequate response is achieved (usually after several months), the dosage is decreased to 50 IU SC 3 times a week. If resistance to salmon calcitonin develops, **human calcitonin**, 0.5 mg SC or IM qd, is often effective. Calcitonin is indicated for treatment of fractures and lytic disease of weight-bearing bones. Side effects include flushing, nausea, and, rarely, allergic reactions. Other drawbacks include the high cost and need for injections.

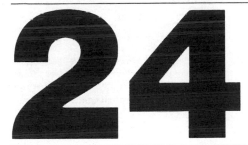

Arthritis and Rheumatologic Diseases

Leslie E. Kahl

Approach to the Patient with a Single Painful Joint

The first step in diagnosis for a patient with a single painful joint is to **identify the structures involved.** Pain arising in periarticular (e.g., tendon, bursa), muscular, and neurologic structures may be perceived as joint pain. If the pain comes from the joint itself and a **single joint** is involved, the differential diagnosis includes **trauma, infection,** and **crystalline arthritis.**

I. **Laboratory studies**
   A. **Radiographs** of the joint may be useful in documenting trauma or preexisting joint disease. The presence of chondrocalcinosis on x-ray film suggests pseudogout but is not diagnostic (see Crystal-Induced Synovitis). Radiographs are usually normal in acute infectious or crystalline arthritis.
   B. **Synovial fluid** (Table 24-1). Aspiration of joint fluid should be performed in all patients with monarticular arthritis who do not have a preexisting diagnosis consistent with the clinical picture. Polyarticular disorders such as rheumatoid arthritis (RA) or systemic lupus erythematosus (SLE) occasionally present as monarthritis, but when a single joint is inflamed out of proportion to the other joints in this setting, infection must be excluded.

II. **Management** is based on the results of radiographs and synovial fluid analysis. **Trauma** or **internal derangement** of the joint can be managed by immobilization of the joint and consultation with an orthopedic surgeon. The treatment of **infectious arthritis** and **crystalline disorders** is detailed below. If the synovial fluid appears to be inflammatory (see Table 24-1) and crystals are not seen, the patient with monarthritis should be presumed to have infectious arthritis and should be treated accordingly.

Joint Aspiration and Injection

I. **Indications.** Joint aspiration should be performed (1) when an effusion is present and its etiology is unclear, (2) for symptomatic relief in a patient with a known arthritis diagnosis, and (3) to monitor the response to therapy in infectious arthritis. Analysis of aspirated synovial fluid should include a cell count, microscopic examination for crystals, Gram's stain, and culture (see Table 24-1). Intraarticular glucocorticoid therapy can be used to suppress inflammation when only one or a few peripheral joints are inflamed and infection has been excluded. The joint should be aspirated to remove as much fluid as possible before glucocorticoid injection.

II. **Contraindications. Infection** overlying the site to be injected is an **absolute contraindication;** significant hemostatic defects and bacteremia are relative contraindications to joint aspiration and injection.

III. **Complications** following proper joint aspiration and injection are rare. However, the patient should be cautioned to report any increase in pain, swelling, or warmth

Table 24-1. Classification of synovial fluid

	Normal	Noninflam- matory	Inflammatory	Septic
Color	Colorless	Straw	Yellow	Variable
Clarity	Transparent	Transparent	Translucent	Opaque
WBC/mm^3	<200	200–2,000	2,000–75,000	>75,000
PMN	<25%	<25%	40–75%	>75%
Culture	—	—	—	May be +
Crystals	—	—	May be +	—
Examples		Osteoarthritis	RA	Bacterial
		Trauma	Gout	infection
		Aseptic	Pseudogout	Tuberculosis
		necrosis	SLE	
		SLE	Seronegative	
			spondyloar-	
			thropathies	

PMN = polymorphonuclear leukocyte; SLE = systemic lupus erythematosus.

following arthrocentesis. **Infection** occurs in less than 0.1% of patients when sterile technique is used. **Postinjection synovitis** may occur as a result of phagocytosis of glucocorticoid ester crystals. Such reactions usually resolve within 48–72 hours, and more persistent symptoms suggest the possibility of iatrogenic infection. Localized skin **depigmentation and atrophy** may occur after glucocorticoid injection, particularly when fluorinated steroids such as triamcinolone are used. Accelerated **deterioration of bone and cartilage** may occur when frequent injections are administered over an extended period. Therefore, any single joint should be injected no more frequently than every 3–6 months.

IV. **Intraarticular medications**
   A. **Glucocorticoid preparations** include methylprednisolone acetate, triamcino-lone acetonide, and triamcinolone hexacetonide. The dose used is arbitrary, but the following guidelines are useful.
      1. Large joints, such as the knee, ankle, and shoulder: 20–40 mg of any of the glucocorticoid preparations mentioned above.
      2. Wrists and elbows: 10–20 mg of any of the glucocorticoid preparations mentioned above.
      3. Small joints of the hands and feet: 5–15 mg of any of the glucocorticoid preparations mentioned above.
   B. **Lidocaine** (or its equivalent), up to 1 ml of a 1% solution, can be mixed in a single syringe with the glucocorticoid to promote immediate relief.
V. **Technique.** Gloves should be worn. The site of aspiration should be cleansed with povidone/iodine solution. Topical ethylchloride spray can be used as a local anesthetic. Local infiltration with 1% lidocaine can also be used.
   A. **Knee** (Fig. 24-1). The patient's leg should be positioned by gently flexing the knee 10–15 degrees. A rolled towel can be placed in the popliteal fossa to support the knee and allow the quadriceps to relax. The joint is then entered either medially or laterally, immediately beneath the undersurface of the patella. If the suprapatellar bursa is distended and contiguous with the joint space, it may be aspirated directly, without manipulating the needle beneath the patella.
   B. **Ankle** (Fig. 24-2). Aspiration should be performed with the patient supine and the foot perpendicular to the leg. Medial aspiration is performed immediately medial to the extensor hallucis longus tendon, which can be identified by alternately extending and flexing the great toe. A lateral approach can also be used by introducing the needle just distal to the fibula.
   C. **Wrist** (Fig. 24-3). Aspiration is performed on the dorsum of the wrist in the

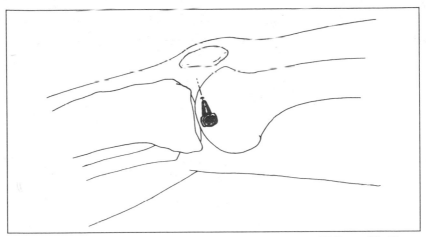

Fig. 24-1. Arthrocentesis of the knee: medial approach. (From JF Beary III, CL Christian, NA Johanson [eds]. *Manual of Rheumatology and Outpatient Orthopedic Disorders* [2nd ed]. Boston: Little, Brown, 1987.)

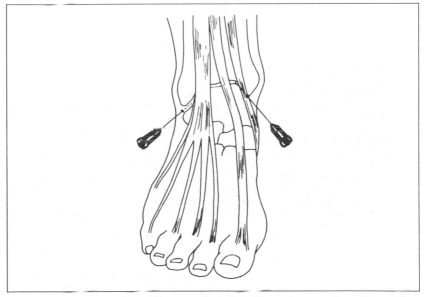

Fig. 24-2. Arthrocentesis of the ankle: medial and lateral approaches. (From JF Beary III, CL Christian, NA Johanson [eds]. *Manual of Rheumatology and Outpatient Orthopedic Disorders* [2nd ed]. Boston: Little, Brown, 1987.)

intercarpal space just distal to the radius, with the wrist joint slightly flexed.

D. **Joints of the hands and feet.** Small joints of the hands and feet are entered similarly by introducing the needle from the dorsal surface immediately beneath the extensor tendon from either the lateral or medial side. Because these joints yield only small amounts of fluid, flushing the aspirate from the syringe with saline may increase the yield when attempting analysis for crystals.

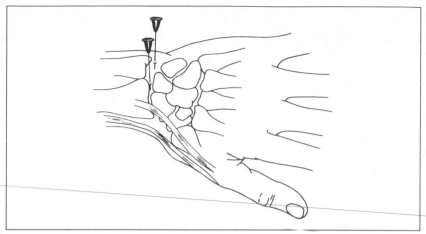

Fig. 24-3. Arthrocentesis of the wrist: medial and lateral approaches. (From JF Beary III, CL Christian, NA Johanson [eds]. *Manual of Rheumatology and Outpatient Orthopedic Disorders* [2nd ed]. Boston: Little, Brown, 1987.)

Infectious Arthritis and Bursitis

Infectious arthritis is generally divided into gonococcal and nongonococcal disease. The usual presentation is with fever and an acute monarticular arthritis, although multiple joints may be affected by hematogenous spread of pathogens. **Nongonococcal infectious arthritis** in adults tends to occur in patients with previous joint damage or compromised host defenses. In contrast, **gonococcal arthritis** causes one-half of all septic arthritis in otherwise healthy, sexually active young adults.

I. **General principles of treatment**
   A. **Joint fluid examination,** including Gram's stain of a centrifuged pellet and culture, is mandatory to make a diagnosis and to guide management. A joint fluid leukocyte count is useful diagnostically and as a baseline for serial studies to evaluate response to treatment. Cultures of blood and other possible extraarticular sites of infection should also be obtained.
   B. **Hospitalization** is indicated to ensure drug compliance and careful monitoring of the clinical response.
   C. **IV antimicrobials** provide good serum and synovial fluid drug concentrations. Oral or intraarticular antimicrobials are not appropriate as initial therapy.
   D. **Repeated arthrocenteses** should be performed daily or as often as necessary to prevent reaccumulation of fluid. Arthrocentesis is indicated to (1) remove destructive inflammatory mediators, (2) reduce intraarticular pressure and promote antimicrobial penetration into the joint, and (3) monitor response to therapy by documenting sterility of synovial fluid cultures and decreasing leukocyte counts.
   E. **Surgical drainage** is indicated for (1) septic hip; (2) joints in which either the anatomy, large amounts of tissue debris, or loculation of pus prevents adequate needle drainage (most commonly the shoulder); (3) septic arthritis with coexistent osteomyelitis; (4) joints that do not respond in 5–7 days to appropriate therapy and repeated arthrocenteses; and (5) prosthetic joint infection. Arthroscopic drainage may also be used in these situations.
   F. **General supportive measures.** Splinting of the joint may relieve pain, but prolonged immobilization can result in stiffness. A nonsteroidal antiinflamma-

tory drug (NSAID) (see Rheumatoid Arthritis, sec. I.A) is often useful to reduce pain and increase joint mobility but should not be used until response to antimicrobial therapy has been demonstrated by symptomatic and laboratory improvement.

II. **Nongonococcal septic arthritis** is most often caused by *Staphylococcus aureus* (60%) and *Streptococcus* species. Gram-negative organisms are less common, except with IV drug abuse, neutropenia, concomitant urinary tract infection, and postoperatively. Initial therapy is based on the clinical situation and a carefully performed Gram's stain, which will reveal the organism in approximately 50% of patients (*N Engl J Med* 330:769, 1994) (see also Chap. 13). IV antimicrobials are usually given for at least 2 weeks, followed by 1–2 weeks of oral antimicrobials, with the course of therapy tailored to the patient's response.

   A. **Gram-positive cocci.** Antistaphylococcal therapy (e.g., nafcillin, 1–2 g IV q4–6h, or vancomycin, 1g IV q12h) is appropriate.

   B. **Gram-negative bacilli.** Empiric therapy must reflect the clinical setting. A third-generation cephalosporin (e.g., ceftriaxone, 2 g IV q24h) is appropriate initial coverage. Patients at high risk of *Pseudomonas* infection (IV drug abusers, neutropenic or postoperative patients) should receive an antipseudomonal beta-lactam agent (e.g., piperacillin, 2–3 g IV q4–6h) plus an aminoglycoside (e.g., gentamicin, 1 mg/kg IV q8h).

   C. **Nondiagnostic Gram's stain**
      1. In an **otherwise healthy adult,** empiric coverage should include an antistaphylococcal agent. If the patient is at risk for gonococcal disease, ceftriaxone, 1 g IV q24h, or penicillin G, 2 million units IV q4h, should be added (see Chap. 13).
      2. In the **immunocompromised host,** antimicrobial coverage must be individualized but should include agents with activity against staphylococci and gram-negative bacilli.

III. **Gonococcal arthritis** is more common than nongonococcal septic arthritis. The clinical spectrum of disease often includes migratory or additive polyarthralgias, followed by tenosynovitis or arthritis of the wrist, ankle, or knee, and dermatitis on the extremities or trunk. In contrast to nongonococcal septic arthritis, Gram's stain of synovial fluid and cultures of blood or synovial fluid are often negative. **Throat, cervical, urethral,** and **rectal cultures** should also be obtained. Treatment includes ceftriaxone, 1 g IV qd for at least 3 days, unless the organism is known to be sensitive to penicillin, along with splinting of the affected joint. Clinical response is usually noted after 2–3 days, when treatment can be switched to cefuroxime axetil, 500 mg PO bid, or, for sensitive organisms, amoxicillin, 500 mg PO qid for 7 days (see Chap. 13).

IV. **Nonbacterial septic arthritis.** Transient arthralgias and arthritis are common with many viral infections, especially hepatitis B, rubella, mumps, infectious mononucleosis, parvovirus, enterovirus, and adenovirus. They are usually self-limited, last for less than 6 weeks, and respond well to a conservative regimen of rest and NSAIDs. A variety of fungi and mycobacteria can cause septic arthritis and should be considered in patients with chronic monarticular arthritis.

V. **Septic bursitis,** usually involving the olecranon or prepatellar bursa, can be differentiated from septic arthritis by localized, fluctuant superficial swelling and by relatively painless joint motion (except with full flexion or extension). Most patients have a history of previous trauma to the area or an occupational predisposition (e.g., "housemaid's knee," "writer's elbow"). *Staph. aureus* is the most common pathogen. The principles of management are similar to those for septic arthritis, although outpatient therapy can be used for otherwise healthy individuals (e.g., dicloxacillin, 500 mg PO qid for 10 days). Preventive measures (e.g., knee pads) should be used in patients with occupational predispositions.

VI. **Lyme disease** is caused by the tick-borne spirochete *Borrelia burgdorferi*. Arthritis is usually preceded by an erythematous annular rash called erythema chronicum migrans. Diffuse arthralgia or an asymmetric oligoarticular arthritis, commonly involving the knees, may be present and may recur. Systemic symptoms, meningoencephalitis, peripheral neuropathy, and cardiac conduction abnormalities may be associated with this disease. The diagnosis is based on the clinical picture, exposure in an endemic area, and serologic studies. Unfortunately, serologic studies often give false-negative or false-positive results (*JAMA* 268:891, 1992). Oral doxycycline, 100 mg PO bid for 4 weeks, or amoxicillin and probenecid, 500 mg of each qid, may be curative in most patients (*Arthritis Rheum* 32:32, 1989). NSAIDs are a useful adjunct for arthritis.

Crystal-Induced Synovitis

Deposition of microcrystals in joints and periarticular tissues results in **gout, pseudogout, and apatite disease.** A definitive diagnosis of gout or pseudogout is made by finding **intracellular crystals in joint fluid** examined with a compensated polarized light microscope. Urate crystals, which are diagnostic of gout, are needle-shaped and strongly negatively birefringent. Calcium pyrophosphate dihydrate (CPPD) crystals seen in pseudogout are pleomorphic and weakly positively birefringent. Hydroxyapatite complexes, diagnostic of apatite disease, and basic calcium phosphate complexes can be identified only by electron microscopy and mass spectroscopy. In most cases, the arthritides associated with these compounds are suspected clinically but never confirmed.

I. **Primary gouty arthritis** is characterized by hyperuricemia caused by either overproduction (10% of cases) or underexcretion (90% of cases) of uric acid. Urate crystals may deposit in the joints, subcutaneous tissues (tophi), and kidneys. Men are much more commonly affected than women; most premenopausal women with gout have a family history of the disease. The clinical phases of gout can be divided into (1) asymptomatic hyperuricemia, (2) acute gouty arthritis, and (3) chronic arthritis.

A. **Asymptomatic hyperuricemia** (uric acid levels >8 mg/dl in men and >7 mg/dl in women) is not routinely treated because of expense, potential drug toxicity, and the low risk for adverse outcome from the hyperuricemia itself (*Am J Med* 82:421, 1987).

B. **Acute gouty arthritis** occurs as an excruciating attack of pain, usually in a single joint of the foot or ankle. Occasionally, a polyarticular onset can mimic RA. Attacks may be precipitated by surgery, dehydration, fasting, binge eating, or heavy ingestion of alcohol. Although the acute gouty attack will subside spontaneously over several days, prompt treatment can abort the attack within hours. **The serum uric acid level is normal in 30% of patients with acute gout and, if elevated, should not be manipulated until an attack has resolved.**

1. **NSAIDs** are effective in acute gout, although clinical response may require 12–24 hours (Table 24-2). Initial doses should be high, followed by rapid tapering over 2–8 days. For example, indomethacin is begun at 50 mg PO q6h for 2 days, followed by 50 mg PO q8h for 3 days, and then 25 mg PO q8h for 2–3 more days. The long-acting NSAIDs are generally not recommended for acute gout (see Rheumatoid Arthritis, sec. I.A). Ease of administration and lower toxicity of NSAIDs make them the **drugs of choice** in most settings.

2. **Colchicine** is most effective if given in the first 12–24 hours of an acute attack and usually brings relief in 6–12 hours.

a. **Oral administration** is often associated with severe GI toxicity. The dosage is 0.5–0.6 mg (1 tablet) q1–2h or 1.0–1.2 mg q2h until symptoms abate, GI toxicity develops, or the maximum dose of 6 mg in a 24-hour period is reached. The dosage should be reduced in elderly patients and patients with renal or hepatic impairment. No more than 1.2 mg/day should be used thereafter during that attack.

b. **IV colchicine** produces faster relief with fewer GI side effects but can cause severe myelosuppression. A rapid response to IV colchicine is relatively specific for crystal-induced arthritis. The drug is diluted in 10–20 ml of normal saline and given slowly over 3–5 minutes through a freely flowing IV to **avoid extravasation** and tissue necrosis. **Colchicine should not be**

diluted with or injected into IV tubing containing 5% dextrose because precipitation will occur. The initial dose is 2 mg, followed by another 1–2 mg in 6 hours if necessary, to a maximum dose of 4 mg in 24 hours. The dosage should be reduced in the elderly, if the patient has been receiving chronic oral colchicine, or if the patient has significant renal or hepatic disease (*J Rheumatol* 15:495, 1988). No further colchicine should be given PO or IV for 7 days.

3. **Glucocorticoids** are useful when colchicine or NSAIDs are contraindicated. An intraarticular injection of glucocorticoids produces rapid dramatic relief. Alternatively, prednisone, 40–60 mg PO qd, can be given until a response is obtained, then tapered rapidly.

C. **Hyperuricemia with recurrent gouty arthritis.** With time, acute gouty attacks occur more frequently, asymptomatic periods are shorter, and chronic joint deformity may appear. Colchicine (0.5–0.6 mg PO qd or bid) can be used prophylactically for acute attacks. Aspirin (uricoretentive), diuretics, large alcohol intake, and foods high in purines (sweetbreads, anchovies, sardines, liver, and kidney) should be avoided. The serum uric acid level should be lowered if arthritic attacks are frequent, renal damage is present, or serum or urine uric acid levels are consistently elevated. **Maintenance colchicine, 0.5–0.6 mg PO bid, should be given a few days before manipulation of the uric acid level to prevent precipitation of an acute attack.** If no attacks occur after the uric acid has been maintained in the normal range for 6–8 weeks, colchicine can be discontinued.

1. **Allopurinol,** a xanthine oxidase inhibitor, is effective therapy for hyperuricemia in most patients.

   a. **Dosage and administration.** The initial dose is usually 300 mg PO qd, but should be reduced in patients with renal or hepatic impairment (Table 24-3). Daily dosages can be altered by 100–200 mg every 2–4 weeks to achieve the minimum maintenance dosage that will keep the uric acid level within the normal range. The concomitant use of a uricosuric agent may hasten the mobilization of tophi. If an acute attack occurs during treatment with allopurinol, it should be continued at the same dosage while other agents are used to treat the attack.

   b. **Toxicity. Hypersensitivity reactions** from a minor skin rash to a diffuse exfoliative dermatitis associated with fever, eosinophilia, and a combination of renal and hepatic injury occur in up to 5% of patients. Patients with mild renal insufficiency who are receiving diuretics are at greatest risk. **Severe cases are potentially fatal** and usually require glucocorticoid therapy. Allopurinol may potentiate the effect of oral anticoagulants. Allopurinol blocks metabolism of 6-mercaptopurine and azathioprine, necessitating a 60–75% reduction in dosage of these cytotoxic drugs.

2. **Uricosuric drugs** lower serum uric acid levels by blocking renal tubular reabsorption of uric acid. A 24-hour measurement of creatinine clearance and urine uric acid should be obtained before starting therapy. Uricosuric agents are ineffective with glomerular filtration rates of less than 50 ml/minute. They are not recommended for patients who already have high levels of urine uric acid (800 mg/24 hours) because of the risk of urate stone formation. This risk can be minimized by maintaining a high fluid intake and alkalinizing the urine. If these drugs are being used when an acute gouty attack begins, they should be continued while other drugs are used to treat the acute attack.

   a. **Probenecid** is given at an initial dosage of 500 mg PO qd, which can be raised in 500-mg increments every week until serum uric acid levels normalize or urine uric acid levels exceed 800 mg/24 hours. The maximum dose is 3,000 mg daily. Most patients require 1.0–1.5 g/day in 2–3 divided doses. **Salicylates and probenecid are antagonistic** and should not be used together. Probenecid decreases renal excretion of penicillin, indomethacin, and sulfonylureas. Side effects are minimal.

   b. **Sulfinpyrazone** has uricosuric efficacy similar to probenecid, but sulfinpyrazone also inhibits platelet function. The initial dosage of 50 mg

Table 24-2. Nonsteroidal antiinflammatory drugs

Generic name	Trade name (partial listing)	Tablet size (mg)	Starting dosage (mg)	Maximum daily dose (mg)	Comments
Salicylates					
Aspirin[a] (acetylsalicylate)	Aspirin	325	650–1,300 q4–6h	b	Serum salicylate levels of 20–30 mg/dl have maximum antiinflammatory effect; levels ≥40 mg/dl may produce salicylism.
	Zorprin	800	1,600 q12h	b	
Magnesium salicylate[a,c]	Mobidin	600	600–1,200 tid–qid	b	
	Magan	545	545–1,090 tid–qid	b	
Choline salicylate[c]	Arthropan liquid	1 tsp = 870		b	
Choline magnesium trisalicylate[a,c]	Trilisate	500, 750, 1,000 1 tsp = 500	1,000–1,250 bid	b	
Salsalate[c]	Disalcid	500	1,000 bid–1,500 tid	b	
Nonsalicylates					
Diclofenac sodium	Voltaren	25, 50, 75	50–75 bid	200	
Diflunisal	Dolobid	250, 500	250 bid	1,500	
Etodolac	Lodine	200, 300	400 bid–tid	1,200	
Fenoprofen calcium	Nalfon	200, 300, 600	300–600 qid	3,200	
Flurbiprofen	Ansaid	50, 100	50–100 tid	300	
Ibuprofen	Motrin, Rufen	400, 600, 800	400 qid	3,200	
Indomethacin	Indocin	25, 50, 75	25 tid–qid	200	
	Indocin SR	75	75 qd	200	May cause severe headache.

Generic	Brand	Dose forms (mg)	Dosing	Maximum dose (mg)	Comments
	Indocin suppositories	50	50 bid	200	
Ketoprofen	Orudis	50, 75	75 tid	300	
Meclofenamate sodium	Meclomen	50, 100	50 tid–qid	400	Causes little dyspepsia but causes diarrhea.
Nabumetone	Relafen	500, 750	1,000–2,000 qd	2,000	
Naproxen[a]	Naprosyn	250, 375, 500	250–500 bid	1,250	
Naproxen sodium	Anaprox	275	275 q6–8h	1,375	
Oxaprozin	Daypro	600	600–1,200 qd	1,200	
Phenylbutazone	Butazolidin	100	100 tid	600	Causes severe marrow toxicity.
Piroxicam	Feldene	10, 20	20 qd	20	
Sulindac	Clinoril	150, 200	150–200 bid	400	Potentially less nephrotoxic than other nonsalicylates.
Tolmetin sodium	Tolectin	200, 400, 600	400 tid	1,600	

a Available as a suspension.
b Determined by measurement of serum salicylate level.
c Nonacetylated salicylate.

Table 24-3. Maintenance doses of allopurinol for adults based on individual creatinine clearance measurements*

Creatinine clearance (ml/min)	Maintenance dose of allopurinol
0	100 mg every 3 days
10	100 mg every 2 days
20	100 mg daily
40	150 mg daily
60	200 mg daily
80	250 mg daily
100	300 mg daily
120	350 mg daily
140	400 mg daily

* This table is based on a standard maintenance dose of 300 mg/day of allopurinol for a patient with a creatinine clearance of 100 ml/minute.
Source: KR Hande, RM Noone, WJ Store. Severe allopurinol toxicity. *Am J Med* 76:47, 1984.

PO bid can be increased in 100-mg increments weekly until serum uric acid levels normalize, to a maximum dose of 800 mg daily. Most patients require 300–400 mg/day in 3–4 divided doses.
   D. Chronic tophaceous gout results from chronic hyperuricemia. Recurrent attacks of arthritis and tophaceous deposits in the joints lead to bone erosions, remodeling of the joint surface, and impaired joint motion. Colchicine, 0.5–0.6 mg PO bid, may prevent new attacks; NSAIDs can decrease existing inflammation; and allopurinol or uricosuric agents will help resorb tophi. Rehabilitation includes physical and occupational therapy as well as corrective surgery.
II. Secondary gout, like primary gout, may be caused by either defective renal excretion or overproduction of uric acid. Intrinsic renal disease, diuretic therapy, low-dose aspirin, nicotinic acid, cyclosporine, and ethanol all interfere with renal excretion of uric acid. Starvation, lactic acidosis, dehydration, preeclampsia, and diabetic ketoacidosis can also induce hyperuricemia. Overproduction of uric acid occurs in myeloproliferative and lymphoproliferative disorders, hemolytic anemia, polycythemia, and cyanotic congenital heart disease. Management includes treatment of the underlying disorder and allopurinol therapy.
III. Pseudogout results when CPPD crystals deposited in bone and cartilage are released into synovial fluid and induce acute inflammation. **Risk factors** include older age, advanced osteoarthritis, neuropathic joint, gout, hyperparathyroidism, hemochromatosis, diabetes mellitus, hypothyroidism, hypomagnesemia, and hypophosphatasia. Chondrocalcinosis is seen on x-ray films in 75% of patients, although its presence is not diagnostic. The disease may present as an acute monarthritis or oligoarthritis mimicking gout, or as a chronic polyarthritis resembling RA or osteoarthritis. The knee is usually affected, although any synovial joint may be involved. Dehydration, acute illness, and surgery (especially parathyroidectomy) are common precipitants of an acute attack of pseudogout. As in gout, a brief, high-dose course of an NSAID (see Table 24-2) is the therapy of choice for most patients. Colchicine (PO or IV; see sec. **I.B.2**) may also relieve symptoms promptly. Maintenance colchicine may diminish the number of recurrent attacks. Aspiration of the inflammatory joint fluid often results in prompt improvement, and intraarticular injection of glucocorticoids may hasten the response.
IV. Apatite disease may present with periarthritis or tendinitis, particularly in patients with chronic renal failure. An episodic oligoarthritis may also occur, and apatite disease should be suspected when no crystals are present in the synovial

fluid. Erosive arthritis may be seen, particularly in the shoulder ("Milwaukee shoulder"). The treatment of apatite disease is similar to that for pseudogout.

Rheumatoid Arthritis

Rheumatoid arthritis (RA) is a systemic disease of unknown etiology, characterized by symmetric inflammation of synovial tissues. Serum rheumatoid factor is usually present. Extraarticular manifestations include, in order of decreasing frequency, (1) rheumatoid nodules, (2) pulmonary fibrosis, (3) serositis, and (4) vasculitis. **Felty's syndrome**—the triad of RA, splenomegaly, and granulocytopenia—occurs in a subset of patients who are at risk for recurrent bacterial infections and nonhealing leg ulcers. **Sjögren's syndrome,** characterized by failure of exocrine glands, also occurs in a subset of patients with RA, producing sicca symptoms (dry eyes and mouth), parotid gland enlargement, dental caries, and recurrent tracheobronchitis. The course of RA is variable but tends to be chronic and progressive. Most patients can benefit from a combined program of medical, rehabilitative, and surgical services designed with three distinct goals: (1) suppression of inflammation in the joints and other tissues, (2) maintenance of joint and muscle function and prevention of deformities, and (3) repair of joint damage to relieve pain or improve function. **Patients with RA and a single joint inflamed out of proportion to the rest of the joints must be evaluated for coexistent septic arthritis.** This complication occurs with increased frequency in RA and carries a 20–30% mortality rate (*Am J Med* 88:503, 1990).

I. **Medical management** is usually provided in a "stepped" approach.
 A. **NSAIDs** (see Table 24-2), including salicylates, are inhibitors of cyclooxygenase (prostaglandin synthetase). Individual responses to these agents are variable; if one drug is not effective during a 2–3 week trial at full dosage, another should be tried.
    1. **Side effects.** The major side effects of the NSAIDs include dyspepsia, nausea, and, less commonly, headaches, tinnitus, dizziness, and confusion. Localized **GI irritation** may be minimized by administration after food or the use of enteric-coated preparations. However, all NSAIDs have a systemic effect on gastric or duodenal mucosa, resulting in increased membrane permeability to gastric acid. Misoprostol, a synthetic prostaglandin analogue, decreases the risk of NSAID-induced gastric or duodenal ulceration (*N Engl J Med* 327:1575, 1992). All NSAIDs **inhibit platelet aggregation** reversibly (except aspirin, which is irreversible) and should be used cautiously in patients with bleeding tendencies or those taking warfarin (*Br J Rheumatol* 28:46, 1989). Reversible elevations of **serum transaminases** may occur. Serum transaminase levels should be monitored periodically. Patients known to have **hypersensitivity to aspirin** (asthma, angioedema, urticaria, and nasal polyps) should avoid all NSAIDs except nonaspirin salicylates (see Table 24-2). These agents also cause less gastric irritation than aspirin.
    2. **Toxicities. Serious renal toxicity,** including acute renal failure, nephrotic syndrome, and acute interstitial nephritis, may occur. Prerenal azotemia with increased serum creatinine and hyperkalemia occurs more commonly, particularly in individuals whose renal function is already compromised (*N Engl J Med* 310:563, 1984). Periodic monitoring of renal function is recommended, particularly in elderly patients. **NSAIDs should not be given to patients with acute renal or hepatic failure and should be used with caution in patients with chronic renal or hepatic disease.** These agents can also cause sodium retention and edema. Other toxicities, including a variety of rashes, blood dyscrasias, and aseptic meningitis, have been reported.
    3. **Other precautions.** Although combinations of NSAIDs are generally not used, the addition of a long-acting drug at bedtime may significantly decrease morning stiffness. Long-acting preparations improve compliance but should

be used with caution in elderly patients. None of the NSAIDs is recommended for use during pregnancy or lactation. Specific precautions regarding individual NSAIDs are noted in Table 24-2.

B. Glucocorticoids. Although glucocorticoids are not curative and probably do not alter the natural history of RA, they are among the most potent antiinflammatory drugs available. Unfortunately, once systemic glucocorticoid therapy has been initiated, few RA patients are able to discontinue it completely.

1. **Indications** for systemic glucocorticoids include
   a. Persistent synovitis in multiple joints despite adequate trials of several NSAIDs and disease-modifying antirheumatic drugs (DMARDs) (see sec. **I.C**).
   b. Severe constitutional symptoms (e.g., fever and weight loss) or extraarticular disease (vasculitis, episcleritis, or pleurisy).
   c. Occasionally, glucocorticoids are used temporarily for symptomatic relief while waiting for a response to slower-acting, disease-modifying agents (see sec. **I.C**).
2. **Metabolism** (see Systemic Lupus Erythematosus, sec. **II.B**).
3. **Systemic administration.** In non–life-threatening situations, alternate-day glucocorticoid therapy is preferred, because it reduces the incidence of undesirable side effects (except cataracts and osteopenia). A cumulative 2-day dose of a short-acting glucocorticoid preparation (see Table 24-3) is given q48h in the morning. For RA, prednisone, 10–15 mg PO qod, is usually effective. Some patients do not tolerate the increase in symptoms that may occur on the off day and need 5–10 mg prednisone PO qd.
4. **Intraarticular administration.** This technique may provide temporary symptomatic relief when only a few joints are inflamed (see Joint Aspiration and Injection for preparations, dosages, and techniques). The beneficial effects of intraarticular steroids may persist for days to months. This approach may delay or negate the need for systemic glucocorticoid therapy.
5. **Contraindications and side effects** (see Systemic Lupus Erythematosus, sec. **III.C**).

C. Disease-modifying antirheumatic drugs (DMARDs). These drugs appear to alter the natural history of RA by retarding the progression of bony erosions and cartilage loss, unlike the NSAIDs, which only relieve symptoms. DMARDs are characterized by a delayed onset of action and the potential for serious toxicity and should be prescribed with the guidance of a rheumatologist or other physician experienced in their use.

Indications for DMARD use include (1) active synovitis not responding to conservative management, including salicylates or other NSAIDs; and (2) rapidly progressive, erosive arthritis. Clinical response, which is often delayed, can take 2–4 months. An NSAID should be used for symptomatic treatment in the interim. Once a clinical response to a DMARD has been achieved, the drug is usually continued at the lowest effective dosage indefinitely to prevent relapse.

1. **Methotrexate,** a folic acid antagonist, is the initial DMARD prescribed by many rheumatologists. It has also been used successfully in psoriatic arthritis and may improve the leukopenia of Felty's syndrome.
   a. **Dosage and administration.** Although methotrexate can be given parenterally (either IV or IM), the initial dose is usually 7.5 mg PO, taken as a single dose, **once a week.** Toxicity is related to both the total weekly dose and the frequency of administration. Clinical response is usually noted in 4–8 weeks, which is considerably earlier than with other DMARDs. If no response is attained after 6–8 weeks of therapy, the dosage can be increased by 2.5-mg increments every other week to a maximum of 20 mg weekly or until improvement is observed.
   b. **Contraindications and side effects. Methotrexate is teratogenic** and should not be used during pregnancy. It should be avoided in patients with significant hepatic or renal impairment. Major side effects include **GI**

intolerance, bone marrow toxicity, liver damage, and **hypersensitivity pneumonitis.** Stomatitis, rashes, headache, and alopecia may also occur. Blood and platelet counts should be obtained monthly during the first 3–4 months and every 6–8 weeks thereafter. Macrocytosis may herald serious hematologic toxicity (*Arthritis Rheum* 32:1592, 1989). AST, ALT, and serum albumin levels should be measured every 4–8 weeks. Liver biopsy should be performed if there are elevations in the AST in 5 of 9 determinations, or if the serum albumin level falls below the normal range (*Arthritis Rheum* 37:316, 1994). Alcohol consumption increases the risk of methotrexate hepatotoxicity. Patients with preexisting pulmonary parenchymal disease may be at increased risk of methotrexate pneumonitis. Folic acid supplementation may reduce methotrexate toxicity without impeding its efficacy in RA (*Arthritis Rheum* 33:9, 1990).

2. **Gold salts** produce significant improvement in approximately one-half of the patients with RA who can tolerate them. Gold has also been used successfully for juvenile RA, psoriatic arthritis, and Felty's syndrome.

   a. **Metabolism.** Whereas **parenteral gold** salts are absorbed rapidly from IM injection sites, **oral gold** is only approximately 25% absorbed.

   b. **Dosage and administration**

      (1) **Parenteral gold salts**, including Gold sodium thiomalate (Myochrysine) and aurothioglucose (Solganal), are given by deep IM injection. A test dose of 10 mg should be given first and, if tolerated, 50 mg should be given weekly thereafter. After a total cumulative dose of 1,000 mg, the interval between injections can be gradually increased to every 4–8 weeks.

      (2) **Oral gold** (auranofin) is somewhat less effective than parenteral gold but is also less toxic. The recommended initial dosage is 3 mg PO bid. If the response is inadequate after 6 months of therapy, an increase to 3 mg tid may be attempted.

   c. **Contraindications and side effects. Gold is contraindicated** in patients with a known gold allergy or history of a severe toxic reaction and should be used cautiously, if at all, in patients with impaired renal or hepatic function. Adverse reactions can occur at any time during therapy and, with the exception of diarrhea, are much more common with parenteral therapy.

      (1) **Dermatitis** is the most common manifestation of parenteral gold toxicity. This symptom requires discontinuation of injections, which may be restarted carefully at a lower dosage.

      (2) **Gold nephropathy** is usually manifested by proteinuria and occurs in up to 25% of patients receiving IM gold and 1% of patients receiving oral gold. A urinalysis should be performed before each gold injection and monthly in patients taking oral gold. Gold therapy should be discontinued for patients with proteinuria of greater than 1.5 g/24 hours.

      (3) The most serious adverse effects of parenteral gold are **thrombocytopenia, leukopenia, agranulocytosis, and aplastic anemia.** Blood and platelet counts should be performed every 1–2 weeks for the first few months of parenteral therapy and at increasing intervals up to every 6–8 weeks thereafter. Gold therapy should not be restarted in patients who develop cytopenias.

      (4) **GI side effects** including diarrhea, abdominal pain, nausea, and vomiting are common (up to 50%) with auranofin and usually require dosage reduction, discontinuation of therapy, or a change to parenteral gold therapy.

3. **Penicillamine** has benefit and toxicity profiles similar to those of parenteral gold. **Gold and penicillamine should not be used together.**

   a. **Dosage and administration.** Penicillamine is begun at a dosage of 250 mg PO qd for 4–6 weeks and is increased by 125 or 250 mg every 4–8 weeks until clinical improvement occurs or a daily dose of 1,000 mg is reached.

b. Contraindications and side effects
   (1) Penicillamine is teratogenic and should not be used during pregnancy. Allergy to penicillin does not predict potential reactions to penicillamine.
   (2) Dermatitis is the most common side effect of treatment. When rash occurs with fever, rechallenge should be avoided.
   (3) Hematologic toxicity and proteinuria occur as in gold therapy and require the same close laboratory monitoring.

4. **Sulfasalazine** is useful for moderately severe RA.
   a. Dosage. The initial dosage is 500 mg PO qd, with increases in 500-mg increments weekly until a total daily dose of 2,000–3,000 mg is reached. Sulfasalazine should not be used in patients with glucose-6-phosphate dehydrogenase (G6PD) deficiency.
   b. Side effects (see Chap. 15, Inflammatory Bowel Disease, sec. I.A).

5. **Hydroxychloroquine** (Plaquenil) is an antimalarial agent with moderate antiinflammatory and disease-modifying effects in RA. It is generally used in patients with mild or moderately severe RA and has also been used successfully in discoid and systemic lupus erythematosus.
   a. Dosage and administration. Therapy is usually initiated at a dosage of 400 mg PO qd, given after meals to minimize dyspepsia and nausea.
   b. Contraindications and side effects. Hydroxychloroquine should not be used in patients with porphyria, glucose-6-phosphate dehydrogenase deficiency, or significant hepatic or renal impairment. It should be avoided during pregnancy. The most common side effects are allergic skin eruptions and GI disturbances. Serious ocular toxicity occurs but is rare with currently recommended dosages.

D. **Other immunosuppressive agents.** Two other immunosuppressive drugs have been used successfully as DMARDs in patients with RA: the purine antagonist azathioprine and the alkylating agent cyclophosphamide. These drugs are indicated only for patients with severe disabling RA (active synovitis or systemic manifestations) who are refractory to, or intolerant of, standard DMARD therapy. Because of the potential for serious toxicity, these medications should be prescribed with the guidance of a rheumatologist or other physician experienced in their use and given only to well-informed, cooperative patients who are willing to comply with meticulous follow-up.

II. **Surgical management.** Corrective surgical procedures including synovectomy, total joint replacement, and joint fusion may be indicated in patients with RA to reduce pain and improve function. Carpal tunnel syndrome is common. Surgical repair may be curative if local injection therapy is unsuccessful. **Synovectomy** may be helpful if major involvement is limited to one or two joints and if a 6-month trial of medical therapy has failed, but it is usually only of temporary benefit. Prophylactic synovectomy and debridement of the ulnar styloid should be considered for patients with severe wrist disease to prevent rupture of the extensor tendons. Other procedures that may be beneficial include **total joint replacement** of the hip, shoulder, and knee joints and resection of metatarsal heads in patients with bunion deformities and subluxation of the toes. Reconstructive hand surgery may be useful in carefully selected patients. **Surgical fusion of joints** usually results in freedom from pain but also in total loss of motion; this is well tolerated in the wrist and thumb. Cervical spine fusion of C1 and C2 is indicated for significant subluxation (>5 mm) with associated neurologic deficits.

III. **Adjunctive measures**
   A. **Reactive depression and sleep disorders** are often encountered in patients with rheumatic diseases. Judicious use of antidepressants and sedatives may greatly improve the functional status of selected patients.
   B. **Rehabilitative therapy** should be managed by a team of physicians, physical and occupational therapists, nurses, social workers, and psychologists.
      1. **Acute care of arthritis** involves joint protection and pain relief. Proper joint positioning and splints are important elements in joint protection. Heat is a useful analgesic.

2. **Subacute disease therapy** should include a gradual increase in passive and active joint movement.

3. **Chronic care** encompasses instruction in joint protection, work simplification, and performances of activities of daily living. Adaptive equipment, splints, and mobility aids may be useful. Specific exercises designed to promote normal joint mechanics and strengthen affected muscle groups are useful. Overall cardiac conditioning also improves functional status.

C. **Patient education** about the disease process is helpful. Pamphlets and support groups are available in many communities through the Arthritis Foundation.

Osteoarthritis

Osteoarthritis (OA), or degenerative joint disease, is characterized by deterioration of articular cartilage, with subsequent formation of reactive new bone at the articular surface. The disease is more common in the elderly but may occur at any age, especially as a sequel to joint trauma, chronic inflammatory arthritis, or congenital malformation. The joints most commonly affected are the distal and proximal interphalangeal joints of the hands, hips, and knees, and the cervical and lumbar spine. OA of the spine may lead to spinal stenosis (neurogenic claudication), with aching or pain in the legs or buttocks on standing or walking.

I. **Medical management.** The objectives of therapy include relief of pain and prevention of disability. Acetaminophen and low-dose NSAIDs usually provide some relief. However, because this patient population is often elderly and may have concomitant renal or cardiopulmonary disease, NSAIDs should be used with caution. GI bleeding secondary to NSAIDs is also increased in the elderly population. Intraarticular glucocorticoid injections are often beneficial but should probably not be given more than every 3–6 months. Systemic steroids and narcotic analgesics should be avoided.

II. **Adjunctive measures.** Nonpharmacologic approaches may complement drug treatment for arthritis. Brief periods of rest for the involved joint relieve pain. Activities that involve excessive use of the joint should be identified and avoided. Similarly, poor body mechanics can be corrected, and malalignments such as pronated feet may be aided by orthotics. When weight-bearing joints are affected, support in the form of a cane, crutches, or a walker can be helpful, and weight reduction may be advised. An exercise program to prevent or correct muscle atrophy can also provide pain relief. Consultation with occupational and physical therapists may be helpful. When serious disability results from severe pain or deformity, surgery may be indicated. Total hip or knee replacement usually relieves pain and increases function in selected patients. **OA of the spine** may cause radicular symptoms from pressure on nerve roots and often produces pain and spasm in paraspinal soft tissues. Physical supports (cervical collar, lumbar corset), local heat, and exercises to strengthen cervical, paravertebral, and abdominal muscles may provide relief in some patients. Laminectomy and spinal fusion should be reserved for severe disease with intractable pain or neurologic complications. Lumbar spinal stenosis may require extensive decompressive laminectomy for relief of symptoms.

Fibrositis

Fibrositis (fibromyositis, fibromyalgia) is a common nonarticular musculoskeletal disorder that consists of muscle pain and stiffness, fatigue, and nonrestorative sleep. Commonly associated disorders include tension headache, irritable bowel syndrome, and dysmenorrhea. Pain is poorly localized but spares the joints. The physical examination is notable for characteristic tender points occurring bilaterally over the trapezius ridge, second costochondral junction, posterior cervical musculature, and upper gluteal area, and at the anserine and trochanteric bursae. Fibrositis is a diagnosis of exclusion and does not usually respond to NSAIDs or glucocorticoids. **Tricyclic antidepressants** can be given in low doses at bedtime (e.g., amitriptyline, 10–50 mg PO, or cyclobenzaprine, 5–30 mg PO) to correct the disorder of stage 4 sleep, which is characteristic of fibrositis (*Arthritis Rheum* 29:1371, 1986). **Physical therapy** and **aerobic fitness** programs may also be helpful.

Tendinitis, Tenosynovitis, and Bursitis

Inflammation of periarticular soft-tissue structures may result from trauma induced by strain or direct injury and from various rheumatic processes (e.g., RA, Reiter's syndrome, gout). Infection, particularly gonorrhea, must also be considered. Common sites of inflammation include the shoulder (supraspinatus or bicipital head tendinitis), elbow (epicondylitis—"tennis elbow" or "golfer's elbow"), thumb (de Quervain's disease), hip (trochanteric bursitis), knee (prepatellar bursitis), and heel (Achilles or calcaneal bursitis). Rest and immobilization provide adequate relief for most patients; joint rest is essential when weight-bearing tendons (patellar, Achilles) are involved. A local injection of 10–40 mg triamcinolone plus 1 ml of 1% lidocaine usually provides immediate relief that may last indefinitely in some patients. **Weight-bearing tendons should not be injected** because of the risk of rupture. NSAIDs are useful, particularly if multiple areas are involved. Physical therapy may also be beneficial.

Spondyloarthropathies

The spondyloarthropathies are an interrelated group of disorders characterized by one or more of the following features: (1) spondylitis, (2) sacroiliitis, (3) inflammation at sites of tendon insertion (enthesopathy), and (4) asymmetric oligoarthritis. Extraarticular features of this group of disorders may include: (1) inflammatory eye disease, (2) urethritis, and (3) mucocutaneous lesions. The spondyloarthropathies aggregate in families, where they are associated with human leukocyte antigen (HLA)–B27.

I. **In ankylosing spondylitis (AS),** the major clinical problem is inflammation and ossification of the joints and ligaments of the spine and of the sacroiliac joints. Hips and shoulders are the most commonly involved peripheral joints. Because progressive fusion of the apophyseal joints of the spine cannot be predicted or prevented, the therapeutic goal is to maximize the likelihood that fusion will occur in a straight line, which will minimize possible late postural defects and respiratory compromise. Patients should be instructed to sleep supine on a firm bed without a pillow and to practice postural and deep-breathing exercises regularly. Cigarette smoking should be strongly discouraged. Although high-dose salicylate therapy is usually ineffective in controlling pain, other NSAIDs may provide symptomatic relief; indomethacin is the NSAID most commonly used (see Table 24-2). Methotrexate and sulfasalazine also appear to be of benefit in some patients (see Rheumatoid Arthritis, sec. I.C) (*Arthritis Rheum* 31:1111, 1988). Glucocorticoids and immunosuppressive therapy have occasionally been used in patients who do not respond to other agents. Surgical procedures to correct some spine and hip deformities may result in significant rehabilitation in carefully selected patients. Acute anterior uveitis occurs in up to 25% of patients with AS and should be managed by an ophthalmologist. This problem is generally self-limited, although glaucoma and blindness are unusual secondary complications.

II. **Arthritis of inflammatory bowel disease.** In 10–20% of patients with Crohn's disease or ulcerative colitis, an arthritis develops that is similar to that of ankylosing spondylitis. Clinical features include spondylitis, sacroiliitis, and peripheral arthritis, particularly in the knee and ankle. Although peripheral joint disease may correlate with the activity of the colitis, spinal disease does not. **Extraarticular features** of the disease including erythema nodosum, stomatitis, uveitis, and pyoderma gangrenosum are also more closely related to peripheral joint disease. Joint aspiration may be useful to exclude an associated septic arthritis, but antimicrobials are not effective in the management of sterile synovitis associated with colitis. As in ankylosing spondylitis, NSAIDs (other than aspirin) are the treatment of choice, although GI intolerance of NSAIDs appears to be increased among this group of patients. Sulfasalazine may also be of benefit for this form of arthritis (see Rheumatoid Arthritis, sec. **I.C.4**). Local injection of glucocorticoids and physical therapy are useful adjunctive measures.

III. **Reiter's syndrome and reactive arthritis.** Reiter's syndrome occurs predominantly in young men and may occur with increased frequency in patients infected with HIV (*Ann Intern Med* 106:19, 1987). The clinical syndrome consists of asymmetric oligoarthritis, urethritis, conjunctivitis, and characteristic skin and mucous membrane lesions. The syndrome is usually transient, lasting from one to several months, but recurrences associated with varying degrees of disability are common. A reactive enteropathic arthritis may follow dysentery caused by *Shigella flexneri, Salmonella* species, or *Yersinia enterocolitica* infections. Articular manifestations are identical to those of Reiter's syndrome; extraarticular manifestations may occur but tend to be mild. **Conservative therapy is indicated** for control of pain and inflammation in these diseases. Spontaneous remissions are common, making evaluation of therapy difficult. High-dose salicylates are usually ineffective, but other **NSAIDs (especially indomethacin)** are often useful (see Rheumatoid Arthritis, sec. **I.A**). Sulfasalazine or methotrexate may provide symptomatic relief in some patients. In unusually severe cases, glucocorticoid therapy may be required to prevent rapid joint destruction. Conjunctivitis is usually transient and benign, but ophthalmologic referral and treatment with topical or systemic glucocorticoids are indicated for iritis.

IV. **Psoriatic arthritis.** Seven percent of patients with psoriasis have some form of inflammatory arthritis. Four major patterns of joint disease occur: (1) asymmetric oligoarticular arthritis, (2) distal interphalangeal joint involvement in association with nail disease, (3) symmetric rheumatoid-like polyarthritis, and (4) spondylitis and sacroiliitis. High-dose salicylates or NSAIDs (see Rheumatoid Arthritis, sec. **I.A**), particularly indomethacin, are used to treat the arthritic manifestations of psoriasis, in conjunction with appropriate measures for the skin disease (see Chap. 1). Intraarticular glucocorticoids may be useful in the oligoarticular form of the disease, but injection through a psoriatic plaque should be avoided. Gold, sulfasalazine, and hydroxychloroquine (see Rheumatoid Arthritis, sec. **I.C**) may have disease-modifying effects in polyarthritis, but the latter has been reported to cause exacerbation of psoriasis in some patients. Severe skin and joint disease generally responds well to low-dose methotrexate (see Rheumatoid Arthritis, sec. **I.C.1**). When reconstructive joint surgery is performed for patients with psoriatic arthritis, the risk of wound infection is increased approximately fivefold because of colonization of psoriatic skin with *Staph. aureus*.

Systemic Lupus Erythematosus

Systemic lupus erythematosus (SLE) is a multisystem disease of unknown etiology that primarily affects women of childbearing age. The course of this disease is highly variable and unpredictable. Disease manifestations are protean, ranging in severity from fatigue, malaise, weight loss, arthritis or arthralgias, fever, photosensitivity, and serositis to potentially life-threatening thrombocytopenia, hemolytic anemia, nephritis, cerebritis, vasculitis, pneumonitis, myositis, and myocarditis.

I. **The diagnosis of SLE** is made by a combination of physical and historical findings and laboratory testing.

A. Virtually all SLE patients have a positive **antinuclear antibody (ANA)** test. Low-titer ANAs (e.g., <1:640) are somewhat nonspecific and may be seen in a variety of connective tissue and other inflammatory diseases and in some normal elderly people. A positive screening ANA in the proper clinical setting should be followed by further testing to determine the antigenic target of the ANA. For example, anti-SSA/Ro and SSB/La are seen in SLE and Sjögren's syndrome. Anti-Smith (SM), while only present in 10–30% of SLE patients, is pathognomonic for the disease. Antiribonuclear protein (anti-RNP) may be seen in mixed connective tissue disease or overlap syndromes. Antibodies to double-stranded DNA are also diagnostic of SLE. Although they only occur in 20–50% of patients, their presence is usually correlated with severe or active disease, particularly nephritis.

B. Serum complement levels can also be useful in diagnosing SLE. Reduced C3, C4, or CH50 are rarely seen in conditions other than immune complex diseases, so their presence in a patient whose history and physical examination suggest SLE is strongly supportive of that diagnosis. Complement levels often fall during flares of disease and, like anti-DNA antibodies, they may be useful in monitoring disease activity in patients with an established diagnosis of SLE.

C. Other laboratory findings in SLE include leukopenia (which is usually lymphopenia), false-positive syphilis serology, positive direct Coombs' test (even in the absence of overt hemolysis), and a prolonged activated partial thromboplastin time. In patients for whom the diagnosis of SLE is being considered, a urinalysis, serum creatinine, and CBC should be performed to search for potentially silent disease manifestations.

II. Conservative therapy should be used if the patient's manifestations are mild.

A. General supportive measures. Mild disease exacerbations may subside after a few days of bed rest. Adequate sleep, midafternoon naps, and avoidance of fatigue are strongly recommended. For patients with photosensitive rashes, sunscreens with a sun protection factor of 20 or greater are recommended, along with avoidance of sun exposure. These patients should also wear a hat and long sleeves. Isolated skin lesions may respond to topical glucocorticoids (see Chap. 1).

B. NSAIDs usually control arthritis, arthralgias, fever, and serositis, although they are less effective than glucocorticoids. Fatigue, malaise, and major organ system involvement usually do not respond to NSAIDs. Hepatic and renal toxicities of the NSAIDs appear to be increased in SLE (see Rheumatoid Arthritis, sec. I.A), and rare cases of aseptic meningitis have also been reported. NSAIDs should be avoided in patients with active nephritis and should be used carefully if at all in patients with renal insufficiency.

C. Hydroxychloroquine (see Rheumatoid Arthritis, sec. I.C.5) in a dosage of 200–400 mg daily may be effective in the treatment of rash, photosensitivity, arthralgias, arthritis, alopecia, and malaise associated with SLE, and in the treatment of discoid and subacute cutaneous lupus erythematosus. Skin lesions may begin to improve within a few days, but joint symptoms may take 6–10 weeks to subside. The drug is not effective for treating fever or renal, CNS, and hematologic problems.

III. Glucocorticoid therapy

A. Indications for the use of systemic glucocorticoids include life-threatening or debilitating manifestations of SLE such as glomerulonephritis, CNS involvement, thrombocytopenia, and hemolytic anemia.

B. Preparations, dosages, and routes of administration (see Table 24-4). The goal of glucocorticoid therapy is to suppress disease activity with the minimum effective dosage of drug. Prednisone (PO) and methylprednisolone (IV) are generally the preferred drugs because of cost and half-life considerations. Oral forms of hydrocortisone and its synthetic analogues are well absorbed by the intestine. Intramuscular absorption is quite variable and is not advised. The route and frequency of administration are determined by the severity of disease manifestations.

1. Patients with severe or potentially life-threatening complications of SLE should be treated with prednisone, 60–100 mg PO qd, which is often given

Table 24-4. Glucocorticoid preparations

Generic name	Approxmiate equivalent dose (mg)	Usual starting dose (mg/day)	
		Moderate illness	Severe illness
Short-acting			
Hydrocortisone[a] (cortisol)	20.0	80–160	
Cortisone[a]	25.0	100–200	
Prednisone	5.0	20–40	60–100
Prednisolone[a]	5.0	20–40	60–100
Methylprednisolone[a]	4.0	16–32	48–80[b]
Intermediate-acting			
Triamcinolone[a]	4.0	16–32	48–80
Paramethasone	2.0	8–16	24–40
Long-acting			
Dexamethasone[a]	0.75	3–6	9–15
Betamethasone[a]	0.6	2.4–4.8	7.2–12.0

[a] Parenteral forms available. Dosages of oral and parenteral preparations are generally comparable.
[b] High-dose parenteral therapy is often used for severe illness (see Systemic Lupus Erythematosus, sec. III.B.2).

initially in divided doses. After the disease is controlled, therapy should be consolidated to a single daily dose, then slowly tapered, reducing the dosage by no more than 10% every 7–10 days; a more rapid reduction may result in relapse.

2. **IV pulse therapy** has been used in SLE in such life-threatening situations as rapidly progressive renal failure, active CNS disease, and severe thrombocytopenia. IV infusion of 500 mg methylprednisolone in 0.9% saline or 5% D/W is given over 30 minutes q12h for 3–5 days. Patients who do not show improvement with this regimen are probably unresponsive to steroids, and other therapeutic alternatives must be considered. Prednisone, 50 mg PO bid, is begun after completing pulse therapy and is slowly tapered when clinically feasible.

3. **Alternate-day schedules** (see Rheumatoid Arthritis, sec. I.B.3) markedly reduce many of the adverse effects of long-term glucocorticoid therapy, particularly the infectious complications. This approach is not indicated in the initial management of patients with severe, active disease but may be used once the disease is controlled.

C. **Side effects.** All glucocorticoid preparations have similar side effects, which are related to both dosage and duration of administration.

1. **Adrenal suppression.** Glucocorticoids suppress the hypothalamic-pituitary-adrenal axis. Patients who have received more than 10 mg of prednisone (or the equivalent) daily for several weeks may have some degree of axis suppression for up to 1 year following cessation of therapy (see Chap. 21). Adrenal suppression is minimized by using a single daily low dose of a short-acting preparation such as prednisone for a short period of time. In patients receiving chronic glucocorticoid therapy, hypoadrenalism (anorexia, weight loss, lethargy, fever, and postural hypotension) may occur at times of severe stress (e.g., infection, major surgery, serious intercurrent illnesses) and should be treated with stress doses of glucocorticoids (see Chap. 21). Mineralocorticoid activity, however, is preserved. These patients should wear a medical alert bracelet or carry identification.

2. **Immunosuppression.** Glucocorticoid therapy reduces resistance to infections. Bacterial infections, in particular, are related to the dosage of glucocorticoids and are a major cause of morbidity and mortality in SLE. Thus, minor

infections may become systemic, quiescent infections may be activated, and organisms that are usually nonpathogenic may cause disease. Local and systemic signs of infection can be partially masked, although fever associated with infection is generally not completely suppressed by glucocorticoids. Immunizations with influenza and pneumococcal vaccines do not appear to activate SLE and are advised as prophylactic measures. When possible, a skin test for tuberculosis should be placed before glucocorticoid therapy is instituted.

3. **Endocrine abnormalities** may include a cushingoid habitus and hirsutism. **Hyperglycemia** may be induced or severely aggravated by glucocorticoids but is usually not a contraindication to therapy. Insulin therapy may be required, although ketoacidosis is rare. **Fluid and electrolyte abnormalities** include hypokalemia and sodium retention, which may induce or aggravate **hypertension.**

4. **Musculoskeletal problems. Osteopenia** with vertebral compression fractures is common among patients receiving long-term glucocorticoid therapy. Supplemental calcium, 1.0–1.5 g/day PO, should be given. Estrogen therapy may be indicated in postmenopausal women at high risk for osteopenia, but its use is controversial in SLE. Vitamin D, thiazide diuretics, calcitonin, and diphosphonates can also be considered (see Chap. 23). A judicious exercise program may be beneficial in stimulating bone formation. **Steroid myopathy** generally involves the hip and shoulder girdle musculature. Muscles are weak but not tender and, in contrast to inflammatory myositis, muscle enzymes and EMG are normal. The myopathy should resolve slowly with a reduction in glucocorticoid dosage and an aggressive exercise program. **Ischemic bone necrosis** (aseptic necrosis, avascular necrosis) caused by glucocorticoid use is often multifocal, affecting the femoral head, humeral head, and tibial plateau most commonly. Early changes may be demonstrated by bone scan or MRI. Early surgical intervention with core decompression may be beneficial but remains controversial (*Medicine* 59:143, 1980).

5. **Other adverse effects** include changes in mental status that may range from mild nervousness, euphoria, and insomnia to severe depression or psychosis (which can be confused with the CNS manifestations of SLE). **Ocular effects** include increased intraocular pressure (sometimes precipitating glaucoma) and the formation of posterior subcapsular cataracts. Hyperlipidemia, menstrual irregularities, increased perspiration with night sweats, and pseudotumor cerebri may also occur.

IV. **Immunosuppressive agents** are used in patients who are refractory to or intolerant of glucocorticoid therapy or as steroid-sparing agents. These medications should be prescribed with the guidance of a rheumatologist or other physician experienced in their use. Drug dosages must be individualized to avoid toxicity, especially myelosuppression. Peripheral blood counts must be monitored closely: 10–14 days after each dosage change and monthly while the patient is on a stable dosage. The dosage is usually adjusted to maintain a WBC count of 3,500–4,500 cells/mm^3, with at least 1,000 neutrophils. The lowest dosage of medication producing adequate disease control should be used. Objective evidence of improvement may begin after 2–4 weeks of therapy. Potential short-term benefit must be weighed against the possible increased risk of malignancy (lymphoma, leukemia) with long-term use. Chronic or intermittent therapy may be required to control disease activity.

A. **Azathioprine** is initiated at approximately 1.5 mg/kg/day PO, given as a single dose or in 2 divided doses. The dosage can be increased (8- to 12-week intervals) to a maximum of 2.5–3.0 mg/kg/day to obtain the desired WBC count. The dosage of azathioprine should be reduced by 60–75% if it is given concomitantly with allopurinol, which blocks its metabolic degradation.

B. **Cyclophosphamide** is initiated at a **daily morning dose** of 1.0–1.5 mg/kg PO. The dosage can be increased to a maximum of 2.5–3.0 mg/kg/day to obtain the desired WBC count. Patients should be encouraged to take the medication with a lot of fluid, to void frequently, and to void before going to bed to minimize the risk of **hemorrhagic cystitis**. In addition, monthly pulse IV cyclophosphamide (0.5–1.0 g/m^2 IV) for active lupus nephritis may offer a better outcome for renal function than glucocorticoids alone. The blood count should be checked at 10–14 days to determine the degree of bone marrow suppression (see Chap. 19 for contraindications and side effects). The goal of therapy is to achieve a nadir total WBC count of 3,500–4,500 cells/mm^3, with at least 1,000 neutrophils. The dosage for the subsequent pulse or oral therapy should be adjusted accordingly.

V. **Plasmapheresis** has been used on an investigational basis in life-threatening situations to control disease until concomitant therapy with glucocorticoids or immunosuppressives has taken effect. It is an impractical long-term therapy, and its short-term use remains controversial.

VI. **Transplantation and chronic hemodialysis** have been used successfully in SLE patients with renal failure. Clinical and serologic evidence of disease activity often disappear when renal failure ensues. The survival rate in these patients is equivalent to that of patients with other forms of chronic renal disease. Recurrence of nephritis in the allograft occurs rarely.

VII. **Pregnancy in SLE** may be complicated by an increased incidence of spontaneous abortion, fetal death in utero, and prematurity. The correlation between fetal wastage and antibodies to cardiolipin or the lupus anticoagulant is unclear. SLE patients may experience an exacerbation in the activity of their disease in the third trimester or peripartum period. Differentiation between active SLE and preeclampsia is often difficult.

Scleroderma

Scleroderma (systemic sclerosis) is a systemic illness of unknown cause characterized by thickening and hardening of the skin and visceral organs. Most of the manifestations of scleroderma have a vascular basis (Raynaud's phenomenon, telangiectasias, nailfold capillary changes, early edematous skin changes, nephrosclerosis), but frank vasculitis is rarely seen. The label scleroderma includes both diffuse scleroderma and limited scleroderma (**CREST syndrome**: Calcinosis, Raynaud's phenomenon, Esophageal dysmotility, Sclerodactyly, Telangiectasias). Diffuse scleroderma is characterized by extensive skin disease, the potential for hypertensive "renal crisis," and shortened survival. The CREST variant has limited skin involvement but may be associated with primary pulmonary hypertension or biliary cirrhosis. Anticentromere antibodies are found almost uniquely in CREST. No curative therapy for scleroderma exists; instead, treatment focuses on particular organ involvement in a problem-oriented manner.

I. **Raynaud's phenomenon.** This reversible vasospasm of the digital arteries can result in ischemia of the digits. Patients must be instructed to avoid exposure of the entire body to cold, protect the hands and feet from cold and trauma, and discontinue cigarette smoking. Most pharmacologic approaches have had limited success. Vasodilating drugs, such as **calcium channel antagonists**, prazosin, phenoxybenzamine, reserpine, and guanethidine, are occasionally helpful, but significant side effects, especially orthostatic hypotension, may preclude their use. Sympathetic ganglion blockade with a long-acting anesthetic agent may be useful when a patient has progressive digital ulceration that fails to improve with conservative therapy.

II. **Skin and periarticular changes.** Used early in diffuse scleroderma, penicillamine (see Rheumatoid Arthritis, sec. I.C.3) may soften skin and improve joint contractures and may prolong survival. Physical therapy is important to retard and reduce joint contractures.

III. **GI involvement.** Reflux esophagitis generally responds to a vigorous antacid regimen and elevation of the head of the bed during sleep. H$_2$-receptor antagonists and sucralfate are also useful in some patients. Calcium channel antagonists used for Raynaud's phenomenon may worsen esophageal reflux. Mechanical esophageal dilatation may occasionally be necessary for strictures. Decreased motility of bowel segments can occur, leading to bacterial overgrowth, malabsorption, and weight loss. Treatment with broad-spectrum antimicrobials such as tetracycline or metronidazole often improves the malabsorption (see Chap. 15), and metoclopramide may reduce bloating and distention.

IV. Renal involvement. The appearance of hypertension and renal insufficiency, often associated with a microangiopathic hemolytic anemia, signals a poor prognosis. Aggressive BP control with **angiotensin-converting enzyme inhibitors** may delay or prevent the onset of uremia, particularly in patients with a serum creatinine of less than 3 mg/dl (*Ann Intern Med* 113:352, 1990).

V. Cardiopulmonary involvement. Patchy myocardial fibrosis can result in congestive heart failure or arrhythmias. Standard therapies for these conditions are used. Coronary artery vasospasm can cause angina pectoris and may respond to calcium channel antagonists. **Pulmonary involvement** includes pleurisy with effusion, interstitial fibrosis, pulmonary hypertension, and cor pulmonale. Standard therapies for these conditions are used.

Necrotizing Vasculitis

Necrotizing vasculitis is characterized by inflammation and necrosis of blood vessels. This entity includes a broad spectrum of disorders having various causes and involving vessels of different types, sizes, and locations. The immunopathogenic process often involves immune complexes, but in most cases the specific antigen and antibody involved have not been identified. Clinical features are diverse and include systemic manifestations such as fever and weight loss and localized problems including rash, arthritis, myositis, neuropathies, CNS disease, nephritis, pulmonary infiltrates, and GI hemorrhage or perforation. The response to therapy and long-term prognosis of these disorders are highly variable. In the differential diagnosis of most multisystem disorders, vasculitis, infection, and occult emboli (e.g., atrial myxoma, cholesterol emboli) should all be considered.

I. Specific disorders. Hypersensitivity vasculitis affects small vessels, presenting with rash and, occasionally, nephritis. It may occur with infection, connective tissue disease, drug reaction, and malignancy. **Polyarteritis nodosa (PAN)** usually attacks medium-sized vessels in major organs such as kidney, liver, GI tract, and peripheral nerves. **Wegener's granulomatosis** is typified by involvement of small- to medium-sized vessels in upper and lower airways and kidney disease. **Rheumatoid vasculitis,** which often presents when arthritis is clinically inactive, may produce skin ulcers, nailfold infarcts, scleritis, pericarditis, and peripheral neuropathy. Diagnosis of a specific form of vasculitis usually requires both clinical features and a biopsy of clinically involved organs. In PAN, angiography may be diagnostic.

II. Management should include consultation with a physician experienced in the treatment of these disorders. Treatment should be tailored to the severity of organ system involvement.

   A. Glucocorticoids are the usual initial therapy and are beneficial in most vasculitides. Although vasculitis that is limited to the skin may respond to lower dosages, the initial dosage for visceral involvement should be high (60–100 mg/day prednisone). If life-threatening manifestations are present, a brief course of high-dose pulse therapy with methylprednisolone, 500 mg IV q12h for 3–5 days, should be considered (see Systemic Lupus Erythematosus, sec. **II.C.2**).

   B. Immunosuppressive agents. The addition of cyclophosphamide, 1.5–2.0 mg/kg PO qd, to glucocorticoid treatment regimens should be considered when major organ system involvement (e.g., lung, kidney, or nerve) is rapidly progressive. **Early addition of cyclophosphamide is appropriate in Wegener's granulomatosis and polyarteritis nodosa.** Immunosuppressive agents should also be considered for patients who are unresponsive to glucocorticoid therapy or intolerant of glucocorticoid side effects.

Polymyalgia Rheumatica
and Temporal Arteritis

Polymyalgia rheumatica (PMR) presents in elderly patients as proximal limb girdle pain (without weakness or elevated muscle enzymes), morning stiffness, fatigue, weight loss, low-grade fever, anemia, and an erythrocyte sedimentation rate (ESR) of greater than 50 ml/hour. **Temporal arteritis (TA)** is a form of giant-cell arteritis also seen primarily in the elderly. Up to 40% of patients with PMR also have TA. TA can present with symptoms of PMR, as well as with headache, scalp tenderness, claudication of jaw muscles, visual disturbances (including blindness), stroke, and an ESR greater than 50 ml/hour. Less commonly, major branches of the thoracic and abdominal aorta are affected.

I. **Management of PMR.** If PMR is present without evidence of TA, prednisone, 10–15 mg PO qd, usually produces dramatic clinical improvement within a few days. The ESR should return to normal during initial treatment, but subsequent therapeutic decisions should be based on both ESR and clinical status. Glucocorticoid therapy can be gradually tapered to a maintenance dosage of 5–10 mg PO qd and continued for a minimum of 1 year to minimize the risk of relapse. NSAIDs may facilitate reduction in prednisone dosage.

II. **Management of TA.** Patients suspected of having TA should be treated promptly with prednisone, 60–80 mg PO qd, to prevent irreversible blindness. Alternate-day therapy has no role in the initial management of this disease. The diagnosis of TA should be confirmed by temporal artery biopsy, which will not be altered by 3–5 days of prednisone therapy. High-dose steroid therapy should be continued until symptoms have abated and the ESR has returned to normal. The dosage should then be gradually tapered by not more than 10%/week and should be continued for 1–2 years with close monitoring of the ESR and clinical status. A maintenance dosage of prednisone, 10–20 mg PO qd, may be required for years.

Cryoglobulin Syndromes

Cryoglobulins are serum proteins that reversibly precipitate in the cold. More than half of cryoglobulinemic patients have an underlying disease such as an immuno-proliferative process, autoimmune disorder, or underlying infection such as hepa-titis B or C; the remainder are idiopathic (essential cryoglobulinemia). Clinical manifestations of cryoglobulins may be mediated by immune complex deposition (arthralgias, purpura, Raynaud's phenomenon, glomerulonephritis, and neuropa-thy) or by hyperviscosity (headache, lethargy, blurred vision).

I. **Diagnosis requires the proper collection of serum** for the detection of cryoglobu-lins. Blood should be collected in prewarmed tubes and kept at 37°C while clotting occurs. Serum should be promptly harvested after centrifugation at 37°C and then incubated at 4°C for at least 72 hours. Normal values vary considerably among laboratories, but trace amounts of cryoglobulins may be found in normal persons. Whenever cryoglobulins are identified, immunoelectrophoresis should be performed to identify the proteins as monoclonal (associated with immunoproliferative dis-eases) or polyclonal.

II. **Therapy** of secondary cryoglobulinemic states is directed at the underlying disease. Essential cryoglobulinemia may respond to prednisone or immunosuppressive agents. Hyperviscosity responds dramatically to plasmapheresis.

Polymyositis and
Dermatomyositis

Polymyositis (PM) is an inflammatory myopathy that presents as weakness and, occasionally, tenderness of the hip and shoulder girdle musculature. **Dermatomy-**

ositis (DM) is, by definition, PM with a concomitant rash. PM-DM can occur in three forms: (1) alone, (2) in association with any of the other autoimmune diseases, or (3) with a variety of neoplasms. Men with DM, cutaneous vasculitis, and disease onset after the age of 50 years are at greatest risk of having an associated malignancy (*J Rheumatol* 10:85, 1983).

I. **Diagnosis.** Abnormal EMG patterns and elevated muscle enzyme levels (creatine kinase, aldolase, SGOT, and lactate dehydrogenase) are usually present. Although the diagnosis is confirmed by muscle biopsy, the disease is patchy, and a biopsy may miss involved areas or show nonspecific changes.

II. **Treatment.** When PM-DM occurs without associated disease, it usually responds well to prednisone, 60–100 mg PO qd. Alternate-day therapy (see Rheumatoid Arthritis, sec. **I.B.3**) can also be successful and should be tried if the patient is not severely ill. Systemic complaints such as fever and malaise respond to therapy first, followed by muscle enzymes, and, finally, muscle strength. Once serum enzyme levels normalize, the prednisone dosage should be slowly reduced to maintenance levels of 10–20 mg PO qd or 20–40 mg PO qod. The appearance of steroid-induced myopathy and hypokalemia may complicate therapeutic assessment. PM-DM associated with neoplasia tends to be less responsive to glucocorticoid therapy but may improve following removal of an associated malignant tumor. Patients who fail to respond or cannot tolerate the side effects of glucocorticoids may respond to methotrexate (0.1–0.3 mg/kg/week) or azathioprine (2–4 mg/kg/day) (*Ann Intern Med* 111:143, 1989) (see Rheumatoid Arthritis, sec. **I.C** and Systemic Lupus Erythematosus, sec. **III**). Complications of severe disease include interstitial lung disease, cardiomyopathy, and respiratory failure caused by aspiration pneumonia or diaphragmatic weakness. Physical therapy is essential in the management of myositis. Bed rest with active-assisted range of motion is appropriate during very active disease, with more active exercise prescribed to improve strength once inflammation has been controlled.

Neurologic Emergencies in Internal Medicine

Sylvia Awadalla,
S. Kathleen Doster, and
Kelvin A. Yamada

Coma

Coma is a state of unresponsiveness to external stimulation. Because some causes of coma may rapidly lead to irreversible brain damage, resuscitation and treatment must proceed concurrently with assessment.

I. **Pathophysiology.** Stupor and coma result from diseases that affect (1) **both cerebral hemispheres** or (2) the **brainstem.** Unilateral cerebral lesions (e.g., stroke, tumor, subdural hematoma) rarely impair consciousness unless they have sufficient mass effect to compress the opposite hemisphere (midline shift or subfalcine herniation) or the brainstem (transtentorial herniation). Mass lesions in the posterior fossa cause coma by compressing the brainstem. Metabolic disorders impair consciousness by diffuse effects on both cerebral hemispheres.

II. **Causes of stupor and coma** in patients whose initial diagnosis is unclear are shown in Table 25-1.

III. **Diagnosis and treatment of the comatose patient.** A systematic, expeditious approach should lead to a prompt diagnosis and determine if neurosurgical management is necessary.

   A. **The airway** should be secured, ventilation and circulation should be supported, and body temperature should be maintained.

   B. **The neck** must be immobilized if there is any possibility of trauma until cervical spine films exclude injury or instability.

   C. **IV access** should be established. **Initial blood tests,** including glucose, electrolytes, urea, CBC, calcium, arterial blood gas, drug/alcohol/toxin screen, cultures, liver enzymes, prothrombin time (PT) and partial thromboplastin time (PTT), should be performed. A type and crossmatch should be included if an operative lesion is anticipated.

   D. **Thiamine,** 100 mg, followed by **dextrose,** 1 g/kg, should be given by IV push.

   E. **Naloxone,** 0.01 mg/kg IV push to a maximum of 2 mg, and **flumazenil,** 0.2 mg IV push, repeated at 1-minute intervals up to a 1-mg total dose, should be given.

   F. **Initial assessment**

   1. **The patient's history** should be obtained from relatives, friends, ambulance drivers, police, or anyone with recent contact with the patient regarding trauma, seizure activity, alcohol or drug use, diabetes, or other systemic disease.

   2. **General physical examination** may reveal a systemic illness associated with coma (e.g., cirrhosis, hemodialysis shunt, rash consistent with meningococcemia) or signs of head trauma (e.g., lacerations, periorbital or mastoid ecchymosis, hemotympanum).

   3. **Neurologic examination** (see sec. **IV**) is focused on determining the patient's level of consciousness, location of the lesion, and whether herniation is occurring. Repeated examinations are necessary to detect and intervene if clinical deterioration occurs.

   G. **Herniation** (see sec. **V**) must be recognized and treated immediately. Treatment consists of temporary measures to lower intracranial pressure until neurosurgical intervention can take place if indicated. If herniation is occurring, the following steps should be taken.

   1. **Hyperventilation** with a target PCO_2 of 25–30 mm Hg will reduce intracra-

Table 25-1. Causes of stupor and coma

Metabolic and diffuse disorders (60%)
Drugs or toxins
Encephalitis
Meningitis
Cerebral ischemia
Hypertensive encephalopathy
Subarachnoid hemorrhage
Disseminated intravascular coagulation
Thiamine deficiency
Hepatic encephalopathy
Uremia
Electrolyte abnormalities
   Hyponatremia
   Hypernatremia
   Hypercalcemia
Hypoxemia
Hypercapnia
Hypocapnia
Acidosis or alkalosis
Hypo- or hyperglycemia
Adrenal insufficiency
Hyperadrenalism
Panhypopituitarism
Hypo- or hyperthermia
Seizure or postictal state
Increased intracranial pressure
Closed head trauma

Supratentorial lesions (30%)
Intracerebral hemorrhage
Subdural or epidural hematoma
Pituitary apoplexy
Cerebral infarction
Venous sinus occlusion
Tumor
Abscess
Hydrocephalus

Infratentorial lesions (10%)
Brainstem hemorrhage or infarction
Basilar migraine
Cerebellar hemorrhage or infarction
Tumor
Abscess
Subdural or epidural hematoma
Basilar aneurysm

Psychogenic conditions mimicking coma (<1%)
Depression
Catatonia
Malingering
Conversion reaction
Hysteria

Source: Adapted from F Plum, JB Posner. *The Diagnosis of Stupor and Coma* (3rd ed).
Philadelphia: Davis, 1980.

nial pressure, with the peak effect occurring within 2–30 minutes. Reduction of PCO_2 below 25 mm Hg is inadvisable because cerebral blood flow may be reduced excessively.

    2. Mannitol (100 g in 500 ml of 5% D/W) should be infused as a bolus of 1–2 g/kg IV over 10–20 minutes, followed by a maintenance dose of 50–300 mg/kg IV q6h. Therapeutic effect begins within minutes, reaches a peak within 90 minutes, and decreases over several hours.

    3. Glucocorticoids reduce the edema surrounding a tumor or abscess; dexamethasone, 10 mg, is given by IV push, followed by 4 mg IV q6h.

    4. A head CT scan should be performed as soon as the patient is stable to determine if neurosurgical intervention is possible. Inoperable lesions require supportive care.

H. If herniation is not occurring, a careful examination for focal neurologic signs and a CT scan of the head should be obtained.

    1. Operable lesions require neurosurgical consultation.

    2. Inoperable lesions require supportive care.

    3. If the head CT is not diagnostic and laboratory tests do not suggest a diagnosis, a lumbar puncture should be considered.

I. Lumbar puncture should not be performed if a mass lesion or midline shift is present on the CT scan. **If meningitis is suspected, antimicrobial coverage should be started without waiting for the lumbar puncture.** CSF should be sent for cell count, protein, glucose, Gram's stain, acid-fast stain, India ink stain, fungal and bacterial cultures, and cryptococcal and bacterial antigens (particularly if antimicrobials have been given), and an extra tube should be saved in the refrigerator.

    1. Infections should be treated with appropriate antimicrobials immediately (see Chap. 13).

    2. Subarachnoid hemorrhage requires neurosurgical consultation.

    3. An EEG may be helpful if CSF and laboratory studies are not diagnostic.

J. The EEG is abnormal in almost all conditions of impaired consciousness but may point to otherwise unsuspected diagnoses. Some conditions such as hepatic encephalopathy, herpes encephalitis, and barbiturate or other anesthetic intoxications have characteristic (but not necessarily diagnostic) EEG findings. Electrical seizures (nonconvulsive status epilepticus) may be diagnosed by EEG. A normal awake EEG suggests psychogenic coma.

K. Coagulopathy must be corrected immediately with fresh-frozen plasma, cryoprecipitate, or platelet transfusion in any patient with hemorrhage or an operable lesion determined on CT scan. Hemorrhages may progress until the coagulopathy is reversed, and neurosurgical intervention cannot take place until coagulation is normal.

L. If there is no diagnosis after the initial evaluation, the most likely cause of coma is a metabolic or toxic etiology or a brainstem stroke. The patient should be hospitalized for close monitoring of his or her neurologic and respiratory status while further diagnostic studies are performed, including studies of thyroid, adrenal, and pituitary function.

IV. Neurologic examination of the comatose patient

    A. Level of consciousness can be assessed and monitored with the **Glasgow coma scale** (Table 25-2).

    B. Respiratory rate and pattern should be noted.

        1. Cheyne-Stokes respiration occurs in metabolic coma, supratentorial lesions, chronic pulmonary disease, and congestive heart failure.

        2. Hyperventilation is usually a sign of metabolic acidosis, hypoxemia, pneumonia, or other pulmonary disease but may also be caused by upper brainstem injury.

        3. Apneustic breathing (long pauses after inspiration), **cluster breathing** (breathing in short bursts), and **ataxic breathing** (irregular breaths without pattern) are signs of brainstem injury. **These patterns may suggest impending respiratory arrest.**

Table 25-2. Glasgow coma scale

Points are assigned and totaled based on patient response to stimuli.
Total range = 3 (unresponsive) to 15 (normal).

Eye opening
Spontaneous	4
To voice	3
To painful stimulation	2
Never	1

Verbal responses
Oriented	5
Confused	4
Inappropriate words	3
Unintelligible sounds	2
None	1

Motor responses
Follows commands	6
Localizes pain	5
Withdraws from pain	4
Flexor response	3
Extensor response	2
None	1

C. **Pupil size and light reactivity** are very useful for evaluating the comatose patient.
   1. **A unilateral dilated and fixed pupil in a patient with altered mental status requires that uncal herniation be excluded and treated, if present.** Mydriatics (e.g., scopolamine, atropine) may produce asymmetric pupils and cycloplegia.
   2. **Small but reactive pupils** are seen in narcotic overdose, metabolic encephalopathy, and thalamic or pontine lesions.
   3. **Midposition, fixed pupils** imply a midbrain lesion and occur in central herniation.
   4. **Bilateral fixed and dilated pupils** are seen with severe anoxic encephalopathy or intoxication with drugs such as scopolamine, atropine, glutethimide, or methyl alcohol.
D. **Eye movements.** The **oculocephalic** (doll's eyes) test can be performed **if no cervical injury is present** by quickly turning the patient's head laterally or vertically. If the brainstem is intact, the eyes move conjugately in a direction opposite of the head movement. The more potent **oculovestibular** (cold caloric) test is used if cervical trauma is suspected or if no eye movements are elicited by the oculocephalic test. The patient's head is elevated 30 degrees above the horizontal while the tympanic membrane is lavaged with 10–50 ml of ice water. The eyes should move conjugately toward the ear being stimulated. Vertical gaze can be assessed with simultaneous stimulation of both ears.
   1. **Absence of all eye movements** indicates a bilateral pontine lesion or drug-induced ophthalmoplegia (e.g., sedatives, phenytoin, tricyclic antidepressants).
   2. **Dysconjugate gaze** suggests a brainstem lesion.
   3. **A horizontal gaze preference** (both eyes conjugately to one side) indicates either a unilateral pontine or frontal lobe lesion. Eye deviation **toward** the side of a hemiparesis suggests a pontine lesion contralateral to the hemiparesis. Eye deviation **away** from a hemiparesis suggests a lesion in the frontal lobe, contralateral to the hemiparesis. Oculocephalic and oculovestibular maneuvers (passive head rotation and ice water irrigation of ear, respectively) help distinguish between these possibilities; in frontal lobe lesions eyes move conjugately to the side opposite the stimulation whereas in

unilateral pontine lesions the eyes move toward the opposite side but do not cross the midline.

4. **Loss of vertical gaze** occurs in midbrain lesions, central herniation, and acute hydrocephalus.

E. **Motor responses,** both spontaneous and in response to painful stimulation, should be observed for symmetry and purpose.

1. **Preferential use of the limbs** on one side indicates hemiparesis of the unused limbs.

2. **Stereotyped posturing,** rather than purposeful protective movements, is not of localizing value and can occur in metabolic coma.

3. **External rotation** of one leg at rest may be caused by hemiparesis of that side or by a dislocated or fractured hip.

V. **Herniation** occurs when mass lesions cause shifts in brain tissue. It must be recognized and treated immediately to prevent irreversible brain damage or death. Treatment consists of temporary measures to lower intracranial pressure until neurosurgical intervention can take place (see sec. III.G).

A. **Nonspecific signs and symptoms of increased intracranial pressure** include headache, nausea, vomiting, hypertension, bradycardia, papilledema, sixth nerve palsy, transient visual obscurations, and alterations in consciousness.

B. **Uncal herniation** is caused by unilateral, supratentorial lesions and may progress rapidly. Signs include alteration of consciousness, a dilated pupil ipsilateral to the mass, and hemiparesis or posturing on either side.

C. **Central herniation** is caused by medial or bilateral supratentorial lesions. Signs include progressive alteration of consciousness, Cheyne-Stokes or normal respirations followed by central hyperventilation, midposition and unreactive pupils, loss of upward gaze, and posturing of the extremities.

D. **Tonsillar herniation** occurs when pressure in the posterior fossa forces the cerebellar tonsils through the foramen magnum compressing the medulla. Signs include altered level of consciousness and respiratory irregularity or apnea.

Acute Confusional States

I. **Acute confusional states (delirium)** are characterized by abnormal attention, fluctuations of consciousness, disorientation, incoherent speech, memory impairment, agitation, and altered circadian rhythms.

II. **Causes** include septicemia, drug intoxication, drug or alcohol withdrawal, thiamine deficiency, hepatic or renal failure, thyrotoxicosis or hypothyroidism, hypoxia, hypoglycemia, electrolyte abnormalities, CNS infections (e.g., meningitis, encephalitis), subarachnoid hemorrhage, head trauma, and (rarely) stroke. A relatively mild systemic illness may produce delirium in a demented patient. Psychiatric illness generally does not cause severe confusion, disorientation, or an altered level of consciousness.

III. **Evaluation**

A. **Initial blood tests** should include glucose, electrolytes, urea, CBC, calcium, magnesium, ammonia, arterial blood gas, cultures, and thyroid-stimulating hormone (TSH). **Toxicologic screening** of urine and blood should be performed, including alcohol level.

B. **History** should include a careful review of all medications. **General physical and neurologic examination** may reveal systemic illness or focal neurologic signs.

C. **A CT scan** of the head should be performed when a structural lesion is suspected by the history (e.g., sudden onset) or neurologic examination (e.g., focal signs).

D. **Lumbar puncture** is indicated if fever, elevated WBC, or meningismus are present, or the cause of delirium is unclear. A CT scan should be performed prior to lumbar puncture if signs of increased intracranial pressure or focal neurologic signs are present (see Coma, sec. V).

IV. **Treatment** depends on the etiology and often consists of stopping or replacing a medication.

A. **Thiamine,** 100 mg, followed by **dextrose,** 1 g/kg, should be given by IV push, and **oxygen** by nasal cannula should be administered while awaiting initial results.
B. **Close observation of the patient in a quiet, well-lighted environment** is necessary.
C. **Sedatives** can aggravate symptoms. If sedation is necessary, low doses of short-acting benzodiazepines or haloperidol may be used with caution. Haloperidol and phenothiazines may cause hypotension, especially in the elderly, and may lower the seizure threshold.
D. **Restraints** are occasionally needed for patient safety. Care should be taken to avoid circulatory compromise from tight restraints.

Alcohol Withdrawal

Alcohol withdrawal has a significant risk of death and requires a high index of suspicion for diagnosis. **Manifestations** include tremulousness, hallucinosis, seizures, and delirium tremens. Often, an illness (e.g., trauma, infection, pancreatitis, gastritis) has interfered with alcohol intake, precipitating an episode of withdrawal.

I. **Minor withdrawal** is characterized by tremulousness, irritability, anorexia, and nausea. Symptoms usually appear within a few hours after reduction or cessation of alcohol consumption and resolve within 48 hours. A well-lighted room, the presence of friends or relatives, and reassurance are important aspects of treatment. Many of the symptoms can be treated with **benzodiazepines,** including chlordiazepoxide, 25–100 mg PO q6h; diazepam, 5–20 mg PO q6h; or **lorazepam,** 1–2 mg PO q6h. The goal of therapy is to sedate the patient until he or she is calm. The dosage must be titrated to the patient's clinical state. **Thiamine,** 100 mg IM or IV qd for 3 days, followed by 100 mg PO qd, and multivitamins containing folic acid should be given. The patient should be observed for signs of major alcohol withdrawal; social circumstances dictate whether this should be done at home or in the hospital.

II. **Delirium tremens** is manifested by tremulousness, hallucinations, agitation, confusion, disorientation, and autonomic hyperactivity, including fever, tachycardia, and diaphoresis. It usually occurs 72–96 hours after cessation of drinking and generally starts to resolve within 3–5 days. It is seen in 5–10% of cases of alcohol withdrawal and carries a mortality rate of 5%. Other causes of delirium must be considered in the differential diagnosis (see Acute Confusional States). Supportive management is identical to that for minor withdrawal. Physical restraints should be avoided if possible, but self-inflicted injury must be prevented.
A. **Chlordiazepoxide,** 100 mg IV or PO, repeated q2–6h as needed, with a maximum dose of 500 mg in the first 24 hours, is an effective sedative in this situation. One-half the initial 24-hour dose may be administered over the next 24 hours; the dosage may be reduced by 25–50 mg/day each day thereafter. **Lorazepam,** 1–2 mg IV, IM, or PO q6–8h, or **oxazepam,** 15–30 mg PO, repeated q6–8h, may be used instead of chlordiazepoxide in patients with severe hepatic dysfunction because there is decreased potential for delayed clearance. Specifications for holding benzodiazepines (e.g., sleeping, nystagmus) should be clearly written.
B. **Clonidine and atenolol** may be used to attenuate withdrawal symptoms caused by central noradrenergic overactivity (*Alcoholism* 9:238, 1985; *N Engl J Med* 313:905, 1985). Care must be taken to avoid hypotension. An initial dosage of clonidine, 0.1 mg PO tid, can be increased gradually to 0.2–0.4 mg tid if symptoms persist and BP is stable. Atenolol is used in dosages of 50–100 mg PO qd.
C. **Maintenance of fluid and electrolyte balance** is important, because these patients are susceptible to hypomagnesemia, hypokalemia, and hypoglycemia. Fluid losses may be considerable because of fever, diaphoresis, and vomiting.

III. **Alcohol withdrawal seizures** occur 12–48 hours after cessation of intake and are usually generalized motor seizures. Seizures are usually few in number and responsive to PO or IV benzodiazepines; if they are acute and frequent, phenytoin or barbiturates can be effective (see Seizures, secs. **II.B** and **II.C**). **Treatment of alcohol** withdrawal seizures with chronic anticonvulsant drugs is not indicated. Neurologic and systemic illnesses that present with seizures, including **head trauma, meningitis, and metabolic abnormalities, are common in alcohol abusers and must always be considered.**

Head Injury

Management of head injury depends on the extent of brain injury and the presence of fractures, hematoma, and associated injuries.

I. **Initial assessment**
   A. **Airway, ventilation, and circulation** must be assessed in any patient with altered consciousness or significant trauma. Severe head trauma usually causes hypoventilation, which raises intracranial pressure. Systemic hypotension causes secondary brain injury from ischemia. Nasal intubation should be avoided in patients with facial fractures.
   B. **Cervical spine films** should be obtained for all patients, and **the neck should be immobilized** until cervical fracture or dislocation is ruled out.
   C. **History** should document the temporal course of all symptoms, particularly loss of consciousness, occurrence of a lucid interval (which suggests expanding hematoma), and amnesia (which is related to the severity of the blow).
   D. **General physical examination** must establish whether the patient's vital signs are stable. The presence of penetrating wounds and other significant trauma should be determined.
   E. **Neurologic examination** should assess the level of consciousness and Glasgow coma score (see Table 25-2), focal deficits, and signs of herniation, and should be repeated at frequent intervals to document any progression of neurologic deficits.

II. **Management** is determined by the severity of brain injury.
   A. **Mild head trauma.** Awake, alert patients with **concussion** (transient loss of consciousness, confusion, agitation, or amnesia) but without focal neurologic deficits require skull films, cervical films, and close observation for 24 hours to rule out delayed deterioration. **If fractures are not suspected,** the patient may be observed at home by a reliable adult with instructions for frequent mental status assessment and criteria for return. **Fractures or the absence of a reliable observer require hospital admission.**
   B. **Moderate head trauma** or focal neurologic deficits require cervical films and a head CT scan. Patients with contusion or a normal head CT should be observed in the hospital for at least 24 hours or until he or she is stable. **Hematoma** requires neurosurgical consultation.
   C. **Severe head trauma** requires immediate neurosurgical consultation. Cardiopulmonary resuscitation is the first priority, and the patient should be intubated and hyperventilated to a PCO_2 of 35 mm Hg. Herniation (see Coma, secs. **III.G and V**) must be recognized and treated immediately, with more vigorous hyperventilation to a PCO_2 of 25 mm Hg and mannitol until surgery is possible. Steroids are not indicated. A CT scan of the head and cervical spine radiographs should be performed as soon as the patient is stable. The patient's head should be elevated 30 degrees. Intravascular volume expansion and hypoosmolar fluids should be avoided.
   D. **Penetrating head trauma,** even with a normal neurologic examination, requires an immediate head CT and neurosurgical consultation. Foreign objects (e.g., knives) should not be moved.
   E. **Delayed neurologic deterioration** requires an immediate head CT to rule out expanding hematoma, even if a prior CT was negative.
   F. **Intracranial hematoma** requires neurosurgical evaluation.
      1. **Epidural hematoma** is caused by skull fractures crossing a meningeal artery and may cause precipitous deterioration after an asymptomatic period. Pupil asymmetry occurs in 30–50% of patients with epidural hematoma. Without immediate surgical evacuation, brain herniation will occur.

2. **Acute subdural hematoma** is a neurosurgical emergency. The mortality risk is 20–50% and may be reduced by surgical evacuation within 4 hours.

3. **Chronic subdural hematoma** is most common in the elderly, debilitated patients, alcoholics, and patients receiving anticoagulants. Antecedent trauma is often minimal. Symptoms tend to be nonspecific (e.g., headache, confusion, lethargy) and can fluctuate markedly. Need for surgical evacuation depends on symptoms and mass effect.

4. **Intracerebral hematomas** may be present initially or develop in a contused area. The decision to surgically evacuate or observe them depends on the location and size of the hematoma and on the patient's neurologic status.

G. **Skull fractures** increase the risk of epidural hemorrhage and infection. They may be diagnosed by skull radiographs or head CT or inferred by the presence of otorrhea, rhinorrhea, hemotympanum, postauricular hematoma, and periorbital hematoma. Fractures require a CT scan of the head and neurosurgical evaluation.

Acute Spinal Cord Dysfunction

Spinal cord syndromes may result from trauma, compression by mass lesions, or noncompressive etiologies such as inflammation, infection, or infarction. Early recognition and treatment may reverse or prevent progression of neurologic deficit.

I. **Cord compression** often presents with back pain at the level of compression, increasing difficulty walking, and a loss of sensation in a dermatomal distribution, followed by rapid deterioration and urinary retention with overflow incontinence. However, some lesions are painless. An etiology may be suggested by patient history in known malignancy, by fever and elevated WBC in epidural abscess, or by coagulopathy in hematoma.

A. **Examination** should determine the level of compression; however, there may be many lesions. There may be tenderness to spinal percussion over the lesion. Radicular signs caused by nerve root involvement may be found at the level of compression, with myelopathic signs secondary to cord dysfunction below the lesion. Sensory loss often localizes the lesion within 2 dermatomal levels.

1. **Radicular signs** include lancinating pain, paresthesias, and numbness in the dermatomal distribution of the sensory nerve root. Weakness, decreased tone, and decreased reflexes occur in the muscles supplied by the motor nerve root.

2. **Myelopathic signs** include a band of dysesthesia at the level of compression, with bilateral loss of all sensory modalities and bilateral weakness below the level of the lesion. In acute lesions (spinal shock), tone and reflexes are diminished below the lesion, whereas in more slowly progressive lesions, tone and reflexes are increased below the lesion and plantar responses are extensor. Urinary retention commonly accompanies spinal cord compression.

3. **Incomplete cord lesions** may result in contralateral pain and temperature loss below the lesion, with ipsilateral weakness and proprioceptive loss (**Brown-Séquard syndrome**).

4. **Cauda equina syndrome** results from compression of the lower lumbar and sacral roots, causing sensory loss in a saddle distribution, flaccid weakness of the legs, decreased reflexes, and urinary and fecal incontinence.

B. **Imaging studies. Plain radiographs of the spine** may reveal metastatic disease, osteomyelitis, diskitis, or pathologic fractures. **MRI scanning** should be obtained urgently to determine the exact level and extent of the lesion(s). **Myelography with CT scan** can be performed if MRI is unavailable or contraindicated. MRI and myelography should include the entire spine. Neurosurgical consultation should be obtained prior to myelography, as acute decompensation requiring urgent decompressive laminectomy may occur.

C. **Dexamethasone,** 10 mg IV, followed by 4 mg IV q6h, should be started immediately. Higher doses may result in better pain relief but do not affect motor outcome (*Neurology* 39:1255, 1989).

D. **Emergency radiation therapy** combined with high-dose glucocorticoids is usually recommended for cord compression caused by metastatic malignancy. A tissue diagnosis (from the cord lesion or elsewhere) is usually required prior to radiation.

E. **Neurosurgical consultation** should be obtained early. Surgical decompression is indicated for cord compression caused by abscess, hematoma, herniated disk, primary tumors, and for some metastatic tumors: (1) radiation-resistant cancer; (2) patients who have already received maximal radiation; (3) patients without a tissue diagnosis; and (4) patients with rapid and relentless deterioration of neurologic function despite medical and radiation therapies.

II. **Noncompressive spinal cord lesions,** such as transverse myelitis or infarction, present with the same symptoms as cord compression. MRI or myelography must be obtained to rule out a mass lesion.

A. **Lumbar puncture** should be performed to identify infection or inflammation **after** a compressive lesion is excluded.

B. **Treatable infections** such as syphilis and herpes require appropriate antimicrobials (see Chap. 13).

C. **High-dose glucocorticoids** (dexamethasone, 10 mg IV, then 4 mg IV q6h) can be administered for transverse myelitis or cord infarction but have not proved beneficial in all etiologies.

III. **Traumatic spinal injury** may be obvious from the history or initial examination but may present with only minimal weakness. It must be ruled out in patients who are unconscious, confused, or inebriated and have a history of head or other trauma.

A. **Immobilization of the neck** with collars, backboards, and logrolls is essential to prevent further injury until spine radiographs are reviewed.

B. **Examination** may reveal local and radicular pain, weakness, absent tone and reflexes, extensor plantar responses, or urinary retention. Cervical injuries may present with torticollis, paradoxical ventilation (normal diaphragmatic function with absent intercostals), hypoventilation, or respiratory arrest. Shock with hypotension, bradycardia, or priapism may occur secondary to loss of sympathetic innervation.

C. **Respiratory compromise** in cervical lesions must be carefully sought and requires immediate intubation. If the patient cannot be orally or nasally intubated easily, cricothyroidotomy or emergent tracheostomy is indicated.

D. **Hypotension** and bradycardia secondary to sympathectomy in cervical injury require cardiac support with beta-adrenergic agonists (dopamine, 5–15 μg/kg/minute, or dobutamine, 3–20 μg/kg/minute). Alpha-adrenergic agonists will increase BP but reduce cardiac output and impair spinal cord perfusion. Fluid resuscitation alone usually results in pulmonary edema (see Chap. 9).

E. **A Foley catheter** should be placed to relieve bladder distention, preventing reflex vagal stimulation and sudden fluctuations in cardiac function and BP.

F. **Methylprednisolone,** 30 mg/kg IV bolus, followed by an infusion of 5.4 mg/kg/hour for 23 hours, improves neurologic recovery when administered within 8 hours of injury (*N Engl J Med* 322:1405, 1990).

G. **Immediate neurosurgical or orthopedic consultation, or both,** should be obtained.

Cerebrovascular Disease

I. **Ischemic cerebrovascular disease.** Insufficient cerebral perfusion produces signs and symptoms referable to the distribution of the vessel or vessels involved. In a transient ischemic attack (**TIA**), the symptoms resolve within 24 hours. Reversible ischemic neurologic deficits (**RIND**) resolve within 1 week. TIAs and RINDs usually reflect atherosclerotic disease of the cerebral arteries and are risk factors for subsequent cerebral infarction (**stroke**). Systemic hypotension typically presents with syncope and rarely causes focal ischemia or infarction. However, when systemic hypotension is prolonged, ischemic damage occurs in zones between major vascular territories (**watershed infarction**).

A. Assessment

1. **History** should establish the pattern of onset and duration of symptoms. The abrupt onset of a focal deficit without a change in level of consciousness is characteristic of ischemia and infarction but may also occur with intracranial hemorrhage, tumor, or migraine. Systemic diseases, such as cardiac embolic disease, connective tissue disease, carcinoma, or IV drug abuse, can also cause stroke.

2. **General physical examination** should search for cardiac etiologies of cerebral embolism, such as atrial fibrillation, rheumatic valvular disease, infective endocarditis, recent anteroseptal myocardial infarction, or ventricular aneurysm. Approximately one-fifth of cerebral infarctions result from cardiogenic embolism (*Arch Neurol* 46:727, 1989). Acute systemic illnesses commonly cause focal neurologic signs from a previous stroke to recur, mimicking acute ischemia. **Carotid bruits alone are unreliable indicators of clinically significant atherosclerosis.**

3. **Neurologic examination** is the most accurate means of determining the location of a cerebral infarction.

   a. **Carotid circulation** lesions produce various signs, including contralateral hemiparesis, hemisensory loss, homonymous hemianopsia, ipsilateral monocular visual loss (**amaurosis fugax**), aphasia, and dysarthria.

   b. **Vertebral-basilar circulation ischemia** produces unilateral or bilateral weakness, sensory loss, diplopia, ataxia, nystagmus, dysarthria, hoarseness, dysphagia, hearing loss, and vertigo. Cranial nerve signs contralateral to somatic signs occur secondary to brainstem lesions. **Syncope** or near-syncope is usually secondary to a disorder of the cardiovascular system, rather than brainstem ischemia. Vertigo without other brainstem signs is usually caused by labyrinthine or eighth nerve disease.

4. **Diagnostic tests** useful in the evaluation of cerebrovascular disease are described below.

   a. **CT or MRI** of the head is necessary to clarify the structural abnormalities responsible for the patient's symptoms (e.g., tumor, abscess, intracerebral hematoma, subdural hematoma, subarachnoid hemorrhage). Although an ischemic infarction may not be evident on a noncontrast CT within the first 36 hours, intracerebral hemorrhages are easily seen and may affect therapeutic decisions. Hemorrhage into an infarct can develop 1–7 days following the infarction.

   b. **Lumbar puncture** should be performed on all patients with suspected septic embolism from bacterial endocarditis. Meningeal infections with a variety of bacterial, spirochetal, and fungal agents can produce an inflammatory vasculitis that may present as a stroke. A CSF leukocytosis may precede fever, positive blood cultures, and other clinical clues of these diagnoses (*Stroke* 17:332, 1986; *Stroke* 18:544a, 1987).

   c. **Laboratory tests** should include CBC, platelet count, clotting studies (PT, aPTT), VDRL, and erythrocyte sedimentation rate (ESR) to screen for systemic causes of stroke such as polycythemia, blood dyscrasias, or connective tissue disease. Serum chemistries, including glucose and sodium, are mandatory.

   d. **An ECG and chest radiograph** should be obtained for all patients. Two-dimensional echocardiography should be obtained if a cardiac source is suspected. Transesophageal echocardiography and contrast echocardiography may be indicated when a cardiac source is suspected but cannot be adequately evaluated by transthoracic echocardiogram.

   e. **Noninvasive Doppler ultrasound** studies of the carotid arteries are often used as a screening test for significant stenosis that should be further evaluated by angiography.

   f. **Angiography** may be useful to evaluate intracranial atherosclerosis and is essential for the preoperative evaluation of candidates for carotid endarterectomy (see sec. **I.B.2.b**). Angiography may also demonstrate intracranial vasculitis, and it is indicated when the diagnosis is unclear.

B. Treatment depends on the underlying cause of stroke and the general condition of the patient.

1. **Cardiogenic embolus** is an indication for systemic anticoagulation. The aim of anticoagulant therapy is to prevent subsequent CNS emboli; the timing for its use in acute stroke remains controversial and depends on the size of the infarct, associated hemorrhage, the presence of systemic hypertension, and the risk of recurrent embolism (*Arch Neurol* 46:727, 1989). Therapy should be continued for as long as the embolic source is present. Heparin is used acutely to prolong the aPTT to 1.5–2.0 times normal. Warfarin is used for chronic anticoagulation with a target international normalized ratio of 2–3 (*J Am Coll Cardiol* 8:41b, 1986) (see Chap. 17). Systemic hypertension is a relative contraindication to long-term anticoagulation, because the risk of intracranial hemorrhage is increased. A history of hemorrhagic complications (e.g., peptic ulcer disease) is also a relative contraindication to anticoagulation. Dipyridamole and warfarin in combination are more effective than warfarin alone in the prevention of embolism from prosthetic cardiac valves (*Mayo Clin Proc* 56:265, 1981; *Am J Cardiol* 51:1537, 1983). Mitral valve prolapse may be an embolic source, but appropriate treatment has not been defined.

2. **TIAs and RINDs.** Approximately one-third of patients with TIA or RIND will experience cerebral infarction within 5 years. This risk is greatest immediately following the event and diminishes with time. When cardiac disease and other systemic illnesses are not causal, TIAs in patients older than 50 years are usually caused by atherosclerotic disease of the cerebral vasculature and are treated with the therapeutic measures described below.

   a. **Aspirin** has been shown to reduce the incidence of stroke and death in prospective, randomized studies. Dosages ranged from 300 mg PO tid to 325 mg PO qid. Lower dosages (300 mg qd) have fewer adverse side effects (*Br Med J* 296:316, 1988), but benefit has not been proved. Other antiplatelet agents (e.g., dipyridamole, sulfinpyrazone), alone or in combination with aspirin, are not effective. Ticlopidine, 250 mg PO bid, is an alternative to aspirin for stroke prophylaxis in patients who cannot tolerate it or in whom aspirin therapy has failed (*N Engl J Med* 321:501, 1989).

   b. **Carotid endarterectomy** decreases the risk of stroke and death in patients with recent TIAs or nondisabling strokes and ipsilateral high-grade (70–99%) carotid stenosis (*Stroke* 22:816, 1991; *N Engl J Med* 325:445, 1991). Benefit has not yet been documented for patients with either moderate symptomatic stenosis or asymptomatic stenosis of any degree. **Cerebral angiography** is the standard method for viewing extracranial and intracranial vessels before surgery. The combination of extracranial and intracranial Doppler for detecting high-grade stenosis and occlusion may prove useful as a preliminary, low-risk screening assessment.

   c. **Anticoagulant therapy** in the treatment of TIA and RIND caused by atherosclerosis is controversial. Randomized prospective studies have failed to show that long-term anticoagulation prevents stroke or death, and it may increase the risk of intracerebral hemorrhage as well as non-CNS hemorrhagic complications.

3. **Stroke in evolution** refers to progression of neurologic signs caused by ischemia. Patients with evolving stroke can deteriorate quickly; thus, they require repeated neurologic assessment. IV heparin may be beneficial in the treatment of ischemic, nonhemorrhagic, progressive stroke (*Stroke* 19:10, 1988).

4. **Completed stroke** is a stable, nonprogressing neurologic deficit that is completed within the first 96 hours following onset of stroke. No therapy reduces the extent of a completed event, and the goal of treatment is rehabilitation and prevention of recurrent stroke.

   a. **Risk factors, especially hypertension,** should be treated long term. However, **in acute stroke, reduction of BP should be avoided** because vascular autoregulation is disturbed. Even very high levels of BP should be left untreated, unless evidence of systemic end-organ damage is present such as proteinuria, hematuria, papilledema, or heart failure (see Chap. 4). BP elevation secondary to brain ischemia usually returns to normal levels within days without treatment.

  b. **Aspirin and ticlopidine** reduce the incidence of subsequent strokes in patients with completed stroke.

  c. **Endarterectomy** is indicated in some circumstances (see sec. I.B.2.b).

  d. **Cerebral edema** following large infarctions is maximal at **24–72 hours** and may cause late deterioration. Medical therapy is usually not effective. Surgical decompression is indicated for cerebellar infarctions when edema causes brainstem compression. Surgical decompression is rarely helpful for infarctions of the cerebral hemispheres.

5. **Intraarterial thrombolysis** is experimental therapy available in some centers for treatment of major intracranial vascular thrombosis.

II. Intracranial hemorrhages arise in the intracerebral, subarachnoid, epidural, or subdural spaces (see Head Injury).

  A. **Intracerebral hemorrhage** usually presents with the acute onset of focal neurologic deficits. Signs of sudden increase in intracranial pressure, including alteration in mental status, headache, and vomiting, are present when the hemorrhage is extensive. Focal deficits depend on the location and size of the hemorrhage. With massive bleeding, brain herniation may occur (see Coma, sec. V). Intracerebral hemorrhage may not be clinically distinguishable from cerebral ischemia without the aid of a CT scan.

    1. **Chronic systemic hypertension** is the most common cause. The locations of hypertensive intracerebral hemorrhage are the basal ganglia (70%), pons (10%), cerebellum (10%), and cerebral white matter (10%). Less commonly, intracerebral hemorrhage results from trauma, anticoagulant therapy, saccular aneurysm, arteriovenous malformation, tumor, blood dyscrasia, angiopathy, or vasculitis.

    2. **Treatment** consists of supportive care and correction of precipitating factors.

      a. **Systemic BP** should be lowered gradually, over days, with close observation for evidence of cerebral ischemia. Normal vascular autoregulatory mechanisms are unpredictably impaired in chronically hypertensive patients.

      b. **Surgical consultation** should be obtained for patients with cerebellar hematomas, because brainstem compression or obstructive hydrocephalus may develop, requiring immediate surgical treatment. Superficial cerebral hematomas causing significant mass effect can be evacuated, sometimes with clinical improvement. Evacuation of deep cerebral hematomas is rarely beneficial.

  B. **Subarachnoid hemorrhage (SAH)** can result from intracerebral hemorrhage, ruptured aneurysm, arteriovenous malformation, blood dyscrasia, head trauma, cocaine or amphetamine abuse, or tumor. Rupture of a saccular (**berry**) **aneurysm,** caused by defects in the arterial media and internal elastic membrane, is the most common cause. Other types of aneurysm include the fusiform aneurysm, thought to be secondary to atherosclerosis, and the mycotic aneurysm, from septic embolism. Sudden onset of severe **headache** may be the only symptom of subarachnoid hemorrhage. **Altered mental status,** fever, vomiting, nuchal rigidity, low back pain, focal neurologic deficits, seizures, and retinal hemorrhages (subhyaloid hemorrhages) also occur. ECG abnormalities are common (70%). **Complications** of SAH include rebleeding (20% at 2 weeks), vasospasm with ischemia (days 4–14), hydrocephalus, seizures, and hyponatremia.

    1. **Early diagnosis is essential** when the history and physical examination suggest SAH.

      a. **Head CT** will show blood in the subarachnoid spaces of the sulci and cisternae in 90% of patients within the first 24 hours. Parenchymal and intraventricular hemorrhage can accompany SAH following the rupture of a saccular aneurysm, but suspicion of another etiology should be raised. The source of SAH, especially arteriovenous malformation, may be demonstrated by CT or MRI after IV administration of contrast material, but most patients require angiography for definitive diagnosis.

b. **Lumbar puncture** should be performed when the clinical impression of SAH is not confirmed by imaging studies. Hemorrhagic CSF should be centrifuged immediately to look for a xanthochromic (yellow) supernatant. Xanthochromia, resulting from RBC lysis, takes several hours to develop and indicates SAH rather than a traumatic lumbar puncture. Comparison of the first and last specimens of CSF may show a significant decline in RBC count when the blood is from traumatic puncture, but not when it is from SAH. In general, an increase of 1 WBC is expected for every 700 RBCs, and 1,000 RBCs correspond with an increase of 1 mg/dl of protein.

c. **Angiography** is needed preoperatively to determine aneurysm size and location.

2. **The treatment of choice** for saccular aneurysm is surgical repair. Timing is controversial and depends on the clinical condition of the patient. Supportive measures to be used while awaiting surgery include bed rest, sedation, analgesia, and laxatives to prevent sudden increases in intracranial pressure or BP. Only extreme elevations in BP (diastolic >130 mm Hg) should be treated. **Hypotension must be avoided,** as it may exacerbate ischemic deficits. Any reduction in BP should be performed slowly and carefully, preferably with a short-acting agent (see Chap. 4). Cardiac monitoring is advised. **Nimodipine,** a calcium channel antagonist, improves outcome in patients with subarachnoid hemorrhage and appears to reduce the incidence of associated cerebral infarction (*N Engl J Med* 308:619, 1983; *Br Med J* 298:636, 1989). The recommended dosage is 60 mg PO q4h for 21 days, initiated within 4 days of presentation. Volume expansion and induced hypertension can occasionally be used to reverse neurologic deterioration caused by vasospasm. Aminocaproic acid (Amicar) increases the risk of complications without improving outcome (*N Engl J Med* 311:432, 1984; *Neurology* 37:1586, 1987).

Seizures

Prolonged generalized convulsions (**convulsive status epilepticus**) may be life-threatening and require prompt medical attention. Recurrent generalized seizures without recovery of consciousness between seizures also constitutes status epilepticus, but if the seizures are brief and supportive care is adequate, maximal combinations of parenteral anticonvulsants may not be necessary. Prolonged or recurrent seizures of other types such as complex, absence, or simple partial seizures (**nonconvulsive status epilepticus**) are not acutely life-threatening and do not require as immediate or aggressive therapy as convulsive status epilepticus. The goals of treatment of convulsive status epilepticus are to (1) support vital functions, (2) stop the seizures, (3) identify and treat the precipitating causes, (4) anticipate and treat complications, and (5) ensure long-term protection against subsequent seizures with long-acting anticonvulsants. Patients who do not have status epilepticus should be given oral anticonvulsants (see sec. **V**).

I. **Initial measures.** Vital signs should be monitored closely. A soft, plastic oral or nasal airway should be placed atraumatically, and maximal supplemental oxygen should be provided by mask. If necessary, the patient should be intubated. One and preferably two (one dextrose-free) large-bore peripheral IV lines should be placed. Venous blood should be obtained for glucose, electrolytes, calcium, magnesium, BUN, CBC, and anticonvulsant levels if indicated, and 25–50 ml of 50% dextrose should be administered IV. Serum and urine should be obtained in case toxicologic analysis is necessary. Gastric contents should be removed via a nasogastric tube, and padding should be provided to reduce traumatic injury.

II. **Parenteral anticonvulsants.** Parenteral anticonvulsants are used to stop convulsive seizures rapidly, but they may have adverse effects that must be anticipated and minimized. There are a variety of therapeutic approaches to treating persistent convulsive seizures and choices may be influenced by the patient's current medications or drug allergies.

   A. **Benzodiazepines** stop seizures quickly and allow supportive and diagnostic measures to be performed easily while loading doses of long-acting anticonvulsants are administered. Because of the short duration of action of benzodiazepines, long-acting agents (e.g., phenytoin) should be administered concomitantly. **Diazepam** (5–10 mg IV) or **lorazepam** (2–4 mg IV) should be administered directly into the vein (to avoid adherence to IV tubing) at a rate of 1–2 mg/minute. **Respiratory depression may require intubation.**

   B. **Phenytoin** is the long-acting anticonvulsant of choice for treating convulsive status epilepticus. **Phenytoin must be administered via a glucose-free IV line to avoid precipitation in the tubing.** The loading dose is 20 mg/kg. A large-bore IV infusing saline solution at a high rate minimizes local irritation. **The infusion rate of phenytoin (injected into the IV line as close as possible to the vein) should not exceed 50 mg/minute. Transient hypotension and heart block** may occur during IV phenytoin administration, particularly in elderly and debilitated patients. Close monitoring of BP and cardiac rhythm is necessary. These effects are usually related to the infusion rate and do not necessarily limit the total dose of phenytoin. Anticonvulsant effects are observed within approximately 20 minutes of administration. A total dose of 30 mg/kg may be required to stop seizures in some patients.

   C. **Phenobarbital** should be administered if phenytoin does not stop the seizures after a complete loading dose. Respiratory depression caused by the combination of benzodiazepines and phenobarbital may require intubation. There is no recommended loading dose for phenobarbital when it is used to stop recalcitrant seizures, but it is administered in 5- to 10-mg/kg increments until the seizures are controlled. In general, an IV loading dose of 20 mg/kg achieves a serum level of approximately 20 μg/ml, which is sufficient to stop most seizures. The infusion rate should not exceed 50 mg/minute. Arrhythmias and hypotension may occur, and the ECG and BP should be continuously monitored during administration of phenobarbital. Peak plasma levels are achieved within 1 hour of IV administration.

   D. **Barbiturate coma or general anesthesia** with neuromuscular blockade may be required when seizures persist despite the preceding measures. ICU support and appropriate consultations should be obtained.

III. **Determination and treatment of the underlying cause.** A specific metabolic or structural etiology can be identified in most cases of generalized status epilepticus. Identifying such causes is important because status epilepticus may be difficult to abort if a specific etiology is causative but untreated. Structural abnormalities include primary or metastatic CNS tumors, posttraumatic injury, CNS infection, CNS inflammatory process (e.g., lupus), cerebral infarction (more commonly embolic), and preexisting brain injury. Nonstructural precipitants include hypoglycemia, electrolyte abnormalities (including hyponatremia and hypocalcemia), uremia, anoxia, alcohol and sedative drug withdrawal, drug intoxication (e.g., theophylline, amphetamines, cocaine, isoniazid), and epilepsy. The most common precipitants of status epilepticus in epileptic patients are subtherapeutic anticonvulsant levels (e.g., noncompliance, drug interaction) or an acute febrile illness.

IV. **Complications,** such as aspiration, rhabdomyolysis, myoglobinuria, and hyperthermia, must be anticipated and treated as they arise.

V. **Preventing subsequent seizures** requires maintenance doses of long-acting anticonvulsants. In general, the drug or drugs required to abort status epilepticus should be maintained (excepting benzodiazepines) until causative factors can be identified and treated and until the patient is well enough to capably institute a long-term drug regimen. Both phenytoin (4–7 mg/kg/day) and phenobarbital (1–5 mg/kg/day) can be given IV or PO either as a single dose or divided into 2 doses and used for long-term management of epilepsy. Other anticonvulsants may be desirable for long-term management, and monotherapy should be practiced if possible.

Headache

Headache is a common complaint requiring emergency evaluation when it is debilitating or associated with neurologic deficits.

I. **Etiology**

A. **Primary headache syndromes** include migraines with or without aura, tension headaches, and cluster headaches. Posttraumatic, exertional, cough- and cold-induced, and fleeting ice pick headaches are also considered within the same category after underlying structural lesions have been excluded. The etiology of primary headache syndromes is poorly understood. A disturbance in serotonergic neurotransmission may be the etiology (*Headache*. New York: Churchill-Livingstone, 1988; *Neurology* 43:[Suppl 3], 1993).

B. **Secondary headache syndromes** can be caused by many disease processes (see sec. **II.D**).

II. **Evaluation**

A. **Migraines** are commonly unilateral, pulsating, or throbbing, with associated nausea, vomiting, and phonophotophobia. Duration varies from 4–72 hours. They tend to build over minutes to hours. Longer spells constitute intractable migraines or "status migrainosus." The aura of **classic migraine** is a transient visual, motor, sensory, cognitive, or psychic disturbance that usually lasts minutes and precedes or coincides with the headache. **Provoking factors** may be identified and include stress, hunger, fatigue, sleep deprivation or excess, physical exertion, bright light, alcohol, menstruation, pregnancy, oral contraceptives, foods (cheese, chocolate), food additives (monosodium glutamate, nitrites), and nitroglycerin. Migraines occur more commonly in females, and the first episode usually occurs before 30 years of age.

B. **Muscle contraction or tension headache** is often diagnosed when headaches are chronic, bilateral, constricting, nonpulsatile, and associated with neck muscle rigidity. Stress and anxiety are common aggravating factors. Migrainous symptoms often overlap and can be difficult to separate from tension headache. Tension headaches typically occur daily, begin later in the day, and wax and wane in intensity.

C. **Cluster headaches** are more common in males, excruciatingly painful, unilateral, orbital and periorbital or temporal in location; last 0.5–2.0 hours; and are associated with unilateral autonomic dysfunction (lacrimation, ptosis, miosis, nasal congestion, or conjunctival injection). Alcohol and nitroglycerin are known precipitants of cluster headaches. Most sufferers assume an upright position to alleviate the discomfort (as opposed to napping in a darkened room as with migraines). Periodicity is a hallmark of cluster headache, with pain often recurring daily at about the same hour. "Clusters" last days to weeks and recur at intervals of months to years. In contrast, **chronic cluster headaches** recur at intervals of 4–5 years.

D. **Secondary headache syndromes** vary depending on the underlying pathologic process (Table 25-3). For example, subarachnoid hemorrhage causes the abrupt onset of severe pain, whereas cerebral tumors tend to cause a fluctuating, less severe pain of gradual onset, sometimes affected by posture. Age at onset can also be helpful in that the headache of temporal arteritis rarely begins before age 50, whereas the onset of migraines is uncommon after age 50. Persistent neurologic signs suggest an underlying neurologic disorder. Signs preceding a headache and resolving before or during the headache suggest classic migraine. **Examination** should reveal normal findings during asymptomatic intervals in patients with primary headache syndromes. Persistent neurologic deficits require investigation to rule out an underlying disorder.

Table 25-3. Secondary causes of headache

Intracranial causes
Subdural hematoma
Intracerebral hematoma
Subarachnoid hemorrhage
Arteriovenous malformation
Brain abscess
Meningitis
Encephalitis
Vasculitis
Obstructive hydrocephalus
Lumbar puncture
Cerebral ischemia or infarction

Extracranial causes
Sinusitis
Disorders of the cervical spine
Temporomandibular joint syndrome
Giant-cell arteritis
Glaucoma
Optic neuritis
Dental disease

Systemic causes
Fever
Viremia
Hypoxia
Hypercapnia
Systemic hypertension
Allergy
Anemia
Caffeine withdrawal
Vasoactive chemicals (e.g., nitrites, carbon monoxide)
Depression

III. Treatment
  A. Acute treatment is aimed at aborting a headache.
  1. Nonnarcotic analgesics. Aspirin, acetaminophen, and nonsteroidal anti-inflammatory agents may abort a migraine or tension headache if taken early. Ketorolac tromethamine, 30–60 mg IM, naproxen sodium, 550 mg PR or PO bid or tid, or flurbiprofen, 100 mg PO bid, are effective for migraine and tension headache. Indomethacin, 50 mg PR or PO bid–tid, may be helpful for cluster, cough, and "ice pick" headache. Drugs with sedative and analgesic properties including isometheptene and butalbital with aspirin or acetaminophen are helpful in migraine and tension headache.
  2. Ergotamine is a vasoconstrictive agent effective in aborting primary vascular headaches, particularly if administered during the prodromal phase. Ergotamine should be taken at symptom onset in the maximum dose tolerated by the patient; nausea often limits the dose. The maximum dose is best determined during a headache-free interval. Rectal preparations are better absorbed than oral agents, but the oral form is most convenient; an initial dose of 2–3 mg PO is appropriate. Additional doses of 1–2 mg can be taken every 30 minutes, up to a total dose of 8–10 mg, but these rarely succeed when an initial dose has failed. Rectal (2-mg) administration should be tried in patients who do not respond to oral delivery or when emesis prevents oral administration. Dosages exceeding 16 mg/week should be used cautiously to avoid toxicity, which includes angina pectoris, limb claudication, ergotamine headache, and dependency.

3. **Dihydroergotamine (DHE)** is a potent venoconstrictor with minimal peripheral arterial constriction. **Cardiac precautions** are indicated for those with a history of angina, peripheral vascular disease, or age greater than 60 years. A dose of 1–2 mg IM or SC may abort a vascular headache before it reaches peak intensity. If an attack has climaxed, 5 mg of prochlorperazine may be given IV, followed immediately by 0.75 mg of DHE IV given over 3 minutes. If there is no relief in 30 minutes, another 0.5 mg of DHE IV is given. This treatment relieves the primary headache in most cases. For intractable migraines (status migrainosus), DHE can be given 1–2 mg SC or IV q8h in combination with IV metoclopramide (*Neurology* 36:995, 1986; *Neurol Clin* 8:587, 1990).

4. **Sumatriptan** is also effective for acute management of vascular headaches, even after the attack has been under way for several hours. An initial dose of 6 mg SC can be repeated in 1 hour, but studies have not demonstrated additional benefit from a second dose. In approximately one-third of users, the headache can recur within 24 hours after effective suppression (*Neurology* 43 [Suppl. 3]: S43, 1993).

5. **Chlorpromazine,** 0.1 mg/kg IV q15min (up to 3 doses), or **prochlorperazine,** 10 mg IV, may terminate a migraine headache. Acute dystonic reactions and hypotension are potential side effects (see Chap. 1). These drugs are especially useful in patients with severe nausea and emesis. Suppository forms are also available. Intravenous chlorpromazine should not be used with intravenous meperidine because of an increased risk of hypotension.

6. **Opioid analgesics,** such as codeine and meperidine, are sometimes required to abort severe headaches. To prevent habituation and loss of efficacy (see Chap. 1), chronic, daily headaches should not be treated with narcotic analgesics.

7. **Caffeine,** given as coffee, tea, or a tablet in combination with ergotamine (Cafergot), is a useful adjunct to migraine therapy.

8. **Environment** plays an important role in alleviating headache. A quiet, dark, noise-free environment can speed recovery. Sleep is often effective in aborting migraine.

B. **Prophylaxis** is used for recurrent headaches, particularly those that are not responsive to acute therapy.

1. **Tricyclic antidepressants** are effective in preventing migraine and tension headaches. The dose is titrated to patient tolerance and response, with an initial dosage of 10–25 mg of amitriptyline PO qhs. The effective dosage varies from 10–175 mg/day. Efficacy does not depend on the presence of depressive symptoms.

2. **Propranolol** and beta-adrenergic antagonists can decrease the frequency of recurrent vascular headaches. The initial dosage of propranolol is 20 mg PO bid; the effective dosage ranges widely among patients. Heart failure and bronchospasm are contraindications.

3. **Low-dose ergot preparations** may be used for migraine prophylaxis if amitriptyline and propranolol are ineffective or contraindicated. Ergonovine, 0.2 mg PO bid, or a combination of ergotamine, belladonna, and phenobarbital (Bellergal, 1–2 tablets PO bid) may be used.

4. **Prednisone** is a first-line drug in the treatment of cluster headache and is effective in most cases. An initial PO dosage of 60–80 mg/day for the first week should be followed by a rapid taper.

5. **Methysergide,** 2 mg PO qd–qid, is effective in the prevention of migraine and cluster headache. Retroperitoneal, pleural, and endocardial fibrosis are severe but reversible complications of long-term methysergide treatment. These complications occur uncommonly (1 in 5,000 cases).

6. **Other pharmacotherapy** for refractory migraine includes phenelzine, a monoamine oxidase inhibitor (45 mg/day); valproate (average dosage, 1,200 mg/day); and calcium channel antagonists (sustained-release verapamil, 90–360 mg/day as tolerated and needed). Indomethacin and verapamil are useful medications for cluster headache prophylaxis. Lithium and verapamil may be used for chronic cluster headache.

7. Environmental prophylaxis includes avoidance of precipitating foods, chemicals, activities, and situations. Relaxation training should be attempted for sufferers of recurrent stress-induced headaches.

Weakness

Weakness is a common complaint that may be caused by dysfunction at any of 5 levels: muscle, neuromuscular junction, peripheral nerve, lower motor neuron, or upper motor neuron. Identification of the level involved is useful for identifying the specific etiology. Several specific disorders may present as rapidly progressing, generalized weakness. Maintenance of respiration is essential (see Chap. 9), and aggressive supportive measures should be used if necessary.

I. **Myasthenia gravis (MG)** is a disorder of the neuromuscular junction resulting from autoimmune damage to the nicotinic cholinergic receptor. It is often associated with abnormalities of the thymus and is characterized by weakness and fatigability. The weakness is typically worse after exercise and better after rest, but a constant weakness may occur. **Presenting signs** include ptosis, diplopia, dysarthria, dysphagia, extremity weakness, and respiratory difficulty. Women outnumber men with the disease; it tends to occur in young women (third decade) and older men (fifth–sixth decade). The clinical course is variable, and spontaneous remissions and exacerbations may occur. Progressive deterioration is more likely to occur in the first 3 years. The differential diagnosis includes botulism and the Eaton-Lambert syndrome, a neuromuscular defect associated with carcinoma.

A. **Diagnosis** is usually evident from the history and physical examination. Ancillary tests may be useful in confirming the diagnosis.

1. **Edrophonium (Tensilon) test.** Edrophonium often produces a marked temporary improvement of strength in myasthenic patients. To use edrophonium to diagnose MG, a clearly defined and objectively quantifiable neurologic deficit must exist (e.g., extraocular muscle palsy). **A test dose** of 2 mg IV is given; if no reaction occurs after 45 seconds, an additional 3 mg is injected. If no reaction occurs after 45 seconds, the remaining 5 mg is given for a total dose of 10 mg. The response to edrophonium lasts approximately 5 minutes. Because edrophonium may produce **severe bradycardia**, atropine should be available for treatment, and vital signs should be monitored during the test. Muscarinic side effects should be anticipated.

2. **Electromyogram.** The myasthenic muscle action potential shows a decremental response to repetitive nerve stimulation. In botulism and the Eaton-Lambert syndrome, the response is incremental.

3. **Antibody levels** (antiacetylcholine receptor and antistriatal) lend further support to the diagnosis. A chest radiograph or CT scan is necessary to exclude thymoma.

B. **Treatment of MG** follows no specific protocol. The clinician must choose among modalities based on symptoms, life-style, and response to treatment. A rapid deterioration in respiratory and swallowing functions necessitates aggressive support, therapy, and correction of precipitating causes (e.g., infection, thyroid dysfunction).

1. **Anticholinesterase drugs** can produce symptomatic improvement in all forms of MG. Pyridostigmine should be started at 30–60 mg PO tid–qid and subsequently titrated to the minimum amount providing symptom relief. Occasionally, patients require dosing as frequently as q2–3h. Neostigmine methylsulfate, 0.5 mg IM q3–4h, can also be used.

2. **Immunosuppressive drugs** are often effective when cholinesterase inhibitors alone fail. **Prednisone** is often used to alter the natural course of the disease. Improvement is more rapid with high-dose daily regimens, but an initial exacerbation of weakness occurs in many patients and hospitalization is advised. A dosage of 60–80 mg qd for 1–2 weeks, followed by an alternate-day regimen and slow (months) taper to the lowest effective dose, may be used.

Initiation of therapy with alternate-day low-dose regimens may also be used; dosages of prednisone are then gradually increased as needed; onset of beneficial effect may be delayed, but there is reduced risk of early exacerbation. Hospitalization and close observation are advised when initiating steroids. Potential risks of steroid treatment (see Chap. 24) need to be weighed against observed clinical benefit on an individual basis. **Azathioprine**, 1–2 mg/kg PO qd, is an alternative drug for those who do not respond to steroids or cannot tolerate steroids. Onset of benefit is usually delayed for at least 2 months. **Side effects** include leukopenia, pancytopenia, infection, GI irritation, and abnormal liver function tests (see Chap. 24). Cyclophosphamide, cyclosporine, and IV gamma globulin have been beneficial in select refractory patients.

3. **Thymectomy** is effective treatment for generalized or disabling ocular MG and produces complete remission in many patients. Transsternal thymectomy should be carried out in patients with moderate to marked generalized myasthenia, early in the course of their disease, and especially if response to medical treatment is unsatisfactory. Thymoma is an absolute indication for surgery. Thymectomy is controversial in children, adults older than 60 years, and purely ocular MG.

4. **Plasmapheresis** is used in the treatment of acute exacerbations, impending crisis, disabling myasthenia refractory to other therapies, and before surgery when postoperative deterioration is possible. Benefits are temporary, and there is a lack of general agreement about exact indications and protocol. Hypotension and thromboembolism are potential complications.

5. **Precipitating factors** should be treated. These include infection, pregnancy, thyroid dysfunction, and drug reaction. Quinidine, quinine, aminoglycosides, polymyxin, bacitracin, colistin, procainamide, phenytoin, propranolol, curare, and ether can worsen weakness in patients with MG.

C. **Myasthenic crisis,** the need for assisted ventilation or airway protection, or both, occurs in approximately 10% of patients with MG. Patients with bulbar and respiratory muscle weakness are particularly prone to respiratory failure. Respiratory infection and surgery (e.g., thymectomy) can precipitate crisis. Patients at risk should have pulmonary function closely monitored. Respiratory support follows the guidelines given in Chap. 9. Anticholinesterases should be temporarily withdrawn from patients receiving ventilatory support; this avoids uncertainties about overdosage ("cholinergic crisis") and avoids cholinergic stimulation of pulmonary secretions. A 2-mg test dose of edrophonium IV should worsen symptoms caused by cholinergic oversupply if this is a concern. Steroids or plasmapheresis may be helpful. Thymectomy is not part of emergency treatment of MG.

II. **Guillain-Barré syndrome (GBS)**
A. **Presentation** is typically a rapidly progressive, ascending paralysis. Proximal weakness may be pronounced. Cranial nerves, especially the facial nerves, may be involved. Sensory symptoms may be present, but objective sensory loss is uncommon. Reflexes are usually hypoactive or absent. CSF protein is usually elevated (especially immunoglobulin G), typically without pleocytosis. Lymphocytes, usually less than 20/mm^3, may be seen. The differential diagnosis includes arsenic exposure, acute porphyria, collagen vascular disease, tick paralysis, botulism, AIDS, and postdiphtheritic paralysis. A viral or diarrheal illness or exposure to Epstein-Barr virus, cytomegalovirus, *Campylobacter*, hepatitis, or HIV may precede this acute polyneuritis.

B. **Treatment** is supportive. Plasmapheresis is beneficial when carried out early in those who are severely compromised or experiencing progression of symptoms. Indications for plasmapheresis in mild forms of stable and improving GBS are less clear (*Ann Neurol* 22:753, 1987; *Ann Neurol* 23:347, 1988). IV immune globulin (HIG, IVIg) was as effective as plasmapheresis in one study (*N Engl J Med* 326:1123, 1992), but there may be more relapses using this form of therapy (*Neurology* 43:872, 1993; *Neurology* 43:1034, 1993). Glucocorticoids, immunosuppressive drugs, and other agents are not of proved value in acute idiopathic demyelinating polyneuropathy.

1. **Respiratory function** must be closely monitored. Ventilatory assistance may be necessary and should be anticipated.
2. **Autonomic neuropathy** can cause fatal overactivity or underactivity of autonomic functions. There is no uniform approach to the treatment of autonomic dysfunction; only general therapeutic guidelines can be given.
   a. **Paroxysmal hypertension** should be managed with short-acting agents that can be titrated against the patient's BP (see Chap. 4). Hypotension is usually secondary to decreased venous return and peripheral vasodilatation. Ventilated patients, who already have compromised venous return, are particularly prone to hypotension. Treatment consists of intravascular volume expansion with IV fluids. Occasionally, vasopressors may be required (see Chap. 9 and Appendix C).
   b. **Cardiac arrhythmias** have been implicated as a significant cause of mortality in GBS; thus, cardiac monitoring is necessary. Bradyarrhythmias (sinus arrest or complete heart block) and tachyarrhythmias are common. Hypoxia and electrolyte abnormalities should be excluded as causes of cardiac arrhythmias.

III. **Polymyositis and dermatomyositis** may present with rapidly progressive, proximal muscle weakness. Less than one-half of patients with polymyositis have associated muscle pain, and approximately one-third have an elevated ESR. Other causes of acquired myopathies should be considered. In the initial evaluation, it is important to measure electrolytes, particularly potassium, calcium, and phosphate. Thyroid function, BUN, creatine kinase, and antinuclear antibodies should also be determined (see Chap. 24).

IV. **Botulism** is a disorder of the neuromuscular junction caused by ingestion of an exotoxin produced by *Clostridium botulinum*. The exotoxin interferes with release of acetylcholine from presynaptic terminals at the neuromuscular junction as seen with Eaton-Lambert syndrome.
   A. **Symptoms** begin within 12–36 hours of ingestion and include **autonomic dysfunction** (xerostomia, blurred vision, bowel and bladder dysfunction) followed by **cranial nerve palsies** and weakness.
   B. **Management** includes removing nonabsorbed toxin with **cathartics,** neutralizing absorbed toxin with **equine trivalent antitoxin,** 1 vial IV in addition to 1 vial IM (after normal intradermal horse serum sensitivity test), and **supportive care.**

Tetanus

I. **Definition.** Tetanus is characterized by generalized or localized muscle spasm (e.g., trismus) caused by the exotoxin (tetanospasmin) of *Clostridium tetani*. The incubation period ranges from 2–54 days. In most patients, the date of onset is within 14 days from the time of injury. Tetanus often follows puncture wounds, lacerations, and crush injuries but may also occur without a demonstrable wound. Tetanus may be seen in parenteral drug abusers, particularly heroin addicts who inject SC. The mortality rate may be as high as 50–60%; most deaths occur in the first 10 days.

II. **Management.** The goals of therapy are to remove the source of toxin, neutralize toxin not yet affixed to the nervous system, prevent respiratory compromise, and treat muscle spasm. The intensity of muscle spasms begins to diminish during the second week. Complete recovery may take several months.
   A. **Toxin production** is eliminated by cleaning and debriding the infected site. Penicillin G, 2 million units IV q6h for 10 days, should be given. Metronidazole may be effective in patients who are allergic to penicillin (*Br Med J* 291:648, 1985).
   B. **Toxin neutralization** is achieved by administration of 3,000–10,000 units of human tetanus immune globulin distributed IM among several sites proximal to the suspected source of exotoxin. Active immunization is needed after the acute illness (see Appendix E).
   C. **Muscle spasms** are managed with diazepam or barbiturates, or both, or with

chlorpromazine. The patient should be kept in quiet isolation. The optimum level of continuous sedation is achieved when the patient remains sleepy but can be aroused to follow commands. Refractory spasms may necessitate curariform drugs and ventilatory support. Painful tonic contractures require analgesia.

D. Supportive measures include ECG monitoring, because cardiac arrhythmias and fluctuations in BP occur. Endotracheal intubation or tracheostomy is needed to prevent asphyxiation during laryngospasm.

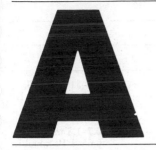

Barnes Hospital Laboratory Reference Values

Scott R. Burger

Reference values for the more commonly used laboratory tests are listed in the following table. The reference values are given in the units currently used at Barnes Hospital and in Systeme International (SI) units, which are used in many areas of the world. Individual reference values can be population- and method-dependent. Footnotes and a key to abbreviations appear on pages 556–557.

Test	Current units	Factor[a]	SI units
Common Serum Chemistries			
Albumin	3.6–5.0 g/dl	10	36–50 g/L
Ammonia (plasma)	19–43 μmol/L	1	19–43 μmol/L
Bilirubin			
Total[b]	0.2–1.3 mg/dl	17.1	3.4–22.2 μmol/L
Direct	0–0.2 mg/dl	17.1	0–3.4 μmol/L
Blood gases (arterial)			
pH	7.35–7.45	1	7.35–7.45
PO_2	80–105 mm Hg	0.133	10.6–14.0 kPa
PCO_2	35–45 mm Hg	0.133	4.7–6.0 kPa
Calcium			
Total	8.9–10.3 mg/dl	0.25	2.23–2.57 mmol/L
Ionized	4.6–5.1 mg/dl	0.25	1.15–1.27 mmol/L
CO_2 content (plasma)	22–31 mmol/L	1	22–31 mmol/L
Ceruloplasmin	21–53 mg/dl	0.063	1.3–3.3 μmol/L
Chloride	97–110 mmol/L	1	97–110 mmol/L
Cholesterol[c]			
Desirable	<200 mg/dl	0.0259	<5.18 mmol/L
Borderline high	200–239 mg/dl	0.0259	5.18–6.19 mmol/L
High	≥240 mg/dl	0.0259	≥6.22 mmol/L
HDL cholesterol[b]	27–98 mg/dl	0.0259	0.70–2.54 mmol/L
Copper (total)	70–155 μg/dl	0.157	11.0–24.3 μmol/L
Creatinine[b]	0.5–1.7 mg/dl	88.4	44–150 μmol/L
Ferritin			
Male adult	36–262 ng/ml	2.25	81–590 pmol/L
Female adult	10–155 ng/ml	2.25	23–349 pmol/L
Folate			
Plasma	1.7–12.6 ng/ml	2.27	3.9–28.6 nmol/L
Red cell	153–602 ng/ml	2.27	347–1367 nmol/L
Glucose, fasting (plasma)	65–110 mg/dl	0.055	3.58–6.05 mmol/L
Glycated hemoglobin	4.4–6.3%	0.01	0.044–0.063
Haptoglobin	44–303 mg/dl	0.01	0.44–3.03 g/L

Test	Current units	Factor[a]	SI units
Common Serum Chemistries (continued)			
Iron (total)	50–175 µg/dl	0.179	9.0–31.3 µmol/L
Binding capacity	250–450 µg/dl	0.179	44.8–80.6 µmol/L
Transferrin saturation	20–50%	0.01	0.20–0.50
Lactate (plasma)	0.7–1.3 mmol/L	1	0.7–1.3 mmol/L
Magnesium	1.3–2.2 mEq/L	0.5	0.65–1.10 mmol/L
Osmolality	270–290 mOsm/kg	1	270–290 mmol/kg
Phosphate	2.5–4.5 mg/dl	0.323	0.81–1.45 mmol/L
Potassium (plasma)	3.3–4.9 mmol/L	1	3.3–4.9 mmol/L
Protein, total	6.2–8.2 g/dl	10	62–82 g/L
Sodium	135–145 mmol/L	1	135–145 mmol/L
Triglycerides, fasting[c]	<200 mg/dl	0.113	<2.83 mmol/L
Urea nitrogen	8–25 mg/dl	0.357	2.9–8.9 mmol/L
Uric acid[b]	3–8 mg/dl	59.5	179–476 µmol/L
Vitamin B$_{12}$	200–800 pg/ml	0.738	148–590 pmol/L
Common Serum Enzymatic Activities			
Aminotransferases			
Alanine (ALT, SGPT)	7–53 IU/L	0.01667	0.12–0.88 µkat/L
Aspartate (AST, SGOT)	11–47 IU/L	0.01667	0.18–0.78 µkat/L
Amylase	35–118 IU/L	0.01667	0.58–1.97 µkat/L
Creatine kinase			
Male	30–220 IU/L	0.01667	0.50–3.67 µkat/L
Female	20–170 IU/L	0.01667	0.33–2.83 µkat/L
MB fraction	0–12 IU/L	0.01667	0–0.20 µkat/L
Gamma-glutamyl transpeptidase (GGT)			
Male	20–76 IU/L	0.01667	0.33–1.27 µkat/L
Female	12–54 IU/L	0.01667	0.2–0.9 µkat/L
Lactate dehydrogenase[b]	90–280 IU/L	0.01667	1.50–4.67 µkat/L
Lipase	2.3–20.0 IU/dl	0.1667	0.38–3.33 µkat/L
5′-Nucleotidase	2–16 IU/L	0.01667	0.03–0.27 µkat/L
Phosphatase, acid	0–0.7 IU/L	16.67	0–11.6 nkat/L
Phosphatase, alkaline[d]	38–126 IU/L	0.01667	0.63–2.10 µkat/L
Common Serum Hormone Values[e]			
ACTH, fasting (8 A.M., supine)	<60 pg/ml	0.22	<13.2 pmol/L
Aldosterone[f]	10–160 ng/L	2.77	28–443 mmol/L
Cortisol (plasma, morning)	8–25 µg/dl	0.027	0.22–0.68 µmol/L

Test	Current units	Factor[a]	SI units
Common Serum Hormone Values[e] (continued)			
FSH			
Male	2.4–19.9 IU/L	1	2.4–19.9 IU/L
Female			
Follicular	3.1–19.7 IU/L	1	3.1–19.7 IU/L
Luteal	1.7–11.2 IU/L	1	1.7–11.2 IU/L
Midcycle	10.4–23.1 IU/L	1	10.4–23.1 IU/L
Postmenopausal	18–126 IU/L	1	18–126 IU/L
Gastrin, fasting	0–130 pg/ml	1	0–130 ng/L
Growth hormone, fasting	<8 ng/ml	1	<8 µg/L
17-Hydroxyprogesterone			
Prepubertal	3–90 ng/dl	0.03	0.1–2.7 nmol/L
Male adult	27–199 ng/dl	0.03	0.8–6.0 nmol/L
Female			
Follicular	15–70 ng/dl	0.03	0.5–2.1 nmol/L
Luteal	35–290 ng/dl	0.03	1.1–8.8 nmol/L
Insulin, fasting	5–25 mU/L	7.18	36–180 pmol/L
LH			
Male	0–8.9 IU/L	1	0–8.9 IU/L
Female			
Follicular	1.4–11.5 IU/L	1	1.4–11.5 IU/L
Luteal	0.1–16.1 IU/L	1	0.1–16.1 IU/L
Midcycle	20.1–73.9 IU/L	1	20.1–73.9 IU/L
Postmenopausal	8.4–46.5 IU/L	1	8.4–46.5 IU/L
Parathyroid hormone	10–55 pg/ml		
Progesterone			
Male	<0.5 ng/ml	3.18	<1.6 nmol/L
Female			
Follicular	0.1–1.5 ng/ml	3.18	0.32–4.80 nmol/L
Luteal	2.5–28.0 ng/ml	3.18	8–89 nmol/L
1st trimester	9–47 ng/ml	3.18	29–149 nmol/L
3rd trimester	55–255 ng/ml	3.18	175–811 nmol/L
Postmenopausal	<0.5 ng/ml	3.18	<1.6 nmol/L
Prolactin			
Male	3–16 ng/ml	1	3–16 µg/L
Female	3–26 ng/ml	1	3–26 µg/L
Renin activity (plasma)[g]	0.9–3.3 ng/ml/hr	0.278	0.25–0.91 ng/(L × s)
Testosterone, total			
Male	350–1030 ng/dl	0.0346	12.1–35.6 nmol/L
Female	10–55 ng/dl	0.0346	0.4–1.9 nmol/L
Testosterone, free			
Male	52–280 pg/ml	3.46	180–970 pmol/L
Female	1.1–6.3 pg/ml	3.46	4–22 pmol/L
Thyroxine, total (T_4)	4.5–12.0 µg/dl	12.9	58–155 nmol/L
Thyroxine, free	0.8–2.7 ng/dl	12.9	10.3–34.8 pmol/L
T-uptake[h]	21–32%	0.01	0.2–0.3
Triiodothyronine (T_3)	80–200 ng/dl	0.0154	1.2–3.1 nmol/L

Test	Current units	Factor[a]	SI units
Common Serum Hormone Values[e] (continued)			
T_4 index[i]	1.2–3.6	1	1.2–3.6
TSH	0.35–6.20 μU/ml	1	0.35–6.20 mU/L
Vitamin D, 1,25 dihydroxy	20–76 pg/ml	2.40	48–182 pmol/L
Vitamin D, 25 hydroxy	10–55 ng/ml	2.49	25–137 nmol/L
Common Urinary Chemistries			
Delta-amino-levulinic acid	1.3–7.0 mg/day	7.6	9.9–53.0 μmol/day
Amylase	0.04–0.30 IU/min	16.67	0.67–5.00 nkat/min
Calcium	0–250 mg/day	0.025	0–6.25 mmol/day
Catecholamines	<540 μg/day		
Dopamine	100–440 μg/day		
Epinephrine	<15 μg/day	5.5	<82 nmol/day
Norepinephrine	11–86 μg/day	5.9	65–507 nmol/day
Copper	15–50 μg/day	0.0157	0.24–0.78 μmol/day
Cortisol, free	20–90 μg/day	2.76	55–248 nmol/day
Creatinine			
Male	1.0–2.0 g/day	8.84	8.8–17.7 mmol/day
Female	0.6–1.5 g/day	8.84	5.3–13.3 mmol/day
5-Hydroxyindole-acetic acid	<9 mg/day	5.23	<47 μmol/day
Hydroxyproline, total	25–77 mg/day	7.63	191–588 μmol/day
Metanephrine	<0.9 mg/day	5.46	<4.9 μmol/day
Oxalate			
Male	7–44 mg/day	11.4	80–502 μmol/day
Female	4–31 mg/day	11.4	46–353 μmol/day
Porphyrins			
Coproporphyrin	0–72 μg/day	1.53	0–110 nmol/day
Uroporphyrin	0–27 μg/day	1.2	0–32 nmol/day
Protein	0–150 mg/day	0.001	0–0.150 g/day
Vanillylmandelic acid (VMA)	2–10 mg/day	5.05	10–51 μmol/day
Common Hematologic Values			
Coagulation			
Bleeding time[j]	2.5–9.5 min	60	150–570 sec
Fibrin degradation products	<8 μg/ml		
Fibrinogen[k]	150–360 mg/dl	0.01	1.5–3.6 g/L
Partial thromboplastin time (activated)	25–33 sec	1	25–33 sec

Test	Current units	Factor[a]	SI units
Common Hematologic Values (continued)			
Prothrombin time	10.7–13.0 sec	1	10.7–13.0 sec
Thrombin time	11.3–18.5 sec	1	11.3–18.5 sec
Complete blood count			
Hematocrit			
Male	40.7–50.3%	0.01	0.407–0.503
Female	36.1–44.3%	0.01	0.361–0.443
Hemoglobin			
Male	13.8–17.2 g/dl	0.620[l]	8.56–10.70 mmol/L
Female	12.1–15.1 g/dl	0.620	7.50–9.36 mmol/L
Erythrocyte count			
Male	$4.5–5.7 \times 10^6/\mu l$	1	$4.5–5.7 \times 10^{12}/L$
Female	$3.9–5.0 \times 10^6/\mu l$	1	$3.9–5.0 \times 10^{12}/L$
Mean corpuscular hemoglobin	26.7–33.7 pg/cell	0.062	1.66–2.09 fmol/cell
Mean corpuscular hemoglobin concentration	32.7–35.5 g/dl	0.620	20.3–22.0 mmol/L
Mean corpuscular volume	$80.0–97.6 \ \mu m^3$	1	80.0–97.6 fl
Red cell distribution width	11.8–14.6%	0.01	0.118–0.146
Leukocyte profile			
Total	$3.8–9.8 \times 10^3/\mu l$	1	$3.8–9.8 \times 10^9/L$
Lymphocytes	$1.2–3.3 \times 10^3/\mu l$	1	$1.2–3.3 \times 10^9/L$
Mononuclear cells	$0.2–0.7 \times 10^3/\mu l$	1	$0.2–0.7 \times 10^9/L$
Granulocytes	$1.8–6.6 \times 10^3/\mu l$	1	$1.8–6.6 \times 10^9/L$
Platelet count	$140–440 \times 10^3/\mu l$	1	$140–440 \times 10^9/L$
Erythrocyte sedimentation rate	0–30 mm/hr		
Reticulocyte count	0.5–1.5%	0.01	0.005–0.015
Immunology Testing			
Complement (total hemolytic)[m]	118–226 U/ml		
C3	77–156 mg/dl	0.01	0.71–1.56 g/L
C4	15–39 mg/dl	0.01	0.15–0.39 g/L
Immunoglobulin			
IgA	91–518 mg/dl	0.01	0.91 5.18 g/L
IgM	61–355 mg/dl	0.01	0.61–3.55 g/L
IgG	805–1,830 mg/dl	0.01	8.05–18.30 g/L
Therapeutic Agents			
Amitriptyline (+ nortriptyline)	100–250 μg/L		
Carbamazepine	4–10 mg/L	4.23	17–42 μmol/L
Clonazepam	10–80 μg/ml	3.17	32–254 nmol/L
Cyclosporine (whole blood)	183–336 ng/ml		

Test	Current units	Factor[a]	SI units
Therapeutic Agents (continued)			
Digoxin	0.5–2.0 µg/L	1.28	0.6–2.6 nmol/L
Disopyramide	2–5 mg/L	2.95	6–15 µmol/L
Ethosuximide	40–100 mg/L	7.08	283–708 µmol/L
Imipramine			
Imipramine	150–300 µg/L	3.57	536–1071 nmol/L
Desipramine	100–300 µg/L	3.75	375–1125 nmol/L
Lithium	0.6–1.2 mmol/L	1	0.6–1.2 mmol/L
Nortriptyline	50–175 µg/L	3.80	190–665 nmol/L
Phenobarbital	10–40 mg/L	4.30	43–172 µmol/L
Phenytoin (diphe-nylhydantoin)	10–20 mg/L	3.96	40–79 µmol/L
Primidone			
Primidone	5–15 mg/L	4.58	23–69 µmol/L
Phenobarbital	10–40 mg/L	4.30	43–172 µmol/L
Procainamide			
Procainamide	4–10 mg/L	4.23	17–42 µmol/L
Procainamide + N-Acetyl-procainamide	6–30 mg/L		
Quinidine	2–5 mg/L	3.08	6.2–15.4 µmol/L
Salicylate[n]	20–290 mg/L	0.0072	0.14–2.10 mmol/L
Theophylline	10–20 mg/L	5.5	55–110 µmol/L
Valproic acid	50–100 mg/L	6.93	346–693 µmol/L
Antimicrobials			
Amikacin			
Trough	5–10 mg/L	1.71	8.6–17.0 µmol/L
Peak	20–30 mg/L	1.71	34–51 µmol/L
5-Fluorocytosine			
Trough	20–60 mg/L		
Peak	50–100 mg/L		
Gentamicin			
Trough	<2 mg/L	2.09	<4.2 µmol/L
Peak	6–8 mg/L	2.09	12.5–16.7 µmol/L
Ketoconazole			
Trough	≤1 mg/L		
Peak	1–4 mg/L		
Sulfamethoxazole			
Trough	75–120 mg/L		
Peak	100–150 mg/L		
Tobramycin			
Trough	0.5–1.5 mg/L	2.14	1.1–3.2 µmol/L
Peak	6–8 mg/L	2.14	12.8–17.0 µmol/L
Trimethoprim			
Trough	2–8 mg/L		
Peak	5–15 mg/L		
Vancomycin			
Trough	5–10 mg/L		
Peak	20–35 mg/L		

[a] A more complete list of multiplication factors for converting conventional units to SI units can be found in *Ann Intern Med* 106:114, 1987, and in *The SI for the Health Professions,* World Health Organization, 1977.

[b] Variation occurs with age and sex. This range includes both sexes and persons older than 5 years.

[c] NIH Consensus Development Panel on Triglycerides, HDL, and Coronary Artery Disease (*JAMA* 269:505, 1993).

[d] Higher values (up to 250 mU/ml) can be normal in persons younger than 20 years.

[e] Since most hormones are measured by immunologic techniques and because hormones may vary in molecular weight (e.g., gastrin), most are expressed as mass/liter. The reference ranges are highly method-dependent.

[f] Supine, normal salt diet; in the upright position, the reference range is 40–310 ng/liter.

[g] High-sodium diet, supplemented with sodium 3 g/day.

[h] Replaces T_3 resin uptake.

[i] $T_4 \times$ (T-uptake).

[j] Template modified after Ivy.

[k] Determined by the Clauss method (see Chap. 17).

[l] This factor assumes a unit molecular weight of 16,000; assuming a unit molecular weight of 64,500, the multiplication factor is 0.155.

[m] CH_{50} = reciprocal of dilution of sera required to lyse 50% of sheep erythrocytes.

[n] Therapeutic range for treatment of rheumatoid arthritis (see Chap. 24).

Key to abbreviations
ACTH = adrenocorticotrophic hormone
dl = deciliter
fl = femtoliter
fmol = femtomole
FSH = follicle-stimulating hormone
hr = hour
g = gram
Hg = mercury
IU = international unit
katal = mole/sec
kPa = kilopascal
kg = kilogram
L = liter
LH = luteinizing hormone
μg = microgram
μkat = microkatal
μl = microliter
μm^3 = cubic micron
μmol = micromole
μU = microunit
mEq = milliequivalent
mg = milligram
min = minute
ml = milliliter
mm = millimeter
mmol = millimole
mOsm = milliosmole
mU = milliunit
ng = nanogram
nkat = nanokatal
nmol = nanomole
pg = picogram
pmol = picomole
sec = second
SGOT = serum glutamic oxaloacetic transaminase
SGPT = serum glutamic pyruvic transaminase
U = unit

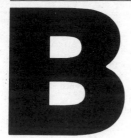

Drug Interactions of Commonly Prescribed Medications

Robyn A. Schaiff and
Lesley Ann Watson

Medication	Increases level or effect of:	Decreases level or effect of:	Potentiates side effect or toxicity of:
Acetazolamide	Quinidine		Phenytoin
Allopurinol	Azathioprine, cyclophosphamide, 6-mercaptopurine, warfarin		Ampicillin
ACE inhibitors	Potassium salts		NSAIDs
Aminoglycosides	Neuromuscular blocking drugs		Loop diuretics
Amiodarone	Digoxin, quinidine, warfarin, cyclosporine, phenytoin, procainamide		
Anabolic steroids	Warfarin		
Antacids	Quinidine	Cimetidine, iron salts, isoniazid, quinolone antibiotics, salicylates, tetracycline	
Antithyroid agents		Warfarin	
Aspirin	Methotrexate	ACE inhibitors	
Barbiturates	CNS depressants	Chloramphenicol, beta-adrenergic antagonists, glucocorticoids, estrogens, oral contraceptives, quinidine, theophylline, tricyclic antidepressants, warfarin	
Benzodiazepines	CNS depressants		
Beta-adrenergic antagonists	Chlorpromazine, epinephrine (pressor effect)		
Cefamandole	Warfarin		
Cefoperazone	Warfarin		
Cefotetan	Warfarin		
Cefoxitin	Warfarin		

Medication	Increases level or effect of:	Decreases level or effect of:	Potentiates side effect or toxicity of:
Carbamazepine	Isoniazid, lithium	Theophylline, warfarin, tricyclic antidepressants	
Chloral hydrate	Ethanol, warfarin		
Chloramphenicol	Barbiturates, phenytoin, oral hypoglycemic agents		
Chlorpromazine	Beta-adrenergic antagonists		
Cimetidine	Benzodiazepines, beta-adrenergic antagonists, CNS depressants, felodipine, procainamide, quinidine, theophylline, tricyclic antidepressants, verapamil, warfarin		
Clofibrate	Oral hypoglycemics, warfarin		
Clarithromycin			Astemizole, terfenadine
Clonidine			Beta-adrenergic antagonists
CNS depressants	Anticonvulsants, barbiturates, benzodiazepines, beta-adrenergic antagonists, cimetidine, ethanol, MAO inhibitors, opiate analgesics, phenothiazines		Lithium, muscle relaxants
Digoxin	Amiodarone		
Diltiazem	Cyclosporine, theophylline		
Disulfiram	Phenytoin, warfarin		
Erythromycin (macrolides)	Carbamazepine, cyclosporine, theophylline, warfarin		Astemizole, terfenadine
Fluoxetine	Phenytoin, tricyclic antidepressants		
Furosemide (loop diuretics)			Digoxin

Medication	Increases level or effect of:	Decreases level or effect of:	Potentiates side effect or toxicity of:
Griseofulvin		Warfarin	
HMG CoA reductase inhibitors			Gemfibrozil
Iron		Quinolones	
Isoniazid	Phenytoin, carbamazepine		
Ketoconazole	Warfarin		Astemizole, terfenadine
Lidocaine			Phenytoin
Lovastatin			Gemfibrozil
MAO inhibitors	CNS depressants, oral hypoglycemic agents, sympathomimetics		Meperidine
Methotrexate		Vaccines	
Methyldopa	Lithium, MAO inhibitors		
Metronidazole	Disulfiram, warfarin		
Muscle relaxants	CNS depressants		
Nicardipine	Cyclosporine		
NSAIDs	Lithium, methotrexate	ACE inhibitors, diuretics, beta-adrenergic antagonists	Triamterene, warfarin
Phenytoin		Quinidine, theophylline, warfarin	
Probenecid	Penicillins, methotrexate, zidovudine (AZT)	Salicylates	
Propafenone	Beta-adrenergic antagonists, digoxin, warfarin		
Propoxyphene	Carbamazepine		
Propylthiouracil	Warfarin		
Quinidine	Dextromethorphan, digoxin, neuromuscular blocking drugs, warfarin		
Quinolone antimicrobials	Theophylline, warfarin		

Medication	Increases level or effect of:	Decreases level or effect of:	Potentiates side effect or toxicity of:
Rifampin		Beta-adrenergic antagonists, benzodiaz-epines, calcium channel antago-nists, cyclospo-rine, digoxin, disopyramide, methadone, oral contraceptives, oral hypoglyce-mics, pheny-toin, quinidine, theophylline, warfarin	
Salicylates	Acetazolamide, methotrexate, oral hypoglyce-mics, warfarin		
Sertraline	Tricyclic antide-pressants		
Spironolactone	Digoxin		
Sucralfate	Aluminum salts	Digoxin, ketocon-azole, pheny-toin, quino-lones, quini-dine, warfarin	
Sulfonamides	Oral hypoglyce-mics, meth otrexate, pheny-toin, warfarin		
Theophylline		Adenosine, lith-ium	
Thiazide diuretics	Lithium, digoxin		
Thyroid hormone	Warfarin		
TMP/SMX	Warfarin		
Trazodone		Clonidine	
Triamterene	NSAIDs, potas-sium		ACE inhibitors
Tricyclic antide-pressants	Catecholamines	Clonidine	
Verapamil	Beta-adrenergic antagonists, carbamazepine, cyclosporine, digoxin, quini-dine, theophyl-line		
Zidovudine (AZT)			Ganciclovir

ACE = angiotensin-converting enzyme; MAO = monoamine oxidase; NSAIDs = nonsteroidal antiinflammatory drugs.

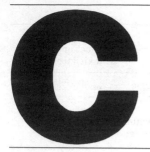

Intravenous Admixture Preparation and Administration Guide*

Dino Recchia and
Robyn A. Schaiff

Aminophylline
Diluent: D5W, NS
Concentration: 1 g/500 ml = 2 mg/ml
Initial dosage: Loading dose 6 mg/kg over 20 min
Infusion rate:
  Adult nonsmokers: 0.4 mg/kg/hr (28 mg or 14 ml/hr for 70-kg patient)
  Adult smokers: 0.7 mg/kg/hr (49 mg or 25 ml/hr for 70-kg patient)
  In CHF: 0.2 mg/kg/hr (14 mg or 7 ml/hr for 70-kg patient)
Amrinone (Inocor)
Diluent: **NS only**
Concentration: 200 mg/100 ml = 2 mg/ml
Initial dosage: Loading dose 0.75 mg/kg over 2 min
Infusion rate: Usually starting at 5 μg/kg/min (10 ml/hr for a 70-kg patient)
Bretylium (Bretylol)
Diluent: NS, D5W
Concentration: 2 g/500 ml = 4 mg/ml
Drip rate:
  1 mg/min = 15 ml/hr
  2 mg/min = 30 ml/hr
  3 mg/min = 45 ml/hr
  4 mg/min = 60 ml/hr
Diltiazem (Cardizem)
Diluent: NS, D5W
Concentration: 125 mg/125 ml = 1 mg/ml
Initial dosage: 20-mg bolus followed by 25-mg bolus if necessary
Infusion rate: Usually starting at 5–10 mg/hr
Dobutamine (Dobutrex)
Diluent: NS, D5W
Concentration: 250 mg/250 ml = 1,000 μg/ml
Drip rate: Usually starting at 3 μg/kg/min
  (Example: For a 70-kg patient to receive 3 μg/kg/min, the drip rate should be
  13 ml/hr)
Dopamine (Intropin)
Diluent: NS, D5W
Concentration: 800 mg/500 ml = 1,600 μg/ml
Drip rate: Usually starting at 3 μg/kg/min
  (Example: For a 70-kg patient to receive 3 μg/kg/min, the drip rate should be
  8 ml/hr)
Esmolol (Brevibloc)
Diluent: NS, D5W
Concentration: 2.5 g/250 ml = 10 mg/ml
Initial dosage: 500 μg/kg loading dose over 1 min
Infusion rate: Usually starting at 50 μg/kg/min (21 ml/hr for a 70-kg patient)
Heparin
Diluent: NS, D5W
Concentration: 25,000 units/250 ml = 100 units/ml
Initial dosage: 5,000-unit bolus
Infusion rate: Usually starting at 1,300 units/hr (13 ml/hr)

Isoproterenol (Isuprel)
Diluent: NS, D5W
Concentration: 2 mg/500 ml = 4 μg/ml
Drip rate:
    1 μg/min = 15 ml/hr
    2 μg/min = 30 ml/hr
Lidocaine
Diluent: NS, D5W
Concentration: 2 g/500 ml = 4 mg/ml
Drip rate:
    1 mg/min = 15 ml/hr
    2 mg/min = 30 ml/hr
    3 mg/min = 45 ml/hr
Nicardipine (Cardene)
Diluent: NS, D5W
Concentration: 25 mg/250 ml = 0.1 mg/ml
Initial dosage: 2 mg/hr (20 ml/hr)
Nitroglycerin
Diluent: NS, D5W (glass or polyolefin containers only)
Concentration: 50 mg/250 ml = 200 μg/ml
Drip rate:
    10 μg/min = 3 ml/hr
    20 μg/min = 6 ml/hr
    30 μg/min = 9 ml/hr
    40 μg/min = 12 ml/hr
Nitroprusside (Nipride)
Diluent: **D5W only**
Concentration: 50 mg/250 ml = 200 μg/ml
Drip rate:
    10 μg/min = 3 ml/hr
    20 μg/min = 6 ml/hr
    30 μg/min = 9 ml/hr
Norepinephrine (Levophed)
Diluent: **D5W only**
Concentration: 8 mg/500 ml = 16 μg/ml
Drip rate:
    2 μg/min = 8 ml/hr (usual starting dose)
    3 μg/min = 11 ml/hr
    4 μg/min = 15 ml/hr
Phenylephrine (Neo-Synephrine)
Diluent: NS, D5W
Concentration: 10 mg/250 ml = 0.04 mg/ml
Drip rate:
    0.04 mg/min = 60 ml/hr
    0.06 mg/min = 90 ml/hr
    0.08 mg/min = 120 ml/hr

Procainamide (Pronestyl)
  Diluent: NS, D5W
  Concentration: 2 g/500 ml = 4 mg/ml
  Drip rate:
    1 mg/min = 15 ml/hr
    2 mg/min = 30 ml/hr
    3 mg/min = 45 ml/hr
Theophylline (see Aminophylline)

* To determine drip rate:

$$\text{Concentration of solution} \left(\frac{\mu g}{ml}\right) \times \text{drip rate} \left(\frac{ml}{min}\right) = \text{desired concentration of infusion} \left(\frac{\mu g}{min}\right)$$

$$\text{Drip rate} \left(\frac{ml}{min}\right) = \frac{\text{Desired concentration infused } (\mu g/kg/min) \times \text{ weight (kg)}}{\text{Concentration of solution } (\mu g/ml)}$$

Drip rate (gtt/min) = (60 gtt/ml) × (drip rate ml/min) **(if using microtubing)**

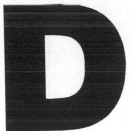

Dosage Adjustments of Drugs in Renal Failure

Steven B. Miller and
Kathryn Vehe

Name	Route	Adjusted dosing interval (hr) or dose % GFR (ml/min)			Supplement after dialysis
		>50	10–50	<10	
Aminoglycosides					
Amikacin*	R	12	12–18	>24	HD, PD
Gentamicin*	R	8–12	12	>24	HD, PD
Tobramycin*	R	8–12	12	>24	HD, PD
Penicillins					
Amoxicillin/clavulanate	R, H	8	8–12	12–24	HD
Ampicillin	R, H	6	6–12	12–16	HD
Carbenicillin	R, H	8–12	12–24	24–48	HD, PD
Dicloxacillin	R, H	N	N	N	N
Mezlocillin	R, H	4–6	6–8	8–12	HD
Oxacillin	R, H	N	N	N	N
Penicillin G	R, H	N	75%	25–50%	HD
Piperacillin	R, H	4–6	6–8	8	HD
Ticarcillin	R	8	8–12	24	HD
Cephalosporins					
Cefadroxil	R	12	12–24	24–48	HD
Cefamandole	R	6	6–8	8–12	HD
Cefpodoxime	R	12	16	24–48	HD
Cefprozil	R	12	16	24	HD
Cefazolin	R	8	12	24–48	HD
Cefixime	R	12–24	75%	50%	N
Cefoperazone	H	N	N	N	N
Cefotaxime	R, H	6–8	8–12	24	HD
Cefotetan	R	12	24	24	HD, PD
Cefoxitin	R	8	8–12	24–48	HD
Ceftazidime	R	8–12	24–48	48–72	HD
Ceftizoxime	R	8–12	36–48	48–72	HD
Ceftriaxone	R, H	N	N	24	N
Cefuroxime	R	N	12	24	HD
Cephalexin	R	6	6	8–12	HD, PD
Cephalothin	R	6	6–8	12	HD, PD
Quinolones					
Ciprofloxacin	R	N	12–24	24	N
Lomefloxacin	R	N	75%	50%	N
Norfloxacin	R	N	12–24	A	N
Ofloxacin	R	N	12–24	24	N
Other antibacterial agents					
Azithromycin	H	N	N	N	N
Aztreonam	R	N	50–75%	25%	HD, PD
Chloramphenicol	R, H	N	N	N	N
Clarithromycin	R, H	N	75%	50%	N

| Name | Route | Adjusted dosing interval (hr) or dose % GFR (ml/min) | | | Supplement after dialysis |
		>50	10–50	<10	
Other antibacterial agents (continued)					
Clindamycin	H	N	N	N	N
Doxycycline	R, H	12	12–18	18–24	N
Erythromycin	H	N	N	N	N
Imipenem	R	N	50%	25%	HD
Metronidazole	R, H	N	N	50%	HD
Minocycline	H	N	N	N	N
Pentamidine	?	N	N	24–48	N
Sulfamethoxazole	R, H	12	18	24	HD
Sulfisoxazole	R	6	8–12	12–24	HD, PD
Tetracycline	R, H	12	12–18	18–24	N
Trimethoprim	R, H	12	18	24	HD
Vancomycin* (IV)	R	24–72	72–240	240	N
Antifungal agents					
Amphotericin B	N	24	24	24–36	N
Fluconazole	R, H	N	50%	25%	HD
Flucytosine	R	6	24	24–48	HD, PD
Itraconazole	H, R	N	N	50%	N
Ketoconazole	H	N	N	N	N
Miconazole	H	N	N	N	N
Antimycobacterial agents					
Ethambutol	R	24	24–36	48	HD, PD
Isoniazid	H, R	N	N	N	HD, PD
Pyrazinamide	H, R	N	N	50%	HD, PD
Rifabutin	H, R	N	?	?	?
Rifampin	H	N	N	N	?
Antiviral agents					
Acyclovir (IV)	R	8	24	48	HD
Acyclovir (PO)	R	N	12–24	24	HD
Amantadine	R	12–24	24–72	72–168	N
Didanosine	R	12	24	48	N
Foscarnet	R	25 mg/kg q8h	15 mg/kg q8h	6 mg/kg q8h	HD
Ganciclovir	R	12	24	24	HD
Zidovudine	H	N	N	N	HD
Nonsteroidal antiinflammatory drugs					
Acetaminophen	H	4	6	8	HD
Aspirin	H, R	4	4–6	A	HD
Diclofenac	H	N	N	N	N
Ibuprofen	H	N	N	N	N
Indomethacin	H, R	N	N	N	N
Ketoprofen	H	N	N	N	N
Ketorolac (IM)	H, R	N	N	50%	N
Nabumetone	H	N	N	N	N
Naproxen	H	N	N	N	N
Oxaprozin	H	N	N	N	N
Piroxicam	H	N	N	N	N
Sulindac	H, R	N	N	50%	N

Name	Route	Adjusted dosing interval (hr) or dose % GFR (ml/min) >50	10–50	<10	Supplement after dialysis
Opioid analgesics					
Codeine	H	N	75%	50%	N
Meperidine	H	N	75%	50%	N
Morphine	H	N	75%	50%	N
Antihypertensives (see Angiotensin-converting enzyme inhibitors, Beta-adrenergic antagonists, and Calcium channel antagonists)					
Clonidine	R	N	N	N	N
Doxazosin	H	N	N	N	N
Guanfacine	H	N	N	N	N
Hydralazine (PO)	H	8	8	8–16	N
Methyldopa	R, H	8	8–12	12–24	HD, PD
Minoxidil	H	N	N	N	HD
Nitroprusside	N	N	N	N	N
Prazosin	H, R	N	N	N	N
Terazosin	R	N	N	N	N
Angiotensin-converting enzyme inhibitors					
Benazepril	H, R	N	75%	50%	N
Captopril	R, H	N	N	50%	HD
Enalapril	H	N	N	50%	HD
Fosinopril	H	N	N	N	N
Lisinopril	R	N	50%	25%	HD
Quinapril	H, R	N	75%	50%	N
Ramipril	R, H	N	50%	50%	HD
Beta-adrenergic antagonists					
Acebutolol	R, H	N	50%	25%	N
Atenolol	R	N	50%	25%	HD
Betaxolol	H, R	N	N	50%	N
Labetalol	H	N	N	N	N
Metoprolol	H	N	N	N	HD
Nadolol	R	N	50%	25%	HD
Pindolol	H, R	N	N	N	?
Propranolol	H	N	N	N	N
Timolol	H	N	N	N	N
Calcium channel antagonists					
Amlodipine	H	N	N	N	N
Diltiazem	H	N	N	N	N
Felodipine	H	N	N	N	N
Isradipine	H	N	N	N	N
Nicardipine	H	N	N	N	N
Nifedipine	H	N	N	N	N
Verapamil	H	N	N	50–75%	N
Diuretics					
Acetazolamide	R	6	12	A	
Bumetanide	R, H	N	N	N	
Furosemide	R	N	N	N	
Indapamide	H	N	N	N	
Metolazone	R	N	N	N	
Spironolactone	R	6–12	12–24	A	
Thiazide	R	N	N	A	
Torsemide	H	N	N	N	

Name	Route	Adjusted dosing interval (hr) or dose % GFR (ml/min)			Supplement after dialysis
		>50	10–50	<10	
Antiarrhythmics					
Amiodarone	H	N	N	N	N
Bretylium	R, H	N	25–50%	A	?
Digoxin*	R	24	36	48	N
Disopyramide*	R, H	75%	25–50%	10–25%	HD
Flecainide*	R, H	N	50%	50%	N
Lidocaine*	H, R	N	N	N	N
Mexiletine	H, R	N	N	50–75%	HD
Moricizine	H	N	N	50–75%	N
Procainamide*	R, H	4	6–12	12–24	HD
Propafenone	H	N	N	50–75%	N
Quinidine*	H, R	N	N	N	HD, PD
Sotalol	R	N	30%	15%	N
Tocainide*	R, H	N	N	50%	HD
Sedatives					
Alprazolam	H	N	N	N	N
Chlordiazepoxide	H	N	N	50%	N
Diazepam	H	N	N	N	N
Flurazepam	H	N	N	N	N
Lorazepam	H	N	N	N	N
Midazolam	H	N	N	50%	N
Temazepam	H	N	N	N	N
Zolpidem	H	N	?	?	N
Antidepressants					
Amitriptyline	H	N	N	N	N
Doxepin	H	N	N	N	N
Fluoxetine	H	N	N	N	N
Imipramine	H	N	N	N	N
Nortriptyline	H	N	N	N	N
Paroxetine	H	N	?	?	?
Sertraline	H	?	?	?	?
Trazodone	H	N	N	N	?
Venlafaxine	H	N	75%	50%	N
Other psychoactive drugs					
Buspirone	H, R	N	N	25–50%	HD
Chlorpromazine	H	N	N	N	N
Haloperidol	H	N	N	N	N
Lithium*	R	N	50–75%	25–50%	HD, PD
Anticonvulsants					
Carbamazepine*	H, R	N	N	75%	N
Ethosuximide*	H, R	N	N	75%	HD
Phenobarbital*	H, R	N	N	12–16	HD, PD
Phenytoin*	H	N	N	N	N
Primidone*	H, R	8	8–12	12–24	HD
Valproic acid*	H	N	N	75%	N
Gastrointestinal drugs					
Cimetidine	R	6	8	12	N
Cisapride	H	N	N	N	N
Famotidine	R, H	N	N	50%	?
Mesalamine	H	N	N	?	N

Name	Route	Adjusted dosing interval (hr) or dose % GFR (ml/min)			Supplement after dialysis
		>50	10–50	<10	
Gastrointestinal drugs (continued)					
Metoclopramide	R, H	N	75%	50%	N
Misoprostol	R	N	N	N	N
Nizatidine	H	N	24	48	N
Omeprazole	H	N	N	N	?
Ranitidine	R	N	18–24	24	HD
Sucralfate	N	N	N	N	N
Antilipemic drugs					
Cholestyramine	N	N	N	N	N
Clofibrate	H	6–12	12–24	24–48	N
Fluvastatin	H	N	N	?	N
Gemfibrozil	R, H	N	50%	25%	N
Lovastatin	H	N	N	N	N
Pravastatin	R, H	N	N	50%	N
Simvastatin	H	N	N	50%	N
Hypoglycemic drugs					
Acetohexamide	H	12–24	A	A	N
Chlorpropamide	?	24–36	A	A	N
Glipizide	H	N	N	N	N
Glyburide	H	N	N	N	N
Insulin	H	N	75%	50%	N
Tolazamide	H	N	N	N	N
Tolbutamide	H	N	N	N	N
Anticoagulants					
Heparin	H	N	N	N	N
Warfarin	H	N	N	N	N
Other drugs					
Allopurinol	R	N	50%	10–25%	?
Colchicine (PO)	R, H	N	N	50%	N
Glucocorticoids	H	N	N	N	?
Dipyridamole	H	N	N	N	?
Finasteride	H, R	N	N	N	N
Nitrates	H	N	N	N	N
Pentoxifylline	H	N	N	N	N
Terbutaline	H, R	N	50%	A	?
Theophylline	H	N	N	N	HD, PD
Ticlopidine	H	N	N	N	?

GFR = glomerular filtration rate; R = renal; HD = hemodialysis; PD = peritoneal dialysis; H = hepatic; N = none; % = percentage of the normal dose; A = should be avoided.
* Serum levels should be used to determine exact dosing.
Source: Data from GK McEvoy (ed). *American Hospital Formulary Service Drug Information.* Bethesda, MD: American Society of Hospital Pharmacists 1991; WM Bennett. Guide to drug dosing in renal failure. *Clin Pharmacokinet* 15:3226, 1988; RW Schrier, JG Gambertoglio (eds). *Handbook of Drug Therapy in Liver and Kidney Disease.* Boston: Little, Brown, 1991.

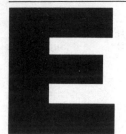

Immunizations

Victoria J. Fraser

Table E-1. Routine adult immunization information

Vaccine	Indicated for	Dosage	Adverse effects	Contraindications
Tetanus-diphtheria (adult Td)[a] Adsorbed tetanus and diphtheria toxoids	Everyone	Unimmunized; 2 doses 0.5 ml IM 1–2 mos apart, then 1 dose 6–12 mos later; booster every 10 yrs	Local pain and swelling, rare hypersensitivity	Neurologic or hypersensitivity reaction to previous dose
Influenza Inactivated subunit or whole virus grown in chick embryo cells	High-risk patients[b], health care workers, and everyone >65 years of age	1 dose 0.5 ml IM annually in the fall	Fever, chills, myalgia, malaise	Anaphylactic hypersensitivity to eggs
Pneumococcal Capsular polysaccharides from 23 types	High-risk patients[c] and everyone >65 years of age	1 dose 0.5 ml IM	Local soreness	Previous pneumococcal vaccine
Hepatitis B Recombinant HBsAg	High-risk patients[d] and health care workers	3 doses each 1 ml IM *in the deltoid*, at 0, 1, and 6 mos, higher doses for dialysis patients and immunocompromised patients[e]	Local soreness	None
Measles[f] Attenuated live virus	Unimmunized born after 1956 Previously immunized: entering college, health care workers, foreign travel	2 doses 0.5 ml SC at least 1 mo apart 1 dose 0.5 ml SC	Low-grade fever	Pregnancy, history of anaphylaxis to eggs or neomycin, significant immunosuppression (except those with HIV)

Table E-1. Routine adult immunization information (continued)

Vaccine	Indicated for	Dosage	Adverse effects	Contraindications
Rubella[f] Attenuated live virus	Nonimmune health care workers and women of child-bearing age	1 dose 0.5 ml SC	Low-grade fever, rash, arthralgia, and arthritis in up to 40% of nonimmune adults	Pregnancy, significant immunosuppression (not HIV), hypersensitivity to neomycin

[a] Guidelines for tetanus prophylaxis in wound management are given in Table E-2.

[b] The population at risk for severe influenza includes those with acquired or congenital heart disease, chronic lung disease, chronic renal disease or nephrotic syndrome, sickle cell disease, diabetes mellitus, and immunocompromised patients.

[c] Populations at increased risk for pneumococcal pneumonia or complications thereof include people with diabetes mellitus; people with anatomic or functional asplenia; and people with chronic lung, cardiac, renal, or hepatic disease or cerebrospinal fluid leaks.

[d] High-risk patients for hepatitis B include IV drug users, sexually active adults with multiple partners, homosexual/bisexual men, dialysis patients, and sex partners or household contacts of hepatitis B carriers.

[e] Compromised hosts or dialysis patients should receive *twice* the recommended dose of plasma-derived HB vaccine.

[f] Available as a monovalent (measles only) or in combination (measles-rubella [MR] and measles-mumps-rubella [MMR]) vaccines.

Table E-2. Guidelines for tetanus (Td) prophylaxis in wound management

History of tetanus immunization (doses)	Clean minor wounds		Other wounds	
	Give Td	Give TIG*	Give Td	Give TIG*
Unknown or <3 doses	Yes	No	Yes	Yes
≥3 doses	No (yes if > 10 yrs since last dose)	No	No (yes if > 5 yrs since last dose)	No

* TIG (tetanus immune globulin) given concurrently with toxoid at separate sites, 250 units IM.

Table E-3. Passive immunization

Disease	Dosage
Diphtheria	Diphtheria antitoxin (DAT), equine source; 20,000–120,000 units IV as specific therapy for diphtheria
Hepatitis A	Immunoglobulin, 0.02 ml/kg IM as soon as possible after exposure to household or sexual contacts
Hepatitis B	Hepatitis B immune globulin (HBIG); 0.06 ml/kg IM as soon as possible after exposure; second dose 1 mo later unless vaccine given
Measles	Immunoglobulin, 0.25 ml/kg IM (maximum dose 15 ml) when live virus vaccine cannot be given to persons exposed to measles, or when close exposure has occurred within 6 days; especially immunocompromised persons
Rabies	Rabies immune globulin (RIG); 20 IU/kg (one-half dose IM and one-half infiltrated at wound site)
Tetanus	Tetanus immune globulin, human (TIG); 3,000–6,000 units IM with part of dose infiltrated around the wound Equine tetanus antitoxin (TAT); 50,000–100,000 units (20,000 IV and the rest IM) if TIG unavailable

Table E-4. Postexposure antirabies treatment guide[a]

Species	Condition of animal at time of attack	Treatment of exposed person
Domestic cat, dog	Healthy and available for 10 days of observation	None unless animal develops rabies[b]
	Rabid or suspected rabid Unknown	RIG and HDCV[c] Contact Public Health Department
Wild skunk, bat, fox, coyote, raccoon, or other carnivore	Regard as rabid unless proved negative by laboratory tests	RIG and HDCV

RIG = rabies immune globulin; HDCV = human diploid cell vaccine.
[a] This guide should be applied in conjunction with knowledge of the animal species involved, circumstances of the bite, vaccination status of the animal, and prevalence of rabies in the region.
[b] Begin RIG and HDCV at first sign of rabies in animal under observation.
[c] Discontinue vaccine if fluorescent antibody test results in the animal are negative.

Table E-5. Rabies immunization and treatment recommendations

Vaccine/passive immunization	Indications	Dosage	Adverse effects
HDCV inactivated virus	Preexposure: veterinarians, animal handlers, people staying > 1 mo in endemic rabies areas	3 doses of HDCV (0.1 ml ID or 1 ml IM) day 0, 7, and 28; booster every 2 yrs	Rare anaphylactic and allergic reactions
	Postexposure: combined passive (RIG) and active (HDCV) treatment recommended for those exposed to animals suspected of being rabid (see Table E-4)	RIG, 20 IU/kg (½ dose IM and ½ infiltrated at wound site) Five 1-ml doses of HDCV IM; first dose immediately with RIG at different site; then day 3, 7, 14, and 28 after first dose If previously immunized, give booster HDCV on days 0 and 3	

HDCV = human diploid cell vaccine; ID = intradermal.

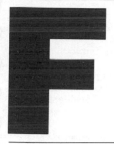

Infection Control and Isolation Recommendations

Marilyn Jones and
Victoria J. Fraser

I. **Body substance isolation (BSI)** should be practiced on **all patients at all times.** All moist body substances should be considered potentially infectious. **Barrier protection (gloves, masks, goggles) should be used to prevent direct contact with moist body substances** based on specific interaction with patient. The use of BSI for all patients eliminates the need for disease-specific categories of isolation except for airborne or respiratory precautions. BSI helps prevent transmission of hospital infections and helps protect health care workers from communicable diseases (*Am J Infect Control* 18:1, 1990).

Specific recommendations:

A. **Wear gloves** when direct contact with moist body substances (e.g., pus, sputum, urine, feces, blood) from any patient is anticipated.

B. **Wear a gown** when clothing is likely to be soiled by any patient's body fluids.

C. **Wear masks and goggles/glasses** when splashes from any patient's body fluids are anticipated.

II. **Respiratory isolation** should be provided for patients with communicable diseases with airborne transmission. Infection Control should be notified, and the patient should be admitted to a private room. Tight-fitting, high-efficiency masks are required. **Tuberculosis** (TB) is of particular concern. Early identification, isolation, and treatment of patients suspected of having TB is critical to limit nosocomial infections. Rooms should be monitored to ensure negative pressure ventilation and special masks should be used. Patients should be kept in the room until they are no longer contagious. Health care workers should be periodically skin tested to monitor for TB infection.

Diseases	Duration of Airborne Precautions
Anthrax	Duration of illness
Chickenpox (varicella)*	Until all lesions are crusted
Diphtheria	Until cultures are negative (at least 24 hours after stopping antibiotics)
Hemorrhagic fevers	Duration of illness
Herpes zoster (varicella)* **localized in immuno-compromised patients or disseminated disease**	Until all lesions are crusted
Influenza	Duration of illness
Measles (rubeola)*	For 4 days after rash starts Immunocompromised patients may remain contagious for the duration of illness
Meningitis (*Haemophilus influenzae* or *Neisseria meningitidis;* known or suspected)	For 24 hours after start of effective antibiotic therapy
Meningococcal pneumonia or sepsis	For 24 hours after start of effective antibiotic therapy
Mumps*	For 9 days after onset of swelling

Pertussis (whooping cough)	For 7 days after start of effective antibiotic therapy
Rubella (German measles)*	For 7 days after rash appears
Tuberculosis, pulmonary (confirmed or suspected) or with draining wounds	Usually 2–3 weeks after therapy begins; duration may be guided by clinical response and a reduction in number of acid-fast bacilli on smears

* People who are not immune to these diseases should not enter the room.

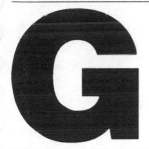

Critical Care Parameters and Formulas

Marin Kollef

Hemodynamic parameters

Systemic arterial pressure (SAP)   100–140/60–90 mm Hg
Pulse pressure (PP) = systolic SAP − diastolic SAP   30–50 mm Hg
Mean SAP (MAP) = (systolic SAP + 2 × diastolic   70–100 mm Hg
SAP)/3
Right arterial pressure (RAP)   0–6 mm Hg
Mean RAP   3 mm Hg
Right ventricular pressure (RVP)   17–30/0–6 mm Hg
Pulmonary artery pressure (PAP)   15–30/5–13 mm Hg
Mean PAP   10–18 mm Hg
Mean pulmonary artery occlusive pressure (PAoP)   2–12 mm Hg
(i.e., pulmonary capillary wedge pressure [PCWP])
Heart rate (HR)   60–100 beats/min
Body surface area (BSA) (in m^2) = [height (cm)]$^{0.718}$
× [weight (kg)]$^{0.427}$ × .007449
Stroke volume (SV)   60–120 ml/contraction
Stroke volume index = SV/BSA   40–50 ml/contraction/
                                                               m^2
Cardiac output (CO) = SV × HR   3–7 liters/min
Cardiac index = CO/BSA   2.5–4.5 liters/min/m^2
Systemic vascular resistance (SVR) = (MAP − mean   800–1,200 dynes/
RAP) × 80/CO   sec/cm^{-5}
Pulmonary vascular resistance (PVR) = (mean PAP −   120–250 dynes/
PAoP) × 80/CO   sec/cm^{-5}

Blood gas values

pH   7.35–7.45
Arterial oxygen tension (PaO$_2$)   75–100 mmHg
Arterial carbon dioxide tension (PaCO$_2$)   35–45 mm Hg
Mixed venous oxygen tension (PvO$_2$)   38–42 mm Hg
Arterial oxygen saturation (SaO$_2$)   95–100%
Mixed venous oxygen saturation (SvO$_2$)   70–75%

Mixed acid-base equations

Henderson-Hasselbalch equation:
$pH = pk + log ([HCO_3^-]/0.03\ PaCO_2)$
Henderson's equation for concentration of
H^+: $[H^+]$ (nM/liter) = 24 × (PaCO$_2$/[HCO$_3^-$])
Metabolic acidosis:
Bicarbonate deficit (mEq/liter) = [0.5 × body
weight (kg)] × (24 − [HCO$_3^-$])
Expected PaCO$_2$ = 1.5 × [HCO$_3^-$] + 8 ± 2
Metabolic alkalosis:
Bicarbonate excess = [0.4 × body weight (kg)] ×
([HCO$_3^-$] − 24)

Expected: $PaCO_2 = 0.7 \times [HCO_3^-] + 21 \pm 1.5$
(when $HCO_3^- \leq 40$ mEq/
liter)
$PaCO_2 = 0.75 \times [HCO_3^-] + 19 \pm 7.5$
(when $HCO_3^- > 40$ mEq/
liter)

Respiratory acidosis:
Acute Δ pH/$\Delta PaCO_2$ = 0.008
Chronic Δ pH/$\Delta PaCO_2$ = 0.003
Respiratory alkalosis:
Acute Δ pH/$\Delta PaCO_2$ = 0.008
Chronic Δ pH/$\Delta PaCO_2$ = 0.002

Oxygen transport

Arterial oxygen content (CaO_2) = $(1.39 \times SaO_2 \times$ $Hb) + (0.0031 \times PaO_2)$	18–21 ml O_2/dl
Mixed venous oxygen content (CvO_2) = $(1.39 \times$ $SvO_2 \times Hb) + (0.0031 \times PvO_2)$	14.5–15.5 ml O_2/dl
Capillary oxygen content ($C_{cap}O_2$ = $(1.39 \times S_{cap}O_2 \times Hb) \times (0.0031 \times PaO_2)$: ($S_{cap}O_2$ is assumed to = 1.00)	21 ml O_2/dl
Arterial-mixed venous oxygen content difference ($C_{a-v}O_2$)	3.5–5.5 ml O_2/dl
Oxygen consumption ($\dot{V}O_2$) = CO $\times$ ($C_{a-v}O_2$)	200–250 ml/min
Oxygen delivery ($\dot{D}O_2$) = CO $\times$ CaO_2	1,000 ml/min
Oxygen extraction ratio = $\dot{V}O_2/\dot{D}O_2$	22–32%
Fick equation: CO = 10 $\dot{V}O_2$/[Hg $\times$ 1.39 ($SaO_2 -$ SvO_2)]	3–7 liters/min

Respiratory parameters

Respiratory quotient (RQ) = $\dot{V}CO_2/\dot{V}O_2$	0.7–1.0
Alveolar oxygen tension (P_AO_2) = F_IO_2 ($P_{atm} - P_{H_2O}$) $-$ $PaCO_2$/RQ (alveolar air equation)	
Alveolar-arteriolar oxygen gradient (P_{A-a} O_2) for F_IO_2 = 21%	5–25 mm Hg
for F_IO_2 = 100%	<150 mm Hg
Physiologic shunt (Qs/Qt) = $(C_{cap}O_2 - CaO_2)/(C_{cap}O_2 - CvO_2)$ where $S_{cap}O_2$ is assumed to be 1.0	<5%
Minute ventilation ($\dot{V}_E$) = k $\dot{V}CO_2/PaCO_2$ = $(0.863 \times \dot{V}CO_2)/[PaCO_2 (1 - \dot{V}_D/\dot{V}_t)]$	4–6 liters/min
Bohr equation of dead space (V_D/V_t) = $(P_ACO_2 - P$ expiratory $CO_2)/P_ACO_2$	0.2–0.3
Physiologic dead space (V_D/V_t) = $(PaCO_2 - P$ expiratory $CO_2)/PaCO_2$	0.2–0.3
Respiratory system compliance (Crs) during mechanical ventilation:	
Static Crs (Cst, rs) = $\dot{V}T$/(Pplateau – PEEP)	70–100 ml/cm H_2O*
Dynamic Crs (Cdyn, rs) = $\dot{V}T$/(Ppeak – PEEP)	60–100 ml/cm H_2O

* Pplateau is obtained by inserting a 0.3-second pause at end inspiration to give a plateau-pressure value.

Index

Index

calcium channel antagonists, 231
cocaine, 227-228
cyclic antidepressants, 11, 228-229
dialysis, 214
diethylene glycol, 221-222
diuresis, 214
ethanol, 219-220
ethylene glycol, 221-222
gastric emptying, 211, 214
hemoperfusion, 214
hydrocarbons, 222
isopropyl alcohol, 220
methanol, 220-221
methemoglobinemia, 222-223
opioids, 223-224
organophosphates, 223
patient discharge, 214
phencyclidine (PCP), 224
phenothiazines, 224
salicylates, 224-225, 226
serotonin reuptake inhibitors, 229-230
supportive care, 211
toxic syndromes and causes, 212-213
Oxacillin, 282
dosage in renal failure, 565
for erysipelas and cellulitis, 313
for infective endocarditis, 308
for meningitis, 306
for *Staphylococcus aureus,* 301
Oxalate
and renal calculi, 278
restriction of, 278
urinary levels of, 554
Oxaprozin, 513
dosage in renal failure, 566
Oxazepam. *See also* Benzodiazepines
for alcohol withdrawal, 534
Oxycodone, 5
Oxygen
in asthma, 237
in chronic obstructive pulmonary disease, 242, 244-245
delivery systems, 188-189
hyperbaric, 233
Oxygen consumption (VO₂), parameters for, 578
Oxygen delivery (DO₂), parameters for, 578
Oxygen extraction ratio, parameters for, 578
Oxygen therapy, 188-189
for adult respiratory distress syndrome, 250
for carbon monoxide poisoning, 233
for chronic obstructive pulmonary disease
acute, 243
long-term, 244-245
in cystic fibrosis, 247
in high-altitude illness, 210

Pacemaker. *See* Pacing, cardiac
Pacemaker-mediated tachycardia (PMT), 169
Pacing
cardiac, 167-169

in children, 168
defibrillation with, 172
dual-chamber, in hypertrophic cardiomyopathy, 134
indications, 167-168
modalities, 167
permanent, 168
complications, 168-169
pacemaker-mediated tachycardia, 169
temporary, 167-168
pacemaker syndrome, 169
transcutaneous, in cardiac arrest, 175, 177, 179
transvenous
in cardiac arrest, 175, 179
in myocardial infarction, 106
preoperative placement of, 23
Paget's disease of bone, 503-504
Pain relief
with acetaminophen, 3-4
with aspirin, 4
in cancer patients, 418
with nonsteroidal antiinflammatory drugs, 4
with opioid analgesics, 4-5
Pamidronate, for hypercalcemia, 492
Pancreatic enzyme supplements, 362
Pancreatitis, 361-362
acute, 361-362
antimicrobial therapy in, 313
chronic, 362
complications, 362
Ranson criteria in, 361
supportive treatment, 361-362
total parenteral nutrition for, 40
Pancuronium, in endotracheal intubation and mechanical ventilation, 204
PAOP, 108-109, 191, 196
Papilledema, 27
Paracentesis, for ascites with hepatic insufficiency, 378
Paralysis. *See* Weakness
Paramethasone, for systemic lupus erythematosus, 523
Parapneumonic effusions, 259, 260
Parathyroid disorders. *See* Hyperparathyroidism; Hypoparathyroidism
Parasitic infections, as cause of diarrhea, 337
Parathion poisoning, 223
Parathyroidectomy
for chronic hypercalcemia, 493-494
for renal osteodystrophy, 273
Parathyroid hormone
in hypercalcemia, 490-493
laboratory values for, 553
in nephrolithiasis, 277
in secondary hyperparathyroidism, 273
Paregoric, for diarrhea, 338
Parenteral nutrition, 34-40
complications, 36, 39-40
in Crohn's disease, 359